Exercise in Rehabilitation Medicine

Second Edition

Editor-in-Chief

Walter R. Frontera, MD, PhD
Chairman and Earle P. and Ida S. Charlton Professor,
Department of Physical Medicine and Rehabilitation, Harvard Medical School
Chief, Physical Medicine and Rehabilitation, Spaulding Rehabilitation Hospital
Massachusetts General Hospital, and Brigham and Women's Hospital

Associate Editors

David M. Slovik, MD
Associate Professor of Medicine
Harvard Medical School
Chief of Medicine, Spaulding Rehabilitation Hospital

David M. Dawson, MD
Professor of Neurology
Harvard Medical School

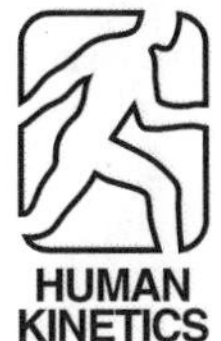

Library of Congress Cataloging-in-Publication Data

Exercise in rehabilitation medicine / editor-in-chief, Walter R. Frontera ; associate editors, David M. Slovik, David M. Dawson. --2nd ed.
p. ; cm.
Includes bibliographical references and index.
ISBN 0-7360-5541-X (hard cover)
1. Exercise therapy. 2. Medical rehabilitation. I. Frontera, Walter R., 1955- . II. Slovik, David M., 1945- . III. Dawson, D.M. (David Michael), 1930- .
[DNLM: 1. Exercise Therapy--methods. 2. Primary Prevention --methods. 3. Rehabilitation--methods. WB 541 E9541 2006]
RM725.E926 2006
615.8'2--dc22

2005010110

ISBN: 0-7360-5541-X

The Web addresses cited in this text were current as of October 21, 2005, unless otherwise noted.

Acquisitions Editor: Loarn D. Robertson, PhD; **Developmental Editor:** Elaine H. Mustain; **Assistant Editor:** Sandra Merz Bott; **Copyeditor:** Joyce Sexton; **Proofreader:** Red Inc.; **Indexer:** Robert Howerton; **Permission Manager:** Dalene Reeder; **Graphic Designer:** Nancy Rasmus; **Graphic Artist:** Kathleen Boudreau-Fuoss; **Photo Manager:** Kareema McLendon; **Cover Designer:** Keith Blomberg; **Photographer (interior):** Tom Roberts, unless otherwise noted; **Art Manager:** Kelly Hendren; **Illustrator:** Al Wilborn; **Printer:** Sheridan Books

Printed in the United States of America 10 9 8 7 6 5 4 3 2 1

Human Kinetics
Web site: www.HumanKinetics.com

United States:
Human Kinetics
P.O. Box 5076,
Champaign, IL 61825-5076
800-747-4457
e-mail: humank@hkusa.com

Canada:
Human Kinetics
475 Devonshire Road Unit 100
Windsor, ON N8Y 2L5
800-465-7301 (in Canada only)
e-mail: orders@hkcanada.com

Europe:
Human Kinetics
107 Bradford Road, Stanningley
Leeds LS28 6AT, United Kingdom
+44 (0) 113 255 5665
e-mail: hk@hkeurope.com

Australia: Human Kinetics
57A Price Avenue
Lower Mitcham, South Australia 5062
08 8277 1555
e-mail: liaw@hkaustralia.com

New Zealand:
Human Kinetics
Division of Sports Distributors NZ Ltd.
P.O. Box 300 226 Albany
North Shore City, Auckland
0064 9 448 1207
e-mail: info@humankinetics.co.nz

CONTENTS

FOREWORD

You should get more exercise! This is perhaps the advice patients most frequently hear from their physicians—as well as from friends, spouses, and their own "inner voices." Yet, without greater specificity, a recommendation for "exercise" is as useless as advice to "take some pills" or "try a little surgery." What kind of exercise? For how long? At what intensity? Which technique? What apparatus? Without these and a host of other details, few will perform well or be motivated to persevere.

While the use of exercise in medical practice remains haphazard, an "exercise craze" has swept over the general public in recent years. In the United States, concern about poor physical fitness began to grow in the 1950s, when the Krause-Weber Test of school of children evidenced dismal performance on the part of American children compared to European. Both Presidents Eisenhower (1952-1960) and Kennedy (1960-1963) brought physical fitness to the forefront as a national concern.

Educators, fitness writers, and exercise crusaders such as Bonnie Pruden and Kenneth Cooper began to offer specific exercise and fitness guidelines for lay readers. Cooper's "Aerobics" exercise program became immensely popular. Health clubs and fitness centers grew in number and popularity as the "baby boom" generation came of age in the 1960s and 1970s.

Meanwhile, medically supervised exercise regimens introduced in the 1940s and 1950s for war injuries and polio epidemics expanded to serve patients with stroke, cardiac, pulmonary, and many other disabilities. Today, we find a large network of medical rehabilitation facilities, an equally vibrant health club and fitness center industry, as well as a worldwide sports medicine movement. Yet many health care providers outside these fields remain either uninformed or misinformed about how to prescribe exercise as part of a treatment plan.

The interest in and respect for exercise as an important factor in health enhancement and health maintenance received major backing in recent years from the U.S. Surgeon General. In his 1997 Report on Exercise and Cardiovascular Disease, strong support was given to the positive role of regular exercise in a person's daily and weekly schedules. The 1999 Report, Physical Activity and Health, constituted a milestone in the promotion of regular exercise as an integral part of health maintenance on a national scale. Whereas an attitude of indifference regarding the role of regular exercise on the part of the medical and allied health communities existed in the 1950s, exercise in the 21st century is being touted as a necessity for the well-being of people of all ages.

The beginnings of research on physical exercise date back to the late 1700s. In 1784, the illustrious French chemist, Antoine Lavoissier, published a study on respiratory exchange during one-legged exercise. Lavoissier's methodology for estimating energy cost became standard practice, and present-day laboratory techniques follow his basic principles. However, concerted efforts to investigate acute responses and chronic adaptations to physical exercise did not begin until the early 1900s, and gathered significant impetus only in midcentury. Probably more than 99% of all exercise physiology research in the history of the world has been published since 1960.

During the last 45 years, "exercise science" has generated an impressive but still growing scientific base of objective data on the methods and outcomes of therapeutic exercise. Research has confirmed the important role of regular physical exercise in health development and health maintenance. A carefully prescribed exercise program has emerged as the most important modality employed in rehabilitation medicine. Yet the link between published research and medical practice has developed slowly and still remains weak. *Exercise in Rehabilitation Medicine* organizes the application of this science to physical medicine and rehabilitation in a form that all health care providers can use in their daily patient care.

Following the success of the first edition, Drs. Frontera, Dawson, and Slovik have again assembled a distinguished group of chapter authors for the second edition of this impressive volume. The new edition has kept pace with the rapidly expanding fields of physical medicine and rehabilitation and the accumulated research of recent years. Those chapters that were retained from the first edition have been updated in terms of new research and new information. New chapters have been included relative to the relationship of exercise to cancer, end-stage renal disease, and human immunodeficiency virus. The volume will continue to serve as an indispensable reference for practitioners of rehabilitation and primary care medicine, as well as for individuals in many other medical and allied health specialty areas.

Paul J. Corcoran, MD
Senior Lecturer on Physical Medicine and Rehabilitation
Harvard Medical School

Howard G. Knuttgen, PhD
Senior Lecturer on Physical Medicine and Rehabilitation
Harvard Medical School
Professor Emeritus of Applied Physiology
Pennsylvania State University

PREFACE

Broadly defined, rehabilitation is the development of a person to the fullest physical, psychological, social, vocational, avocational, and educational potential, within his or her physiological or anatomic impairments and environmental limitations (DeLisa et al. 1998). Briefly, rehabilitation can also be defined as the restoration of normal form and function. That approximately 50 million people in the United States, and many times that number in the world, live with a disability demonstrates the importance of rehabilitation.

Clinicians design rehabilitation programs for various reasons including the prevention of complications of chronic illness and injury, to compensate for loss of anatomic or physiologic capacity, and to optimize function. It is appropriate that exercise is one of the most frequently used strategies to achieve these goals, since nearly 70% of disabling conditions limit mobility by interfering with the function of skeletal muscles, joints, endocrine glands, bones, heart, and lungs. It is therefore of utmost importance that rehabilitation professionals have a comprehensive knowledge of the physiology of exercise and its application in the clinical setting.

Many excellent publications have addressed important aspects of the basic science of exercise. Others have discussed various clinical aspects of rehabilitation. However, recent advances in both fields—exercise science and rehabilitation medicine—require an amalgamation of this knowledge. Our objective in the first edition of this book was to present, in a single volume, an organized and in-depth discussion of the basic science and the clinical correlates of exercise as a therapeutic and rehabilitative intervention strategy. The objective of the second edition is to update that discussion with recent research findings and to broaden the scope of the book by including new topics. The new chapters have been designed to provide more comprehensive clinical applications for the reader.

Proper use of exercise in rehabilitating patients with a wide variety of disabling illnesses requires understanding of the basic physiological adaptations to exercise. Only by understanding the nature of the adaptations to training with various kinds of exercise (strength, endurance and flexibility) can a health professional properly match a training program with the impairment, activity, the activity level, and the participation goal appropriate for the patient. Part I takes a detailed look at these basic facts. Relevant clinical examples selected using accepted research criteria have been added to the discussion.

Rehabilitation professionals should have a working knowledge of the various testing devices and protocols used to evaluate a patient's functional capacity. They must understand the relevance of these tests for appropriate exercise prescription. Part II discusses the principles of exercise testing and exercise prescription, ending with a discussion of the importance of exercise in the primary prevention of disease. During the last five years more research has been conducted on the optimal exercise prescription that resulted in updated recommendations for the public. These will be discussed here. Also, the role of exercise in the prevention of chronic illness continues to receive attention and better designed clinical and longitudinal studies have been published to support this role.

In part III, specialists discuss the rationale and the clinical importance of exercise in the rehabilitation of patients with a wide variety of disabling conditions, and address the factors that must be weighed when prescribing exercise for these conditions. The authors discuss diseases that impair the function of the heart, circulation, lungs, joints, endocrine system, bones, and neuromuscular system. Three new chapters will discuss the use of exercise in patients with HIV/AIDS, renal insufficiency, and cancer. Tables summarize published training studies; and authors provide the details of exercise prescriptions for patient populations with specific disabling illnesses.

The scientific and clinical literature increasingly address the aging of the population and the benefits of exercise training in older age groups. Also, more survivors of disabling injuries are developing interest in competitive sports. Part IV considers these two special populations: the elderly and elite athletes with disabilities.

This book should be useful for many different professionals: physicians practicing rehabilitation (including specialists and primary care providers), physical therapists, occupational therapists, recreational therapists, nurses, and exercise physiologists with an interest in clinical applications of exercise. Theoretical, practical, and clinical information is included under one cover. Extensive reference lists serve as additional sources of information. The text is clearly written, so even those with little technical expertise should be able to follow it, yet it is sufficiently advanced that those who are not beginners will significantly improve their understanding.

PART I

BIOLOGICAL CONSIDERATIONS

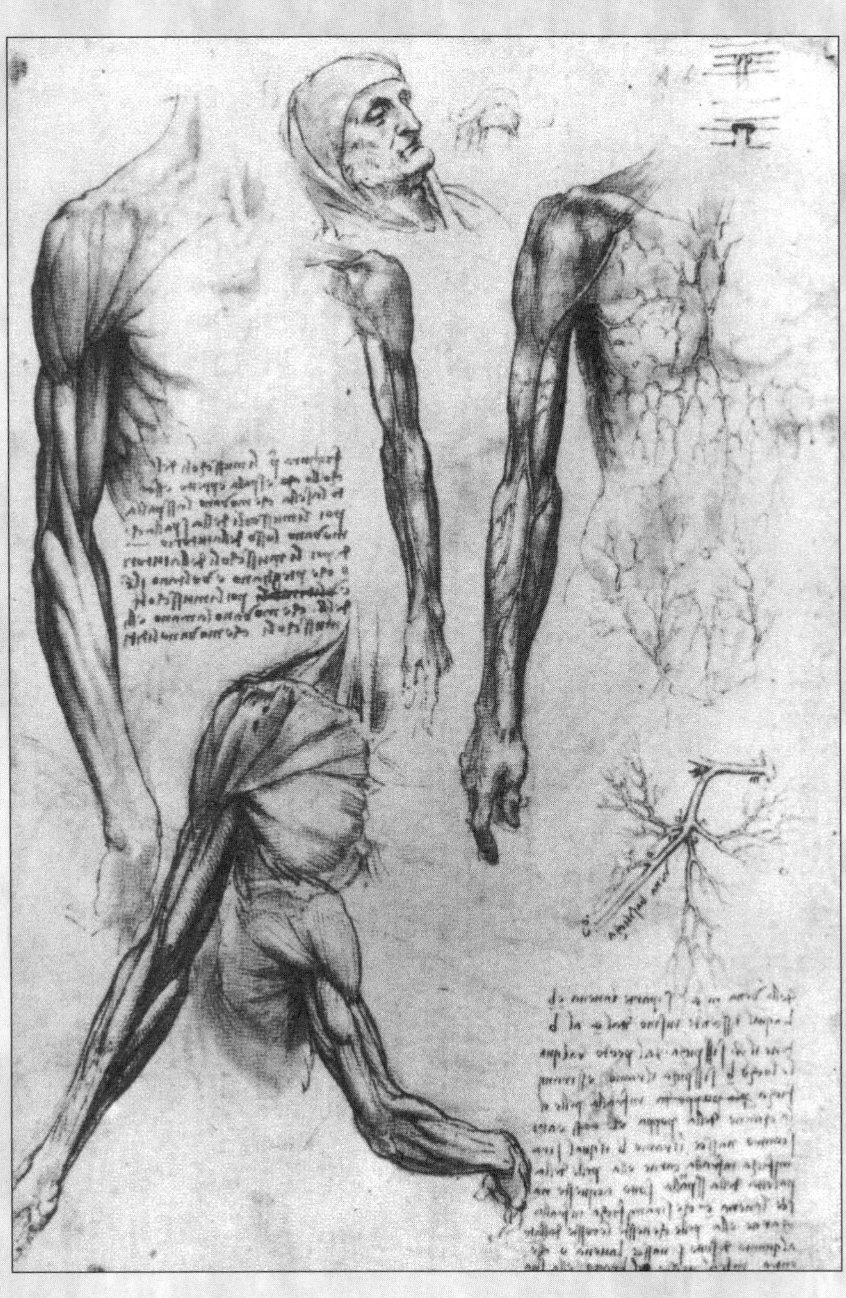

CHAPTER 1

ACUTE PHYSIOLOGICAL RESPONSES TO DYNAMIC EXERCISE

Roger A. Fielding, PhD; and Jonathan Bean, MD, MS

Exercise and increased physical activity improve cardiovascular fitness (Saltin 1985) and, according to several epidemiological studies, decrease mortality from all causes (Blair et al. 1989; Lee et al. 1992; Paffenbarger et al. 1986) and more specifically in individuals with documented metabolic syndrome, adult-onset diabetes mellitus, or both (Katzmarzyk et al. 2004).

Nearly all providers within medical rehabilitation use exercise as an important therapeutic intervention. This chapter reviews acute cardiorespiratory and metabolic responses to dynamic exercise, focusing particularly on the coordination of these responses throughout the body by alterations in specific regulatory processes. We also briefly discuss the roles of exercise training and detraining as they influence physiological responses to acute exercise. At the end of each section, we discuss a specific pathophysiological process that relates to perturbations in the physiological response to exercise.

During dynamic exercise, different organ systems interact to maximize the resynthesis of ATP within active muscle in order to perform physical work. Dynamic exercise induces an increase in oxygen uptake and cardiac output. In explaining the relationships among whole-body measures of oxygen consumption, energy expenditure during exercise, and cellular energy metabolism, we explore the connections between the cardiorespiratory system and peripheral factors linked to oxygen extraction and substrate utilization.

CARDIORESPIRATORY RESPONSE TO DYNAMIC EXERCISE

Whole-body oxygen consumption is the product of maximal cardiac output and maximal peripheral O_2 extraction. These two terms are usually considered the central and peripheral links in the oxygen transport chain, respectively. Oxygen is the final electron acceptor during oxidative phosphorylation. Because researchers cannot conveniently measure rates of **adenosine triphosphate (ATP)** turnover through direct means, they have traditionally used whole-body oxygen consumption to indirectly estimate energy expenditure during exercise (Åstrand 1960). More recently, non-invasive methods using phosphorus nuclear magnetic resonance spectroscopy have increased our ability to directly quantify skeletal muscle high-energy phosphate metabolism during exercise (Smith et al. 2004).

MAXIMAL OXYGEN UPTAKE

Hill and Lupton (1923) first described **maximal oxygen uptake ($\dot{V}O_2max$)** as an upper physiological limit for

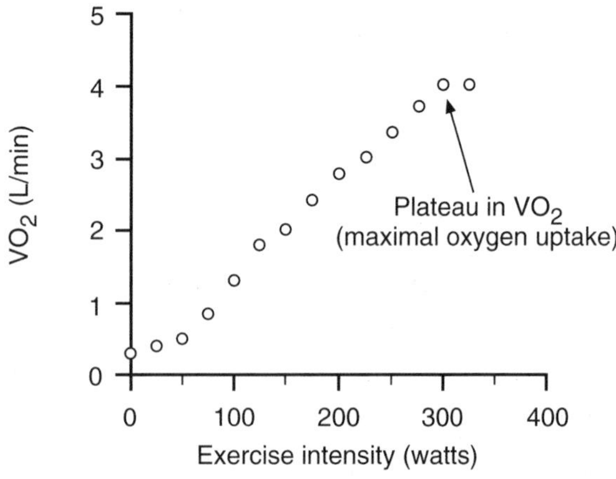

Figure 1.1 Plot of oxygen uptake versus exercise intensity (watts) during an incremental cycling test in a young sedentary individual. Note the linear relationship between power output and $\dot{V}O_2$ up to the plateau and achievement of $\dot{V}O_2$max.
Source: Fielding, 1997, unpublished data.

aerobic exercise; Taylor and colleagues (1955) validated the concept. These studies demonstrated a direct relationship between whole-body oxygen consumption and exercise intensity (figure 1.1). Oxygen consumption increases linearly with the intensity of exercise, until it plateaus at or near the $\dot{V}O_2$max. Across a wide span of individuals, $\dot{V}O_2$max is a reproducible estimate of aerobic exercise capacity and cardiovascular fitness (Rowell 1974). Assessment of $\dot{V}O_2$max has been an important clinical tool used in many settings for determination of an individual's functional capacity.

The Fick equation describes $\dot{V}O_2$max as the product of **maximal cardiac output (CO)** centrally and maximal peripheral arterial-venous oxygen difference (arterial O_2 – venous O_2) (see table 1.1). The Fick equation illustrates the partitioning of the components of $\dot{V}O_2$max into central and peripheral factors (Saltin and Rowell 1980). In healthy individuals, the central and peripheral processes work in tandem to facilitate oxygen delivery and utilization within active skeletal muscle. Cardiac output and peripheral oxygen uptake are coupled in a tight physiological relationship. Differences in maximal cardiac output explain most of the variance in $\dot{V}O_2$max among individuals (Åstrand et al. 1964; Saltin and Strange 1992) and these differences appear to result solely from differences in maximal stroke volume in individuals with a wide range of aerobic capacities (Blackmon et al. 1967). This exceptional linkage of oxygen supply and demand to active muscle occurs through virtually all intensities and conditions of exercise, and represents a remarkable example of the integration of central and peripheral responses during aerobic exercise.

$\dot{V}O_2$MAX AND THE CARDIOVASCULAR SYSTEM

Cardiac output is the product of heart rate and stroke volume. Factors that regulate heart rate include intrinsic autonomic input via sympathetic and parasympathetic pathways, and extrinsic hormonal factors such as circulating catecholamines. Heart rate increases under conditions of sympathetic activation. Conversely, elevated parasympathetic input decreases heart rate. At all exercise intensities, elevations in sympathetic input and release of circulating catecholamines result in increased heart rate (Seals et al. 1988). These same intrinsic and extrinsic neurohormonal factors regulate cardiac function, influencing both heart rate and stroke volume under conditions of stress or relaxation (Stone et al. 1985). Factors that determine stroke volume include venous return and ventricular compliance (related to ventricular filling), plus ventricular contractility and total peripheral resistance (related to ventricular emptying). Elevations in stroke volume with exercise are due to improved filling and emptying of the ventricles (Polinar et al. 1980). Improved filling increases stroke volume via the Frank-Starling mechanism. With increased filling, there is greater ventricular stretch and therefore a stronger resultant contraction of the myocardium. Greater emptying occurs with a larger myocardial contraction regardless of the ventricular volume of blood (Polinar et al. 1980).

$\dot{V}O_2$MAX AND THE ARTERIAL-VENOUS OXYGEN DIFFERENCE

Peripheral factors are those that affect extraction of oxygen from the blood by the metabolically active skeletal muscle (Holloszy 1967). These factors can be intrinsic (intracellular) or extrinsic (extracellular). **Intrinsic factors** within muscle fibers include the absolute quantity and the respiratory capacity of the mitochondria. **Extrinsic factors** include the quality and

Table 1.1 Fick Equation

$\dot{V}O_2$max	= Cardiac output max	×	Arterial-venous oxygen difference
Influenced by:	• Stroke volume maximum		• Blood flow • Muscle capillarization
	• Heart rate maximum		• Skeletal muscle oxidative capacity

quantity of capillarization, red blood cell transit time, and blood flow to active muscle (Saltin 1985). Exercise training can modify these factors, which contribute to $\dot{V}O_2$max and submaximal exercise capacity (Holloszy and Coyle 1984).

Pulmonary System and Oxygen Transport

The lungs are the interface between the central and peripheral factors. They serve the central role of oxygenating the blood under all conditions; yet if arterial O_2 concentration is low, they can profoundly influence peripheral O_2 extraction. Fortunately, in individuals with normal pulmonary functioning this essentially does not occur (Dempsey and Fregosi 1985). However, Dempsey and colleagues have also suggested that in some elite athletes, pulmonary ventilation may limit exercise capacity by inducing arterial desaturation at maximal or near-maximal exercise intensities (Dempsey et al. 2003). The products of metabolism mediate much of the respiratory response to exercise, and the lungs serve as a gateway for metabolism: oxygen enters the body, and carbon dioxide and water (the products of metabolism) exit. **Ventilation (VE)** is quantified in liters of air exchanged per minute. Like cardiac output, it is the product of rate (ventilatory rate) and volume (tidal volume). **Tidal volume** is the volume of air moved in and out of the lungs with a single breath (Guyton 1991).

The brain stem regulates pulmonary ventilation at centers that control both inspiration and expiration. The centers control both the rate and volume of breathing. The primary factors that mediate this control in normal individuals are changes in body temperature, circulating pH, and concentrations of O_2 and CO_2. Stretch receptors within the diaphragm, lung, and intercostal muscles also can modulate inspiration and expiration by feedback through autonomic pathways. CO_2 and pH act centrally within the brain stem through direct means. More peripherally, receptors within the carotid bifurcation and the aortic arch respond primarily to the **partial pressure of oxygen (pO_2)** along with the **partial pressure of carbon dioxide (pCO_2)** and pH (Dempsey et al. 1985). At these sites pO_2 exerts the strongest influence, causing ventilation to increase under conditions of low oxygenation and decrease when pO_2 levels are high. Centrally, it appears that pCO_2 exerts the greatest influence, causing ventilation to increase with rising blood concentrations and to decrease under opposite conditions. Increased temperature increases ventilation through direct central stimulation (Dempsey et al. 1985).

Ventilation is the mechanism by which hemoglobin is saturated with oxygen. **Hemoglobin (Hb)** is the carrier protein for oxygen within the blood. Factors that control ventilatory function will influence Hb saturation. Optimal physiologic functioning during exercise requires maximal binding of oxygen within pulmonary capillaries and release of oxygen within skeletal muscle capillaries. Under such conditions the alveolar environment is characterized by elevated pH, low pCO_2, and reduced temperature; active skeletal muscle exchange sites have a low pH, high pCO_2, and elevated temperature. Under conditions that mirror the chemical environment of alveolar capillaries in exercising lungs, the oxygen dissociation curve for hemoglobin favors higher hemoglobin saturation levels. In contrast, conditions that reflect the environment of the exercising muscle favor oxygen release from hemoglobin (Guyton 1991). This remarkable phenomenon, known as the **Bohr effect,** maintains the strong coupling between central supply and peripheral extraction of oxygen.

To summarize what we have discussed thus far:

- Whole-body oxygen consumption is correlated with exercise intensity.
- Both central and peripheral factors determine oxygen consumption.
- These central supply functions and peripheral demand functions work together. Some processes, such as those in the exercising lung, affect both functions.
- Chemical mechanisms, such as the Bohr effect on Hb saturation, underlie the coupling of oxygen supply and metabolic demand.

Cardiovascular Response to Dynamic Exercise

In untrained individuals, resting heart rate is generally 60 to 100 beats per minute; it increases directly and proportionally with exercise intensity, and, like oxygen consumption, plateaus at maximal exercise intensities (Ekelund and Holmgren 1967). Heart rate and work rate are so intimately linked that, within an individual with known $\dot{V}O_2$max, one can closely predict oxygen uptake at a given submaximal heart rate. Clinicians often use heart rate as an indirect measure of exercise intensity (ACSM 1995). Maximal heart rate varies within individuals and declines with age, typical maximal rates being 190 to 200 in young adults and 140 to 160 in older adults. Because the variance increases significantly as the population ages, however, heart rate is a poor predictor of exercise intensity in the geriatric population (Shephard 1990). Regulation of heart rate occurs via neurohormonal input. The elevation in heart rate with dynamic exercise is mediated intrinsically via elevated sympathetic input and extrinsically via stimulation from circulating catecholamines (Stone et al. 1985).

Table 1.2 Cardiovascular Reponses During Dynamic Exercise

	Rest	Moderate exercise	Maximal exercise
Cardiac output (L/min)	5.0	17.0	25.0
Stroke volume (ml)	71	117	131
Heart rate (beats/min)	70	145	190
Oxygen uptake (L/min)	0.3	2.0	3.4

Human Cardiovascular Control by Rowell, L.B. © 1993 by Oxford University Press, Inc. Reprinted by permission.

Although stroke volume also increases with rising exercise intensity, it tends to plateau prior to maximal work loads at approximately 40% to 60% $\dot{V}O_2$max (Crawford et al. 1985; Hermansen et al. 1970). Interestingly, during exercise in the upright posture, stroke volume may increase continually until achievement of $\dot{V}O_2$max (Krip et al. 1997). Therefore, whereas heart rate is closely linked to intensity of exercise, stroke volume may be more loosely associated. Body position and the form of exercise testing can influence stroke volume, accounting in part for some of the variability researchers have found with stroke volume response (Crawford et al. 1985; Polinar et al. 1980). A number of factors mediate changes in stroke volume. Sympathetic input and circulating catecholamines influence stroke volume through a direct effect on cardiac contractility and compliance (Stone et al. 1985). Increased activity through pumping action of the active skeletal muscle augments venous return, while redistribution of blood to the active muscle reduces total peripheral resistance. These factors increase with heavier levels of exercise (see table 1.2). Together, these changes in heart rate and stroke volume can increase cardiac output two to four times with heavy exercise (Dowell 1983).

Along with the elevation in cardiac output during dynamic exercise, there are dramatic changes in blood flow distribution. In order to maximize delivery of oxygen-rich blood to active skeletal muscle, flow is shunted away from inactive tissues (see table 1.3): active skeletal muscle blood flow increases to 20 times normal levels, and circulation to inactive skeletal muscle declines by approximately one-third. Coronary circulation increases by 400% in order to support the increased myocardial demands; splanchnic blood flow, however, declines by as much as 50% of basal levels, slowing gastrointestinal transit time. Although blood flow to the skin varies with the ambient temperature, overall it increases in order to maximize heat exchange and slow the rise in core body temperature during exercise (Rowell 1986). Lastly, with dynamic exercise, circulation to the brain needs to remain constant and thus does not change appreciably. The combination of input from circulating catecholamines and local metabolites mediates all the above-mentioned changes. Vascular changes influence central factors through a reduction in total peripheral resistance (TPR) and through increased delivery of oxygen-rich arterial blood to the exercising muscle (Blomquist and Saltin 1983; Saltin 1985).

RESPIRATORY RESPONSE TO DYNAMIC EXERCISE

At rest, normal respiratory rate is 8 to 20 breaths per minute. It increases with increasing effort, as does tidal volume, in an effort to maximize ventilation. Like heart rate, pulmonary ventilation increases linearly with oxygen consumption. Again there is close linkage between central supply of oxygen and peripheral demand. In all but highly trained individuals, arterial

Table 1.3 Typical Distribution of Cardiac Output at Rest (CO = 5 L/min)

Tissue	L/min	%
Heart	0.2	4
Skin	0.3	6
Brain	0.7	14
Liver	1.3	27
Kidneys	1.1	22
Skeletal muscle	1.0	20
Other	0.4	7

Typical Distribution of Cardiac Output During Maximal Exercise (CO = 25 L/min)

Tissue	L/min	%
Heart	1.0	4
Skin	0.6	2
Brain	0.9	4
Liver	0.5	2
Kidneys	1.1	3
Skeletal muscle	21.0	83
Other	0.8	2

Human Cardiovascular Control by Rowell, L.B. © 1993 by Oxford University Press, Inc. Reprinted by permission.

pO_2 remains at resting levels even with heavy exercise. This is accomplished through three mechanisms:

1. In the resting state there is a large functional reserve of both alveolar and capillary surface area. These underutilized surfaces for diffusion serve as added sources for oxygen exchange.
2. Pulmonary capillary blood flow increases threefold with maximal exercise, and lymphatic drainage is optimized. These mechanisms speed red blood cell transit time but reduce diffusion distance, respectively.
3. The ratio of ventilation to perfusion increases four to five times over resting levels, maintaining a high gradient for diffusion.

Together, these factors maximize arterial oxygenation (Dempsey et al. 1985). By maximizing oxygenation of hemoglobin during exercise, the lungs balance the increased peripheral extraction of oxygen.

Cardiorespiratory Response to Exercise in Patients With Spinal Cord Injury

Exercise response in spinal cord injury (SCI) patients is particularly interesting. It is the level of spinal injury that dictates the major physiologic differences between individuals who are labeled as SCI and those who are able-bodied. The two most significant factors that influence the exercise response are reductions in active muscle mass and reductions in circulating blood volume. Since large segments of the body are paralyzed in SCI, the amount of active muscle mass declines, thereby reducing $\dot{V}O_2$max, since less muscle is available to consume oxygen (Glaser 1989; Lasko-McCarthey and Davis 1991). This fact significantly limits overall endurance and influences the substrates used for metabolism. For a given task such as propelling a wheelchair, the same level of work represents a much higher percentage of $\dot{V}O_2$max in an SCI patient. Thus, with more challenging tasks, the ratio of anaerobic to aerobic metabolism is higher, leading to early fatigue and reduced endurance.

Reductions in circulating blood volume also impair work capacity in patients with spinal cord injury (Figoni et al. 1991; King et al. 1994), for two reasons: (1) There is a considerably smaller active muscle mass with SCI, resulting in a large increase in venous pooling during exercise and thus reducing venous return. (2) Changes in autonomic control of blood flow also increase venous pooling in SCI. With SCI (especially lesions at higher thoracic levels), cortical control of autonomic pathways is either reduced or absent, preventing the normal redistribution of blood to active muscle (Glaser 1989; Sawka et al. 1989). There is a qualitative reduction in substrate delivery and in disposal of metabolic end products. The reduced venous return due to excessive pooling also reduces cardiac output. In fact, a challenge in prescribing cardiovascular exercises for individuals with SCI is providing exercises that generate large increases in cardiac output. Researchers have explored a variety of exercise techniques to maximize the exercise stimulus in SCI patients, including supine positioning and use of electrical stimulation to inactive muscle (Glaser 1989; Rodgers et al. 1991). Given the physiological circumstances of spinal cord injury, it is not surprising that a leading source of morbidity and mortality in such individuals is cardiac disease (DiTunno and Formal 1994).

Metabolic Response During Dynamic Exercise

Physical exercise profoundly challenges homeostasis of fuel in normal humans. Whole-body energy expenditure can increase ten- to twentyfold from rest to maximal exercise (Taylor et al. 1955). Since quantities of high-energy phosphate compounds such as **creatine phosphate (CP)** and ATP within muscle are relatively limited (26 mM/kg wet wt. for CP; 8 mM/kg wet wt. for ATP), metabolic machinery and oxidizable substrate are necessary for sustained muscular activity. Enzymatically-regulated metabolic pathways in human skeletal muscle produce energy by oxidizing carbohydrate (in the forms of glucose and glycogen), nonesterified fatty acids (transported from adipocytes and derived from intramuscular triglycerides), and, to a small extent, amino acids (Newsholme and Start 1973) (see table 1.4). In order to meet the requirements of exercise and at the same time maintain the fuel supply to vital organs, the body must make major metabolic, hormonal, and cardiovascular adjustments.

Carbohydrate Metabolism

Glucose uptake in skeletal muscle is a carrier-mediated process initiated by the pancreatic hormone insulin (Berger et al. 1976; Ivy et al. 1983). Minimum levels of insulin are necessary for glucose uptake to occur at rest; but during exercise, glucose uptake increases despite declining circulating insulin concentrations (Felig et al. 1982; Felig and Wahren 1975), apparently because of non-insulin-dependent signaling mechanisms (Sakamoto and Goodyear 2002). Blood glucose may account for up to 40% of the total oxidizable substrate during prolonged submaximal exercise (i.e., 40% to 50% $\dot{V}O_2$max). The decline in blood glucose concentrations at the end of prolonged exercise lasting for several hours may be a possible cause of fatigue (Coyle et al. 1983; Coyle et al. 1986; Felig et al. 1982).

Table 1.4 Fuel Reserves and Rates of Utilization Under Different Conditions in Humans

Tissue	Approximate total fuel reserve		Estimated period for which fuel store would provide energy
	g	kcal	Minutes of marathon running
Adipose tissue triacylglycerol	16,000	144,000	7,143
Liver glycogen	90	360	18
Muscle glycogen	350	1,400	71
Blood and extra fluids	20	80	4

Adapted, by permission, from E.A. Newsholme and C. Start, 1973, *Regulation in metabolism* (New York: Wiley), 255.

Under resting conditions, catecholamines, glucagon, cortisol, and growth hormone stimulate hepatic glucose production, balancing the stimulatory action of insulin on glucose uptake. The result is euglycemia, in which glucose production matches glucose utilization (Kemmer and Berger 1986). During exercise, skeletal muscle glucose uptake can increase up to 28-fold, depending on the intensity of the exercise (Katz et al. 1986), despite a decrease in insulin secretion by the pancreas. It appears that catecholamines released from the adrenal medulla, and/or from nerve endings in the liver and pancreas, may suppress both insulin secretion and stimulate hepatic glucose production (Galbo et al. 1977; Wasserman 1995). In addition to the effects of sympathetic nerve endings in the liver, a state of hypoinsulinemia (coupled with relative hyperglucagonemia in the portal blood) further increases hepatic glucose output during exercise (Vranic et al. 1976). The result of these hormonal alterations is that blood glucose levels remain unchanged during exercise of relatively short duration.

Skeletal muscle glucose uptake increases linearly with increasing exercise intensity (Katz et al. 1986). Despite this dramatic increase in glucose uptake by active muscle, plasma glucose concentration remains notably level in normal humans during exercise of low to moderate intensity. Feedback signals from plasma glucose sensors appear to elicit changes in neuroendocrine function that increase hepatic glucose production (Richter et al. 1992). Decreases in plasma glucose may also directly stimulate hepatic glucose production. Feedback mechanisms are less involved during intense exercise as plasma glucose concentrations increase initially, then fall as hepatic glycogen stores are depleted (Richter et al. 1992). Instead, the glycemic response during periods of intense exercise may be subject to a feed-forward regulation elicited by the central command—it changes neuroendocrine function, causing an initial overshoot in hepatic glucose production. For example, at the onset of exercise, impulses from the working muscles and motor centers increase neuroendocrine activity in an intensity-dependent manner (Galbo 1983).

As happens with blood glucose supply, intramuscular stores of glycogen are broken down to enable resynthesis of high-energy phosphate compounds. Muscle glycogen's direct availability to the contractile tissue eliminates the need for a circulatory response for its mobilization. Muscle glycogen utilization appears greatest at the onset of exercise; as other substrates become available, the rate of muscle glycogen utilization slows (Hermansen et al. 1967) (figure 1.2). As with blood glucose uptake, the rate of muscle glycogen utilization increases with exercise intensity, reaching maximal rates well above the maximal oxygen uptake (Hermansen et al. 1967). Animal studies have shown a close relationship between intramuscular availability of glycogen and its rate of utilization during contractile activity (Richter and Galbo 1986). Several researchers have noted a relationship between pre-exercise muscle glycogen concentrations and time to exhaustion during submaximal endurance exercise (Bergstrom et al. 1967; Hermansen et al. 1967). Fatigue during intermittent high-intensity exercise also appears to coincide with low intramuscular glycogen concentra-

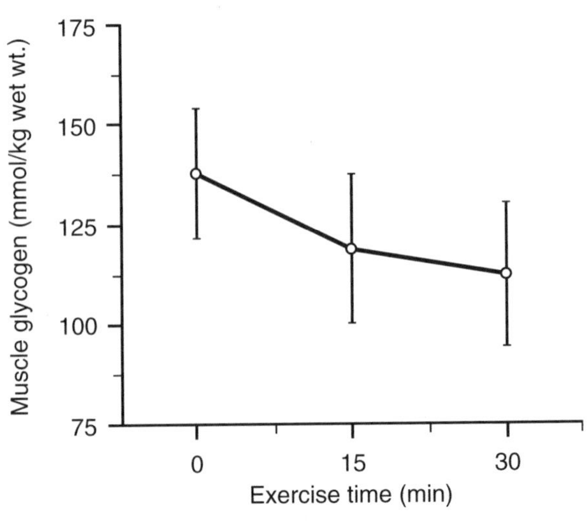

Figure 1.2 Plot of muscle glycogen (mmol/kg wet wt.) versus exercise time during 30 min of treadmill running (70% $\dot{V}O_2max$) in well-trained runners.

tions (Jacobs 1980; Maughan and Poole 1981). It is possible that with the depletion of muscle glycogen, selected muscle fibers may no longer be able to generate the necessary force to maintain a given power output. Sedentary untrained individuals have lower baseline muscle glycogen levels than do active trained people (Costill et al. 1985); reduced substrate availability may be a significant cause of fatigue in patients undergoing exercise training in rehabilitation.

FATTY ACID METABOLISM

Skeletal muscle can derive energy from blood-borne nonesterified fatty acids and intramuscular stores of triglyceride. In an individual of normal body mass and composition, the total body stores of carbohydrate and fat account, respectively, for 2,000 and 140,000 kcal of energy (Newsholme and Start 1973). Because of the enormous difference in the amounts of these substrates available for energy metabolism, a coordinated process of carbohydrate and fat metabolism is essential for prolonged muscular activity. During prolonged exercise and the resultant hypoinsulinemia and increased catecholamine release, **free fatty acids (FFAs)** mobilized from adipose tissue become a more important energy-yielding substrate. The process of lipolysis in adipose tissue results in the breakdown of triglycerides to FFA and glycerol. In addition to its stimulatory effect on hepatic glucose output, epinephrine further stimulates lipolysis in an effort to preserve circulating glucose (Zinman et al. 1977). Transported in the plasma bound to albumin, FFAs are then taken up by contractile tissue independent of insulin, but not necessarily by simple diffusion (Richter et al. 1992). Sorrentino et al. (1988) and Stremmel (1988) have isolated FFA-binding proteins from plasma membranes of adipocytes, hepatocytes, and cardiac myocytes. Because antibodies to these proteins inhibit FFA uptake, it is possible that FFA transport across the plasma membrane is in fact carrier-mediated.

Fatty acid oxidation rates increase progressively during prolonged exercise. The increase appears to be related to increases in circulating nonesterified fatty acid (NEFA) concentrations; however, there appears to be some dissociation between the rate of fatty acid lipolysis from adipose tissue and the increased rates of skeletal muscle fatty acid oxidation (figure 1.3). Interestingly, despite similar increases in adipose tissue lipolysis and fatty acid uptake, rates of fatty acid oxidation are higher during low-intensity exercise in exercise-trained than in untrained men (Klein et al. 1994)—an effect possibly related to increased oxidation of fatty acids derived from intramuscular triglycerides (Hurley et al. 1986) and enhanced fatty acid extraction during exercise by the more trained muscle (Turcotte 1992).

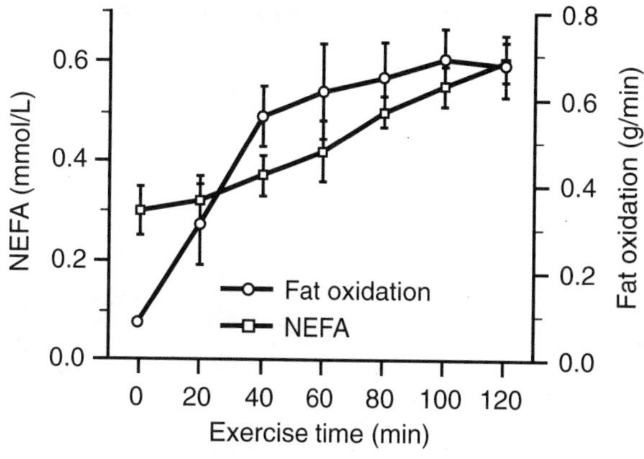

Figure 1.3 Plot of serum NEFA (non-esterified fatty acids) concentration and rates of fat oxidation during 2 hours of cycling exercise (70% $\dot{V}O_2$max).

Source: Fielding, 1995, unpublished observations.

PROTEIN AND AMINO ACID METABOLISM

Oxidation of specific amino acids (e.g., the branched-chain amino acids leucine, isoleucine, and valine) increases during exercise to a smaller extent than oxidation of fat and carbohydrate (10% to 15% of total oxidized substrate) (Rennie et al. 1981). Several researchers have reported that increased amino acid oxidation during prolonged exercise increases the dietary requirement for protein in physically active individuals (Meredith et al. 1989; Tarnopolsky et al. 1992).

Several variables can significantly modify the sequence of metabolic fuel mobilization outlined above; these include the duration of exercise, its intensity, the fitness of the individual, and the previous nutritional state. Carbohydrate and fatty acid oxidation appear to be inversely related: carbohydrate (as muscle glycogen and blood glucose) tends to be preferred early during exercise, and at higher exercise intensities; fat becomes the primary substrate toward the end of prolonged exercise (see figure 1.4).

ACUTE EXERCISE RESPONSE IN DIABETES MELLITUS

Exercise-induced changes in glucose homeostasis in patients with insulin-dependent diabetes mellitus (IDDM) are quite complex (Vitug et al. 1988; Zinman et al. 1984). The metabolic perturbations caused by exercise in diabetic individuals superimpose additional challenges to the normal metabolic response to exercise and provide interesting insights into the control of fuel utilization during exercise.

The method of insulin replacement in patients with IDDM does not duplicate the normal secretion of insulin

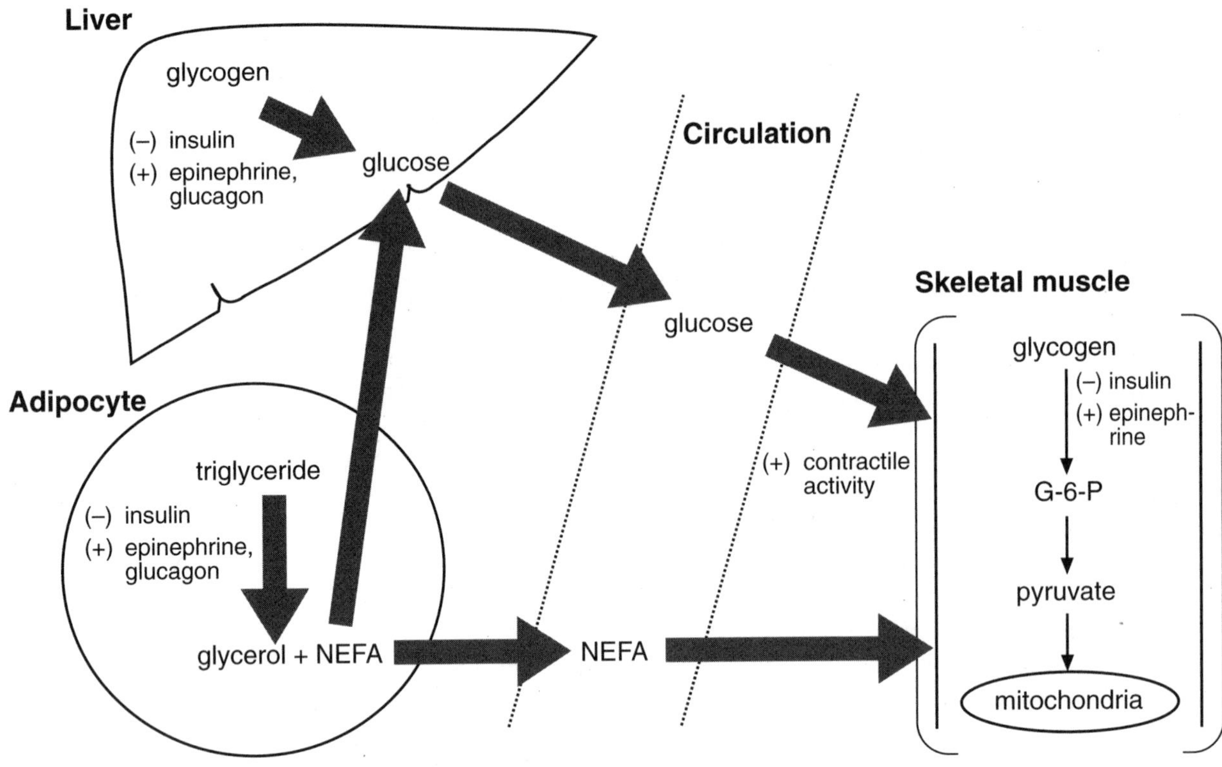

Figure 1.4 Overview of the metabolic response to dynamic exercise: (+) indicates activator, (–) indicates inhibitor. NEFA (non-esterified fatty acids), G-6-P (glucose-6-phosphate).

from the pancreas. Yet insulin and contractile activity constitute the two most instrumental stimulators for membrane transport of glucose in skeletal muscle (Arvill 1967; Helmreich and Cori 1957).

Average whole-body measures of aerobic fitness appear to be reduced in the IDDM population, primarily as a result of a characteristically sedentary lifestyle (Kemmer and Berger 1986). Interestingly, $\dot{V}O_2$max in physically active individuals with IDDM generally is no different from that in nondiabetic individuals; only if individuals with IDDM also have clinical manifestations of autonomic neuropathy will their $\dot{V}O_2$max be lower than in nondiabetic individuals (Veves et al. 1997). The metabolic alterations commonly associated with diabetes have a profound effect on the metabolic response to exercise. Diabetic patients commonly oscillate between states of insulin excess and insulin deficiency—and their metabolic responses to exercise correlate with the metabolic state at the onset of exercise (Giacca et al. 1991; Hilsted 1982; Kawamori and Vranic 1977; Vranic et al. 1990; Vranic and Wrenshall 1969). The most familiar disturbance of glucose homeostasis during exercise in IDDM is hypoglycemia. Hypoglycemia most often occurs during a relatively prolonged session of moderately intense exercise, when hepatic glucose production cannot keep pace with the increased use of glucose by exercising muscle. There is unrestrained peripheral glucose utilization, while portal hyperinsulinemia suppresses an appropriate rise in hepatic glucose output (Kawamori and Vranic 1977; Zinman et al. 1977). Conversely, patients in a state of chronic, moderate insulin deficiency have decreased glycogen stores in the liver and, to a lesser extent, in skeletal muscle (Wasserman and Zinman 1995). Insulin deficiency results in impaired aerobic exercise endurance; more rapid switch of fuels (during prolonged activity) to the utilization of free fatty acids; hyperglycemia; and accelerated formation of ketone bodies by the liver (Wasserman and Zinman 1995). Already increased levels of plasma glucose are further elevated by an exaggerated increase in hepatic glucose production caused by insulin deficiency (Vranic et al. 1976; Vranic and Wrenshall 1969). Elevated muscle glycogen concentrations, along with a rapid rate of glycogen breakdown, lead to high intramuscular concentrations of glucose-6-phosphate, which inhibits hexokinase (Newsholme and Leech 1983). As intracellular muscle glucose concentrations increase, the gradient of glucose from the interstitial space to the cytoplasm decreases; in turn, cells reduce their net uptake of glucose (Hespel and Richter 1990; Richter and Galbo

1986). Furthermore, lactate production is higher when glycogen concentrations are elevated than when they are low. Thus, the metabolic profile of an exercising individual with hyperglycemia after 40 minutes mirrors that of a normal human who has been performing aerobic exercise for 4 hours. This is known as the **accelerated adaptation to exercise** (Wahren et al. 1984).

In non-insulin-dependent diabetes mellitus (NIDDM), the diabetic state (i.e., hyperglycemia concomitant with either insulin deficiency or hyperinsulinemia) causes metabolic changes that affect skeletal muscle glucose transport (Olefsky et al. 1988). Exercise-induced changes in glucose homeostasis in NIDDM result from a positive impact on peripheral insulin action. Enhancement of insulin action in NIDDM with exercise appears to be related to an enhanced efficiency in glucose uptake mediated through increased translocation of the "GLUT-4" glucose transporter (Dohm 2002). The mechanism(s) by which exercise increases GLUT-4 translocation and reduces insulin resistance remains elusive but may be associated with activation of the adenosine monophosphate protein kinase (AMP-kinase) (Winder and Hardie 1999). Insulin resistance in the periphery occurs primarily in the skeletal muscle (the largest insulin-sensitive tissue) and therefore significantly affects overall glucose homeostasis in type 2 diabetic patients (Wallberg-Henriksson 1987).

CARDIORESPIRATORY CHANGES WITH ACTIVITY AND INACTIVITY

Cardiorespiratory fitness varies across different populations of healthy individuals. Generally, $\dot{V}O_2$max is higher in trained than in untrained individuals of both genders (although higher differences tend to be found in men). Yet because considerable variability exists among the four groups (Drinkwater 1984; Hermansen and Anderson 1965), overall means can be misleading when $\dot{V}O_2$max and levels of conditioning are measured across gender lines. As one might expect, $\dot{V}O_2$max values are larger in adults than in children. When controlled for variations in body size, however, these differences tend to diminish (Rowland et al. 1997). Many of the differences noted by gender, age, and training level correlate to increases in cardiac output and body size; increases in cardiac output, in turn, are directly related to elevated levels of stroke volume; and stroke volume is a function of increased cardiac size, left ventricular volume, and blood volume (Dowell 1983). Body size also contributes to differences in $\dot{V}O_2$max since a larger mass of muscle consumes a larger absolute volume of oxygen; one must account for this factor when drawing comparisons across populations.

It is well known among rehabilitation professionals that training improves fitness and can reverse changes induced by inactivity or immobilization. Improvements in $\dot{V}O_2$max vary with initial level of conditioning and intensity of training but range on average between 10% and 30% (Pollack 1973). Central effects of training include increased cardiac size (specifically, elevated left ventricular wall thickness) and left ventricular volume (Dowell 1983). Both circulating blood volume and red blood cell number increase in endurance-trained athletes. These factors collectively contribute to increased cardiac output. Peripherally, training increases levels of oxidative enzymes and positively influences the quantity and concentration of capillaries (Andersen 1975; Hermansen and Wachlova 1971). The net result is that skeletal muscle increases its capacity to utilize oxygen (Saltin and Rowell 1980), paralleling the increased capacity for oxygen delivery.

For over a century, physicians have prescribed immobility and bed rest for a variety of medical conditions. The adverse effects of immobility are a common comorbidity in patients with chronic disease. In large part, exercise rehabilitation aims to reverse the negative effects of prolonged inactivity (DeLisa 1993). Not surprisingly, debility is now a recognized diagnosis for admission to inpatient rehabilitation units (CFAR 1996). Immobility (specifically, bed rest) has detrimental effects on $\dot{V}O_2$max. Saltin and colleagues (1968) demonstrated these effects in a classic study using healthy young males. Twenty-one days of complete bed rest decreased $\dot{V}O_2$max by 25% and reduced stroke volume, cardiac output, and plasma volume by similar levels. Both resting and maximal heart rates increased. Recently, these same individuals were studied 30 years after their initial evaluation (McGuire et al. 2001). Aerobic capacity had declined over the 30 years since the initial study due to an impaired efficiency of peripheral oxygen extraction. Maximal cardiac output was maintained, with a decline in maximal heart rate compensated for by an increased maximal stroke volume. Interestingly, 21 days of bed rest had a more profound impact on exercise capacity than did three decades of aging. Reduced cardiac output appears primarily to be a function of reduced cardiac size and reduced plasma volume (Convertino 1997). The latter, along with changes in stroke volume, reduces cardiac output largely via the Frank-Starling mechanism. Increases in heart rate may represent a physiologic attempt to maintain cardiac output. Peripherally, there is a concomitant reduction in levels of oxidative enzymes and alterations in capillarization. With inactivity or complete cessation of training, the reductions in skeletal muscle oxidative capacity appear to occur sooner than the absolute declines in $\dot{V}O_2$max (Costill et al. 1985; Henriksson and Reitman 1977). All of these changes contribute to impaired extraction of oxygen within active skeletal muscle (Bloomfield 1997; Convertino et al. 1997). The coupling of these central and peripheral factors leads to decline in work capacity (Convertino et al. 1997; Saltin and Rowell 1980). Again, note the close linkage of these physiologic adjustments to decreased physical activity.

Physiological Adjustments to Isometric Exercise

Isometric exercise presents unique physiological demands. Hettenger and Muller first popularized it in the 1950s, describing it as muscle contraction against an immovable object. More specifically, active muscle contraction occurs with an absence of any limb movement or change in muscle length. Isometric muscle actions occur during normal human activity. For example, an individual waiting in line or leaning against a post or wall can have low-level isometric muscle activity within his paraspinal muscles as well as his lower extremity musculature. For people with slight hip and knee contractures, even quiet standing requires extensive isometric activity within lower extremity extensor musculature. All rehabilitation professionals—especially those who work with the elderly and debilitated populations—should understand the physiologic effects of isometric muscular activity.

Significant cardiovascular effects can occur with isometric exercise, including marked elevation of both systolic and diastolic blood pressure. There also can be greatly elevated stress to the left ventricular wall. Patients with hypertension, congestive heart failure, and other forms of cardiovascular disease should perform isometric exercise with caution (Atkins et al. 1976). Blood pressure increases in proportion to the effort exerted: as little as 15% of maximal voluntary contraction can produce changes in blood pressure (Coote et al. 1971). We do not know the specific mechanism by which this occurs, but apparently it is mediated in part through peripheral reflexes, since the phenomenon occurs in both large and small muscle groups (Buck et al. 1980). Heart rate accelerates, compromising diastolic filling time and in turn reducing stroke volume. Total peripheral resistance remains unchanged. The net effect is an elevation in blood pressure (Donald et al. 1967).

Supervision and feedback on technique and breathing can temper these potentially adverse effects (Goldberg et al. 1982; O'Connor et al. 1989)—in fact, even at high levels of isometric contraction, blood pressure response can be indistinguishable from that seen in other forms of strength training (Greer et al. 1984). Isometric exercise programs in appropriate patient populations can even lower resting blood pressure (Wiley et al. 1992).

Not only are isometric training effects generally specific to the joint angles at which they occur (Graves et al. 1989)—pure isometric exercise can reduce maximal limb velocity. Despite these apparent adverse effects, isometric exercise can be very beneficial in many cases. Under conditions where limited limb motion is required, such as acute arthritis or joint injury, isometric exercise can maintain strength and muscle bulk. Depending on the technique, clinicians have reported strength gains of as much as 5% per week in such patients (DeLisa 1993).

Summary

This chapter has introduced several key components of the physiological response to dynamic exercise, including the relationships between oxygen transport and peripheral oxygen extraction. We have highlighted the tight coupling of metabolism to its substrate delivery mechanisms. By illustrating the exercise response to several disease states, we have also illustrated the abundant overriding and compensatory mechanisms that these diverse pathologies call into play. Because exercise is a key component of many treatments in rehabilitation, these fundamental principles underlie nearly every procedure and treatment plan in modern physical rehabilitation. Understanding normal and abnormal responses to exercise may stimulate new and innovative thinking about future roles of exercise and physical activity in the prevention and treatment of chronic diseases.

CHAPTER 2

ADAPTATIONS TO ENDURANCE EXERCISE TRAINING

Martin D. Hoffman, MD

Aerobic or endurance exercise refers to dynamic contractions of large muscle groups at relatively low forces, with sufficient oxygen present to allow continuation of the exercise for several minutes or longer. This type of exercise stimulates many systems of the body, resulting in acute **physiological responses**. Endurance exercise performed regularly, at adequate intensities and durations, is referred to as **endurance exercise training**. The body responds to this training through **physiological adaptations**. Associated with the physiological adaptations are a host of **health benefits** (see chapters 8-18). This chapter focuses on the basic physiological adaptations that result from endurance exercise training. More extensive discussions on this topic can be found in other publications (McArdle et al. 2001; Wilmore and Costill 1999).

It is important that rehabilitation clinicians understand the adaptations that result from endurance training, since their goals are to prevent deterioration of and to restore functional capacity. Since endurance capacity is a major determinant of functional abilities, knowledge of the factors affecting endurance is fundamental for the clinical practice of rehabilitation medicine.

PHYSIOLOGICAL ADAPTATIONS TO ENDURANCE EXERCISE TRAINING

Endurance exercise training results in a wide variety of adaptations that enhance a person's ability to respond to subsequent exercise loads and to the demands of functional activities. Many adaptations involve improved oxygen delivery to the exercising muscles; others serve to reduce the demands on the body in other ways. A description of the most important adaptations to endurance exercise training follows.

MAXIMAL AEROBIC POWER

An important adaptation to endurance exercise training is increased maximal aerobic power ($\dot{V}O_2max$), considered the best single indicator of the cardiorespiratory system's functional capacity. **$\dot{V}O_2max$** is defined as the highest rate of oxygen consumption attainable during maximal exercise. It is determined as the rate of oxygen uptake at which no further increase occurs despite an increase in exercise intensity or power output. The term **peak $\dot{V}O_2$** is referred to when it is realized that the individual did not reach his highest attainable $\dot{V}O_2$ during an exercise test because of the mode of exercise being used, the testing protocol or lack of motivation. Such limitations are frequently an issue in the clinical setting and make it challenging to measure the true extent of improvement in $\dot{V}O_2$ that may result from an exercise training program.

The rate at which the body consumes oxygen is defined by the product of the cardiac output and the arterial-venous oxygen difference. **Cardiac output** is the rate at which blood is pumped by the heart to the tissues of the body. The **arterial-venous oxygen difference** is the difference in oxygen content between arterial and venous blood and indicates how much oxygen has been extracted by the tissues.

Most studies indicate that sedentary people within diverse populations (age, gender, income, ethnic background, health status) experience improvements in $\dot{V}O_2max$ of 15% or more within 3 to 6 months of starting an endurance exercise training program (Clausen 1977; Lavie and Milani 1995; McGuire et al. 2001; NIH 1996; Sheldahl et al. 1993). In youth and early adulthood, this increase is generally about equally due to **peripheral adaptations** that primarily increase the arterial-venous oxygen difference and **central adaptations** that primarily raise maximal cardiac output (Rowell 1974; McGuire et al. 2001).

Central Adaptations

Cardiac output is determined by the product of heart rate and stroke volume. Since maximal heart rate does not rise and may even be slightly reduced with endurance exercise training (Zavorsky 2000), the rise in maximal cardiac output from training results from increased stroke volume. In adapting to endurance exercise training, stroke volume increases not only during maximal exercise, but also at rest and during submaximal exercise where there is a concomitant decrease in heart rate. The mechanisms by which stroke volume increases with training appear to involve increased cardiac preload, enhanced myocardial contractility, and reduced afterload (figure 2.1).

The increased cardiac preload induced by endurance training is partly due to an expansion in plasma volume and total blood volume of approximately 10% within 1 to 4 days of initiation of an exercise training program (Sawka et al. 2000). During exercise, increased release of both antidiuretic hormone and aldosterone causes the kidney to retain water; and increased levels of plasma proteins, particularly albumin, raise the osmotic pressure of the blood and cause intravascular fluid retention.

Increased left ventricular filling time and volume are also important factors that increase cardiac output. Endurance exercise training induces an increase in left ventricular volume, along with some increase in the thickness of the posterior and septal walls of the left ventricle (Ehsani et al. 1991; Landry et al. 1985; Morrison et al. 1986; Rerych et al. 1980). The increased ventricular volume may be due to a chronic stretch of the myocardium at rest from the training-induced plasma volume expansion and to the greater diastolic filling time associated with a slower resting heart rate (Rowell 1986). It has been postulated that the heart adapts to the resultant increase in end-diastolic volume by increasing the left ventricle chamber size.

As a result of the increased left ventricular preload, the greater stretch on the ventricular walls produces greater elastic recoil via the Frank-Starling mechanism. This effect, coupled with the more forceful contraction that occurs from the larger ventricular muscle mass, also serves to increase stroke volume.

Another factor serving to increase maximal stroke volume after endurance exercise training is a reduction in total peripheral resistance, or afterload. Because the increased cardiac output can maintain mean arterial blood pressure, sympathetic vasoconstrictor activity to the arterioles of the trained muscles can be reduced (Rowell 1986).

The autonomic nervous system control of heart function is altered by endurance exercise training (Carter et al. 2003). There is an increase in parasympathetic activity and a decrease in sympathetic activity to the heart at rest, helping to account for the reduction in resting heart rate. Decreases in sympathetic activity to the heart are also associated with the reduction in submaximal exercise heart rates. Such changes in cardiac autonomic regulation have been suggested as part of the explanation for the impairment in orthostatic tolerance that appears to be associated with endurance training (Zhang et al. 1999).

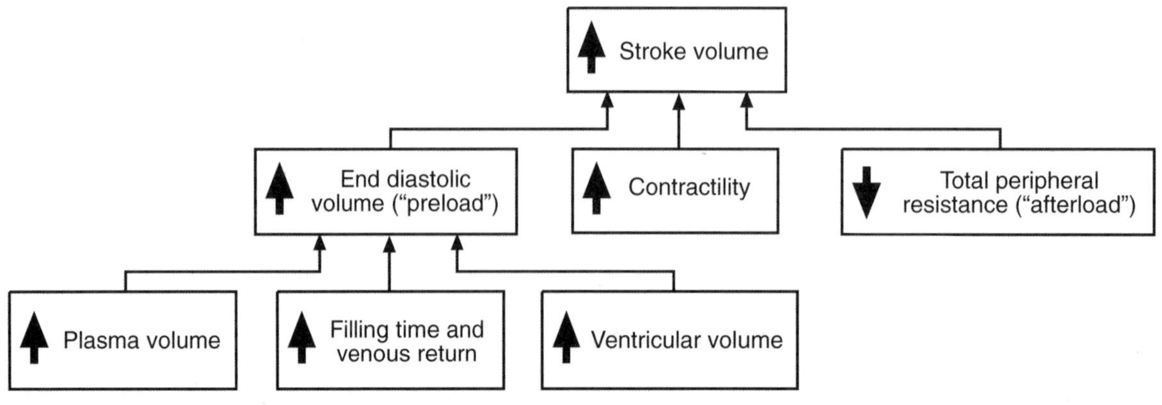

Figure 2.1 Summary of factors causing an increase in stroke volume with endurance exercise training.

Adapted from S. Powers and E. Howley, 1997, *Exercise physiology: Theory and application to fitness and performance,* 3rd ed. (Brown and Benchmark), 234. With permission of The McGraw-Hill Companies.

PERIPHERAL ADAPTATIONS

Some of the training-induced improvements in $\dot{V}O_2max$ generally result from peripheral adaptations that primarily increase the arterial-venous oxygen difference—an increase due to lower mixed venous oxygen content, reflecting both greater oxygen extraction at the tissue level and more effective distribution of total blood volume (McGuire et al. 2001; Rowell 1974). The arterial oxygen content does not increase with training, even though total hemoglobin is increased. The increase in plasma volume is greater than the increase in hemoglobin, so the amount of hemoglobin per volume of blood is the same or slightly reduced. Since the arterial partial pressure of oxygen is usually sufficient to maintain arterial saturation of hemoglobin, the arterial oxygen content does not increase with training.

A variety of structural, functional, and metabolic changes enhance oxygen delivery and extraction within the trained muscle. An increase in the number and size of mitochondria, along with increases in their respiratory enzyme activities, enhances the capacity of trained muscle cells for aerobic energy provision from both fatty acid and carbohydrate oxidation (Hawley 2002; Holloszy and Coyle 1984). There is also an increase in capillary density and capillary-fiber ratio, which promotes efficient metabolic exchange (Prior et al. 2003). The increase in the number of capillaries surrounding each muscle fiber improves the oxygen exchange between capillary and fiber by presenting a greater surface area for the diffusion of oxygen; by shortening the average distance required for oxygen to diffuse into the muscle; and by slowing the rate of blood flow, thereby increasing the length of time for diffusion to occur. The increase in muscle myoglobin observed with endurance training is also important in oxygen delivery. When oxygen enters the muscle fiber, it binds to myoglobin, which shuttles the oxygen to the mitochondria.

Improved blood flow capacity and muscle perfusion also result from training adaptations in the control of vascular tone and enlargement in the caliber of arterial supply vessels. Endurance training induces enhanced vascular responsiveness to endothelium-dependent vasodilators and decreased sensitivity to the vasoconstrictor effects of norepinephrine (Delp 1995; Hambrecht et al. 2000). Structural enlargement of conduit vessels occurs with training, serving to increase blood flow potential (Miyachi et al. 2001; Prior et al. 2003).

Whether endurance training results in conversion of fast type II fibers to slow type I fibers remains unclear. However, there is evidence for a transformation of fast type IIx myosin heavy chain to fast type IIa myosin heavy chain (Fitts and Widrick 1996). Furthermore, the mitochondrial content of type II fibers tends to increase more than in type I fibers in response to very strenuous endurance training, essentially eliminating the difference in mitochondrial enzyme levels between type I and II fibers (Chi et al. 1983; Jansson and Kaijser 1977).

Figure 2.2 summarizes the factors causing an increase in $\dot{V}O_2max$. Besides increasing maximal exercise capacity, endurance training allows one to perform submaximal exercise at a given absolute intensity or power output with less cardiovascular stress—probably providing the broadest therapeutic value of exercise training. Table 2.1 summarizes the cardiorespiratory adaptations to endurance exercise training at rest, during submaximal exercise, and during maximal exercise.

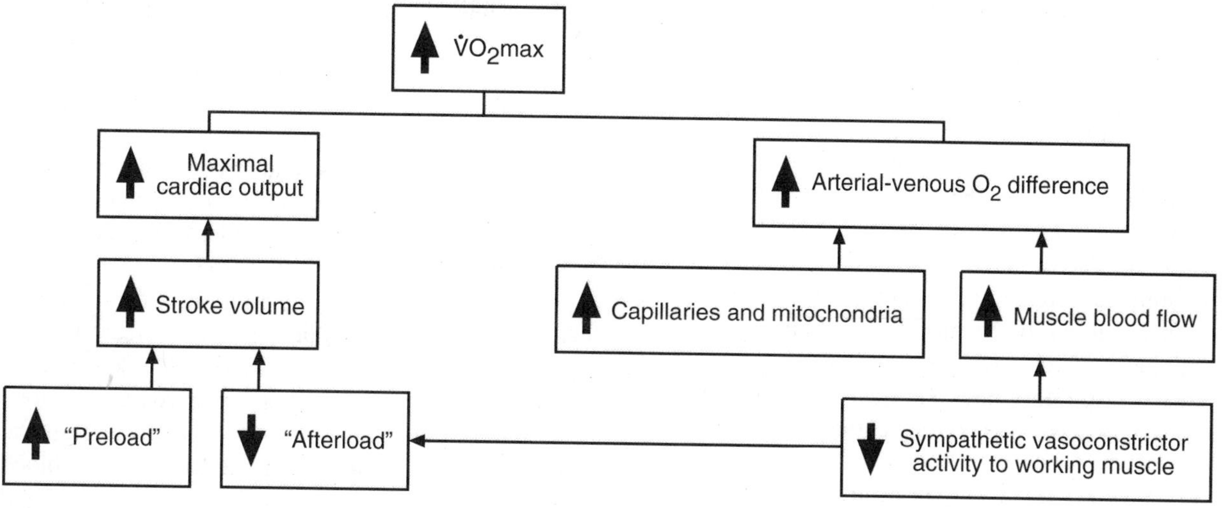

Figure 2.2 Summary of factors causing an increase in $\dot{V}O_2max$ with endurance exercise training.

Adapted from S. Powers and E. Howley, 1997, *Exercise physiology: Theory and application to fitness and performance*, 3rd ed. (Brown and Benchmark), 235. With permission of The McGraw-Hill Companies.

Table 2.1 Cardiorespiratory Adaptations to Endurance Exercise Training As Observed in Resting and Exercise States

	Rest	Submaximal exercise	Maximal exercise
Oxygen uptake	No change*	No change†	Increase
Heart rate	Decrease	Decrease	Decrease
Stroke volume	Increase	Increase	Increase
Cardiac output	No change	No change	Increase
Myocardial oxygen demand	Decrease	Decrease	No change
Ventilation	No change	Decrease	Increase
Arterial-venous oxygen difference	No change	Increase	Increase
Blood lactate concentration	No change	Decrease	Increase
Muscle blood flow	No change	Decrease	Increase
Splanchnic blood flow	No change	No change	Decrease
Systolic blood pressure	Decrease	Decrease	No change
Diastolic blood pressure	Decrease	Decrease	No change

*Or may increase slightly.

†Or may decrease slightly.

RESPIRATORY ADAPTATIONS

The respiratory system usually does not limit endurance exercise capacity. As a result, adaptations to the respiratory system from endurance training have less functional importance than some of the other adaptations. Adaptations to the respiratory system are observed primarily during exercise rather than at rest.

Endurance training may slightly lower respiratory rate and tidal volume and slightly decrease ventilation at light exercise loads (Åstrand and Rodahl 1977; Martin et al. 1979). It is thought that this small reduction in ventilation may be due to reduced sensitivity of the arterial and brain chemoreceptors that respond to carbon dioxide in the blood (Martin et al. 1979). At moderate to heavy exercise intensities, the ventilation for a fixed power output can be reduced by 20% to 30% below pretraining levels (Casaburi et al. 1987; Clanton et al. 1987). This training adaptation is thought to result from a lower accumulation of lactic acid in the blood, which causes less afferent feedback from the working muscles to stimulate breathing. Because of the greater power output that can be produced as a result of endurance training, maximal exercise after such a program induces greater respiratory rates and tidal volumes, causing an overall increase in maximal ventilation.

METABOLIC ADAPTATIONS

Endurance training markedly changes the metabolic responses of muscles to submaximal exercise. There are smaller increases in muscle and blood lactate concentrations, reduced reliance on carbohydrate, and increased utilization of fatty acid oxidation at a given absolute exercise level after training. These interrelated metabolic adaptations are largely responsible for the increased endurance from training.

LACTATE LEVELS

Lactate accumulation has long been suspected to be important in the development of fatigue. While the mechanisms are not clear, it is apparent that there is an association between endurance capacity and the exercise intensity required to elicit a given lactate concentration (Farrell et al. 1979; LaFontaine et al. 1981; Sjodin and Jacobs 1981).

Endurance exercise training allows a higher power output, and higher absolute oxygen consumption, without raising blood lactate concentrations above resting levels (figure 2.3). Intense endurance training can also lead to an increase in the percentage of $\dot{V}O_2max$ at which an individual must exercise in order to induce a given blood lactate level (Hurley et al. 1984).

Lower blood lactate concentrations after endurance exercise training may be due largely to decreased lactate production by the exercising muscles (Henriksson 1977; Saltin et al. 1976), resulting from improvements in blood flow and oxygen extraction. Increased lactate removal may also play a role in accounting for the lower blood lactate concentrations after training, possibly related to improved blood flow to the liver (a major site for lactate removal for gluconeogenesis). Training also induces adaptations within the muscle that minimize

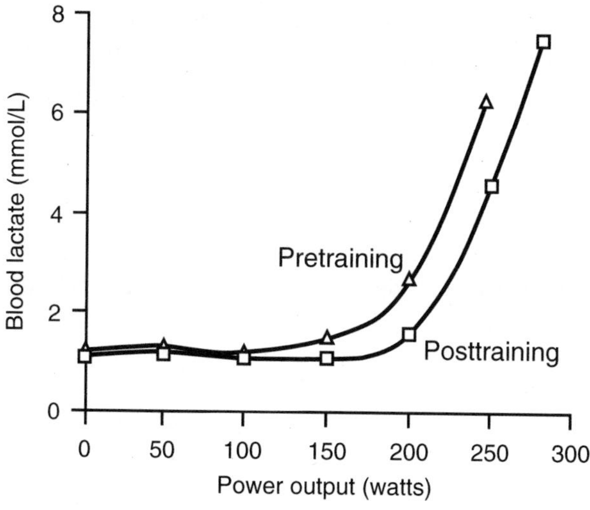

Figure 2.3 Blood lactate concentrations relative to work rate before and after an endurance exercise training program.

the changes in internal pH that occur during intense exercise (Juel 1997).

FUEL UTILIZATION

Biochemical adaptations in trained muscle have metabolic effects that improve endurance during prolonged exercise. The biochemical signals that accelerate metabolism during submaximal exercise are attenuated in trained muscles, reducing the rate of carbohydrate metabolism and tending to spare the use of muscle glycogen in trained individuals (Hermansen et al. 1967; Karlsson et al. 1972). A proportional increase in fatty acid oxidation compensates for the decreased utilization of carbohydrate during submaximal exercise in the trained state, even when the circulating fatty acid concentration is not elevated (Mole et al. 1971; Spriet 2002)—an effect reflected by a lower respiratory exchange ratio at both the same absolute and the same relative exercise intensities after training compared with before training (Holloszy 1973).

There is evidence that depletion of glycogen stores can be important in the development of fatigue during prolonged exercise (Holloszy 1973). The glycogen-sparing effect probably plays a major role in the increase in endurance that occurs with training.

OXYGEN UPTAKE

Oxygen consumption at rest is either unchanged or slightly increased following an endurance exercise training program (Poehlman et al. 1991). The oxygen consumption required for a given submaximal task, which defines the economy for performing the activity (Cavanagh and Kram 1985), is either unchanged or slightly reduced after training, depending on the activity and the mode of training. For activities such as walking, running, and cycling, there is minimal or no improvement in economy with training, since individuals generally are proficient at these activities when they begin a training program. However, when the activity is unfamiliar and requires the development of some skill to perform, economy is improved with training (Vokac and Rodahl 1976). As such, training at activities such as swimming and cross-country skiing will likely result in improvements in economy, as demonstrated by a reduction in oxygen uptake and cardiac output at submaximal speeds after training. From a practical standpoint, an improved economy reduces the physiological demands on an individual when performing a given task.

THERMOREGULATORY ADAPTATIONS

Although full adaptation to heat requires a period of acclimatization, endurance-trained individuals show some of these adaptations without undergoing heat acclimatization (Terrados and Maughan 1995). Endurance-trained individuals therefore have a greater heat-dissipating capacity than sedentary individuals (Wyndham 1973). The beneficial effects of endurance training on heat tolerance appear more closely related to training volume than to aerobic capacity (Pandolf et al. 1988).

Endurance exercise training leads to increased sensitivity of sweating mechanisms and a lowering of the sweating threshold (Nadel et al. 1974). Increased sweating limits the rise in body temperature during exercise. And because trained individuals maintain a higher total blood volume during exercise (Convertino et al. 1983) more blood can be directed to the periphery for heat transfer to the environment.

HORMONAL ADAPTATIONS

Hormones are chemical messengers secreted by endocrine glands and cells throughout the body. Collectively, hormones are involved in the regulation of energy metabolism, fluid and electrolyte balance, circulation, reproductive function, growth and development, and pain perception. Because of the widespread influence of hormones on various body systems, the hormonal adaptations to endurance exercise training have a vast array of effects. In fact, it is probable that the adaptations in hormonal function play a role in many of the physiological adaptations to exercise. Selected hormones will be discussed below.

Exercise stimulates secretion of **catecholamines** (epinephrine and norepinephrine), whose plasma concentrations increase exponentially with exercise intensity (Bloom et al. 1976; Galbo et al. 1975). In addition to their effects on cardiorespiratory function and thermoregulation, catecholamines have a number of important metabolic effects, including the stimulation of lipolysis and hepatic glycogenolysis (Vander et al. 1985). Training reduces plasma epinephrine and norepinephrine concentrations at a given *absolute* exercise intensity; however, at the same *relative* exercise intensity, responses of epinephrine and norepinephrine are unchanged after training (Hartley et al. 1972a, 1972b; Peronnet et al. 1981; Winder et al. 1979). Trained individuals possess an enhanced adrenal medullary secretory capacity, as demonstrated by plasma epinephrine concentrations almost double the pretraining levels for the same relative supramaximal intensity (Kjaer et al. 1986).

Insulin and glucagon are secreted by the pancreas. **Insulin** generally increases fat and glycogen synthesis and lowers blood glucose levels, whereas **glucagon** increases the rate of glycogenolysis. Appropriately, insulin levels decrease as the duration or intensity of exercise increases, and glucagon levels increase to maintain blood glucose levels during exercise. Regular endurance exercise reduces the capacity of pancreatic beta cells to secrete insulin (Dela et al. 1987; Mikines et al. 1987); at the same time, the effect of insulin on muscle cell glucose uptake from plasma is increased (Mikines et al. 1988). This increased insulin sensitivity is partly due to induction of muscle glucose transporter (GLUT4, a cell membrane-spanning protein), along with increased enzyme capacities and muscle capillarization (Borghouts and Keizer 2000; MacLean et al. 2000). Thus, exercise training results in a lower need for insulin to handle a given carbohydrate load. The resting levels of glucagon decrease with training, but the exercise response increases (Galbo et al. 1977).

Growth hormone, produced by the anterior pituitary, enhances lipolysis and gluconeogenesis (Shephard and Sidney 1975). It is thought that growth hormone is important in maintaining blood levels of free fatty acids and glucose during exercise of long duration (Shephard and Sidney 1975). Although training has been reported to generally diminish the growth hormone response (Bloom et al. 1976; Sutton 1978), maintenance of peak growth hormone levels during prolonged exercise durations may be enhanced in trained individuals (Hartley 1975).

Another anterior pituitary hormone that increases with exercise is **adrenocorticotropic hormone (ACTH),** which acts on the adrenal cortex to secrete cortisol. **Cortisol** enhances free fatty acid mobilization and acts to conserve carbohydrates. Like growth hormone, cortisol may be more significant for potentiating than for initiating lipolysis. Training does not change the plasma concentrations of cortisol at the same relative exercise intensity, whereas the levels may be lower for a given absolute exercise intensity after training (Hartley et al. 1972a and 1972b; Sutton 1978; Sutton et al. 1969).

Maintenance of fluid and electrolyte balance is under hormonal control through actions on renal function. **Aldosterone** secretion from the adrenal cortex is elevated during exercise, leading to increased renal reabsorption of sodium. Sodium retention results in a higher plasma osmolarity which, in turn, stimulates **antidiuretic hormone** secretion by the posterior pituitary to increase renal retention of water. Such adaptations help prevent dehydration during exercise. Training reduces the degree to which these hormones increase during exercise at a given absolute intensity (Convertino et al. 1981; Melin et al. 1980).

Reproductive hormones can indirectly (and possibly directly) affect fuel utilization during exercise. However, the bulk of research in recent years has focused on the responses of these hormones to exercise training and the resulting effect on reproductive function. The anterior pituitary hormone **prolactin** increases during exercise, and trained women exhibit an enhanced response (Brisson et al. 1980; Keizer et al. 1987). It is possible that repeatedly elevated prolactin levels suppress ovarian function, which in turn contributes to menstrual dysfunction, including delayed menarche, a shortened luteal phase, and primary and secondary amenorrhea (Prior et al. 1981). While most adaptations to endurance training appear to serve a beneficial role, long-term amenorrhea from intense training has been associated with reduced bone density (Cann et al. 1984; Drinkwater et al. 1984). In men there is evidence that intense training causes a suppression of spermatogenesis and **testosterone** (Hackney 1996), the significance of which is unclear.

Endogenous opioid peptides have been associated with many physiological processes. At least one of these peptides, **beta-endorphin**, appears to act within the central nervous system to produce analgesia (Hosobuchi and Li 1978). Several animal studies have demonstrated that the concentration of beta-endorphin increases in specific regions of the brain following exercise (Blake et al. 1984; Christie and Chesher 1983; Hoffmann et al. 1990; Sforzo et al. 1986), and a number of human studies have shown decreased pain perception immediately after exercise (Droste et al. 1991; Hoffman et al. 2004; Janal et al. 1984; Kemppainen et al. 1990, 1985; Koltyn et al. 1996; Olausson et al. 1986; Pertovaara et al. 1984). While there is good support for the presence of exercise-induced analgesia, the evidence that endogenous opioid peptides are the cause of mood alterations and the "runner's high" frequently attributed to these peptides is inconclusive. Some evidence suggests that exercise training results in an enhanced beta-endorphin output during exercise (Carr et al. 1981; Farrell et al. 1987; Mougin et al. 1987), yet the data are not consistent (Metzger and Stein 1984). It has been suggested that regular exercise may offer protection from the development of chronic pain syndromes (Moldofsky and Scarisbrick 1976), but current evidence indicates that there may be only a modest favorable impact of endurance exercise training on pain intensity from chronic pain states (Busch et al. 2002). It is unclear if endogenous opioid peptides are involved in this process.

NEUROLOGICAL ADAPTATIONS

Little is known about adaptations of the nervous system to exercise, since it is difficult both to measure performance and to examine tissue of the central and peripheral nervous system. Nevertheless, it is evident that adaptations occur to the nervous system from exercise training. For example, exercise training at a skilled activity can result in improved neuromuscular coordination and a reduction in the energy required to perform that activity (i.e., an improvement in economy) (Vokac and Rodahl 1977). Neurological adaptations associated with endurance training have also been demonstrated through the findings of enhanced motor unit recruitment (Lucia et al. 2000).

Exercise training may affect central motor drive. Although it is possible for highly motivated subjects to voluntarily achieve full activation of muscles, under normal conditions the strong desire to reduce the intensity of the motor drive is a limiting factor during physical exertion. It has been suggested that learning to overcome these inhibitory sensations is one of the most important adaptations of exercise training (Bigland-Ritchie 1990).

Animal studies have shown that endurance exercise training may cause changes in neural tissue, including increases in nerve terminal size, an increase in nerve-evoked transmitter release, and an increase in the activity of acetylcholinesterase at the neuromuscular junction (Panenic and Gardiner 1998). While the significance of these changes is not clear, this evidence indicates that there may be important neural adaptations to exercise.

ADAPTATIONS IN COGNITION AND MENTAL HEALTH

Cross-sectional studies have suggested that aerobic capacity is associated with preserved cognitive function in older age (Barnes et al. 2003; van Boxtel et al. 1997). Furthermore, longitudinal studies have demonstrated that endurance exercise training can improve multiple aspects of attention and mental function during aging (Hawkins et al. 1992; Kramer et al. 1999). Endurance exercise has also been demonstrated to be effective in improving general mood and symptoms of depression and anxiety in both healthy individuals and psychiatric patients (Meyer and Broocks 2000).

Exercise is widely believed to improve sleep quality and reduce daytime sleepiness. While there is some scientific evidence to support these beliefs, the evidence is mixed and, as yet, inconclusive (O'Connor and Youngstedt 1995).

ADAPTATIONS OF BONE AND CONNECTIVE TISSUE

Bone and connective tissue adapt to mechanical loading. Mechanical loading, like that experienced with exercise, contributes to an increase in bone mass and can reduce the bone demineralization that occurs with aging (Aloia et al. 1987; Gleeson et al. 1990; Margulies et al. 1986; Williams et al. 1984). Furthermore, the effect on bone density from exercise during the peak bone forming years appears to remain evident years later (Kohrt et al. 1995; Ulrich et al. 1996).

Besides the positive effects on bone, endurance exercise training strengthens ligaments and tendons, as well as the attachments of ligaments and tendons to bones (Tipton et al. 1975). Moreover, damaged ligaments regain strength at a faster rate if physical activity is performed after the injury (Tipton et al. 1975).

ADAPTATIONS IN FUNCTIONAL CAPACITY

While many adaptations result from endurance exercise training, the most important change may relate to function. Since endurance capacity is a major determinant of functional abilities, it should be clear from the preceding discussion that endurance exercise training produces functional benefits. Training increases maximal exercise capacity and the sustainable power output. Perhaps even more importantly, an endurance exercise training program decreases the physiological and psychological demands from an absolute exercise intensity or power output—in other words, the individual performs a given amount of work with less physiological stress and perceives it as being easier.

Enhancing functional capacity can especially benefit those with limited physiological reserve due to age, disease, or disability (Clausen and Trap-Jensen 1976; NIH 1996; Shephard 1993). Greater functional capacity enables one to be more active in normal daily routines; maintain greater independence in older age or with disabilities; and resume activities, including occupational work, sooner after a disabling injury or illness (Fentem 1992; Fries 1996; Fries et al. 1994; Hiatt et al. 1994; Shephard 1993; Strawbridge et al. 1996; Young et al. 1995). There appears to be an obligatory decrease in $\dot{V}O_2max$ of about 5% to 10% for every decade of adult life (Heath et al. 1981; Kasch et al. 1990; Rogers et al. 1990), and it has been estimated that an able-bodied person needs a $\dot{V}O_2max$ of about 12 to 14 $ml \cdot kg^{-1} \cdot min^{-1}$ to sustain independent living (Shephard 1991). Remaining physically active into old age may allow a

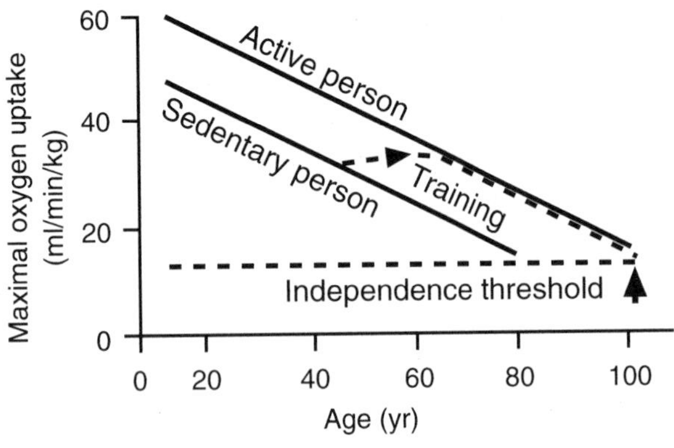

Figure 2.4 Demonstration of the effect of endurance exercise training on improving maximal aerobic power and on delaying its drop to a threshold where independent function can no longer be maintained.

Reproduced, with permission, from *Geriatrics*, Vol. 48, Number 5, May 1993, page 62. Copyright by Advanstar Communications Inc. Advanstar Communications Inc. retains all rights to this article.

person to maintain functional independence for 10 to 20 years longer than if he or she is inactive (figure 2.4).

Psychological Adaptations to Endurance Exercise Training

A large body of evidence indicates that regular exercise produces a variety of psychological benefits. Acutely after endurance exercise, ratings of self-esteem, depression, psychological tension, and mood are significantly improved (Farrell et al. 1987; Janal et al. 1984; Markoff et al. 1982; McCann and Holmes 1984; Sonstroem 1984). Regular physical activity improves the sense of well-being (Blumenthal et al. 1990; Lavie et al. 1993). Endurance exercise, when performed on a regular basis, is associated with acute reductions in anxiety (Morgan 1979) and muscle tension (deVries 1968) in normal individuals. Among those who are mildly or moderately anxious or depressed, positive mood changes are associated with exercise training (Simons et al. 1985). Improvements in psychological well-being from regular physical activity have also been demonstrated during pregnancy (Da Costa et al. 2003), and among patients with fibromyalgia syndrome (Busch et al. 2002).

Factors Affecting Adaptations to Endurance Exercise Training

The adaptations to endurance exercise training, as described above, can occur in all populations—young, old, able-bodied, and disabled. Several factors influence the extent and time course of the adaptations, however, including initial level of fitness, design and duration of the training program, genetics, age and gender.

Initial Level of Fitness

In general, the extent of adaptations to training is greater among individuals who are less conditioned at the beginning of the training program (Sharkey 1970). Sedentary middle-aged men with heart disease may improve their $\dot{V}O_2$max by 50%; a similar training program in normal active adults may lead to a smaller, but significant, 10% to 15% improvement (Cronan and Howley 1974; Ekblom 1969; Hickson et al. 1981; Saltin 1969). Well-conditioned athletes may increase their $\dot{V}O_2$max by only 2% to 3% following an increase in their training (Cronan and Howley 1974).

Intensity, Duration, and Frequency of Exercise

The extent of physiological adaptations to endurance training is highly related to the intensity, duration, and frequency of training. Figure 2.5 shows the effects of these variables on oxidative capacity of muscle. Numerous longitudinal studies have also demonstrated that the intensity, duration, and frequency of training are important determinants of the improvement in $\dot{V}O_2$max (Sharkey 1970; Shephard 1968). Figure 2.6 schematically displays the effects of these variables on $\dot{V}O_2$max. In general, optimal increases in $\dot{V}O_2$max result from

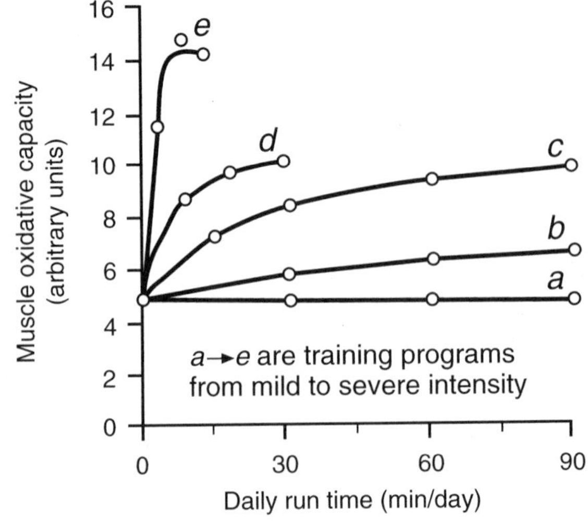

Figure 2.5 Influence of exercise bout duration and intensity on muscle oxidative capacity (as measured by cytochrome *c* concentration) in rats that underwent various treadmill training regimens for 8 weeks.

Adapted, by permission, from G. Dudley, W. Abraham, and R. Terjung, 1982, "Influence of exercise intensity and duration on biochemical adaptations in skeletal muscle," *Journal of Applied Physiology* 53(4):846.

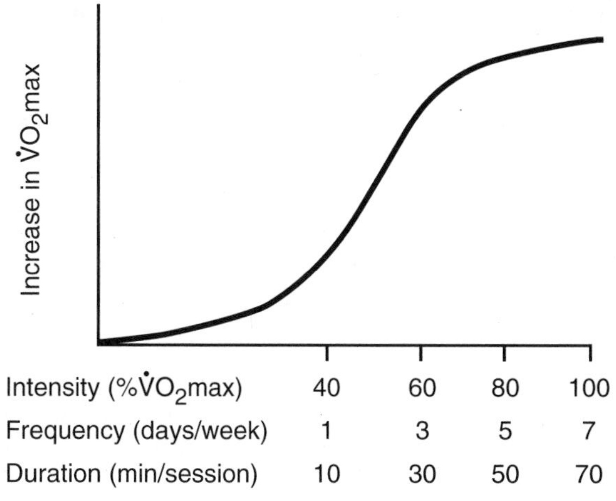

Figure 2.6 Schematic representation of the effect of exercise intensity, frequency, and duration on $\dot{V}O_2$max.

training programs that are 20 to 60 min per session, three to five times per week, at intensities of 50% to 85% $\dot{V}O_2$max (American College of Sports Medicine 1998). Below these levels, little or no gain in $\dot{V}O_2$max occurs. Beyond these levels, the benefits become smaller relative to the additional demands.

Recent reports from both the Surgeon General (1996) and the NIH (1996) have emphasized the importance of regular physical activity for all Americans. These statements stress the health benefits of even moderate levels of physical activity performed on a regular basis.

Using meta-analysis, Londeree (1997) recently examined how training intensity alters the exercise level at which blood lactate concentration begins to rise (**lactate threshold**) or a fixed blood lactate concentration occurs. He concluded that exercise intensity near the lactate threshold is necessary to improve the threshold intensity among sedentary people. Training at higher intensities seems to have minimal benefits in sedentary individuals, but is probably necessary to increase the lactate threshold in conditioned individuals.

GENETICS

The extremely high $\dot{V}O_2$max levels of elite endurance athletes have been ascribed to genetics. While training is necessary for these individuals to reach their upper limit in $\dot{V}O_2$max, genetic factors establish the upper boundaries. The importance of genetics in determining $\dot{V}O_2$max is rather clear: identical (monozygous) twins have much more similar $\dot{V}O_2$max values than fraternal (dizygous) twins (Bouchard et al. 1986; Fagard et al. 1991; Maes et al. 1996; Sundet et al. 1994). In fact, as much as 50% to over 65% of variations in $\dot{V}O_2$max are currently thought to be related to genetic factors (Bouchard et al. 1999, 1998; Fagard et al. 1991; Maes et al. 1996; Sundet et al. 1994). An individual's responsiveness to a training program also seems to have a genetic association (Pérusse et al. 2001). Recent work has demonstrated that the genes and markers that have evidence of linkage with a fitness phenotype, acute responses to exercise, or training-induced adaptations are positioned on the genetic map of all autosomes and the X chromosome (Pérusse et al. 2003).

AGE

$\dot{V}O_2$max typically peaks at 15 to 20 years of age, with women being at the lower end of this range. Cross-sectional analysis suggests that, after this age, $\dot{V}O_2$max gradually declines—typically about 10% per decade (Buskirk and Hodgson 1987). Until recently, it was difficult to determine whether the decline is related to age, disease, or just physical inactivity. It is now clear that maximal heart rate declines with aging regardless of training status (Åstrand 1960; McGuire et al. 2001; Reeves and Sheffield 1971), and that there is an obligate decrease in $\dot{V}O_2$max of about 5% per decade (Heath et al. 1981; Kasch et al. 1990; Rogers et al. 1990). The typical age-related decline in $\dot{V}O_2$max apparently can be slowed through regular endurance training (Bortz and Bortz 1996). Furthermore, it is well documented that the elderly have a capacity similar to that of younger individuals to improve $\dot{V}O_2$max through endurance training (Hagberg et al. 1989; Kohrt et al. 1991; Makrides et al. 1990; Meredith et al. 1989; Saltin et al. 1969; Seals et al. 1984; Sheldahl et al. 1993).

GENDER

$\dot{V}O_2$max values of females and males are similar until puberty. Beyond puberty, the average woman's $\dot{V}O_2$max is only 70% to 75% that of the average man's (Åstrand 1960). The difference is smaller, but still present, among elite endurance athletes (Pollock 1977; Saltin and Åstrand 1967). The higher percentage of body fat and lower percentage of muscle mass in women accounts for a major part of the difference (Cureton and Sparling 1980). To a lesser extent, the gender difference in $\dot{V}O_2$max is related to the lower hemoglobin concentrations of women and the impact this has on oxygen delivery to active muscles (Cureton et al. 1986).

In general, the adaptations to endurance exercise training do not appear to be gender-specific. Except for older adults where there is evidence that women may rely entirely on peripheral adaptations while men rely mostly on an enhanced cardiac output (Spina 1999), similar cardiorespiratory and metabolic adaptations have been found in women and men (Mitchell et al. 1992). As in men, the adaptations to training in women depend on the initial level of fitness; the intensity, duration, and frequency of training sessions; the length of the training program; and genetic factors.

Specificity of Training

Physiological adaptations to exercise training are highly specific to the type of training. Magel and coworkers (1975) examined the change in $\dot{V}O_2max$ after a 10-week swim training program. Subjects performed maximal treadmill running and tethered swimming tests before and after the training program. Whereas the swimming $\dot{V}O_2max$ significantly increased by 11.2%, the mean running $\dot{V}O_2max$ was only 1.5% greater, an amount not statistically different from the pretraining value. Pierce and colleagues (1990) examined the lactate threshold after subjects performed either cycle or running training. Running training increased the lactate threshold by 58% and 20% for running and cycling, respectively. The cycle training increased the lactate threshold for cycling by 39% but induced no change in the lactate threshold during running.

Both of these studies demonstrate that training adaptations are most evident with the activity used in the training. In other words, the adaptations are primarily specific to the type of training. When evidence of adaptations is confined to the exercise used in training, these adaptations are considered to be peripheral in nature; they are specific to the muscles and motor units involved in the activity.

Recognition of the phenomenon of specificity of training has clinical relevance. Specificity should be considered when advising an injured athlete about alternate forms of exercise that may be feasible during recovery from the injury. Similarly, consideration should be given to the goals of any individual when planning a rehabilitation program so there is optimal carry-over of the training effect to prepare the individual for meeting the physiological demands associated with those goals.

Active Muscle Mass Involved in the Exercise Training

Physiological adaptations to exercise are dependent on the mass of muscle involved in the exercise. Endurance training with large muscle groups elicits central and peripheral adaptations; adaptations from training with small muscle groups may be limited to the periphery. In general, a training program induces central and peripheral adaptations in proportion to the degree of stress placed on both the heart and skeletal muscle—an important point to recognize when designing programs for disabled persons whose impairments may limit the muscle groups they can exercise.

Arm endurance exercise training leads to increased arm exercise capacity, according to a number of studies (Clausen et al. 1970; Clausen et al. 1973; Glaser et al. 1981; Magel et al. 1978; Pollock et al. 1974); it may not, however, strongly affect the central cardiovascular system. Magel et al. (1978) found no significant increase in running $\dot{V}O_2max$ after an intensive arm training program; other researchers observed some central adaptations after arm training—including a decrease in heart rate at rest and during submaximal leg exercise (Clausen et al. 1973) and an increase in running $\dot{V}O_2max$ (Pollock et al. 1974). It is likely that peripheral adaptations specific to the trained muscles account for a large component of the training adaptations from arm training. Central adaptations appear to be possible, but less pronounced, when training with small muscle groups such as the arms—presumably because lower blood flow and cardiac output requirements lessen the stimulus for central adaptations.

Specificity of training may yield arm ergometry and wheelchair propulsion to be reasonable exercise modes for wheelchair-dependant individuals. Furthermore, arm ergometry may be a valuable exercise mode for individuals in occupations relying heavily on repetitive use of the upper extremities. Such training can induce peripheral adaptations and improved economy resulting in enhanced functional use of the arms. Yet, since these modes of exercise use a relatively small muscle mass, the potential for central cardiovascular adaptations is limited (Hoffman 1986).

Mode of Exercise Training

An important training issue is the effect of exercising muscle mass on the relationship between oxygen uptake and perceived effort. This comparison is worthy of consideration since most individuals set their exercise intensity by their perception of effort, while many of the benefits of endurance exercise are a function of the absolute exercise intensity. Hoffman and colleagues (1996) compared leg cycling with combined leg cycling and dynamic arm exercise in a group of young healthy subjects. Oxygen uptake at a given perceived effort was higher for the combined arm and leg exercise than for the leg-only exercise. Thus, it appears that individuals are more likely to exercise at higher oxygen uptakes with exercise modes that use a large muscle mass.

When Zeni et al. (1996) compared oxygen uptake at different levels of perceived exertion among six different modes of exercise, they found significant differences in oxygen uptake among the modes of exercise (figure 2.7). Interestingly, the amount of exercising muscle could not always explain the differences between exercise modes. For example, treadmill walking and running induced higher oxygen uptakes at given levels of perceived effort than rowing ergometry and simulated cross-country skiing, both of which might be expected to engage a larger muscle mass than walking and running. Factors related to the movement pattern of the exercise may be important—such as the degree to which eccentric and

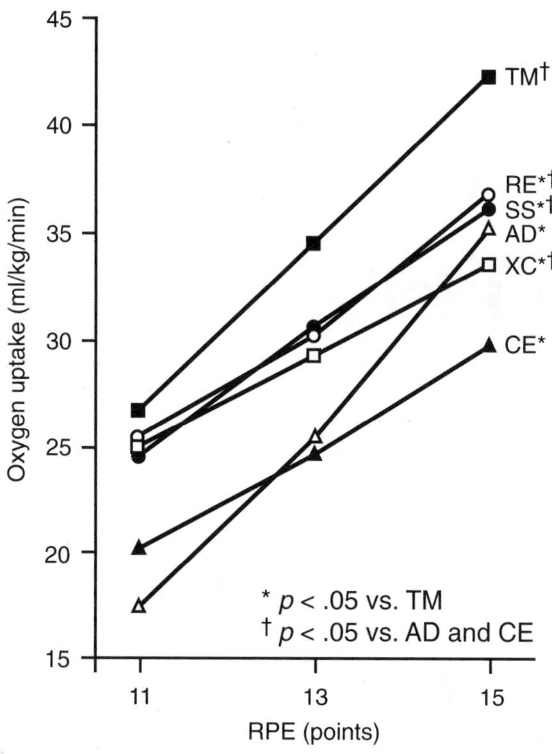

Figure 2.7 Mean oxygen uptakes as a function of rating of perceived exertion (RPE) on the 6- to 20-point scale (Borg 1970) for Airdyne exercise (AD), simulated cross-country skiing (XC), cycle ergometry (CE), rowing ergometry (RE), stair stepping (SS), and treadmill walking/running (TM).

Adapted, by permission, from A.I. Zeni, M.D. Hoffman, and P.S. Clifford, 1996, "Energy expenditure with indoor exercise machines," *Journal of the American Medical Association* 275 (18): 1426.

isometric contractions are required, the incorporation of neural pathways for reciprocal innervation, and the familiarity with the movement pattern.

SIMULTANEOUS STRENGTH AND ENDURANCE EXERCISE TRAINING

Simultaneous performance of endurance exercise training and strength training programs can induce gains in endurance, strength, and power. Concurrent strength and endurance training does not appear to impair improvements in $\dot{V}O_2max$ compared with endurance training alone (Ferketich et al. 1998; Hickson et al. 1988).

SUMMARY

Regular endurance exercise elicits a wide variety of physiological changes that improve an individual's ability to respond to subsequent exercise demands. These adaptations allow the body to send more blood to the tissues and the muscles to extract more oxygen from the blood. The adaptations lead to improved maximal exercise capacity and reduced physiological demands during submaximal exercise, both of which favorably affect functional abilities. Adaptations to endurance exercise training can occur among all populations regardless of age or disability. However, the extent of the adaptations is influenced by a number of factors including the individual's age, gender, genetic makeup, initial level of fitness, and design and duration of the exercise training program.

CHAPTER 3

Adaptations to Strength Training

Bette Ann Harris, DPT, MS; and Mary P. Watkins, DPT, MS

Strength training as an element of physical rehabilitation has an impact on not only skeletal muscle, but also neuromotor excitation, cardiovascular function, immunological activity, integrity and viability of connective tissue, and a sense of well-being. The results may optimize an individual's ability to be an active participant in daily routine and social activities. This chapter describes the rationale for strength training and considers the effects of training and detraining on muscle performance. We discuss the factors that affect muscle strength and present methods for increasing muscle strength, emphasizing those circumstances where immobilization or pathological processes have created a decline in muscle performance. In order to understand this orientation, the impact of these conditions on the anatomy and physiology of muscle will be presented.

In recent years, there have been well-designed studies demonstrating that muscle is very adaptable to the stimulus of training. Positive benefits have been reported over a wide range of subjects including elite athletes, healthy normal people including the very old, and patients with various chronic diseases. Through this literature we have learned about specificity of training, conditioning effects, detraining effects, and the response of aging muscle to exercise. Positive benefits of strength training include increasing muscle mass (Hopp 1993; Kraemer et al. 1996; Starkey et al. 1996); bone mass (Ayalon et al. 1987); tensile strength of connective tissue (Clarkson et al. 1988; Cook et al. 2000); and immunologic (La Pierre et al. 1994; Rowbottom and Green 2000), neurologic (Sale 1988), and cardiovascular well-being (Ades et al. 2003; Leon 1985). These improvements have directly influenced health status with resulting improvements in function and psychological well-being. In order to develop appropriate exercise programs, rehabilitation professionals need an understanding of the effects of immobilization and pathological conditions and, conversely, the potential benefits of strength training.

In *conceptual* terms, our definition of strength is "the ability of skeletal muscle to develop force for the purpose of providing stability and mobility within the musculoskeletal system, so that functional movement can take place" (Harris and Watkins 1994). There are many *operational* definitions of strength. It has been interpreted as "the magnitude of the torque exerted by a muscle or muscles in a single maximal isometric contraction of unrestricted duration" (Enoka 1994). Other definitions include reference to the type of muscle contraction (e.g., concentric, eccentric, or isometric), and specification of velocity. Ultimately, these may be classified as either static or dynamic exercise conditions. Traditionally, strength conditioning programs incorporate high load, low repetition formulas. The challenge for rehabilitation professionals is to select the most appropriate and safe form of strength training of sufficient intensity, frequency, and duration to achieve maximal benefit.

ANATOMICAL AND PHYSIOLOGICAL CONSIDERATIONS

The rationale for strength training is based on an understanding of the structure and function of the musculoskeletal system. The following summary is intended as a review of the important anatomical and physiological factors that have an impact on the individual's response to strengthening exercise.

The amount of force that can be generated by skeletal muscle is dependent on the integrity of both the contractile and non-contractile structural elements, motor units, metabolic support systems, and the central nervous system control mechanisms. The process of voluntary muscular contraction is initiated by the firing of anterior horn cells in the ventral horn of the spinal cord as directed from the higher centers of the central nervous system. Each anterior horn cell innervates a number of individual muscle fibers. The unit of a single anterior horn cell and all of the fibers it innervates is called a **motor unit.** Motor units vary in size reflecting the role of muscles in performance. The innervation ratio, that is, the number of muscle fibers supplied by a single motor neuron, is small for muscles that are required for fine, precision activity, such as the small muscles of the hand. Large motor units supply muscles that perform gross functions such as postural control.

CONTRACTILE ELEMENTS

Muscle fibers are the contractile elements of skeletal muscle. These cells are cylindrically shaped, multinucleated, and encased in a plasma membrane called the **sarcolemma.** The **myofibril** is the subcellular unit of the muscle fiber and is composed of repeated sarcomeres demarcated by dense Z lines. Thin and thick filaments giving skeletal muscle its striated appearance are arranged between Z lines. The thick myosin molecules include projections that when activated form cross-bridges with the thin actin molecules, causing bonds that result in force generation and muscle contraction. This series of events, from the electrical activity of depolarization to the chemical formation of actin-myosin bonds, is called excitation-contraction coupling (Åstrand et al. 2003; Oatis 2004).

The magnitude of force developed in the contractile process is dependent upon not only the number of activated motor units and frequency of motor unit firing but also on the integrity of supporting connective tissue (Stone 1988), metabolic support (Evans 1995), and biomechanical factors of overall muscle length and speed of contraction.

NON-CONTRACTILE ELEMENTS

The non-contractile tissues in skeletal muscle contribute to force production and transmission of force (and stiffness) to the tendon. The continuity of muscle is supported by the **endomysium** that covers each muscle fiber, the **perimysium** that groups fibers into bundles, and the **epimysium** that covers the entire muscle structure. These structures taken together merge at the peripheral ends of muscles to form the **myotendinous** or **aponeurotic junctions** to bone. These attachments complete the structural chain that allows for movement during muscular contraction. A stress is imposed on the connective tissue during muscle contraction. The elastic properties of this connective tissue matrix function to dampen the effects of contraction thereby resulting in smooth translation of force to accomplish functional movement or stabilization.

MUSCLE FIBER TYPES

Skeletal muscle is composed of different fiber types that vary structurally, histochemically, and metabolically (Åstrand et al. 2003; Oatis 2004). Two major categories of fibers have been described. Type I (slow oxidative, or SO) fibers are best suited for sustained or repeated contractions requiring relatively low tension, such as walking, quiet standing, and most activities of daily living. These functions are well supported by a rich blood supply. The major pathway for energy production is oxidative phosphorylation. Type II fibers have been subdivided into types IIa and IIx. Metabolic energy sources for IIx (fast glycolytic or FG) fibers—used for activities that require rapid, high tension development such as heavy lifting—are primarily anaerobic, from glycolosis. The intermediate IIa (fast oxidative glycolytic or FOG) fibers use both aerobic and anaerobic pathways. Type II fibers are more easily fatigued than type I (see chapter 2, page 15, for further details regarding muscle fiber types).

MOTOR UNIT RECRUITMENT

Although each muscle fiber type occurs in all human skeletal muscle, the mix of types varies from muscle to muscle (Saltin et al. 1977; Thorstensson et al. 1976). The grouping of fiber types is directly related to the motor neurons supplying each motor unit. Small alpha motor neurons innervate small type I motor units. Larger, type II motor units are supplied by the larger alpha motor neurons (figure 3.1). The normal sequence of motor unit activation calls upon the smaller units first, because the threshold for firing within the anterior horn cell pool is lowest for the smaller motor neurons. Therefore, with weak effort, the type I motor units are recruited. As the demand for higher force levels increases, the type II motor units become active. This phenomenon, known as the "size principle of recruitment" (Henneman et al. 1965), has implications for strength training. The speed of force development may also affect motor unit recruitment.

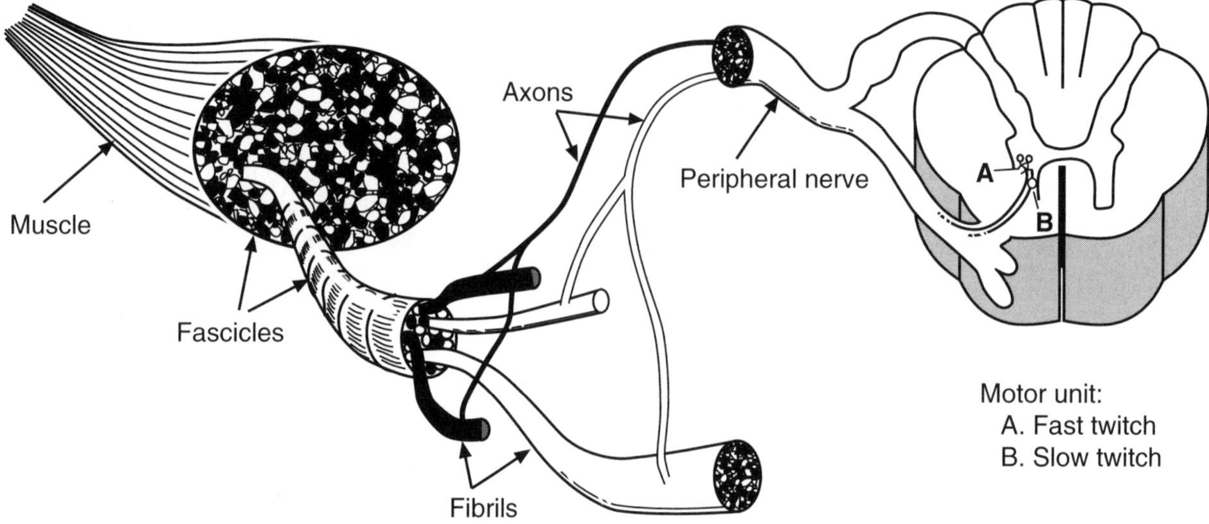

Figure 3.1 Innervation of muscle fibers.

Crowthers and Gronka (2002) have demonstrated that low force, slow contractions recruit primarily slow twitch fibers, whereas high force, rapid contractions recruit both fast and slow twitch fibers. Patients whose exercise program is limited to slow, submaximal effort may be stressing only the type I fibers. Only when the exercise challenge increases above the threshold of the larger motor units will the type II motor units be subjected to a training effect, which is the rationale for progressive resistance exercise programs. Several factors influence the ability of patients to exercise at intensities effective in training the larger motor units. For example, joint pain and swelling interfere with high-intensity levels of exercise, limiting the effectiveness of muscle strengthening programs (Fahrer et al. 1988; Spencer et al. 1984; Young et al. 1987).

Functional Biomechanics

The mechanical factors of muscular contraction type, muscle length, and speed of contraction affect the ability of skeletal muscle to generate force.

Types of Muscle Contraction

Force is generated when muscle is activated. The effect on skeletal levers varies depending upon the amount of force generated in relation to externally applied forces. A **concentric contraction** occurs when the force developed by a muscle exceeds the magnitude of the external force resulting in shortening of the whole muscle. An **isometric** (static) **contraction** occurs when the force developed by a muscle is equal to the external force. An **eccentric contraction** occurs when the external force exceeds the force developed by the muscle resulting in a lengthening of the whole muscle. The purpose of the muscle contraction is to control the moving lever from accelerating as it is being subjected to external forces.

Length–Tension

Muscle length affects the binding capacity between actin and myosin molecules of the component muscle fibers. There is an optimal length at which the greatest number of cross-bridges between these molecules can be formed (Åstrand et al. 2003; Oatis 2004). The length–tension relationship has been documented in situ by maximal voluntary effort performed during isometric, concentric, or eccentric contractions (figure 3.2). Maximal force is generated at some midpoint in the range of motion, while less force is developed at either shortened or lengthened positions (Caiozzo and Green 2002).

Force–Velocity

The binding capacity of actin and myosin is also affected by the speed of contraction. There is an optimal frequency at which the ratchet-like cycling of cross-bridge formation can occur. Figure 3.3 depicts the force–velocity relationship in isolated muscle preparations. This force–velocity relationship can be demonstrated by a series of efforts using changing loads or by controlling the speed of contraction as with "isokinetic" devices.

In *concentric* contractions, greater force is generated as the speed of shortening contractions decreases, becoming maximal at zero velocity—which equates to an isometric contraction. With *eccentric* contraction, increasing speed (to the extent permitted by voluntary and neuromotor control) can generate greater forces than that generated during isometric contractions. These higher forces may reflect the contribution of the passive

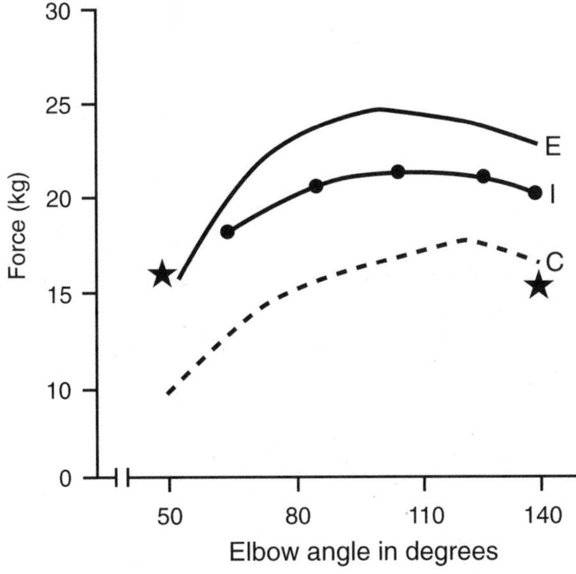

Figure 3.2 Relationship of maximal force of human elbow flexor muscles to elbow position for three types of contraction: eccentric (E), isometric (I), and concentric (C).

Source: Knuttgen 1976.

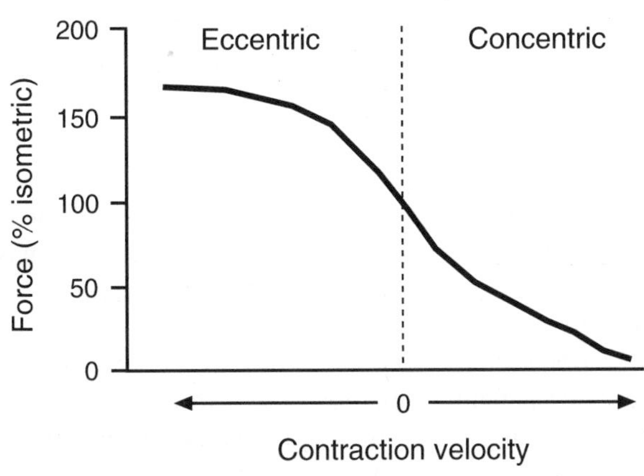

Figure 3.3 The force–velocity relationship for skeletal muscle.

Source: Newham 1993.

elastic components of connective tissues in muscle in addition to the contractile mechanism.

FACTORS INFLUENCING MUSCLE STRENGTH

The ability to generate strength is an interaction between the musculoskeletal system and those systems that provide required neurologic, metabolic, and hormonal support. Psychological well-being, life style, nutrition, level of physical activity and fitness, and general health status directly influence muscle performance. Rehabilitation professionals must consider all of these factors when designing exercise programs. The effects of age, disuse, immobilization, and musculoskeletal trauma are primary considerations because of the immediate and direct impact on muscle function.

AGE

The ability to generate force decreases with age (Hopp 1993; Thompson 1994, 2002). Aging muscle is characterized by decreased muscle mass because of the decline in the number of motor neurons, mainly those innervating type II muscle fibers. This selectivity is clinically supported by the fact that there is little or no change in fatigability with age. Edstrom and Larsson (1987) have documented, in rats, that the remaining motor units are larger secondary to collateral sprouting of active axons from remaining motor units. Sensory and motor conduction velocity and axonal transport are slower, decreasing motor unit recruitment and frequency of action potentials. As a result, reaction time and the ability of older persons to development maximal force rapidly are diminished.

Other factors, such as chronic debilitating disease, altered central nervous system function, poor balance, and frail connective tissue, contribute to diminished muscle performance in the elderly. Chapter 20 provides a full discussion of the effects of aging.

DISUSE AND IMMOBILIZATION

Prolonged bed rest, habitual limited physical activity, and cast immobilization compromise muscular activity. The extent of these changes is dependent on the duration and magnitude of inactivity. Further, the position of limb immobilization influences the type and extent of local muscle weakness. Much of the information about the effects of inactivity comes from animal studies (St. Pierre and Gardner 1987), studies of weightlessness during spaceflight (Akima et al. 2000; Baldwin 1995), studies of patients who have been immobilized secondary to orthopedic injuries (Gossman et al. 1982; Tardieu et al. 1982), and studies of normal healthy and elderly subjects (Bloomfield 1997; Convertino, et al. 1997). Decreased demand for muscular contraction causes generalized structural changes including loss of muscle mass evidenced by decreased muscle fiber size. Metabolic changes include decreases in myofibrillar proteins, phosphocreatine, glycogen, potassium and the enzymes necessary for glycolysis and oxidative phosphorylation. Capillary density and, therefore, oxygen uptake is diminished. There is thinning of the sarcolemma and weakening of other connective tissue with the resultant loss of elasticity of the entire muscular unit. All of these factors reduce both the aerobic and anaerobic capacity of inactive muscle, resulting in compromised muscular performance (Convertino et. al.

1997; St. Pierre and Gardner 1987). Diminished neuromuscular activity and sensory input impairs perception, coordination, and muscle tone.

The impact of fixed immobilization depends on duration and limb position. The rate of atrophy is rapid during the first few weeks of immobilization and then progresses more slowly (Booth 1977). Muscles immobilized in a shortened position will atrophy more than those in a neutral or elongated position. In a shortened position, adult muscle loses sarcomeres, diminishing the capacity to develop tension. In a lengthened position, muscles will adapt by increasing the number of sarcomeres—apparently a response to chronic stretch. These structural alterations change the normal length–tension relationship, causing maximal force to occur at an abnormal point in the physiologic range of motion, and thereby compromising muscle performance (Gossman et al. 1982).

Whether disuse and immobilization selectively affect one muscle fiber type more than others is not clear. Loss of cross-sectional area of both type I and type II fibers has been reported (Haggmark et al. 1981; Sargeant et al. 1977). Studies reporting findings of proportional losses of one or the other fiber type may have been affected by selection of muscles studied, diagnosis, length of immobilization, age, and method of analysis. In general, studies of immobilization in otherwise healthy subjects show initially diminished neural activity (Berg et al. 1997) followed by decreased type I fiber cross-sectional area and, over time, loss of both type I and type II cross-sectional area. Studies involving older subjects report a preferential loss of type II cross-sectional area—possibly a reflection of normal changes with aging and/or of prolonged periods of inactivity (Hopp 1993; St. Pierre and Gardner 1987).

Musculoskeletal Trauma

Trauma involving connective tissue or joint structures can cause atrophy and decreased muscle performance. For example, Stevens et al. (2003) documented diminished voluntary activation and decreased quadriceps force in patients following total knee replacement surgery. During the inflammatory process, pain and swelling inhibit muscle function. Activation of nociceptors inhibits the anterior horn cell pool, thereby diminishing the motor neuron outflow to muscle (Spencer et al. 1984). Mechanical deformation of tissue caused by joint effusion and abnormal afferent firing of joint receptors can inhibit muscle function. Fahrer et al. (1988) measured isometric quadriceps strength in patients with chronic knee effusions. Immediately following aspiration of fluid, quadriceps strength improved. Injecting lidocaine into the aspirated joints brought further improvement.

Events that occur during the healing process also affect muscle performance. Because immature scar tissue has decreased tensile strength, it is vulnerable to reinjury. As scar tissue matures, there is a loss of elasticity in the affected tendon, in the musculotendinous junction, or in the intramuscular connective tissue matrix. The resulting inability to store elastic energy limits production of force (Akeson et al. 1977; Hardy 1989; Williams and Goldspink 1984), especially during eccentric contractions.

Training

Skeletal muscle and neuromotor mechanisms are extremely adaptable to the stresses of activity. The magnitude of change in the capability of muscle is directly related to the intensity, duration, and frequency of exercise. Many methods to increase strength are described in the literature and used by clinicians. In order to achieve a strength benefit, an exercise regimen must be of sufficient frequency, intensity, and duration to challenge the physiologic components of muscle. As described by Hakkinen and Komi (1983) and Komi (1986), the first response to isometric strength training is an increase in neural activation, followed by hypertrophy of individual muscle fibers as documented by cross-sectional area of both slow twitch and fast twitch fibers (Shoepe et al. 2003). Exercise increases stiffness in the noncontractile components of muscle, allowing these passive components of force production to be more efficient. In addition to these general adaptations, there may be specific adaptations based on whether concentric, isometric, or eccentric contractions are emphasized. In prescribing exercise training to increase strength, always keep the patient's functional goals in mind, with full understanding of the underlying causes of his or her strength performance deficits.

Principles of Strength Training

Several strengthening methods are available. The selection of method depends upon the clinical assessment of the magnitude of the muscle impairment, the functional goals of the patient, and the settings in which the patient will conduct the program. Factor into your treatment decisions how the patient's pathology and comorbidities will affect the exercise program. Because adherence to programs is directly linked to success, take care to design a program that the patient understands and is able to perform at the prescribed dosage. We will describe the principles of muscle strengthening based on levels of weakness. Although our descriptions focus on strength training, all rehabilitation programs should include endurance and flexibility training as well. All are necessary for optimal physical function, which is the primary goal of rehabilitation.

THE BASIC PRINCIPLES

Effective strengthening programs are based on overload, specificity, cross training, and reversibility (Enoka 1994).

- **Overload.** Muscle tissue must be challenged beyond its current force capability in order to change both structurally and functionally. The intensity of the exercise program must reach a threshold that exceeds that current capability.
- **Specificity.** Training effects are specific to the mode of exercise stress imposed on the exercising muscle. For example, isometric training at a selected point in the range of motion does not necessarily carry over to concentric or eccentric demands; perhaps a reflection that the adaptations are not limited to changes in muscle (such as hypertrophy) but also include neuromotor adaptation by which the individual learns to use muscle force for specific musculoskeletal functions.
- **Cross training.** To overcome the limitations of specificity and to maximize the broad range of muscle performance, incorporate all modes of training into your programs whenever possible; i.e., include isometric, concentric, and eccentric elements as well as an endurance component.
- **Reversibility.** The benefits of training are not sustained unless muscles remain sufficiently challenged through continuous use of the strength gains. The initial changes that occur with detraining are decreased muscle recruitment, followed by muscle fiber atrophy. These changes take place rapidly, often within a week of inactivity as demonstrated by studies placing normal healthy subjects on bed rest for several weeks (Convertino et al. 1997; Hakkinen et al. 1983).

EXERCISE METHODS

Techniques of muscle re-education are useful in cases of major weakness and diminished neuromotor function, where the goal is to activate a voluntary contraction. The techniques include shortened held resisted contraction, active assisted range of motion, facilitation techniques such as quick stretch, and application of vibratory stimuli (Sullivan and Markos 1995). Ancillary techniques of biofeedback (Krebs 1990) or neuromuscular electrical stimulation (Delitto and Robinson 1989) can be useful. The functional goal in this circumstance is to encourage active voluntary motion within a specified movement pattern. For a patient on bed rest following knee surgery, for example, regaining active control of the quadriceps is a prerequisite for transferring from bed to chair, or for using crutches.

Initially, simply moving against gravity may challenge skeletal muscle. As patients gain strength, they should increase resistance through a variety of methods. Manual resistance applied by the therapist is often the first procedure. In this way, the therapist can judge the capability of muscle to safely meet externally applied forces, and can select appropriate facilitation techniques to optimize the muscle output and to provide feedback to the patient. These techniques are especially useful in postoperative orthopedic patients and in patients who have neuromotor disorders such as a cerebral vascular accident that compromise normal voluntary motor unit recruitment.

When the affected muscles are able to tolerate externally applied resistance, and the patients understand the rules of safe exercise regarding their specific condition, they can choose from several methods to increase resistance. The patients become responsible for carrying out their own programs, with guidance from the therapist. The methods and specific goals of the programs are based on the patients' functional requirements. For example, for an elderly patient who is recovering from a hip fracture and whose goal is walking and light housekeeping, a program using graded weights or resistive elastic bands through a range of motion may be adequate. Such a program would enable the patient to do what he/she needs to do and would also be easy to continue at a maintenance level at home. In contrast, a college soccer player whose lower extremity was immobilized for three months following a tri-malleolar fracture would require much more intense exercise to enable him/her to resume athletic activity. Modes of resistance could include progressive resistance exercise using free weights or isokinetic or hydraulic machines.

The paradigm for strength conditioning programs is based on DeLorme's prescription of high load and low repetition. His original technique, known as progressive resistance exercise, consists of establishing the maximal load a patient can lift through 10 repetitions (10 RM). The program proceeds to a regimen of 10 repetitions at 50% of that maximal value, followed by 10 repetitions at 75%, and finally 10 repetitions at 100% of the 10RM load, with one to two minutes of rest between sets. The usual frequency is three or four times a week. The spacing of sessions permits a recovery period (DeLorme and Watkins 1951). Modifications of this technique have been described, such as the "Oxford" technique (Zinovieff 1951) and the "brief maximal effort or one repetition maximum (1 RM)" (Rose et al. 1957).

Newer methods of strength training are possible with the advent of dynamic variable resistance machines. The "volume" of exercise, was studied by Starkey et al. (1996) who demonstrated using the knee flexors and extensors as a model, that one set of repetitions three times a week was as effective as three sets, three times a week. Taaffe et al. (1999) reported similar results in older subjects. The optimal dosage for eliciting a change in strength requires further study.

Strengthening programs originally used the "open chain" method, whereby the distal segment of the extremity moves and stabilization occurs proximally. Today many programs use a "closed chain" model whereby the distal part is fixed, as in weight bearing, and muscles perform reverse action. Many consider closed chain exercises—particularly with the lower extremities—to be safer because they use normal movement patterns and sensory cues (Falkel and Cipriani 1996; Sullivan and Markos 1995). An example of functional closed chain resistive exercise is weighted stair climbing. Bean et al. (2002) demonstrated strength gains in older men and women following a program of stair climbing wearing a weighted vest.

With the variety of exercise devices available, the therapist can design strengthening programs based on the type of muscle contraction, force, or speed required for optimal therapeutic response. Selecting the "best" mode of strengthening depends upon the patient's particular impairment, medical problem, and requirements for optimal functional performance. The therapist must also consider practical issues. For example, can the patient go to a facility that has a selection of exercise equipment or is she confined to home? Finally, choosing a form of strengthening exercise that is enjoyable to the patient is important in maintaining adherence to the program (Dishman 1988).

There are several variables that must be taken into account when designing a strengthening program, namely, number of repetitions per set, rest between sets, and sequence of training several muscle groups in a single session. In order to give patients a sense of structure, prescribing three sets of 10 repetitions with a 30- to 60-second rest period in between is most commonly recommended (U.S. Department of Health and Human Services 1996). However, care must be taken to ensure that the patient is recruiting the proper muscles with the correct technique. The patient's training effort should be either "hard" or "very hard" while maintaining a normal breathing pattern. The criterion for increasing resistance is the patients' report that the exercise effort is "easy." The frequency of strength training is three to four times a week to allow exercising muscles to recover between sessions. The order of exercising is usually based on practicality. For example, we suggest completing all in each position before changing to another position. Recent data suggest that correctly performing even one set of repetitions as little as once a week can induce a training effect.

Adaptations to Strength Conditioning

The most obvious result of strength conditioning is an increase in the functional capacity of muscle to generate force—an increase stemming from several alterations in morphology and physiology caused by the stresses of exercise. Many studies have described these local and systemic effects of strength training (table 3.1).

Table 3.1 Adaptations to Strength Conditioning

Physiologic adaptations	Positive changes in impairments	Positive changes in function	Quality of life
Increased motor unit recruitment	Strength-force production	Balance and coordination	Athletic performance
Synchronization of motor unit discharge	Bone mass	Gait	Job performance
Hypertrophy Increased fiber size Remodeling of muscle proteins Increase in size and number of myofibrils Increase in sarcomeres	Body composition—improved fat to lean body mass ratio Reaction time Immunologic function Cardiopulmonary status Metabolism	Activities of daily living	Social activity Sense of well-being
Hyperplasia (from animal models, possibly in humans)			
Increased tensile strength of connective tissue			

Neuromuscular Adaptation

Hakkinen and Komi (1983) elucidated the sequence of adaptation to strength training in the neuromuscular system. In the early stages of exercise, the changes as documented by electromyography include increased motor unit recruitment and synchronization of motor unit discharge. These changes reflect more effective activation of anterior horn cells, elicited by improved voluntary motor control. In addition, Deschenes et al. (1993) demonstrated (in rats) hypertrophic alteration of the neuromuscular junction—namely, a broadening of the synaptic area—in response to heavy resistance exercise. As the efficiency of neural elements improves, hypertrophy of skeletal muscle occurs when the exercise challenge is adequate. The changes that result in this increase in muscle fiber size include remodeling of muscle proteins, increase in size and number of myofibrils, and an increase in the number of sarcomeres (Åstrand et al. 2003). Each of the major fiber types may be affected differentially, depending on the intensity of the imposed resistance and the type of contraction. Studies have shown increased cross-sectional area selectively for type II fibers or in both type I and type II fibers (Kraemer et al. 1996; Shoepe et al. 2003). Further, Staron et al. (1994) documented a metabolic response of fiber types with a conversion of type IIb (or IIx) fibers to type IIa, indicating an increase in oxidative capacity following strength training. Exercise studies of subjects who have been immobilized for long periods of time have reported initial increases in type I fiber cross-sectional area, followed by changes in type II fibers. Based on the size order of recruitment, low-intensity exercise may not challenge the large type II fibers sufficiently to cause hypertrophic changes.

Antonio and Gonyea (1993) reviewed evidence that exercise may induce hyperplasia, which is an increase in the number of muscle fibers. The mechanism for hyperplasia may be fiber splitting (Gonyea 1980), or perhaps activation of satellite cells (Darr and Schultz 1987). It may be caused by heavy resistance exercise and overuse (Hall-Craggs 1970) or by weight-induced prolonged stretch (Alway et al. 1989). Several animal studies have demonstrated this phenomenon. Evidence of hyperplasia in humans is less convincing at this time. However, Tesch and Larsson (1982) concluded on somewhat indirect evidence that hyperplasia does occur in humans. They described an increase in muscle mass and limb circumference in body builders in whom there was no evidence of muscle fiber hypertrophy.

The temporal relationship between neural and muscular changes depends on the interaction of several factors: the intensity, frequency, and duration of the exercise program; the age and health status of the patient; and the specific cause of the muscle weakness. With minimal impairment or in healthy subjects, strength changes during the first 6 to 12 weeks of a training program are primarily due to increased motor unit recruitment and motor learning (Komi 1986). However, in patients who have coordination problems or disuse secondary to immobilization, the neural adaptation phase may be prolonged (Buckwalter et al. 1993; Kraemer et al. 1996).

Alterations of connective tissue within skeletal muscle also occur (Stone 1988). Application of an external load stimulates the proliferation of connective tissue. The resultant increase in tensile strength improves the structural and functional integrity of the skeletal muscle unit, allowing for more efficient force production. Clinically, this concept is useful in treating patients with chronic tendinosis. Several studies demonstrate that designing a program of eccentric loading of the affected musculotendinous complex, taking care not to irritate the structures, results in decreased pain and increased function (Alfredson et al. 1998; Cook et al. 2000; Holmich et al. 1999; Khan et al. 2000).

System Benefits

Adaptations to a strength conditioning program include increased bone mass, alterations in body composition, and improved balance and coordination. Adaptations to strength training may also include improved immunologic function (Rowbottom and Green 2000), cardiopulmonary status (Ades et al. 2003), increased metabolism, decreased pain, and improved sleep quality (King 1997). However, the effect on these systems is dependent on many factors, including exercise intensity and duration and health status. There is evidence that overtraining may have a detrimental impact on these systems. For example, evidence indicates that a well-designed strengthening program for patients with fibromyalgia can result in increased strength and decreased pain; however, the converse has been described when the exercise stimulus exceeds the patients' capacity (Jones et al. 2002).

Bone mass increases in response to the stresses imposed during strength training (Stone 1988). The extent of this effect depends on the magnitude of skeletal loading through weight bearing and on the torque applied to bone during muscular contraction. For example, when Smith and Rutherford (1993) compared male rowers, triathletes, and sedentary men, the rowers (whose training included heavy resistive exercise and high mechanical loading) had higher bone mineral density than the triathletes (whose training emphasized lower intensities and endurance). Studies have addressed the effectiveness of exercise in retarding bone loss during menopause and aging. Ayalon et al. (1987) reported site-specific increases in bone mineral density in the forearm in response to dynamic resistance exercise of the forearm in postmenopausal women. In studying the effect of high-intensity strengthening in 50- to 70-year-old women, Nelson et al. (1994) found increased bone mineral density in the femoral neck and lumbar spine. Chapter 15 presents a full discussion of this topic.

Strength training increases lean tissue mass and decreases percent fat. These changes have been documented after resistance training in athletes, normal healthy subjects, and older individuals. The demands of active muscle include the utilization of fatty acids, particularly to support oxidative phosphorylation. Mobilization and utilization of free fatty acids accounts in part for the decrease in adipose tissue (Martin 1996). In highly trained athletes, the ratio of lean body mass to fat is high (Wenger et al. 1996). Treuth et al. (1995) and Nichols et al. (1993) have documented these same benefits in older women as a result of heavy resistance training.

Functional Benefits

Improvement in strength can result in improved balance and coordination, gait speed, ability to perform activities of daily living, and higher-level activity in athletic performance or occupational tasks. The magnitude of functional changes depends on the interaction of baseline strength, the strength requirements to perform specific tasks, and health status factors, such as disorders of metabolism or cardiorespiratory support systems. Psychological state also affects the carryover from strength improvement to actual function.

Several recent studies have measured functional change in response to strength training in older individuals. Lord and Castell (1994) studied the effects of a 10-week strengthening and cardiovascular exercise program in 50- to 75-year-old men and women. They found improvement in the exercised lower extremity muscles, reaction time, and body sway. In a randomized placebo-controlled trial with 100 elderly subjects, Fiatarone et al. (1994) compared high-intensity exercise, nutritional supplement, a combination of both, and no intervention. The exercise regimen improved muscle strength, gait velocity, stair climbing, and the level of spontaneous physical activity. There was no change in the groups who took nutritional supplements. Ettinger et al. (1997) reported positive results in an 18-month home-based resistive exercise program for community-dwelling men and women who had osteoarthritis. Significant, though modest, improvements were noted in subjects' self-reports of physical activity, six-minute walk tests, and timed activities of lifting, stair climbing, and getting in and out of a chair. Jette et al. (1996, 1999) report positive strength gains and modest improvements in gait and function after a home-based strengthening program in frail or disabled elders.

Summary

This chapter has presented an overview of the adaptations to strength training. Over a period of time, strength training elicits significant alterations in morphology and physiology. The magnitude of these changes is affected by the type of stress imposed and the age and general health status of the patient. Specific improvements in functional performance have been demonstrated. These adaptations justify the use of strength training to ameliorate the impairments of muscle weakness and atrophy that result from disuse and immobilization, and to maximize muscle performance in conditions that create permanent dysfunction of muscle. The ultimate goal is to optimize the functional performance of the patient. Given the substantial benefits of strength conditioning, we encourage rehabilitation professionals to include strength conditioning within the patient's tolerance as part of a treatment program regardless of the diagnosis.

CHAPTER 4

TRAINING FLEXIBILITY

Lisa S. Krivickas, MD

Strength, endurance, and flexibility training are integral components of any comprehensive exercise, fitness, or sport-specific training program. While researchers have extensively studied endurance and strength training, they have placed less emphasis on flexibility training. While most professionals and athletes believe that adequate or even above-average flexibility is an asset, scientific work to support this assertion is weak. In this chapter, I will summarize the current scientific literature on flexibility and suggest areas requiring further investigation. I will apply the limited results of existing literature to clinical situations. Topics addressed include the definition of flexibility; factors influencing flexibility; both cellular and macroscopic responses of muscle to stretching; methods of measuring and quantifying flexibility; the relationship between muscle stiffness and flexibility; the relationship between flexibility, ligamentous laxity, and injury; the relationship between flexibility and post-exercise muscle soreness; and the relationship between flexibility and activities of both daily living and athletic performance. I will also discuss stretching techniques, a prescription for developing flexibility, the effect of strength training on flexibility, and the effect of various disease processes on flexibility.

DEFINITION OF FLEXIBILITY

Flexibility is the range of motion of a joint or series of joints. Although flexibility is influenced by muscles, tendons, ligaments, bones, and bony structures, the muscle-tendon unit is by far the greatest contributor. The contribution of muscle fascicle versus tendon elongation to changes in range of motion varies with the geometry of individual muscle-tendon units (Herbert et al. 2002).

Gajdosik (1995) has challenged the preceding definition of flexibility, suggesting that flexibility is a physiologic phenomenon requiring simultaneous measurement of the length–tension relationship of muscles as they are lengthened passively without muscle activation. According to this definition, flexibility must be measured as a ratio of change in muscle length or change in joint angle to change in force or torque; these ratios are actually measures of compliance. Gajdosik's definition does not encompass the concept of dynamic vs. static flexibility, since he requires that the muscle be lengthened without muscle activation. Because there is no consensus as to the definition of flexibility, it is best defined operationally, i.e., as either a change in length or a change in the ratio of length to tension. While reviewing studies that have used both definitions, this chapter focuses primarily on the role of the muscle–tendon unit—and to a lesser extent on that of ligamentous laxity—on joint range of motion and stiffness.

FACTORS INFLUENCING FLEXIBILITY

Flexibility is muscle and joint specific and is influenced by the age, gender, and, possibly, the race of the individual. Static flexibility refers to the ability of a joint to move through a passive range of motion. It differs from dynamic flexibility in that the latter depends on the strength of antagonist muscles to move the limb and on the freedom of the limb to move. A ballet dancer with excellent static hamstring flexibility may perform a split on the floor with ease; however, if she has weak hip flexors or hip pain that impairs her ability to move her leg, she may have poor dynamic flexibility and be

Factors Influencing Flexibility

- Muscle and joint specificity
- Age
- Gender
- Ethnic origin
- Temperature
- Reflex activity
- Central nervous system disease processes
- Antagonist muscle strength (dynamic flexibility)

unable to lift her leg even 90 degrees when standing. Neuromuscular factors (e.g., reflex activity and diseases affecting the central nervous system) influence both static and dynamic flexibility, as does muscle temperature because of its effect on collagen extensibility. See "Factors Influencing Flexibility" above.

Gender, Age, and Race

Scientific literature is scant on the relationship between flexibility and gender, age, or race. No normal values have been established for flexibility of specific joints or muscles in various populations, and clinicians do not agree on what should be considered the optimal degree of muscle flexibility. Laubach and McConville (1966) explored the relationship between flexibility and somatotype in college men and found no significant association. Comparisons of hip flexion and shoulder extension in college students, and of lower extremity flexibility in male and female college athletes, have shown that women generally have greater flexibility than men (Etnyre and Lee 1988; Krivickas and Feinberg 1996). A study of children attending tennis camp found greater hamstring flexibility in girls than in boys, but no difference in soleus, adductor, or shoulder external rotator flexibility (Marshall et al. 1980). In the same study, age was negatively correlated with flexibility for shoulder external rotation ($r = -.68$) and ankle dorsiflexion ($r = -.26$), but was not significantly correlated with hamstring or adductor flexibility.

Before we accept any such associations, we must critically evaluate the methods by which researchers have measured flexibility. For example, one study of male high school athletes concluded that flexibility increased with both age and sexual maturation. However, the measure used for flexibility was the sit-and-reach test, which is influenced by body proportion (both trunk-to-leg length ratio and arm length)—and body proportion changes as children grow (Pratt 1989). I will address specific methods for measuring flexibility in a later section.

Clinicians generally believe that flexibility decreases with age, but no one has systematically studied this relationship. Children tend to lose flexibility during growth spurts, because their bones elongate at a faster rate than their muscles (Micheli 1983)—a major factor in the high number of lower extremity overuse injuries in adolescent athletes (see Case Study below). A longitudinal study performed in Sweden demonstrated a decrease in flexibility in both men and women from age 16 to 34 (Barnekow-Bergkvist et al. 1996). In the elderly, inactivity caused by medical illness, social factors, or environmental factors may contribute to loss of muscle flexibility. In addition, an age-associated cross-linking of collagen molecules may alter the properties of col-

Case Study

An elite 17-year-old male singles figure skater trains 35 hours per week including on-ice and off-ice activities. He recently experienced a growth spurt, adding two inches to his height in nine months. He suffered from jumper's knee (patellar tendinitis) in the right (his landing) leg and had very tight rectus femoris muscles. The flexibility of the rectus femoris is assessed by measuring the quadriceps inhibited knee flexion angle (QFA). The QFA is the difference between (1) the angle of maximal knee flexion with the ipsilateral hip flexed 80 degrees, and (2) the angle of maximal knee flexion with the ipsilateral hip fully extended. A QFA greater than 10 degrees indicates rectus femoris muscle tightness. In elite adolescent skaters, rectus femoris tightness is associated with anterior knee pain overuse syndromes (Smith et al. 1991). When this skater initially came to us with right jumper's knee, he had a QFA of 30 degrees on the right and 38 degrees on the left. We placed him on a quadriceps muscle stretching program and a general rehabilitation program for his jumper's knee. After six months, his jumper's knee had resolved, and QFA was 0 degrees bilaterally. One year later, he presented with bilateral jumper's knee. He had discontinued his quadriceps muscle stretching program, and QFA was now 30 degrees on the right and 18 degrees on the left. This case study demonstrates the importance of flexibility training for both injury prevention and rehabilitation.

lagen and contribute to decreased joint range of motion in the elderly (Liebesman and Cafarelli 1994). No one has formally studied the relationship between race and muscle flexibility, but variations in ligamentous laxity in different ethnic populations have been observed.

In addition, a recent study comparing the viscoelastic properties of muscle in black and white collegiate sprinters showed increased muscle stiffness among black athletes (Fukashiro et al. 2002).

The influence of activity level has not been incorporated into any of the observed associations between age, gender, and flexibility. Training and activity may have a greater influence than genetic factors on muscle flexibility in healthy individuals.

Physiological and Neurological Factors

The cytoskeletal protein titin gives myofibrils their intrinsic elasticity (Lindstedt et al. 2001). We may hypothesize that the quantity and quality of titin in any given muscle influence its flexibility. The third most abundant protein in the sarcomere (after actin and myosin), titin runs the entire length of the half sarcomere. Its major function is to maintain the central position of the myosin filaments in the relaxed sarcomeres. Figure 4.1 illustrates the positioning of titin within the muscle fiber. Fast-twitch muscle fibers have more titin than slow-twitch fibers and are more flexible (Waterman-Storer 1991). The degradation of titin during exercise-induced muscle damage may explain the loss of muscle flexibility sometimes reported in association with a single strenuous bout of heavy resistance training and eccentric exercise (Trappe et al. 2002).

Two spinal reflexes, initiated by the muscle spindle and the Golgi tendon organ, influence muscle flexibility (Proske 1997). The muscle spindle is a muscle stretch receptor composed of 2 to 12 thin intrafusal (within the spindle) muscle fibers arranged in parallel with the extrafusal, or main, muscle fibers. Muscle spindles are composed of three types of intrafusal fibers (dynamic nuclear bag or bag_1, static nuclear bag or bag_2, and nuclear chain), which combine to function as primary and secondary spindles. Primary spindles respond to rate of length change, creating a dynamic response. Secondary spindles respond to a static absolute length change. When muscle stretch activates the spindle reflex, the extrafusal fibers contract, shortening the muscle. The Golgi tendon organ is a braided structure consisting of collagenous fibers and afferent axons in series with several extrafusal muscle fibers at the muscle tendon interface. When the extrafusal fibers contract, a force is applied to the Golgi tendon organ, which sends to the spinal cord a message that results in inhibition of the agonist muscle and contraction of the antagonist. Thus, the Golgi tendon reflex enhances the ability of a muscle to stretch, while the spindle reflex attempts to prevent muscle elongation. The goal of a stretching exercise should be to enhance the Golgi tendon reflex and inhibit the spindle reflex. Figure 4.2 illustrates the complex interaction between these two spinal reflexes. The influence on flexibility of these reflexes and other neural factors appears to be minor in healthy individuals (Krabak et al. 2001; McHugh et al. 1998).

In addition to the spinal reflexes, supraspinal reflexes and other neural pathways influence muscle flexibility. A detailed discussion of these phenomena is beyond

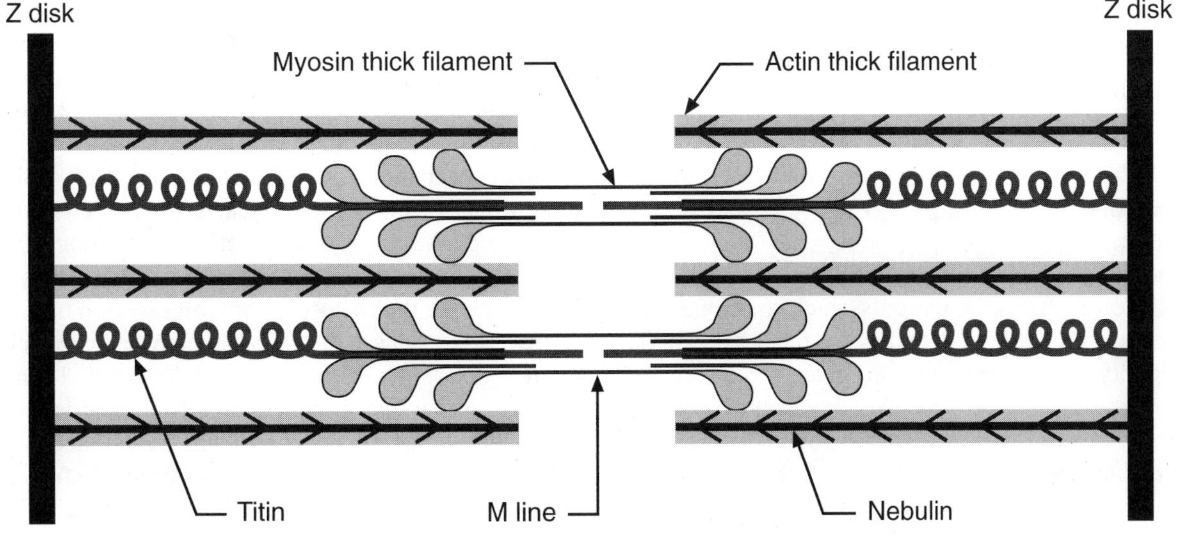

Figure 4.1 An illustration of the position of titin within the sarcomere.

MOLECULAR CELL BIOLOGY 3/E by Lodish, © 1986, 1990, 1995 by W.H. Freeman and Company. Used with permission.

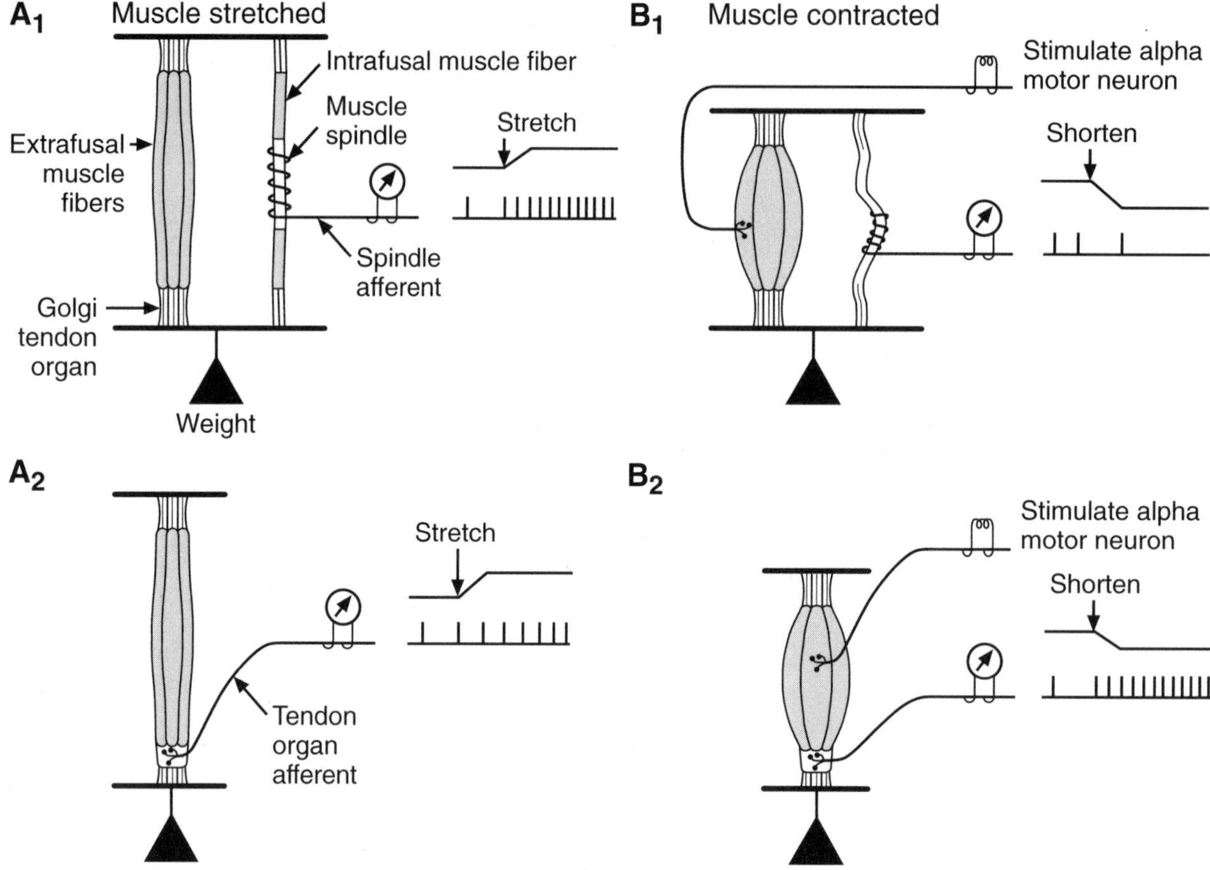

Figure 4.2 The spindle afferent and Golgi tendon organ (GTO) respond differently to muscle stretch and contraction. Both discharge when muscle is stretched (A), the GTO (A_2) less than the spindle (A_1). When the muscle contracts (B), the spindle ceases firing (B_1), and the GTO increases its firing rate (B_2).

Reprinted, by permission, from E.R. Kandel, J.H. Schwartz, and T.M. Jessell, 1991, *Principles of neural science,* 3rd ed. (Norwalk, CT: Appleton & Lange), 568.

the scope of this chapter, but damage to these neural pathways produces spasticity, rigidity, or hypotonia. Spasticity occurs in upper motor neuron lesions, such as cortical stroke and spinal cord injury, because the spinal reflexes are isolated from inhibitory or modulating supraspinal reflexes. Spasticity is defined by three characteristics:

1. Unidirectional resistance to passive movement
2. Velocity-dependent resistance to muscle stretch
3. Hyperactive muscle stretch reflexes

Rigidity occurs in patients, such as those with Parkinson's disease, with damage to the basal ganglia. In rigidity, resistance to muscle stretch is bidirectional and independent of velocity. In addition, muscle stretch reflexes are not hyperactive. Hypotonia, or lack of normal muscle resistance to stretch, is seen in patients with cerebellar lesions, because the baseline alpha motor neuron and muscle spindle activity are decreased, and the firing thresholds of both alpha and gamma motor neurons are increased.

Temperature

Muscle and joint temperature affect flexibility. Heating augments the increase in range of motion achieved by stretching, by increasing the extensibility of collagen, a major component of tendon and joint capsules (Gersten 1955; Lehman et al. 1970). Thus the increased range of motion achieved with heating is probably more related to elongation of the tendon than of the muscle. Heat also facilitates the response of the major spinal reflexes to stretch, by decreasing the sensitivity of muscle spindle reflexes and increasing the firing rate of Golgi tendon organs (Mense 1978). This is the physiologic basis of muscle spasm relaxation with heat application. Animal studies have shown that warming up muscle and tendon by preconditioning with electrically stimulated isometric contractions increases extensibility (Safran et al. 1988). However, human studies using running to warm up muscles have failed to demonstrate a significant change in muscle-tendon viscoelastic properties (Magnusson et al. 2000).

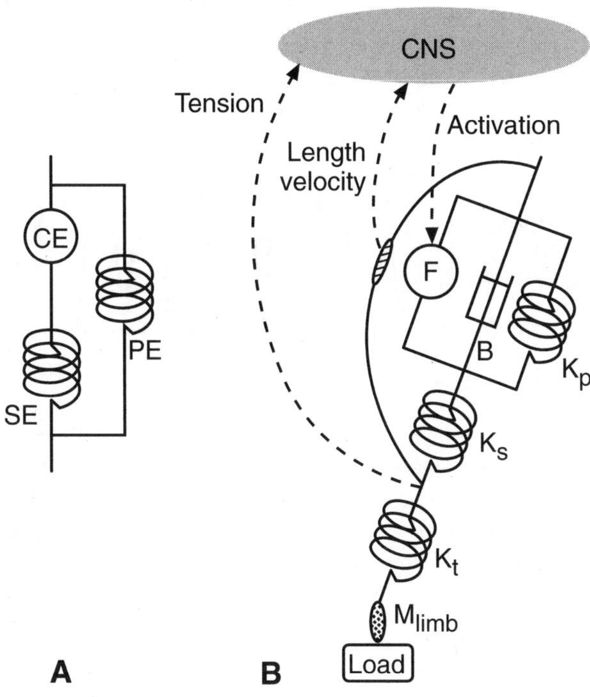

Figure 4.3 *(A)* Three-element muscle model has a complex contractile element (CE) in parallel with a passive elastic element (PE) and in series with another elastic element (SE) that has both passive (tendon/aponeurosis) and active (cross-bridge) components. *(B)* A more complex model of muscle contains elastic (K_s and K_p), viscous (B, a dash pot), and force-generating (F) elements. K_t is a nonlinear elastic element representing tendon and aponeurosis. These elements are modulated by length- and force-sensitive reflexes, which are in turn modulated by the central nervous system (CNS).

Reprinted, by permission, from G. Gottlieb, 1996, "Muscle compliance: Implications for the control of movement," *Exercise and Sport Sciences Reviews* 24: 4.

Response of Muscle to Stretch

Tabary and colleagues (1972) studied the effect of chronic stretch on cat muscle fibers. They found that chronic stretch increased the number of sarcomeres by 20% to 25%, but decreased the sarcomere length by 11% to 16%; the additive effect was a 5% overall increase in muscle fiber length. Presumably, increasing muscle fiber length increases joint range of motion; the extent to which this is true will depend on the architecture of each specific muscle. This type of study has not been performed in humans.

Viscoelastic Muscle-Tendon Behavior

The muscle-tendon unit is viscoelastic in its mechanical behavior. Frequently, a spring and dash pot model is used to describe its behavior. The term "dash pot" describes a disk attached to a plunger that is immersed in a fluid, providing frictional resistance to movement. The spring represents the elastic elements, and the dash pot the viscous elements. Gottlieb (1996) has expanded the classic three-element model of muscle (figure 4.3a) into a more complex five-element model (figure 4.3b). The classic model consists of a contractile element (CE), a series elastic element (SE), and a parallel elastic element (PE) that is passive and comes into play only at longer muscle lengths. The more complex model includes a parallel elastic element (K_p), a viscous element (B), a force generator (F) controlled by neural activation, a series elastic element for muscle (K_s), and a nonlinear series elastic element for tendon (K_t). Under most physiologic conditions, including exercise and sports activity, the muscle-tendon unit behaves like a spring, and the viscous element has minimal influence on its behavior.

In order to understand the viscoelastic behavior of muscle, one must understand several engineering terms that describe the behavior of viscoelastic substances. In general, when a pure elastic material is stretched, it returns to its initial length when the stretch is released. When a purely viscous material is stretched, its rate of deformation is proportional to the force applied, and it does not return to its original length when the stretch is released. Viscoelastic materials combine these properties such that the phenomena of stress relaxation, creep, strain rate dependence, and hysteresis occur. These behaviors are defined in table 4.1.

Table 4.1 Behavior of Viscoelastic Materials

Behavior	Definition
Stress relaxation	Less force is required over time to maintain a given increase in length during a sustained stretch.
Creep	A fixed force is applied to a material, and continued slow deformation occurs.
Strain–rate dependence	A slower stretch (strain) produces greater elongation than a faster stretch.
Hysteresis	More energy is absorbed during a stretch than is released when the stretch is terminated; the material absorbs energy when stretched.

Studies of Viscoelastic Properties

Taylor and his colleagues at Duke University (1990) have studied the viscoelastic properties of the muscle-tendon unit, using a rabbit model consisting of muscle and tendon with an intact neurovascular supply. Stress relaxation was demonstrated by stretching the muscle to 10% greater than its initial length and then immediately releasing it. After 10 repetitions, the tension required to produce the stretch decreased 17%. Most of the stress relaxation occurred during the first four stretches (figure 4.4). Creep was demonstrated by a similar experiment in which muscle was stretched to a given tension, held at that tension for 30 seconds, and then relaxed. After this series of stretches was repeated 10 times, overall muscle length increased by 3.5%; the greatest elongation occurred with the first stretch (figure 4.5). This experiment simulates the static stretching technique. Strain rate dependence and hysteresis were demonstrated by stretching muscle to 10% greater than its initial length at four different velocities. Energy absorption and the tensile force required to achieve elongation were greatest at the highest stretch velocity. Hysteresis may occur either because of heat transfer to the muscle or because of internal changes in the muscle structure.

The experiments of Taylor et al. (1990) have several clinical implications. They demonstrate that muscle length gains achieved by stretching are not rapidly reversible. They help explain why ballistic stretching may be harmful and ineffective—rapid stretching velocity increases tension and energy storage in muscle, which may increase both risk and severity of injury. In addition, ballistic stretches are not held long enough to allow stress relaxation or creep to occur. Most muscle lengthening occurs during the first 12 to 18 seconds of a stretch and during the first four stretch cycles.

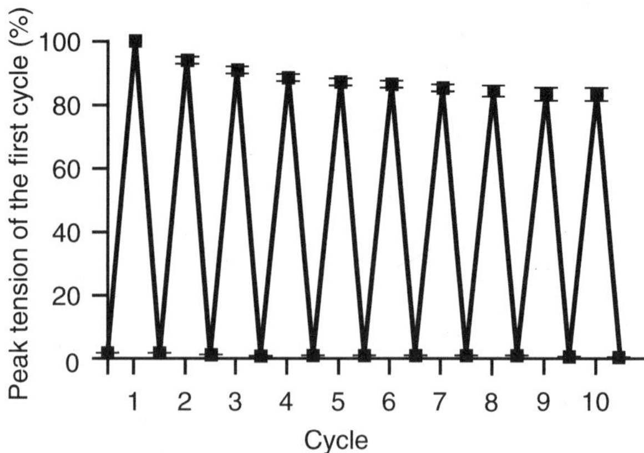

Figure 4.4 The extensor digitorum longus (EDL) muscle of rabbits is repeatedly stretched to 10% beyond its resting length. The overall tension decreases 16.6%, demonstrating the phenomenon of stress relaxation with repeated stretches.

Reprinted, by permission, from D. Taylor, J. Dalton, A. Seaber, and W. Garrett, 1990, "Viscoelastic properties of muscle-tendon units: The biomechanical effects of stretching," *American Journal of Sports Medicine* 18(3):303-309. Reprinted by permission of Sage Publications, Inc.

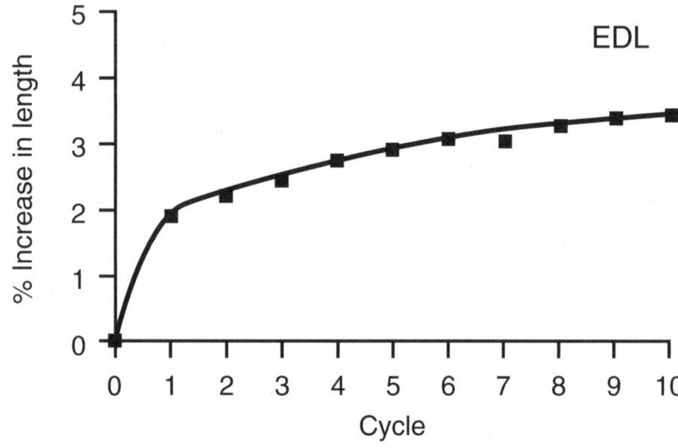

Figure 4.5 Rabbit EDL is repeatedly stretched to the same tension. The progressive increase in muscle length demonstrates the phenomenon of creep in a viscoelastic material.

Reprinted, by permission, from D. Taylor, J. Dalton, A. Seaber, and W. Garrett, 1990, "Viscoelastic properties of muscle-tendon units: The biomechanical effects of stretching," *American Journal of Sports Medicine* 18(3):300-309. Reprinted by permission of Sage Publications, Inc.

Relationship Between Muscle Stiffness and Flexibility

The stiffness of a material describes its ability to resist elongation or stretching. Engineers use Young's modulus (also known as the "modulus of elasticity") to describe stiffness. Young's modulus (Y) is defined as

$$Y = \text{stress/strain} = (F/A)/(\Delta l/l_0)$$

where F = pulling force, A = cross-sectional area, Δl = change in length, and l_0 = initial length. Since A and l_0 are fixed properties of an individual muscle, Y, or stiffness, is proportional to $F/\Delta l$. It may be that muscle stiffness rather than range of motion (which we typically call flexibility) is more properly associated with risk and severity of injury.

Halbertsma and colleagues (1994, 1996) studied the effect of both a single 10-minute stretch and a 4-week stretching program on range of motion and muscle stiffness in neurologically normal individuals with short hamstring muscles. Both the single stretch and the 4-week program increased hamstring flexibility, measured by a passive straight leg raise. However, neither program altered muscle stiffness, measured by Young's modulus. In these subjects, the improvement in flexibility apparently was due to increased stretch tolerance or decreased sensitivity to pain, rather than to a change in mechanical properties of the muscle. Magnusson and colleagues (1998, 2000) have reached similar conclusions from studying the effect of both 45- and 90-second stretches on the hamstring muscles. Other investigators have also failed to find a correlation between muscle flexibility and stiffness (Cornu et al. 2003). In contrast, Gleim and McHugh (1997) demonstrated that stiffness in the central portion of a joint's range of motion is related to the terminal range of motion.

Wilson and his colleagues (1991, 1994) used a more complex model to study active muscle stiffness in weightlifters performing the bench press. Conceptually, it is difficult to relate this measurement of active stiffness to flexibility when the latter is defined either as range of motion or as a length:tension ratio. The model uses a damped oscillation technique in which the weightlifters hold a barbell in a static bench press position 3 cm above the chest. The experimenter manually perturbs the bar (causing it to oscillate), while instructing the subject not to alter his muscle firing pattern. The more rapidly the oscillations are damped, the stiffer the muscles are assumed to be. According to this model, flexibility of the anterior deltoid and pectoralis muscles decreased as muscle stiffness increased. These authors also demonstrated that strength training increases muscle stiffness. Their study of the relationship between power generation and muscle stiffness during the bench pressing exercise showed that increased muscle stiffness was associated with increased power generation during concentric and isometric contractions, but not during eccentric contractions (Wilson et al. 1994). Klinge et al. (1997) demonstrated increased stiffness and energy storage in hamstring muscles trained isometrically.

More research is needed. With our current knowledge we can assume, at best, that changes in muscle stiffness may develop over time but are more likely to be influenced by strength training than by stretching. We must be careful to note how we are defining both stiffness and flexibility when we try to relate one property of muscle to the other.

MEASURING AND QUANTIFYING MUSCLE FLEXIBILITY AND LIGAMENTOUS LAXITY

Most researchers have used goniometers to measure static joint range of motion. Gajdosik and Bohannon (1987) have extensively reviewed this technique's limitations, which affect both its reliability and validity. The measurements are dependent on the amount of force applied to range the joint, the stretch or pain tolerance of the subject, and any contraction of the muscle being stretched. Joint range of motion may be limited by nonmuscular structures or by the inflexibility of more than one muscle. To assess the flexibility of muscles that cross two joints (e.g., the rectus femoris and gastrocnemius), one must position both joints appropriately, properly stabilizing them to insure validity and reliability. For example, in using a passive straight leg raise with the subject supine to assess flexibility of the hamstring muscle group, one must stabilize the pelvis—pelvic rotation can increase hip flexion range of motion (figure 4.6). Flexibility measurements made at two different times, such as before and after initiation of a stretching program, should be made at the same time of day, at the same environmental temperature, and following a similar level of activity (e.g., with no warm-up or after a similar warm-up).

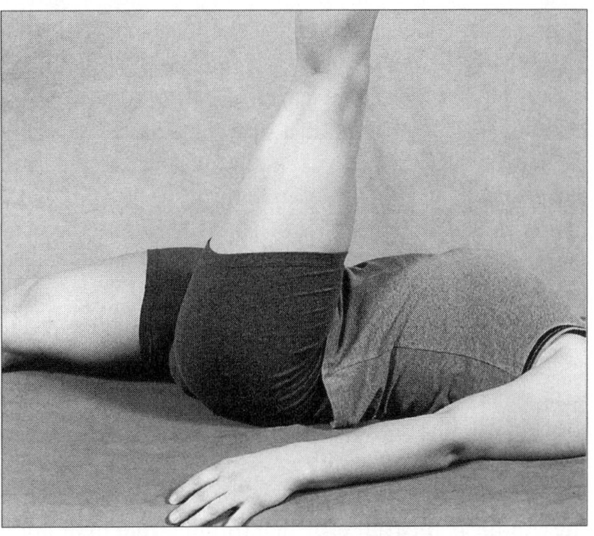

a

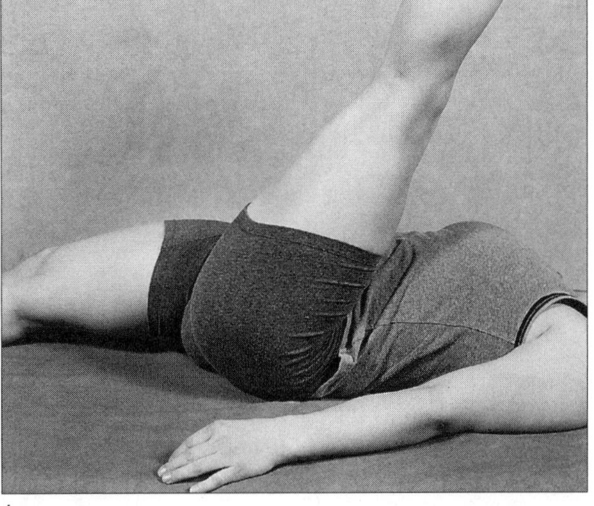

b

Figure 4.6 *(a)* An athlete performing a hamstring stretch in the straight leg raise position with the pelvis squared. *(b)* The same athlete can achieve a much greater arc of motion by rotating the pelvis during the straight leg raise.

A more valid method of measuring flexibility might be to measure a ratio of change in joint range of motion to the force applied to achieve that change (Gajdosik 1995). Although this technique can be applied in research settings, it is not very practical for clinicians, as it requires specialized apparatus not commonly available in the clinic.

A Proposed Composite Scale

There are no widely used composite scales for clinical assessment of flexibility. We have proposed one such scale for assessing the flexibility of lower extremity muscles in which poor flexibility or tightness has been associated with overuse injuries (Krivickas and Feinberg 1996). We derive a composite muscle tightness score by assessing the bilateral flexibility of five muscle groups and classifying each group as either acceptably flexible or excessively tight. Since each tight muscle is given a score of 1, the total score ranges from 0 to 10—a score of 0 indicating adequate flexibility and a score of 10 indicating very poor flexibility. Muscle groups included in this scale are the iliotibial band, the rectus femoris, the hamstrings, the iliopsoas, and the gastrocsoleus; table 4.2 lists the criteria for muscle tightness. We assess flexibility of the iliotibial band with a modified version of the Ober test (figure 4.7), of the iliopsoas with the Thomas test (figure 4.8), and of the hamstrings by measuring popliteal angle (figure 4.9). For rectus femoris flexibility, we measure the difference between knee flexion with the hip flexed and with the hip extended (Ely test, figure 4.10). This difference is called the quadriceps inhibited knee flexion angle (QFA). Gastrocsoleus flexibility is measured by determining maximal ankle dorsiflexion with the knee extended—a position closer to that experienced during ambulation than the 90-degree knee flexion used in many tests. This muscle tightness scale has been used to assess flexibility in collegiate athletes, but requires studies of validity and reliability before use in other populations.

Table 4.2 Lower Extremity Muscle Tightness Score

Muscle	Tightness criterion
Iliotibial band	Positive Ober test
Rectus femoris	QFA* ≥10°
Iliopsoas	Positive Thomas test
Hamstrings	Popliteal angle ≥25°
Gastrocsoleus	Ankle dorsiflexion ≤5°

Evaluate each lower extremity. Score one point for each tight muscle group in each leg, yielding a score ranging from 0 (all muscles flexible) to 10 (all muscles tight).

*QFA = quadriceps inhibited knee flexion angle (see paragraph above for explanation).

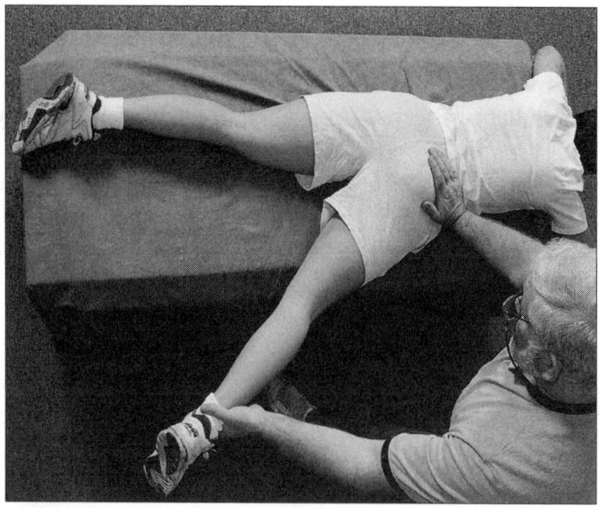

a

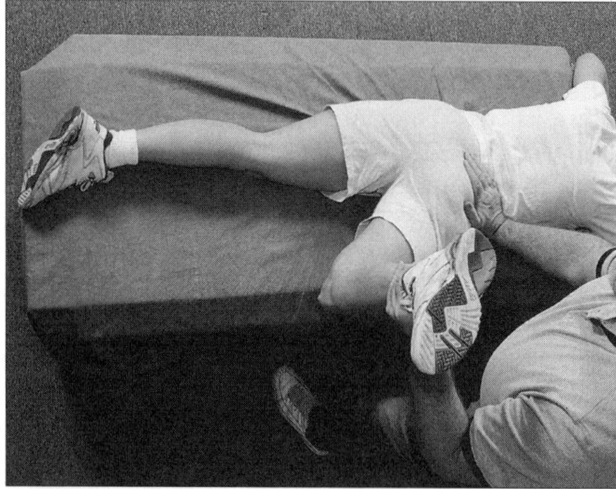

b

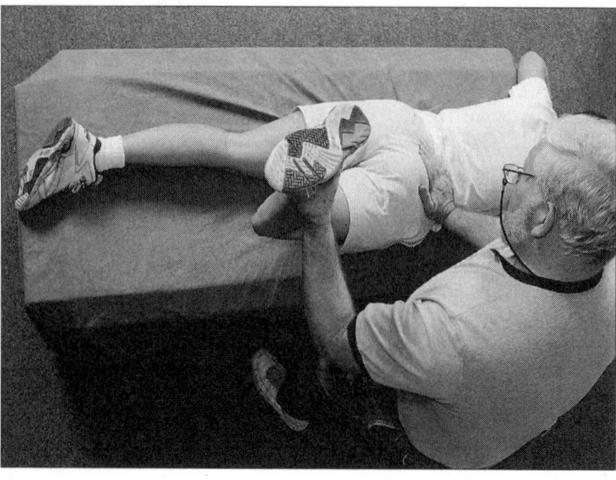

c

Figure 4.7 The Ober test assesses iliotibial band flexibility. A modified form of the traditional test, eliminating the assistance of gravity, is depicted. *(a)* The leg to be tested is abducted while the subject is prone. *(b)* The knee of the abducted leg is flexed 90 degrees and the hip extended. *(c)* The leg should freely adduct to midline from the position in figure 4.7b if the iliotibial band is flexible.

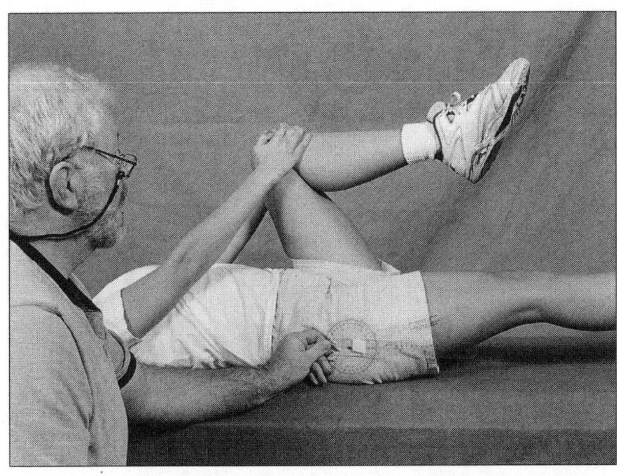

Figure 4.8 The Thomas test assesses iliopsoas flexibility. The subject holds one knee flexed to the chest while extending the other hip and knee. In the absence of iliopsoas tightness, the extended leg should rest comfortably on the examining table.

MEASURING LIGAMENTOUS LAXITY

Ligamentous laxity is widely assessed by using the Beighton scale (Beighton et al. 1973), a modification of a scoring system Carter and Wilkinson (1964) devised to study children with congenital dislocation of the hip (see table 4.3 and figure 4.11). The first four of the five elements in the scale are assessed bilaterally, for a maximum score of 2; the last element is scored either 0 or 1, giving a maximum ligamentous laxity score of 9 points (hyperlax) and a minimum of 0 (tight). Several authors have labeled Beighton scores of 0-3 as normal and scores of 4-9 as representing ligamentous laxity (Al-Rawi et al. 1985; Diaz et al. 1993; Klemp et al. 1984). The spinal forward flexion criterion (palms to floor) differs from the other criteria, in that it measures hamstring flexibility and anatomic proportions in addition to ligamentous laxity (Klemp et al. 1984); some believe it should be dropped from the scale.

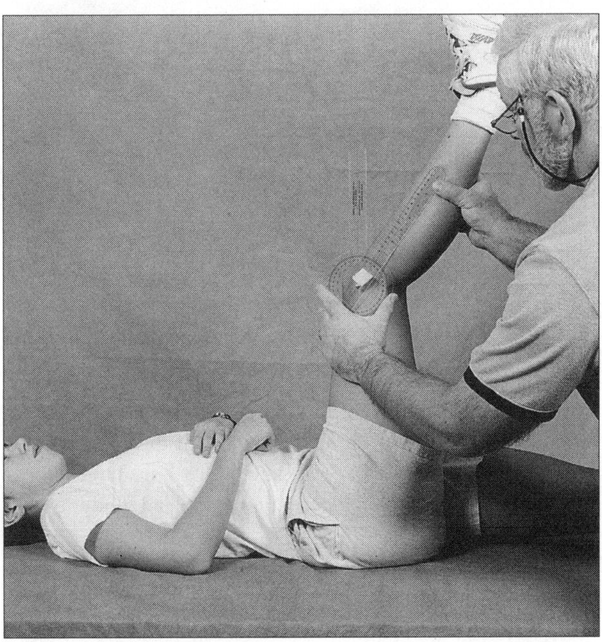

Figure 4.9 Measurement of popliteal angle assesses hamstring flexibility. With the subject supine, the hip is flexed 90 degrees and the knee extended as much as possible. A goniometer is used to measure the angle between the lower leg and vertical.

RELATIONSHIP BETWEEN MUSCLE FLEXIBILITY AND INJURY

Most health care professionals, athletes, and coaches believe that improving flexibility helps prevent musculoskeletal injuries—particularly overuse injuries and muscle strains. Most researchers addressing this issue have studied athletes or other "healthy," relatively young populations, and they have looked only at the relationship between static flexibility and injury. Ideally, of course, one would like to measure flexibility immediately before an injury occurs. Since this is not possible, investigators must measure flexibility at some point prior to the injury, such as at the beginning of an athletic season. Measuring flexibility after an injury has been sustained is not acceptable: either the injury itself or the treatment of the injury may alter flexibility. Theoretically, one can randomize subjects to stretching vs. nonstretching programs and record injuries for each group; but such a study must control for many extraneous variables.

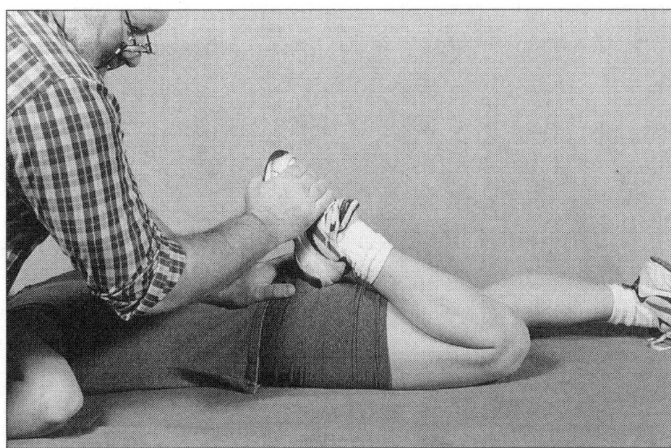

Figure 4.10 The Ely test assesses rectus femoris flexibility. With the subject prone and the pelvis stabilized against the examining table, the knee is flexed until the heel touches the buttock. If this maneuver cannot be performed without flexing the hips and/or lifting the pelvis from the examining table, the rectus femoris muscle is tight.

Table 4.3 Beighton Scale for Ligamentous Laxity

Test element	Maximum score
Thumb to forearm	2
5th MCP* extension > 90°	2
Elbow hyperextension > 10°	2
Knee hyperextension > 10°	2
Palms to floor	1
TOTAL	9

*MCP = metacarpal phalangeal joint

Adapted, by permission, from P.L. Beighton, L. Solomon, and C. Soskolone, 1973, "Articular mobility in an African population," *Annals of the Rheumatic Diseases* 32: 413-418.

Several investigators have observed correlations between flexibility deficits and specific types of injuries. A study of adolescent elite figure skaters found an association between anterior knee pain syndromes and hamstring, rectus femoris, and gastrocsoleus muscle tightness (Smith et al. 1991). Quadriceps muscle tightness is also associated with patellofemoral pain syndrome among Belgian collegiate physical education students (Witvrouw et al. 2000). Witvrouw et al. (2003) found an association between hamstring and quadriceps muscle tightness and muscle strain injuries among professional soccer players. In another group of collegiate physical education students, Lysens et al. (1989) found an association between muscle inflexibility and increased incidence of overuse injuries. Army recruits with gastrocsoleus muscle tightness have an increased incidence of lower leg injuries, particularly ankle sprains (Pope et al. 1998). Knapik et al. (1991) observed that female collegiate athletes with asymmetric lower extremity flexibility developed more lower extremity injuries than those with symmetric flexibility. Table 4.4 shows specific flexibility deficits that have been associated with particular overuse injuries (Krivickas 1997).

We studied the relationship between lower extremity muscle tightness and lower extremity injuries in college athletes using the 10-point muscle tightness scale previously described (Krivickas and Feinberg 1996). Men had significantly tighter muscles than women. For men, each additional point on the muscle tightness scale increased risk of injury by 23%, but muscle tightness was not associated with injury incidence in women. It may be that the women in this study had achieved a threshold flexibility level necessary to avoid increased risk of injury.

Hilyer and colleagues (1990) assigned municipal fire fighters either to a flexibility training program or to no training program. Those in the experimental group performed flexibility exercises for one-half hour per shift for two years. Overall flexibility improved in the trained group, and although the incidence of injury did not differ from that in the control group, those in the trained group sustained less severe and less costly injuries. A similar study of stretching prior to physical training in army recruits also failed to reduce incidence of injury (Pope et al. 2000). In contrast, Hartig and Henderson (1999)

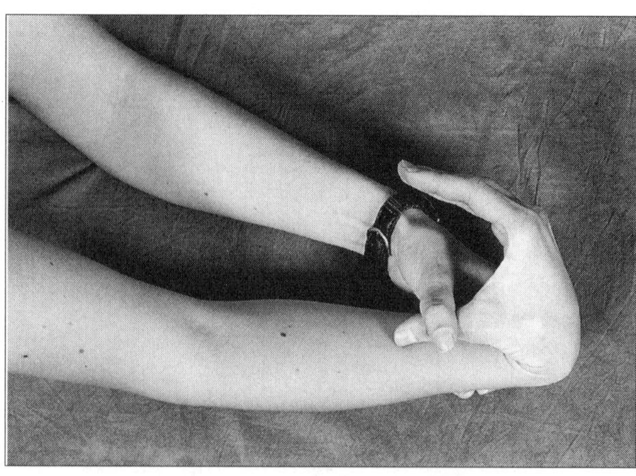

a

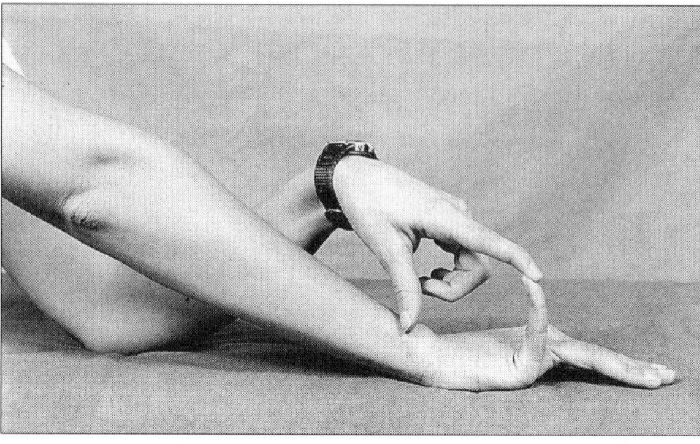

b

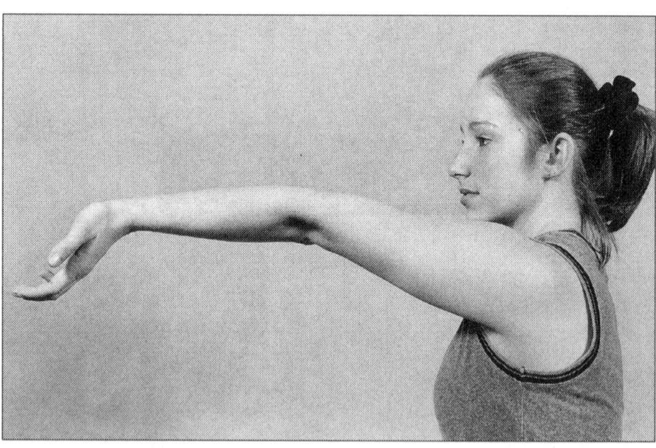

c

(continued)

Figure 4.11 Elements of Beighton scale. *(a)* Passive opposition of the thumb to the flexor aspect of the forearm. *(b)* Passive hyperextension of the 5th metacarpal phalangeal joint beyond 90 degrees. *(c)* Hyperextension of the elbow by 10 degrees or more.

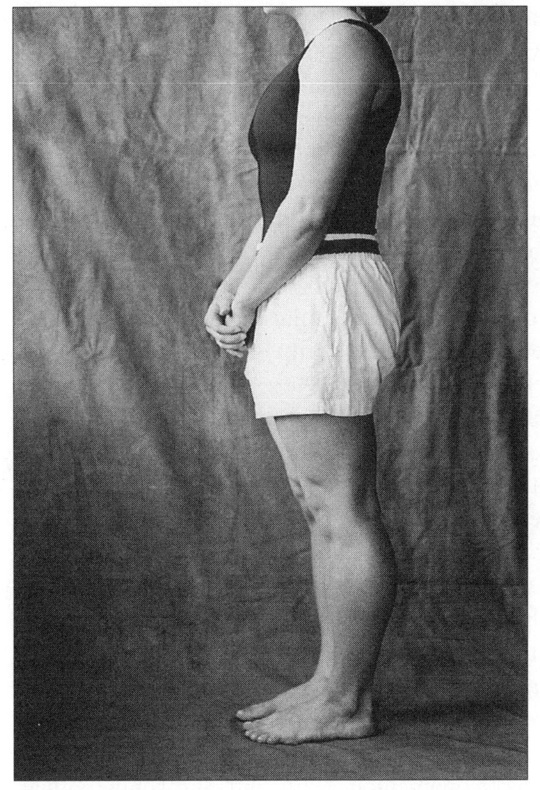

d

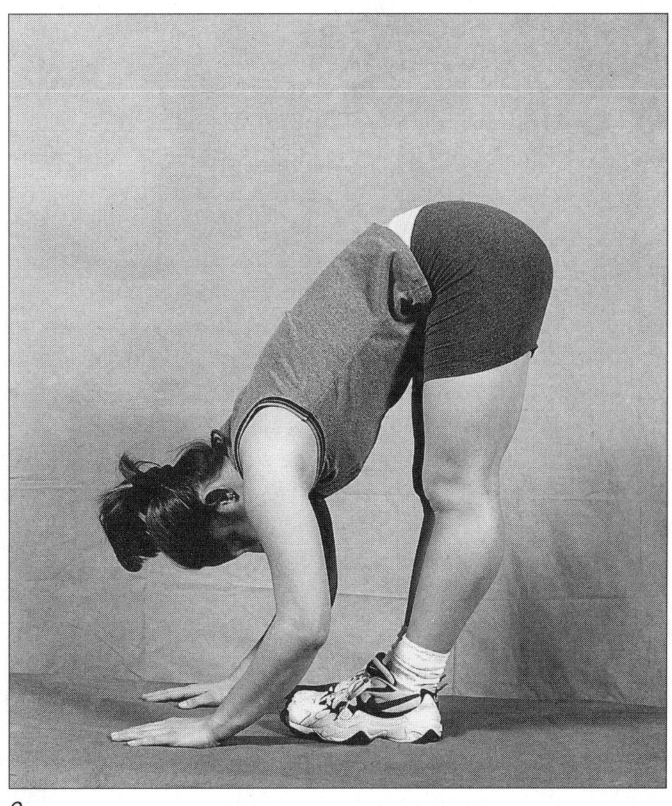

e

Figure 4.11 *(continued)* *(d)* Hyperextension of the knee by 10 degrees or more. *(e)* Forward flexion of the trunk with the knees fully extended and palms flat on the floor.

Table 4.4 Flexibility Deficits Associated With Overuse Injuries

	Lesser trochanter apophysitis	PFSS*	JK*	OS*	MTSS*	ITB* syndrome	Plantar fasciitis
Iliopsoas	X						
ITB*						X	
Rectus femoris		X	X	X			
Hamstrings		X	X	X			
Gastrocsoleus		X			X		X
Tibialis posteriors							

	Sever's	Painful accessory navicular	Anterior impingement
Gastrocsoleus	X	X	
Tibialis posterior		X	
Shoulder external rotators			X

*PFSS = patellofemoral stress syndrome; JK = jumper's knee; OS = Osgood Schlatter's disease; MTSS = medial tibial stress syndrome; ITB = iliotibial band

Adapted, by permission, from L.S. Krivickas, 1997, "Anatomical factors associated with overuse injuries," *Sports Medicine* 24(2): 132-146.

were able to reduce the incidence of lower extremity overuse injuries in a group of army recruits undergoing basic training by implementing a hamstring stretching program. These are the types of prospective studies that need to be done to further explore the relationship between flexibility and injury.

No one has specifically studied the relationship between flexibility and injury in the elderly, but one study found that elderly adults with a history of falls had decreased hip flexion and ankle dorsiflexion range of motion when compared to the "nonfallers" (Gehlsen and Whaley 1990). Falls are a major cause of injury in the elderly, and decreased lower extremity flexibility may increase the risk of injury in the elderly.

Few or no clinical studies have addressed the relationship between flexibility deficits and injury in populations with various disease processes.

Relationship Between Ligamentous Laxity and Injury

The relationship between ligamentous laxity and musculoskeletal injuries is even more confusing than the relationship between flexibility deficits and injury. Some studies have shown associations between ligamentous laxity and an increased injury incidence, while others have found no association or even an association with decreased incidence of injury. Two types of studies have attempted to address this issue. One has looked at generalized ligamentous laxity, as measured by the Beighton scale, while the other type has focused on joint-specific ligamentous laxity, such as knee ligament laxity measured by a KT-100 arthrometer.

Researchers have explored the relationship between generalized ligamentous laxity and injury in ballet dancers, soldiers, football players, female soccer players, and collegiate athletes (Diaz et al. 1993; Godshall 1975; Grana and Moretz 1978; Kalenak and Morehouse 1975; Klemp et al. 1984; Krivickas and Feinberg 1996; Moretz et al. 1982; Nicholas 1970; Soderman et al. 2001). Ballet dancers with hypermobility, defined as a score of 4 or greater on the Beighton scale, sustained significantly more injuries (Klemp et al. 1984). In a group of soldiers undergoing a two-month period of intense military training, those with hypermobility sustained more ankle sprains and knee injuries but fewer muscle strains (Diaz et al. 1993). In contrast, in collegiate athletes there was no association between generalized ligamentous laxity and the incidence of ankle sprains (Baumhauer et al. 1995). Nicholas (1970) found an association between generalized ligamentous laxity and knee ligament rupture in professional football players, but Kalenak and Morehouse (1975) found no such association among collegiate football players. The findings of Moretz et al. (1982), Grana and Moretz (1978), and Godshall (1975) agree with those of Kalenak and Morehouse. Among female soccer players in Sweden, generalized ligamentous laxity and knee ligament laxity are both associated with traumatic leg injuries (Soderman et al. 2001).

In our study of collegiate athletes participating in a variety of sports, male athletes with tight ligaments (i.e., low scores on the Beighton scale) sustained a greater number of lower extremity injuries during a single competitive season than those with higher Beighton scores (Krivickas and Feinberg 1996). Although we saw no such relationship among the female athletes, it should be noted that they had significantly higher Beighton scores than the males (mean ± *SD* = 3.3 ± 2.2, vs. 1.8 ± 2.0). Because very few men had Beighton scores greater than or equal to 4, this study did not have the power to detect an association between true hypermobility and injury in men. One hypothesis that would explain the conflicting results is that either too little or too much ligamentous laxity increases the risk of injury.

Larsson et al. (1993) used the Beighton scale to assess hypermobility in 660 musicians, testing the relationship between ligamentous laxity and injury of individual joints. Unlike in previous studies, individual elements of the scale were correlated with specific injuries, and no composite ligamentous laxity score was correlated with overall injury incidence. Musicians playing instruments requiring repetitive upper extremity motion were less likely to experience hand and wrist symptoms if they had wrist hypermobility; however, hypermobility of joints not involved in repetitive motion was a liability rather than an asset. Those with knee and spine hypermobility suffered more frequently from knee and low back pain.

Effect of Stretching on Delayed Onset Muscle Soreness

Delayed onset muscle soreness (DOMS) occurs following heavy bouts of exercise, particularly those involving eccentric contractions. DOMS peaks 24 to 48 hours after exercise completion and is believed to be caused by exercise induced muscle fiber damage (Friden et al. 1983). Many fitness instructors believe that static stretching before or following exercise can minimize the effects of DOMS. This belief is supported by the work of McHugh et al. (1999), who investigated the relationship between hamstring muscle flexibility and DOMS following eccentric hamstring exercise. Subjects were classified based on the results of an instrumented straight leg raise as having stiff, normal, or compliant hamstrings. All subjects performed the same bout of eccentric exercise. Those with stiff hamstrings experienced greater muscle pain and strength loss than those with compliant hamstrings.

Unfortunately, studies that have directly investigated the effect of stretching on DOMS have all been negative; outcome measures utilized have included various pain scales, serum creatine phosphokinase measurements, and force decrement measurements. Five studies have explored the effect of static stretching before (Johansson et al. 1999; High and Howley 1989; Wessel and Wan 1994) and/or after (McGlynn et al. 1979; Buroker and Schwane 1989; Wessel and Wan 1994) exercise bouts designed to induce DOMS. The muscle groups studied have included the biceps, hamstrings, and quadriceps; and total stretch time has ranged from 80 to 600 seconds. In no instance has the stretching program reduced DOMS. Thus, it does not appear that stretching is an effective means of decreasing DOMS.

Effect of Disease Processes on Flexibility

Several categories of disease processes adversely affect joint range of motion and, when severe, may result in a contracture, which means that muscle cannot be passively extended to its full normal length without pain or soft tissue injury such as a muscle tear. The flexibility of muscles surrounding a joint must be lost in order for a contracture to develop. However, once a contracture has developed, it does not respond readily to a stretching program and is difficult to treat. All of the following conditions decrease flexibility and predispose to the development of contractures: upper motor neuron lesions that produce spasticity, lower motor neuron lesions that produce severe weakness, chronic pain, arthritis, and burns or orthopedic injuries whose treatment requires immobilization.

Spasticity decreases flexibility via hyperactivity of the muscle spindle reflex and of suprasegmental reflexes. If spastic muscles are not stretched regularly, contractures develop. Muscle cooling decreases the firing rate of the spindle, while heat increases its firing rate (DeLateur 1994; Eldred et al. 1960; Mense 1978; Miglietta 1973; Petajan and Watts 1962). Interestingly, individual muscle fibers from muscles with spasticity are stiffer than normal muscle fibers, a finding independent of the neural reflexes associated with spasticity (Friden and Lieber 2003). The etiology of this increase in muscle fiber stiffness is unknown. It is hypothesized that it may be related to variations in titin isoforms or concentration. In individuals whose weakness is related to lower motor neuron dysfunction (e.g., spinal muscular atrophy or a severe myopathy), loss of flexibility and contractures develop despite normal or decreased muscle spindle activity. Muscles are maintained in a shortened position because the patient is too weak to move the joints through a full range of motion. The most common sites for contracture are the shoulders in those with proximal upper extremity weakness, the hip and knee flexors in those who are wheelchair bound, and the ankle plantar flexors of individuals with foot drop. A daily range-of-motion program can easily prevent loss of range of motion in these cases. People requiring immobilization of a joint for a prolonged period of time also lose flexibility in muscles that are chronically shortened. For example, an elbow flexion contracture may develop after an arm has been kept in a sling for 6 weeks to treat a proximal humerus fracture. Similarly, pain—such as that produced by a flare of rheumatoid arthritis—can limit joint range of motion enough to promote contracture.

A few disease processes, such as pentazocine fibrous myopathy, actually cause muscle fibrosis to develop (DeLateur 1994). In these cases, the application of heat increases collagen extensibility and should be used prior to stretching the involved muscles. Burn injuries also result in formation of tissue with excessive collagen content, and heat application facilitates stretching.

A few other disease processes produce excessive flexibility. These are primarily connective tissue diseases such as Ehlers-Danlos syndrome, Marfan's syndrome, and osteogenesis imperfecta. Individuals with diseases of amino acid metabolism, such as homocystinuria and hyperlysinemia, may also have joint hypermobility.

Relationship Between Flexibility and Athletic Performance

Only a few studies have explored the relationship between flexibility and performance. In these studies, researchers have measured both muscle power generation and the VO_2 required to complete a given activity, in order to assess muscle efficiency. Once again, the results conflict with one another, and it is not yet known whether increasing range of motion enhances athletic performance.

Gleim et al. (1990) assessed trunk and lower extremity flexibility in healthy men and women, and then measured VO_2 during treadmill walking and jogging. Those with the tightest muscles were the most efficient, with the lowest VO_2 at any given speed. A similar study by Craib et al. (1996) looked at the relationship between flexibility and running economy in sub-elite male distance runners. Tightness of the hip external rotators and ankle dorsiflexors was associated with lower VO_2 and accounted for 47% of the variance in running economy. One possible explanation for these findings is that those who train more intensely develop both greater cardiovascular fitness and more muscle tightness. The elastic recoil of muscle contributes to energy necessary for movement (Cavagna et al. 1964), and tighter muscles may have greater elastic recoil, enabling them to store more energy. An earlier study by DeVries (1963) did not find any change in VO_2 or speed when runners stretched prior to a 100-yard sprint. In contrast, a study of college students by Godges et al. (1989) demonstrated greater gait economy after a single session of stretching.

Other investigators have attempted to correlate muscle flexibility with force and power production. The findings of various studies are somewhat contradictory. Wilson et al. (1994) found that weightlifters with the greatest stiffness of their upper extremity and chest muscles were able to generate more power during isometric and concentric contractions, but not during eccentric contractions. The same investigators found that flexibility training decreases muscle stiffness. According to their work, increasing flexibility appears to decrease power production. Several investigators have documented a decrease in vertical jump height following an acute bout of stretching (Church et al. 2001; Cornwell et al. 2002). In contrast, Worrell and colleagues (1994) found that a hamstring stretching program in healthy university students increased peak eccentric and concentric hamstring torque. Theoretically, improving flexibility of a muscle should increase its ability to generate concentric force: during stretch, elastic components of muscle absorb mechanical work and store it as potential energy, which is released when the muscle shortens. By increasing muscle length, more energy can be stored and then released during the subsequent concentric contraction. Hortobagyi et al. (1985) found that a hamstring stretching program increased the power of concentric quadriceps contraction by increasing the speed of contraction without altering force production. Thus, it appears that increasing the flexibility of an antagonist muscle can also increase contraction speed of the agonist muscle.

Flexibility and Activities of Daily Living in the Elderly or Disabled

No one has scientifically studied the relationship between flexibility and performance of activities of daily living (ADLs) in the elderly or disabled population. Clinicians caring for the elderly or disabled realize that a certain minimal range of motion is necessary to perform ADLs. Adequate shoulder range of motion is required to reach a glass on an overhead shelf, handle garment closures behind one's back, brush one's hair, and even feed oneself. Table 4.5 shows the necessary joint range of motion for commonly performed ADLs. In a study of patients with elbow flexion contractures associated with spinal muscular atrophy or congenital myopathy, 59% of the patients reported that the contractures interfered with their ADLs, while 12% felt the contractures were beneficial (Willig et al. 1995). Research evaluating the effect of flexibility training on function in the elderly or disabled must be performed before we can draw conclusions about the benefits of flexibility training in these populations.

Stretching Techniques and Prescription of a Flexibility Training Program

The three major forms of stretching are ballistic, static, and proprioceptive neuromuscular facilitation (PNF). Ballistic stretching utilizes rapid bouncing motions that tend to have relatively high force and velocity. Animal studies suggest that ballistic stretching should increase the risk of muscle injury (Taylor et al. 1990). Although it can be effective, ballistic stretching is not recommended. It activates the spindle reflex, which is counterproductive, and it is more likely than other stretching methods to produce muscle soreness.

Table 4.5 Joint Range of Motion Required for Activities of Daily Living

Joint	Range of motion	Activity
Elbow	120° flexion	Eating, grooming, personal hygiene
Shoulder	45° flexion, 90° abduction, 20° external rotation	Eating, grooming, personal hygiene
Ankle	10° dorsiflexion, 20° plantar flexion	Walking
Knee	60° flexion	Walking
	90° flexion	Stair climbing
Hip	30° flexion	Walking
	70° flexion	Sitting

Static stretching is an effective means of improving flexibility. It minimizes activation of the spindle reflex, activates the Golgi tendon reflex if held long enough, does not require a partner, and is unlikely to cause muscle soreness. A static stretch must be held for at least 6 seconds in order to fully activate the Golgi tendon reflex (Shellock and Prentice 1985).

Knott and Voss (1968) popularized PNF stretching. There are several different techniques of PNF, but they all involve isometric contraction and relaxation of the muscle being stretched. Two of the most popular PNF techniques are contract-relax (CR) and contract-relax agonist-contract (CRAC). To stretch the hamstrings using the CR technique, the subject lies supine while a partner passively performs a straight leg raise on the subject. The subject then contracts his hamstrings while the partner resists movement of the leg; when the subject relaxes his hamstrings, the partner pushes the straight leg raise further, increasing hip range of motion. Using the CRAC technique, the subject would contract his quadriceps while the partner assisted the straight leg raise. PNF stretching techniques take advantage of neurophysiologic principles such as autogenic and reciprocal inhibition, which are believed to alter the spinal reflexes. Autogenic inhibition refers to stimulation of the Golgi tendon organ by contraction of the muscle that is being stretched. Reflex inhibition is believed to occur when the CRAC technique is used; contraction of the antagonist muscle induces relaxation in the muscle being stretched. One drawback of PNF techniques is that most require a partner, and some training is necessary for them to be performed properly.

WHICH TECHNIQUE?

Several investigators have compared the efficacy of ballistic, static, and PNF stretching programs (DeVries 1963; Etnyre and Lee 1988; Funk et al. 2003; Godges et al. 1989; Lucas and Koslow 1984; Moore and Hutton 1980; Sady et al. 1982; Wallin et al. 1985). All three methods improve flexibility, but it is not clear which is most effective. Table 4.6 summarizes the studies.

Table 4.6 Comparison Studies of Stretching Techniques

Author	Year	Population	Stretching techniques	Muscle	Result
DeVries	1962	College M	1. Static 2. Ballistic	Multiple	No difference
Moore and Hutton	1980	College F gymnasts	1. PNF—CR 2. PNF—CRAC 3. Static	Hamstrings	CRAC > static > CR; only statistically significant difference between CRAC and CR; CRAC most painful
Sady et al.	1982	College M	1. PNF—CR 2. Static 3. Ballistic	Multiple	PNF best
Lucas and Koslow	1984	College F	1. PNF—CR 2. Static 3. Ballistic	Hamstrings	No difference
Wallin et al.	1985	M, age 19-32	1. PNF—CR 2. Ballistic	Hamstrings, hip adductors, gastrocsoleus	PNF best
Etnyre and Lee	1988	College M and F	1. PNF—CR 2. PNF—CRAC 3. Static	Hamstrings, shoulder flexors	CRAC best in M; CR and CRAC equal in F but better than static
Godges et al.	1989	College M	1. PNF and soft tissue massage 2. Static	Hamstrings	Static best
Funk et al.	2003	College M and F	1. PNF—CR 2. Static	Hamstrings	PNF best

M = male, F = female, PNF = proprioceptive neuromuscular facilitation, CR = contract-relax PNF technique, CRAC = contract-relax agonist-contract PNF technique.

Moore and Hutton (1980) compared static, CR, and CRAC hamstring stretching protocols in college-aged female gymnasts, quantifying muscle contraction by use of surface EMG recordings from the quadriceps and hamstrings. The CRAC method produced the greatest hamstring EMG activity while the hamstrings were supposed to be relaxed. It was perceived as the most painful technique, and was less effective than either static or CR stretches. Overall, the subjects perceived the static stretch as the most effective—it produced the greatest increase in range of motion and was least painful. Three other studies have found the PNF CR technique to be superior to static stretch (Etnyre and Lee 1988; Funk et al. 2003; Sady et al. 1982). If a PNF technique is used, the CR may be preferable to the CRAC method because it is less painful and less likely to produce co-contraction of the muscle being stretched.

Prescription Recommendations

How long and how frequently must one stretch to increase or maintain flexibility? What is the most appropriate prescription for a flexibility training program? Bandy and Irion (1994) studied hamstring stretching programs with prescribed stretches of 15, 30, or 60 seconds. They found no improvement in flexibility with a single daily 15-second stretch, and equal flexibility improvement with a single daily 30- or 60-second stretch, suggesting that 30 seconds may be the ideal length of time to hold a static stretch. Grady and Saxena (1991) also found that a 30-second stretch is adequate to improve flexibility, with minimal additional gains when the stretch is extended to 1 or 2 minutes. McNair et al. (2001) investigated the amount of force drop associated with a fixed static stretch of the ankle plantar flexors and found no significant difference between a 15- and a 60-second stretch. The animal work of Taylor and colleagues (1990) suggests that the greatest muscle elongation occurs during the first 12 to 18 seconds of a static stretch and during the first 4 static stretches in a series of 10. Wallin et al. (1985) studied the frequency with which a stretching program must be performed to improve or maintain flexibility. After flexibility had been increased through a training program, one session of stretching per week was enough to maintain the increases. Three sessions of stretching per week improved flexibility, but even greater gains in flexibility were made when stretching was performed five times per week. At least one investigator has suggested that performing three stretching sessions per day (every 4-6 hours while awake) will maximize flexibility (Schwellnus 2003); for most patients, and for many athletes, compliance with a program of this intensity is likely to be poor.

Based on the few studies that have addressed the appropriate frequency, duration, and intensity of stretching programs, I recommend the following:

1. Prescribe either static, PNF, or a combination of both types of stretches.
2. Use the CRAC PNF technique with caution, as it may be more painful than other techniques and may encourage co-contraction of the muscle being stretched.
3. Do not prescribe ballistic stretching.
4. Have your patients perform stretching exercises at least three times per week to improve flexibility; daily stretching will probably result in greater, faster gains.
5. Have your patients perform each stretch at least three times and hold it for 30 seconds.
6. Because of most patients' tendency to exercise less than prescribed, I suggest that you instruct patients to stretch at least five days per week, hold each stretch 30 seconds, and perform each stretch five times. You will increase compliance by limiting the number of different stretches prescribed, i.e., prescribe only one stretching exercise for each tight muscle.

Patients with neurologic disorders producing spasticity may need to hold stretches for a longer period of time in order to achieve clinically significant increases in range of motion. Thirty minutes of daily stretching of the ankle plantar flexors in patients with spinal cord injury does not significantly increase ankle range of motion (Harvey et al. 2000). It has been suggested that up to 12 hours per day of stretching should be performed in patients with spinal cord injury in order to effectively improve range of motion (Harvey and Herbert 2002), but additional research must be done before any scientifically based recommendations can be made for this patient population.

Effect of Strength Training on Flexibility

In the past, athletes involved in activities requiring extreme flexibility, such as gymnastics and ballet, were discouraged from performing heavy resistance training because they and their coaches believed that it would decrease their flexibility. Unfortunately, few have addressed this issue in a scientific manner. One study of healthy young men found no relationship between strength and flexibility (Laubach and McConville 1965). A nonscientific observation can be made by looking at elite male gymnasts. They

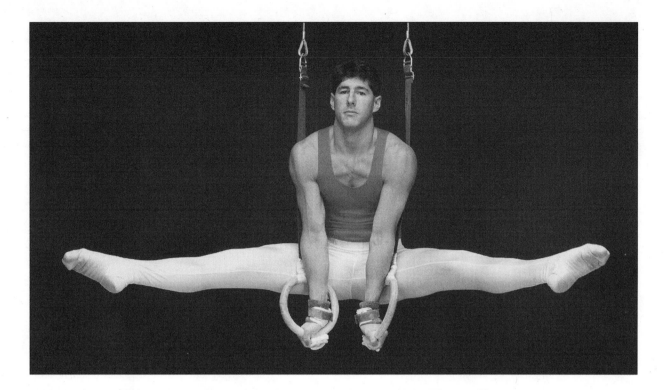

Figure 4.12 This gymnast demonstrates both excellent flexibility and excellent strength.

represent a population with both extreme flexibility and very high strength-to-weight ratios (see figure 4.12). By combining strength and flexibility training, these athletes do not compromise their flexibility with heavy resistance training.

Studying flexibility in older men (mean age 61 years), Girouard and Hurley (1995) compared the effects of either (1) flexibility training alone or (2) a combination of flexibility training and heavy resistance strength training. Those who performed only flexibility training increased their flexibility; while those who performed both types of training had no improvement in flexibility. Although the effect of heavy resistance training alone on flexibility was not studied, these findings suggest that resistance training without flexibility training might actually decrease flexibility in the elderly. The work of Barbosa and colleagues (2002) contradicts this supposition; in their small study, sedentary elderly women who participated in a resistance training program without a flexibility training component actually improved flexibility as measured by the sit and reach test. Fatouros et al. (2002) reported similar findings in elderly sedentary men undergoing strength and aerobic training. However, until further research is conducted in this area, it is prudent to incorporate stretching into any strength training program, particularly in the case of older individuals.

SUMMARY

Flexibility may be defined either as the range of motion of a joint or series of joints, or as a ratio of change in muscle length or joint angle to the force or torque required to passively elicit that change. Flexibility is joint and muscle specific and may differ in static and dynamic situations. Age, gender, race, training, injury history, spinal reflexes, supraspinal neural pathways, temperature, and the cellular composition of muscle all influence flexibility. The muscle–tendon unit is a viscoelastic structure that can be modeled simplistically as a spring and dash pot. It exhibits the viscoelastic properties of stress relaxation, creep, strain rate dependence, and hysteresis when stretched. There are various ways to assess the stiffness of muscle; some feel that measurement of stiffness may have more clinical relevance than measurement of flexibility.

Although there is no universal clinical scale for the measurement of muscle flexibility, many clinicians use the Beighton scale to measure ligamentous laxity. The literature concerning the relationship between flexibility deficits and injury is confusing, with some studies suggesting that flexibility deficits predispose to injury and others showing no relationship between flexibility and injury patterns. The relationship between ligamentous laxity and injury is even more controversial—some studies suggest that ligamentous laxity is beneficial, others suggest it is detrimental. Research addressing the relationship between VO_2, power production, and flexibility is also contradictory. While many disease processes affect flexibility, most research on flexibility training has focused on healthy individuals or athletes rather than on the disabled or elderly. Resistance strength training appears to influence flexibility, but the interaction between these two forms of training requires further study.

At the present time, prescription of a flexibility training program is somewhat empirical: little work has been done to determine the optimal duration, intensity, and frequency of training. Of the three major methods of stretching, it is clear that both static and PNF techniques are superior to ballistic stretching. Of the three major components of a comprehensive training and fitness program—strength, endurance, and flexibility training—flexibility training has received the least scientific attention. The unanswered questions concerning flexibility training are numerous, and opportunities for research in this area abound. What we do not know about flexibility is far greater than what we know.

PART II

SPECIAL CLINICAL CONSIDERATIONS

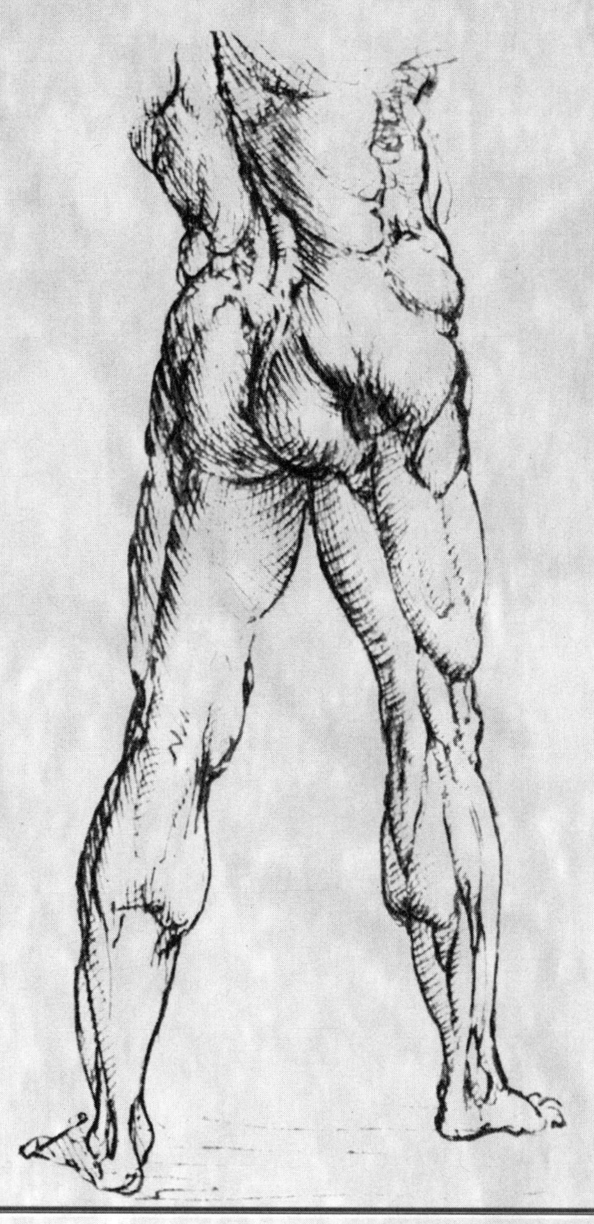

From the Royal Library, Turin.

CHAPTER 5

Testing Exercise Capacity: Cardiopulmonary/ Neuromuscular Models

James C. Agre, MD, PhD

Since the time of the ancient Greeks, physical activity has been acclaimed as an adjunct to good health (Leon and Blackburn 1977). Many research studies of the past half century have confirmed the health-related benefits of regular physical activity (Åstrand and Rodahl 1986; McArdle et al. 1991). The **beneficial physiological adaptations** resulting from regular physical activity have been reviewed (Åstrand et al. 2003; Hahn et al. 1990; Paffenbarger and Hyde 1984; Serfass and Gerberich 1984) and include the following: reduction in heart rate and blood pressure, both at rest and during activity; morphological change in skeletal muscle, resulting in improved physical work capacity; morphological change in cardiac muscle, resulting in improved cardiovascular efficiency; increased muscular endurance; reduced blood coagulability and transient increase in fibrinolysis; reduction in adiposity; increased lean body mass; increased cellular sensitivity to insulin; favorable changes in blood lipids and lipoproteins, including a reduction in plasma triglycerides and an increase in high-density lipoprotein (HDL) cholesterol; reduction in coronary artery disease risk factors; and decreased mortality and morbidity due to primary and secondary prevention. The **beneficial psychological adaptations** of regular physical activity are difficult to measure; however, it is well known that regular physical activity helps relieve muscular tension, makes one feel better and sleep better, and may aid motivation for improving other health habits including dietary changes (such as a reduction in saturated fat consumption and an increase in consumption of fruits, vegetables, legumes, and complex carbohydrates) and cessation of cigarette smoking (Leon and Blackburn 1977). In contrast, **limitation in physical activity** in the form of bed rest results in progressive deterioration of cardiovascular performance and efficiency, metabolic disturbances, difficulty in maintaining normal body weight, disturbed sympathetic nervous system activity, and possible emotional disturbances (Kottke 1966; Leon and Blackburn 1977; Taylor et al. 1949). Unquestionably, the physiological and psychological benefits of regular physical activity improve quality of life.

Yet physical activity carries risks. Regular physical activity increases one's risk for musculoskeletal injury (Buschbacher and Braddom 1994; Prentice 1994), and more serious consequences, such as acute myocardial infarction or cardiac arrest, can occur during the performance of physical activities (American College of Sports Medicine [ACSM] 1995, 2000; Siscovick et al. 1984; Thompson et al. 1982). Fortunately, the incidence of such adverse events is very low (Thompson et al. 1982). The incidence of cardiac arrest during physical activity, for example, is about one event in 18,000 healthy men per year (Siscovick et al. 1984), and pre-participation screening (and appropriate testing where necessary) can lower the risk associated with physical activity (ACSM 1995, 2000).

While there is no nationally accepted standard of guidelines and policies for exercise testing and participation, the American College of Sports Medicine has published very reasonable guidelines for exercise testing and prescription. These guidelines discuss, in detail, many topics concerning exercise testing and prescription—including health screening and risk stratification, pretest evaluation, physical fitness testing, clinical testing, and interpretation of test data. Since it is beyond the scope of this chapter to cover these issues in depth, for more detailed information readers should refer to the *ACSM's Guidelines for Exercise Testing and Prescription, 5th Edition* (ACSM 1995) and the *ACSM's Guidelines for Exercise Testing and Prescription, 6th Edition* (ACSM 2000).

Rationale for Health Screening and Risk Stratification

Health screening and **risk stratification** help physicians to identify individuals who are at risk from physical activity and to stratify individuals according to risk. Screening and stratification also help to determine what (if any) specific medical assessments are needed to assess an individual's response to physical activity, or what supervision (if any) an individual may require to safely participate in a physical activity program. The purposes of a pre-participation health screen include the following:

- Identify and exclude individuals with contraindications to physical activity.
- Identify individuals who need medical evaluation and clearance before starting an activity program.
- Identify individuals who should have medical supervision during physical activity.
- Identify people with other special needs (such as individuals with physical disabilities) (ACSM 1995, 2000).

Health screening can range from completing a simple questionnaire to undergoing very expensive medical testing. The **Physical Activity Readiness Questionnaire (PAR-Q)** (CSEP 2002; Thomas et al. 1992) sets minimal standards for adults who wish to participate in a low- to moderate-intensity physical activity program (ACSM 1995, 2000). This questionnaire helps identify adults with conditions that might require medical evaluation or advice prior to beginning a physical activity program. You may copy and use the PAR-Q, but only if you use the entire questionnaire. Adults who wish to start a physical activity program should also be evaluated for signs and symptoms of coronary artery disease (see "Major Symptoms or Signs Suggestive of Cardiopulmonary and Pulmonary Disease" and "Coronary Artery Disease Risk Factor Thresholds").

The American College of Sports Medicine has suggested that individuals be stratified into one of **three risk categories**, based on the individuals' potential risks for participation in a physical activity program:

1. **Apparently healthy**—individuals with no disease symptoms and no more than one major coronary artery disease risk factor (see "Positive Coronary Artery Disease Risk Factor Thresholds")
2. **At increased risk**—individuals who have signs or symptoms suggestive of serious disease, or two or more major risk factors for coronary artery disease
3. **With known disease**—individuals with known serious medical problems (ACSM 1995, 2000)

Major Symptoms or Signs Suggestive of Cardiovascular and Pulmonary Disease

1. Pain, discomfort (or other anginal equivalent) in the chest, neck, jaw, arms, or other areas that may be due to ischemia
2. Shortness of breath at rest or with mild exertion
3. Dizziness or syncope
4. Orthopnea or paroxysmal nocturnal dyspnea
5. Ankle edema
6. Palpitations or tachycardia
7. Intermittent claudication
8. Known heart murmur
9. Unusual fatigue or shortness of breath with usual activities

Reprinted, by permission, from American College of Sports Medicine, 2000, *ACSM's guidelines for exercise testing and prescription*, 6th ed. (Baltimore: Lippincott Williams & Wilkins), 25.

CORONARY ARTERY DISEASE RISK FACTOR THRESHOLDS

Risk factors	Defining criteria
Positive	
Family history	Myocardial infarction, coronary revascularization, or sudden death before 55 years of age in father or other male first-degree relative (i.e., brother or son), or before 65 years of age in mother or other female first-degree relative (i.e., sister or daughter)
Cigarette smoking	Current cigarette smoker or those who quit within the previous 6 months
Hypertension	Systolic blood pressure of ≥140 mmHg or diastolic ≥90 mmHg, confirmed by measurements on at least 2 separate occasions, or on antihypertensive medication
Hypercholesterolemia	Total serum cholesterol of >200 mg/dL (5.2 mmol/L) or high-density lipoprotein cholesterol of <35 mg/dL (0.9 mmol/L), or on lipid-lowering medication. If low-density lipoprotein cholesterol is available, use >130 mg/dL (3.4 mmol/L) rather than total cholesterol of >200 mg/dL
Impaired fasting glucose	Fasting blood glucose of ≥110 mg/dL (6.1 mmol/L) confirmed by measurements on at least 2 separate occasions
Obesity[†]	Body Mass Index of ≥30kg/m^2, or waist girth of >100 cm
Sedentary lifestyle	Persons not participating in a regular exercise program or meeting the minimal physical activity recommendations[‡] from the U.S. Surgeon General's report
Negative	
High serum HDL cholesterol[§]	>60 mg/dL (1.6 mmol/L)

[†]Professional opinions vary regarding the most appropriate markers and thresholds for obesity; therefore, exercise professionals should use clinical judgment when evaluating this risk factor.

[‡]Accumulating 30 minutes or more of moderate physical activity on most days of the week.

[§]It is common to sum risk factors in making clinical judgments. If high-density lipoprotein (HDL) cholesterol is high, subtract one risk factor from the sum of positive risk factors because high HDL decreases CAD risk.

Reproduced from Expert Panel on Detection, Evaluation, and Treatment of High Blood Cholesterol in Adults. Summary of the second report of the National Cholesterol Education Program (NCEP) expert panel on detection, evaluation, and treatment of high blood cholesterol in adults (Adult Treatment Panel II). *JAMA* 1993; 269:3015-3023.

You can make initial medical decisions after you have stratified an individual into one of the three categories. When you have a medical concern regarding an individual's risk, medically monitored exercise testing and other medical assessments can determine whether the individual can safely exercise.

For individuals with heart disease, the **American Heart Association** has developed a **special classification system** (Fletcher et al. 2001) that divides patients into one of four classes, from Class A (apparently healthy) to Class D (unstable disease with activity restriction) (see "The American Heart Association (AHA) Risk Stratification Criteria," pages 56-57).

Once you have classified an individual's risk category, ACSM guidelines can help determine when diagnostic medical evaluation(s) or exercise test(s), or both, are appropriate, and when a physician should be present for such exercise testing (see ACSM 1995, 2000 and figure 5.1).

RATIONALE FOR EXERCISE TESTING

The following are the major reasons for both cardiopulmonary and neuromuscular exercise testing.

CARDIOPULMONARY EXERCISE TESTING

Most reasons for evaluating a patient's cardiorespiratory condition are related to heart disease, but such evaluation may be appropriate for anyone planning to participate

The American Heart Association (AHA) Risk Stratification Criteria

Class A: Apparently healthy individuals

1. Children, adolescents, men <45 years, and women <55 years who have no symptoms or known presence of heart disease or major coronary risk factors
2. Men ≥45 years and women ≥55 years who have no symptoms or known presence of heart disease and with <2 major cardiovascular risk factors
3. Men ≥45 years and women ≥55 years who have no symptoms or known presence of heart disease and with ≥2 major cardiovascular risk factors

Activity guidelines: no restrictions other than basic guidelines

Supervision required: none

Note: It is suggested that persons classified as class A-2 and particularly class A-3 undergo a medical examination and possibly a medically supervised exercise test before engaging in vigorous exercise.

ECG and blood pressure monitoring: not required

Class B: Known, stable cardiovascular disease with low risk for complications with vigorous exercise, but slightly greater than for apparently healthy individuals

1. CAD (MI, CABG, PTCA, angina pectoris, abnormal exercise test, and abnormal coronary angiograms) whose condition is stable and who have the clinical characteristics outlined below
2. Valvular heart disease, excluding severe valvular stenosis or regurgitation with the clinical characteristics as outlined below
3. Congenital heart disease; risk stratification for patients with congenital heart disease should be guided by the 27th Bethesda Conference recommendations
4. Cardiomyopathy: ejection fraction ≤30%; includes stable patients with heart failure with clinical characteristics as outlined below but not hypertrophic cardiomyopathy or recent myocarditis
5. Exercise test abnormalities that do not meet any of the high-risk criteria outlined in class C below

Clinical characteristics (must include all the following)

1. New York Heart Association (NYHA) class 1 or 2
2. Exercise capacity ≥6 METs
3. No evidence of congestive heart failure
4. No evidence of myocardial ischemia or angina at rest or on the exercise test at or below 6 METs
5. Appropriate rise in systolic blood pressure during exercise
6. Absence of sustained or nonsustained ventricular tachycardia at rest or with exercise
7. Ability to satisfactorily self-monitor intensity of activity

Activity guidelines: Activity should be individualized, with exercise prescription provided by qualified individuals and approved by primary healthcare provider.

Supervision required: Medical supervision during initial prescription session is beneficial.

Supervision by appropriate trained nonmedical personnel for other exercise sessions should occur until the individual understands how to monitor his or her activity. Medical personnel should be trained and certified in Advanced Cardiac Life Support. Nonmedical personnel should be trained and certified in Basic Life Support (which includes cardiopulmonary resuscitation).

ECG and blood pressure monitoring: useful during the early prescription phase of training, usually 6 to 12 sessions

Class C: Those at moderate-to-high risk for cardiac complications during exercise and/or unable to self-regulate activity or to understand recommended activity level

1. CAD with clinical characteristics outlined below
2. Valvular heart disease, excluding severe valvular stenosis or regurgitation with the clinical characteristics as outlined below

3. Congenital heart disease; risk stratification for patients with congenital heart disease should be guided by the 27th Bethesda Conference recommendations
4. Cardiomyopathy: ejection fraction <30%; includes stable patients with heart failure with clinical characteristics as outlined below but not hypertrophic cardiomyopathy or recent myocarditis
5. Complex ventricular arrhythmias not well controlled

Clinical characteristics (any of the following):

1. NYHA class 3 or 4
2. Exercise test results
   - Exercise capacity <6 METs
   - Angina or ischemic ST depression at a workload <6 METs
   - Fall in systolic blood pressure below resting levels during exercise
   - Nonsustained ventricular tachycardia with exercise
3. Previous episode of primary cardiac arrest (i.e., cardiac arrest that did not occur in the presence of an acute myocardial infarction or during a cardiac procedure)
4. A medical problem that the physician believes may be life-threatening

Activity guidelines: Activity should be individualized, with exercise prescription provided by qualified individuals and approved by primary healthcare provider.

Supervision: medical supervision during all exercise sessions until safety is established

ECG and blood pressure monitoring: continuous during exercise sessions until safety is established, usually ≥12 sessions

Class D: Unstable disease with activity restriction

1. Unstable ischemia
2. Severe and symptomatic valvular stenosis or regurgitation
3. Congenital heart disease; criteria for risk that would prohibit exercise conditioning in patients with congenital heart disease should be guided by the 27th Bethesda Conference recommendations
4. Heart failure that is not compensated
5. Uncontrolled arrhythmias
6. Other medical conditions that could be aggravated by exercise

Activity guidelines: No activity is recommended for conditioning purposes. Attention should be directed to treating the patient and restoring the patient to class C or better. Daily activities must be prescribed on the basis of individual assessment by the patient's personal physician.

Reprinted, by permission, from G.F. Fletcher et al., 2001, "Exercise standards for testing and training: A statement for healthcare professionals from the American Heart Association," *Circulation* 104(14):1723-1724.

in a physical activity program. There are five **general indications for clinical cardiopulmonary exercise testing** (ACSM 1995, 2000; Moldover and Bartels 1996):

1. Predischarge status after an acute cardiac event
2. Postdischarge status after a cardiac event
3. Medical diagnosis
4. Disease severity and prognosis
5. Patient's functional status

Determination of Predischarge Status After an Acute Cardiac Event

Cardiorespiratory exercise testing after an acute cardiac event (e.g., **acute myocardial infarction**, **percutaneous transluminal coronary angioplasty**, or **coronary artery bypass graft surgery**) is based upon the patient's specific clinical situation. Some patients have undergone exercise testing—usually submaximal—as soon as three days after an uncomplicated acute myocardial infarction (Topol et al. 1988). Although used primarily to verify that the patient is stable and that the activity level does not cause cardiac ischemia or dysrhythmia, the testing can also help confirm that the patient's medications are adequately controlling the medical condition; in addition it can document the intensity of activity that the patient can safely perform during the recuperative phase (ACSM 1995, 2000; Moldover and Bartels 1996).

ACSM Recommendations for Current Medical Examination* and Exercise Testing Prior to Participation in a Physical Activity Program

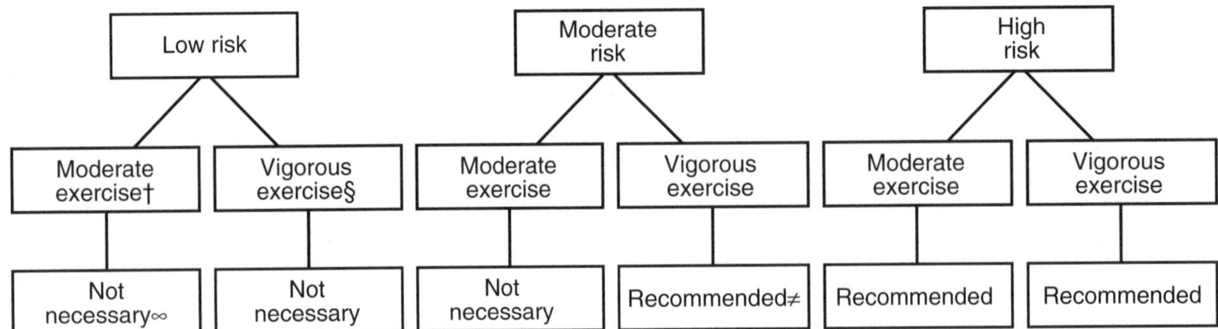

ACSM Recommendations for Physician Supervision of Exercise Tests

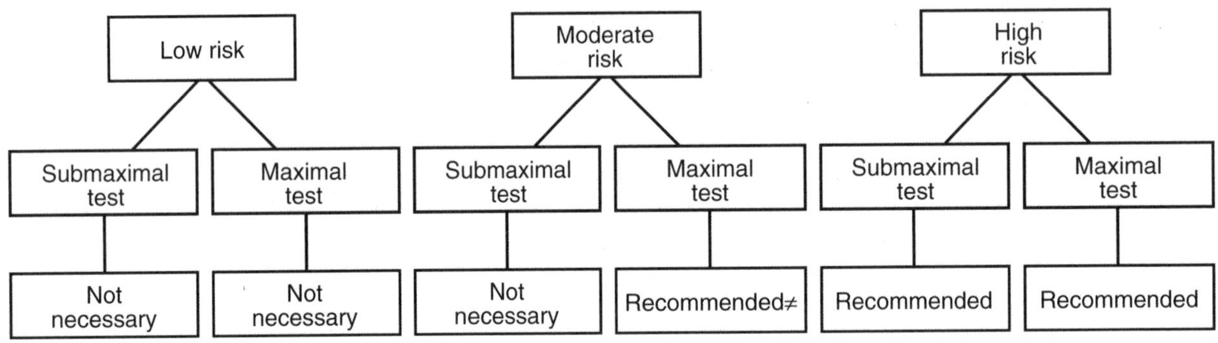

Figure 5.1 ACSM's guidelines for exercise testing.

*Within the past year.

†Absolute moderate exercise is defined as activities that are approximately 1.6 METs or the equivalent of brisk walking at 3 to 4 mph for most healthy adults. Nevertheless, a pace of 3 to 4 mpg might be considered to be "hard" to "very hard" by some sedentary, older persons. Moderate exercise may alternatively be defined as an intensity well within the individual's capacity, one which can be comfortably sustained for a prolonged period of time (~45 min), which has a gradual initiation and progression, and is generally noncompetitive. If an individual's exercise capacity is known, relative moderate exercise may be defined by the range 40%-60% maximal oxygen uptake.

∞The designation of "Not necessary" reflects the notion that a medical examination, exercise test, and physician supervision of exercise testing would not be essential in the preparticipation screening; however, they should not be viewed as inappropriate.

§Vigorous exercise is defined as activities of >6 METs. Vigorous exercise may alternatively be defined as exercise intense enough to represent a substantial cardiorespiratory challenge. If an individual's exercise capacity is known, vigorous exercise may be defined as an intensity of >60% maximal oxygen uptake.

≠When physician supervision of exercise testing is "Recommended," the physician should be in close proximity and readily available should there be an emergent need.

Adapted, by permission, from American College of Sports Medicine, 2000, *ACSM's Guidelines for exercise testing and prescription*, 6th ed. (Baltimore: Lippincott Williams & Wilkins), 27.

Determination of Postdischarge Status After a Cardiac Event

Patients usually perform postdischarge tests when it is believed they are ready to return to normal activities. This exercise test can help determine both the intensity of activity the patient can safely perform and the response of the patient to medication (ACSM 1995, 2000; Moldover and Bartels 1996). Depending on the patient's medical condition, you can perform this test three or more weeks after the acute event (ACSM 1995, 2000).

Determination of Medical Diagnosis

Sometimes a patient's history, physical examination, and other medical evaluations do not lead to a clear medical diagnosis. When there is a concern about the possibility of cardiac ischemia, dysrhythmia, or other adverse problem related to physical activity, a standard exercise tolerance test—with monitoring of the **electrocardiogram (ECG)**, blood pressure, and patient's subjective clinical status—is the best initial diagnostic test (ACSM 1995, 2000).

Determination of Disease Severity and Prognosis

Exercise testing for disease severity and prognosis is used primarily in patients with coronary artery disease. The **size of the ischemic myocardium** is directly proportional to the level of ST segment depression, the number of ECG electrodes that show ST segment depression, and the duration of ST segment depression after an exercise test. It is inversely proportional to the slope of the ST segment; the product of heart rate × systolic blood pressure (double product) at which the ST segment depression occurs; and the maximal heart rate, systolic blood pressure, and maximal exercise intensity attained (ACSM 1995, 2000). The patient's **prognosis** depends on the magnitude of ischemia and the presence or absence of dysrhythmia. The greater the extent of ischemia and the greater the cardiac dysrhythmia, the worse the prognosis.

Determination of Functional Status

Either submaximal or maximal exercise testing can determine a patient's functional status. **Submaximal exercise testing** can help determine a safe level of exertion for a patient's physical activity program. It can also help estimate maximal exercise capacity and maximal aerobic power by performance of several levels of submaximal exertion and use of a nomogram (Åstrand and Rodahl 1986; Åstrand et al. 2003; Morris et al. 1993). Submaximal exercise can help evaluate patients' responses to their physical activity programs. Comparison of heart rate at submaximal levels of exercise before and after an exercise program can provide an indirect assessment of improvement in cardiorespiratory fitness. **Maximal exercise testing** can determine safety for participation in rigorous physical activity programs, and can help estimate an individual's maximal aerobic power when you are unable to directly measure oxygen utilization during the test. As in the submaximal test, nomograms can provide estimates of maximal aerobic power (Åstrand and Rodahl 1986; Åstrand et al. 2003; Morris et al. 1993).

Measurement of respiratory variables permits determination of **oxygen utilization** and **carbon dioxide production**, thereby allowing for the direct measure of an individual's peak oxygen utilization (aerobic power) and determination of the ventilatory threshold. Ventilatory threshold is the point in an individual's ventilation when there is a nonlinear increase in expired carbon dioxide as compared to oxygen utilization; it can be used to estimate the maximal intensity at which an individual can be expected to exercise for prolonged periods of time without accumulating excessive amounts of lactic acid. Exercise at an intensity above the individual's ventilatory threshold will lead to lactic acidosis and fatigue. You can also use ventilatory threshold and peak oxygen utilization to determine an individual's cardiorespiratory functional impairment (see table 5.1) (Weber et al. 1987). Comparison of these variables before and after a physical activity program can determine the individual's level of cardiorespiratory fitness improvement.

Neuromuscular Exercise Testing

The ability to perform activities of daily living depends upon neuromuscular function. In order to stand up out of a chair, for example, people need sufficient strength in the lower limbs and trunk to lift themselves up. To continue with activities, they need muscular endurance and power (the ability to perform an activity at the required work rate). Power is defined as the rate of performing work (work × time^{-1}) (Åstrand et al. 2003). Power is, therefore, measured by the product of the force (F) and the distance moved in the direction of the force (L) per unit of time (s): Power = F × L × s^{-1}. In the metric system the unit of work is the joule (J). One joule of work is done when a force of one newton (N) moves the point of application through the distance of one meter (m). Power in the metric system is measured in watts (W). One watt equals one joule per second (1 W = 1 J × s^{-1} = 1 N × m × s^{-1}). Specific measures of muscular strength,

Table 5.1 Functional Classification of Patients Based on Gas Exchange Criteria

Severity of impairment	Functional class	Peak $\dot{V}O_2$ (ml/kg/min)	Ventilatory threshold (L/min)
None to mild	A	>20	>14
Mild to moderate	B	16-20	11-14
Moderate to severe	C	10-15	8-10
Severe	D	<10	<8

Adapted, by permission, from K.T. Weber, J.S. Janicki, and P.A. McElroy, 1987, "Determination of aerobic capacity and the severity of chronic cardiac and circulatory failure," *Circulation* (Suppl. VI) 76: 40-46.

endurance, and power can help clinicians assess patients' abilities to function in general and design therapeutic exercise programs to improve their patients' capacities to function. Such measures are also useful in assessing the efficacy of a therapeutic exercise program.

Muscle strength can be defined in a number of ways in the clinical setting. With the use of free weights, one can determine the one repetition maximum and ten repetition maximum. The **one repetition maximum** (or **1 RM**) is the maximum amount of weight a person can lift only one time using proper lifting technique. The **ten repetition maximum** (or **10 RM**) is the maximum weight he or she can lift 10 times (but not more) successfully, using proper lifting technique. Special equipment can also measure muscle strength statically, or isokinetically, by measuring the force or torque generated by the muscular activity.

Although strength and endurance are separate neuromuscular factors, they are interrelated. **Muscle strength** may be defined as the maximum force generated by a muscle; endurance as "the ability to continue a prescribed task in the desired manner" (de Lateur 1996); **absolute endurance** as "the time that a subject can sustain a given workload, or the number of seconds a given force can be held, or the number of repetitions of a given load" (de Lateur 1996); and **relative endurance** as the time that a subject can sustain an activity at a certain percentage of maximal force, or the number of seconds a force can be maintained at a certain percentage of maximal force, or the number of repetitions that can be performed at a certain percentage of maximal force. Figure 5.2 shows the relationship between intensity of activity and endurance (defined in figure 5.2a as the total number of muscular contractions, and in figure 5.2b

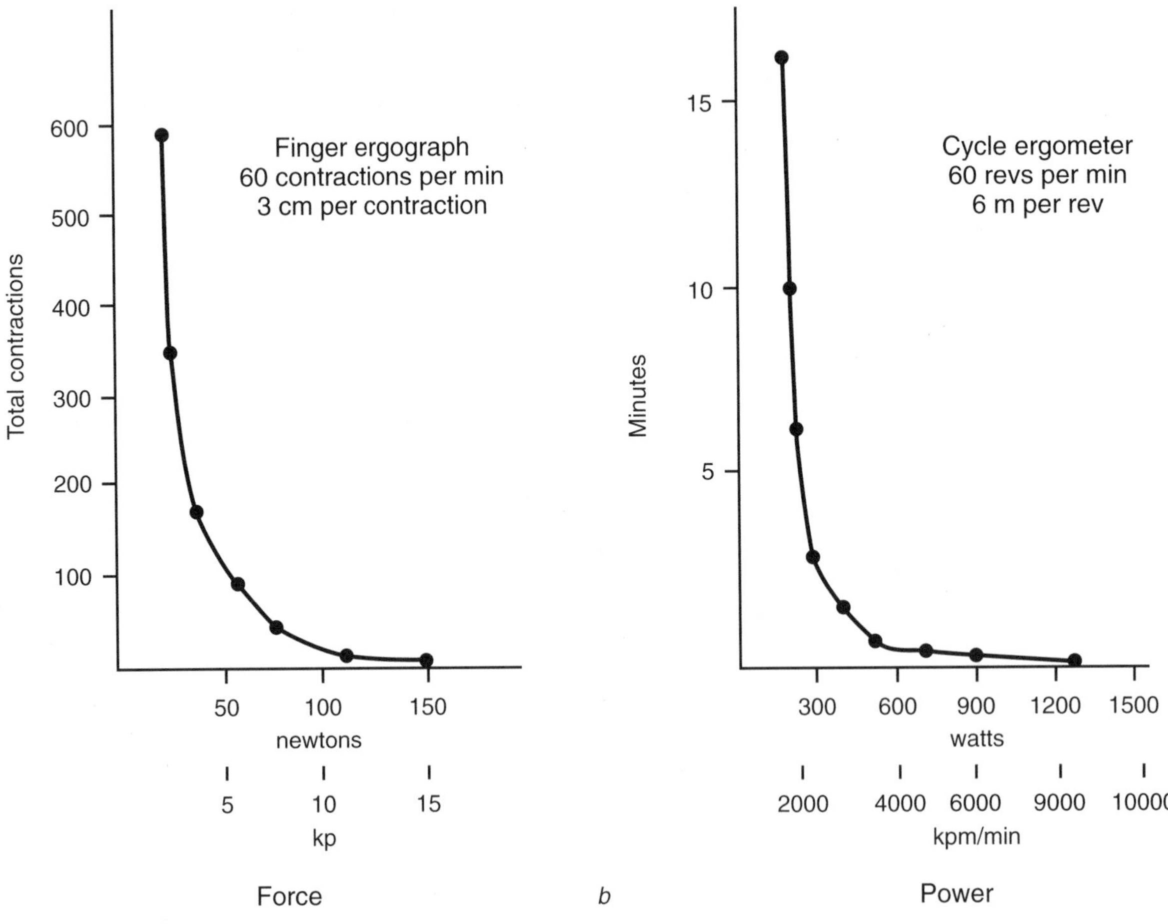

Figure 5.2 *(a)* Relationship of endurance (as total contractions) of repeated flexion of third digit to effective force of contraction. *(b)* Relationship of endurance (as minutes to fatigue) of cycle ergometer exercise to external power production. In both *a* and *b*, the intercept with the abscissa represents the exercise intensity for which the maneuver could be performed only once (and, therefore, the strength of the concentric movement). In both graphs, endurance could be presented as either total contractions or minutes to fatigue, and, as the contraction rate and velocity are designated, either abscissa could be designated as force (per individual repetition) or power (work per unit time).

Reprinted, by permission, from H. Knuttgen, 1976, Development of muscular strength and endurance. In *Neuromuscular mechanisms for therapeutic and conditioning exercises*, edited by H. Knuttgen (Baltimore: University Park Press), 97.

as time in minutes of successful cycling). Both figures 5.2a and 5.2b are examples of absolute endurance, with the absolute units (those that define the assigned workload) recorded on the abscissa. Both the total number of muscular contractions (figure 5.2a) and endurance time (figure 5.2b) decrease as the intensity of effort increases. In figure 5.2a, the total number of muscular contractions that can be successfully repeated is inversely related to the force of contraction—i.e., the greater the force of muscular contraction, the fewer the number of successful muscular contractions. In figure 5.2b, the endurance time on a cycle ergometer is inversely related to the power of cycling—i.e., the greater the power at which the individual cycles, the shorter the endurance time. In figure 5.3, the abscissa reflects relative static force (i.e., the assigned workload is a certain percentage of the individual's maximal static force) from 20% of maximal force to 100% of maximal force. This figure, an example of relative endurance, shows that endurance time (the time that the subject can successfully statically contract the muscle at the assigned relative level of force) is inversely related to the relative workload. When the subject contracts the muscle at 20% of maximal force, the endurance time is approximately 10 minutes, while at 100% of maximal force, the endurance time is well under 1 minute.

In fact, the endurance time of a 100% maximal muscle contraction has been shown to be very short indeed: the time that an individual can hold a maximal static muscle contraction is less than 1 second (see figure 5.4) (Mundale 1970).

The laboratory data in figure 5.3 suggest that muscle strengthening exercise should result in improved endurance in the performance of daily activities—for improvements in strength appear to increase endurance time. Suppose that an individual, prior to an exercise program, performs an activity at an exertion level equal to 40% of her maximal strength. Figure 5.3 shows that the expected endurance time for this activity would be approximately 2 minutes. If this individual doubles her strength through an intensive exercise program, that previous activity would then be performed at only 20% of her maximal strength. Figure 5.3 now shows that the endurance time would now be expected to be approximately 10 minutes.

The data in figure 5.3 may also show why stronger individuals have less difficulty performing certain activities than weaker individuals. In general, the endurance of the stronger individual should be greater than that of the weaker individual when both are performing the same activity (such as a job requiring repeated lifting of 50-pound boxes), because the stronger individual would be working at a lower relative level of effort than the weaker individual. (That is to say, the stronger, more powerful individual will have less difficulty in performing the

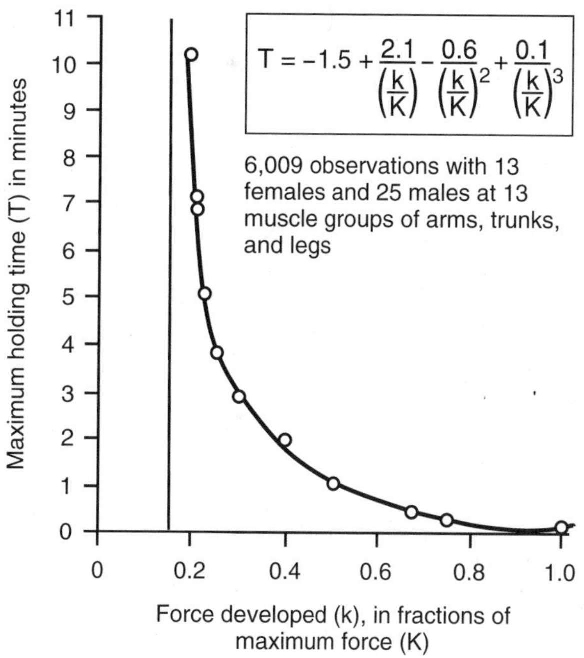

Figure 5.3 Endurance and intensity of work. Static work: tension at fractions of maximum strength.

Reprinted, by permission, from E. Simonson, 1971, Recovery and fatigue. In *Physiology of work capacity and fatigue*, edited by E. Simonson (Springfield, IL: Charles C Thomas), 440.

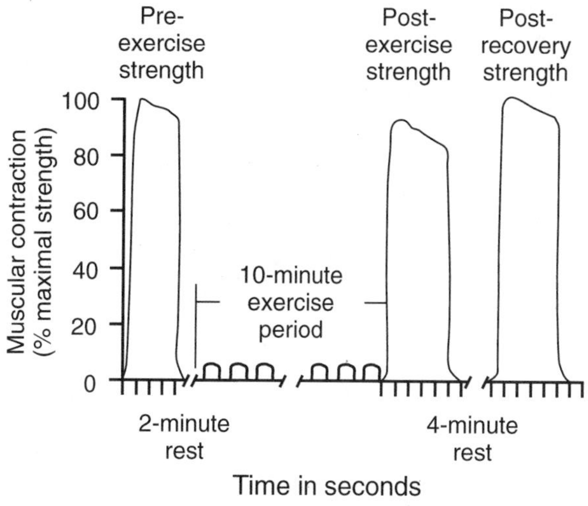

Figure 5.4 Maximal tension can be maintained during a voluntary maximal contraction of hand grip for less than 1 second before evidence of fatigue appears as the available supply of ATP is exhausted. Fatigue (unavailability of ATP) increases in proportion to the intensity of the activity but can be demonstrated following 10 minutes of intermittent contractions at 5% of maximal.

Reprinted from *Archives of Physical Medicine and Rehabilitation*, vol. 51: 532-539, M.O. Mundale, Copyright 1970, with permission from "The American Congress of Rehabilitation Medicine and the American Academy of Physical Medicine and Rehabilitation."

activity than the weaker, less powerful individual. This example has important ramifications for patients with physical disabilities. Many individuals with physical disabilities (e.g., those with post-polio syndrome) are weaker than nondisabled individuals, and therefore they may have less endurance than nondisabled individuals in performing daily activities.

Protocols for Exercise Testing, With Examples

The following section presents common protocols for both cardiopulmonary and neuromuscular exercise testing, followed by some examples.

Cardiopulmonary Testing Protocols

The best way to test the cardiopulmonary system is with dynamic (such as treadmill or bicycle ergometry), rather than static, exercise. Dynamic exercise permits accurate control of the workload and places a volume load on the heart; static exercise is much more difficult to control, and it places a pressor load on the heart (ACSM 1995, 2000). Treadmill and bicycle ergometry are the most common methods for testing the cardiopulmonary system. Although maximal heart rate is similar in the two types of testing (ACSM 1995, 2000), peak oxygen uptake is approximately 10% to 15% higher with treadmill ergometry (Myers et al. 1991).

Measure heart rate and blood pressure prior to, during, and after all cardiopulmonary exercise tests, and monitor the ECG during the test and during the cool-down period until it returns to baseline values (ACSM 1995, 2000). Before the exercise test, take blood pressure and a 12-lead ECG both in the supine position and in the position in which the test will be performed. During the exercise test, continuously monitor the ECG. Record blood pressure and a 12-lead ECG during the last minute of every exercise stage (ACSM 1995). Finally, record blood pressure and a 12-lead ECG immediately after completion of the exercise and every 1 to 2 minutes thereafter, for a minimum of 5 minutes. If you observe changes on the ECG, continue to monitor it until it returns to the baseline level. Similarly, monitor blood pressure till it also stabilizes near the baseline level.

It is possible to evaluate an individual's subjective response to exercise by assessing the **rating of perceived exertion (RPE)** at the end of each stage (Borg 1973). The RPE is a 15-point scale with gradations beginning at 6 (level of exertion less than "very, very light") and progressing to 20 (level of exertion greater than "very, very hard"). This scale can also be of assistance in designing an individual's exercise program. The level of effort usually recommended for an aerobic program is approximately 13 (a level of exertion defined by the individual as "somewhat hard") (ACSM 1995, 2000).

In order to determine oxygen utilization, carbon dioxide production, ventilatory threshold, and **respiratory exchange ratio** (the ratio of expired carbon dioxide to oxygen used) during an exercise test, you must measure expired gases—ideally during the last minute of each exercise stage (ACSM 1995, 2000). These variables can help evaluate an individual's level of fitness. You can also use them to assess the effectiveness of an exercise program by comparing measurements made before and following the program.

Treadmill Ergometry

Treadmill exercise is the most common ergometric test performed in the United States (Moldover and Bartels 1996), and a number of different protocols have been published. Figure 5.5 shows the most commonly used protocols and the predicted oxygen utilization ($\dot{V}O_2$) for each stage. The Bruce protocol is the most commonly used, but has the disadvantage that the exercise stages are large and unequal as they progress. These increments may overestimate the individual's exercise capacity (ACSM 1995, 2000). Protocols that use large increments between exercise stages (such as the Bruce protocol) are probably best suited for younger or more active individuals; those with smaller increments (such as the Balke-Ware) are better for testing older or more deconditioned individuals, patients with cardiovascular or respiratory disease, or individuals with physical disabilities (ACSM 1995, 2000). Another test of cardiorespiratory status is the individualized ramp protocol, in which the workload increases at a constant and continuous rate throughout the exercise test (Myers et al. 1992).

There are no published treadmill exercise protocols specifically for individuals with physical disabilities. Modifications to the above-mentioned protocols may permit testing some populations of physically disabled but ambulatory people. For some individuals with physical disabilities, discontinuous exercise testing may be necessary, with rest breaks between the exercise stages. In any case, the test protocol should be individualized, with the treadmill speed, the inclination, or both speed and inclination based on the individual's physical capabilities. Choose workload increments so that the total exercise time is between 8 and 12 minutes (ACSM 1995, 2000; Buchfuhrer et al. 1983).

Bicycle Ergometry

Bicycle ergometry is the most common alternative to treadmill exercise testing in the United States and is the most common ergometric test performed in Europe (Moldover and Bartels 1996). Figure 5.5 shows the most commonly used protocols and the predicted oxygen utilization ($\dot{V}O_2$) for each stage of bicycle ergometric testing. The initial workload is 150 kiloponds (25 watts) for healthy individuals, with increments of 150 kiloponds (25 watts) for each new stage. In deconditioned, elderly, or physically disabled individuals, the initial workload may be reduced to 60 to 90 kiloponds (10 to 15 watts), with even smaller increments for each new exercise stage. Choose workload increments so that the total exercise time is between 8 and 12 minutes (ACSM 1995, 2000).

Upper Limb Ergometry

Upper limb ergometry can be performed either with a modified bicycle ergometer or with a device specifically designed for upper limb testing. The main advantage is its suitability for patients with impairment of the lower limbs (Moldover and Bartels 1996). Since upper limb ergometry uses a smaller muscle mass than bicycle ergometry, use lower initial workloads and smaller increments than with bicycle ergometry—but still set the workload increments so that total exercise time is between 8 and 12 minutes. Upper limb ergometry has been used to assess paraplegic individuals (Lin et al. 1993), post-polio individuals (Kriz et al. 1992), and men with lower limb disabilities (spinal cord injury or lower limb fracture) (Langbein and Maki 1995; Price et al. 2000).

Wheelchair Ergometry

Wheelchair ergometry is uncommon—the necessary equipment is not readily available commercially, and is often custom-made. Publications concerning wheelchair ergometry are all very individualized, depending upon the equipment available to the experimenters (Bhambhani et al. 1993; Bougenot et al. 2003; Cooper et al. 2001; Eriksson et al. 1988; Hutzler et al. 2000; Janssen et al. 1993; Kerk et al. 1995; Knechtle et al. 2003; Knechtle and Kopfli 2001; Knechtle et al. 2003; Okawa et al. 1999; Pare et al. 1993; Vanlandewijck et al. 1994). The primary advantage of wheelchair ergometry is its most obvious one—it can assess cardiopulmonary fitness in those whose primary means of locomotion is the wheelchair. As in other protocols, set the initial workload as well as incremental increases according to the individual's capabilities, and prescribe increments in the workload so that total exercise time is between 8 and 12 minutes.

Other Ergometry

Other devices are occasionally used to assess the cardiopulmonary system, including **rowing machine ergometers**, simulated cross-country skiing ergometers, and elliptical cross-training ergometers (a hybrid between treadmill and bicycle ergometers). The **simulated cross-country skiing ergometer**, which simulates the motion of diagonal stride cross-country skiing, has separate devices for the poling and kicking motions associated with cross-country skiing. The **elliptical cross-training ergometer**, with pedals that revolve in an elliptical motion, demands movements that are somewhat of a combination between walking and bicycling. The resistance for all of these ergometers can be varied in different ways from low to high. All test protocols using these ergometers must be custom-designed for each individual. As always, select workload increments so that the total exercise time is between 8 and 12 minutes.

Examples of Cardiopulmonary Testing in Physically Disabled Individuals

Below are a few examples of cardiopulmonary assessment in disabled patients. They are not exhaustive, but should help guide your thinking as you evaluate and care for such patients.

Example 1

Treadmill Exercise Testing

A 56-year-old male is admitted to the hospital with acute right hemiparesis due to an ischemic left hemispheral cerebral infarction. The patient smoked one pack of cigarettes per day for the past 40 years, but stopped smoking two years previously; his history includes hypercholesterolemia, hypertension, one myocardial infarction four years ago, and coronary artery bypass graft surgery two years ago. Prior to his recent stroke, he complained occasionally of chest pain with exertion, which resolved with rest. You see the patient two days after admission to evaluate him for possible admission into the acute stroke rehabilitation program. Because the stroke has impaired the patient's walking ability, his maximal velocity is just under two miles per hour.

Given this man's cardiac status and significant past medical history, you are concerned about the safety of his participation in the stroke rehabilitation program. In consultation with the patient's cardiologist, you order a treadmill exercise test to determine (1) his pressor response to exercise, (2) if he has any dangerous arrhythmia associated with exercise, and (3) whether there is evidence of myocardial ischemia during activity.

You choose a modified Bruce protocol for the treadmill test. As the activities in the stroke rehabilitation program will not exceed 3 to 4 METs (i.e., an intensity of exercise equal to three to four times the energy expenditure at rest), the exercise stages for this exercise test are 1.7 miles per hour at a treadmill incline of 0, 5, and 10 degrees, providing a maximum level of 5 METs. Blood pressure, heart rate, and ECG are obtained at rest, in supine and standing positions. The pressor response in both supine and standing positions show that the patient's blood pressure is well controlled with antihypertensive medication. The ECG shows no acute abnormalities at rest. The exercise test begins at 1.7 miles per hour at a zero percent grade. Table 5.2

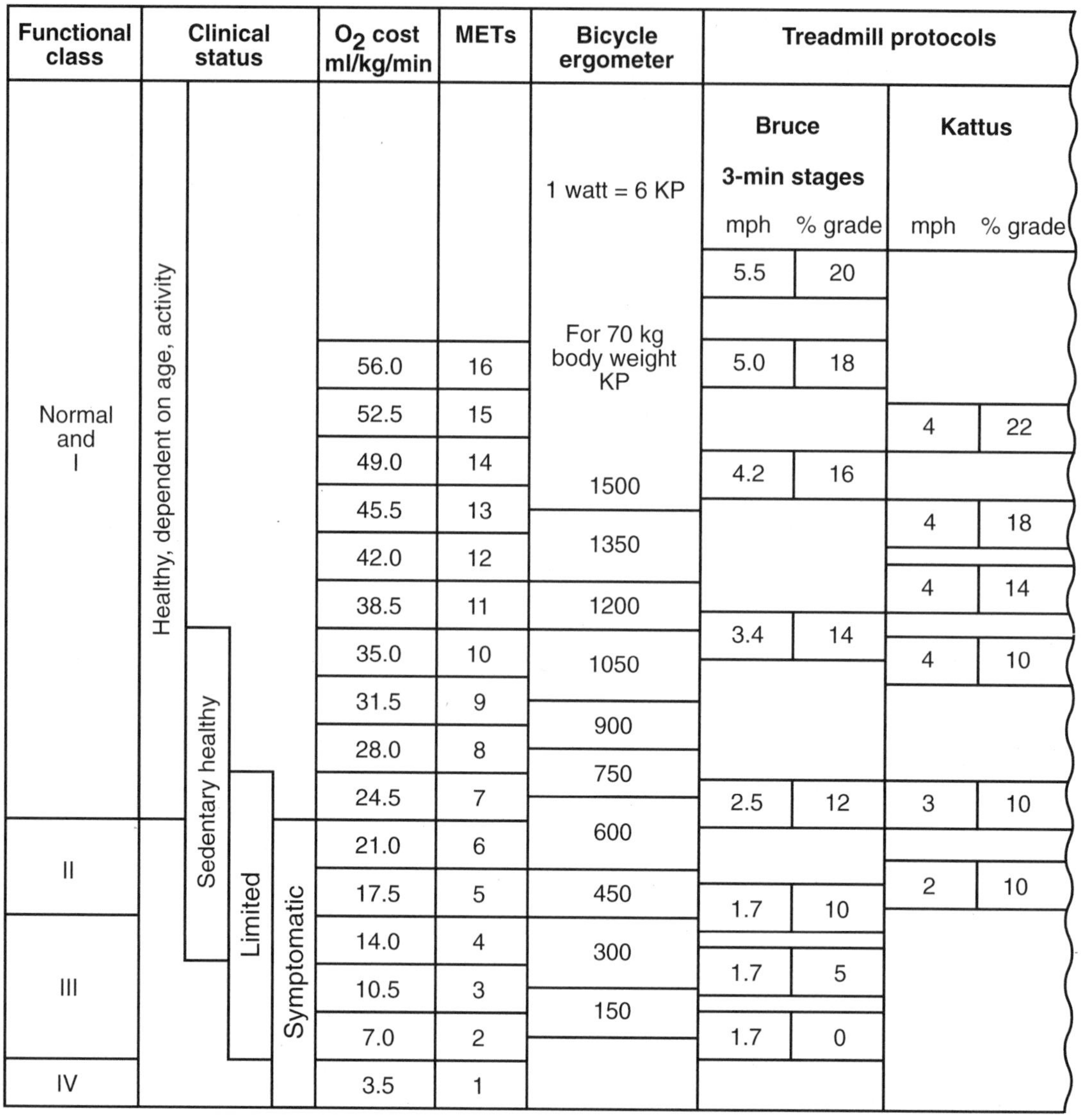

Functional class	Clinical status	O_2 cost ml/kg/min	METs	Bicycle ergometer	Treadmill protocols: Bruce 3-min stages mph	Bruce % grade	Kattus mph	Kattus % grade
				1 watt = 6 KP				
	Healthy, dependent on age, activity				5.5	20		
Normal and I		56.0	16	For 70 kg body weight KP	5.0	18		
		52.5	15				4	22
		49.0	14	1500	4.2	16		
		45.5	13				4	18
		42.0	12	1350				
		38.5	11	1200			4	14
	Sedentary healthy	35.0	10	1050	3.4	14	4	10
		31.5	9	900				
		28.0	8	750				
	Limited	24.5	7		2.5	12	3	10
II	Symptomatic	21.0	6	600				
		17.5	5	450	1.7	10	2	10
III		14.0	4	300				
		10.5	3		1.7	5		
		7.0	2	150	1.7	0		
IV		3.5	1					

Figure 5.5 Common bicycle and treadmill exercise testing protocols.

Reprinted, by permission, from American College of Sports Medicine, 2000, *Guidelines for exercise testing and prescription*, 6th ed. (Baltimore: Lippincott Williams & Wilkins), 98.

summarizes the results of the exercise test including blood pressure, heart rate, ECG response, and rating of perceived exertion (RPE).

The ECG shows no dysrhythmia or ischemic change during the test and cooldown. The maximal heart rate achieved in the test is low at 130 beats per minute (quite high for the 4 MET level of exertion, but consistent with severe deconditioning). The pressure response is normal during and after the test. The patient does not complain of anginal symptoms during the testing or recovery phase, and is able to complete the second stage of the test (at the 4 MET level—the maximal exertion he would need to attain in the stroke rehabilitation program). These results indicate that the patient can safely participate in the

Table 5.2 Treadmill Exercise Testing Results

Stage	Blood pressure	Heart rate	ECG response	RPE
1.7 mph, 0 degrees	120/82	110	Normal rhythm	15
1.7 mph, 5 degrees	140/78	130	Normal rhythm	19
1.7 mph, 10 degrees	Unable due to fatigue			

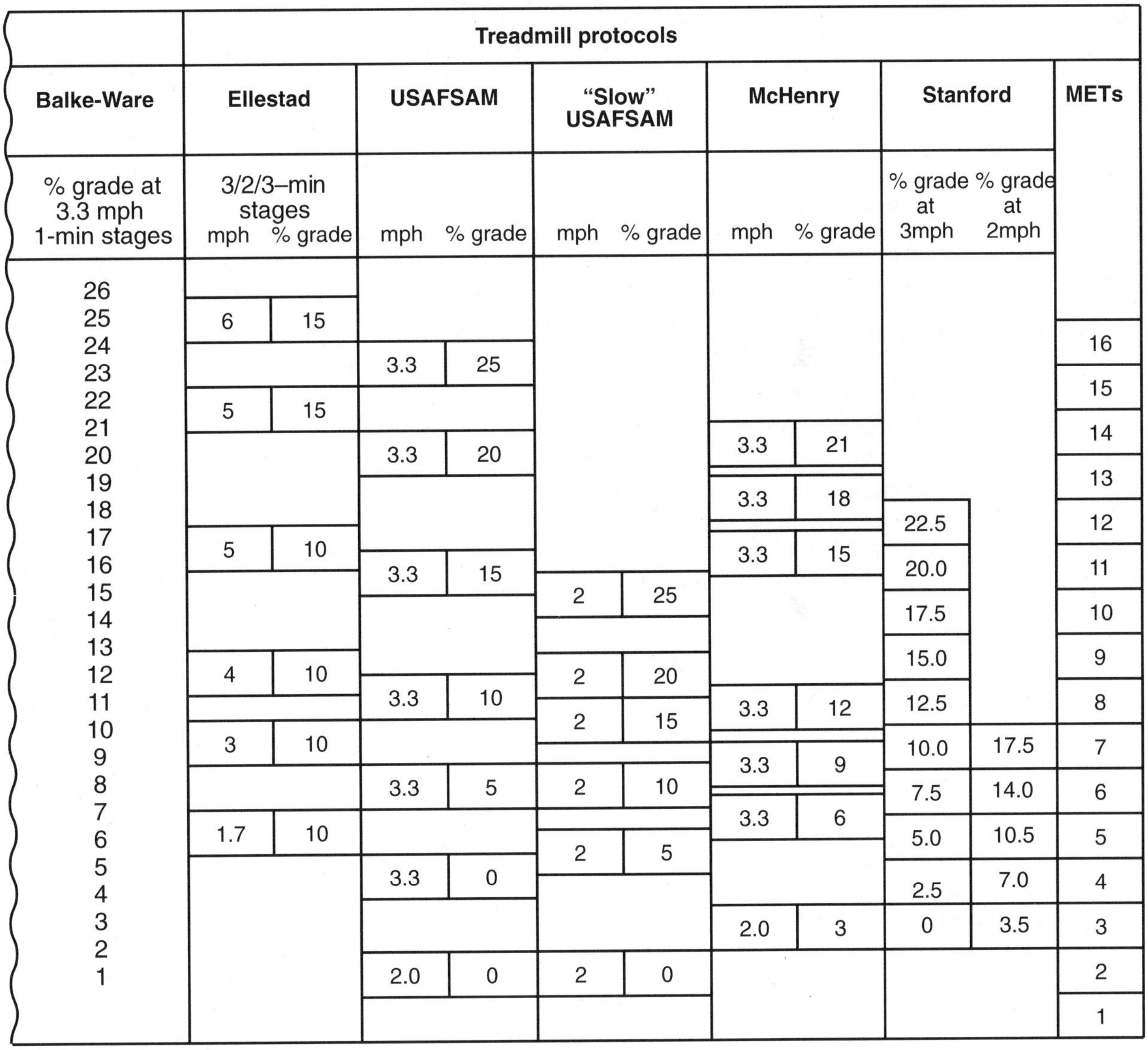

Balke-Ware	Ellestad		USAFSAM		"Slow" USAFSAM		McHenry		Stanford		METs
% grade at 3.3 mph 1-min stages	3/2/3–min stages mph	% grade	mph	% grade	mph	% grade	mph	% grade	% grade at 3mph	% grade at 2mph	
26											
25	6	15									
24											16
23			3.3	25							
22	5	15									15
21							3.3	21			14
20			3.3	20							
19											13
18							3.3	18	22.5		12
17	5	10									
16			3.3	15			3.3	15	20.0		11
15					2	25					
14									17.5		10
13									15.0		9
12	4	10			2	20					
11			3.3	10			3.3	12	12.5		8
10	3	10			2	15					
9							3.3	9	10.0	17.5	7
8			3.3	5	2	10			7.5	14.0	6
7							3.3	6			
6	1.7	10							5.0	10.5	5
5			3.3	0	2	5					
4									2.5	7.0	4
3							2.0	3	0	3.5	3
2											
1			2.0	0	2	0					2
											1

Treadmill protocols

Figure 5.5 *(continued)*

acute stroke rehabilitation program. The RPE demonstrated, however, that he is very deconditioned.

Example 2
Bicycle Ergometer Exercise Testing

The typical post-polio patient is very deconditioned from the cardiovascular standpoint. Owen and Jones (1985) found that the average maximal level of exertion in post-polio individuals was 5 to 6 METs—comparable to a patient shortly after an acute myocardial infarction. Until a few years ago there were no published guidelines for aerobic exercise programs for post-polio patients. Clinicians feared that the exercise might increase overuse weakness rather than aerobic fitness. When Jones et al. (1989) tested this hypothesis, they found it to be without merit; their data form the basis for aerobic exercise programs for many post-polio patients.

A 55-year-old post-polio woman sees you for advice about exercise. She had acute polio at the age of five and has been sedentary for many years. However, she now wants to start an aerobic exercise program. Your initial assessment reveals no cardiovascular disease risk factors other than her age and sedentary life style (see "Coronary Artery Disease Risk Factor Thresholds," page 55). Her neurological examination shows weakness in both lower limbs, but her strength is antigravity or stronger in all muscle groups tested in her hips and thighs. She walks with an ankle foot orthosis on the right because of paresis of the ankle dorsiflexor muscles. You prescribe a cardiovascular exercise test to determine whether she can safely start an exercise program, and, if so, to determine the initial exercise intensity. The resting heart rate, blood pressure, and ECG in the supine and sitting positions are normal. Table 5.3 summarizes results of a bicycle ergometer exercise test (3-minute stages, with rest breaks between the stages).

The patient's blood pressure response to the exercise is normal. The ECG shows no evidence of ST segment depression or dysrhythmia. It appears safe for her to start an exercise program. Her maximal capacity, however, is very low—only 50 watts (or 300 kiloponds or approximately 4 METs; see figure 5.5). Using the exercise program described by Jones and colleagues (1989) above, she starts a bicycle ergometric exercise program. Initially, she exercises for 2 minutes with 1-minute rest breaks, for a total exercise time of 10 minutes. As she progresses, the duration of each bout of exercise gradually increases until she is able to perform six 5-minute bouts of exercise, with 1-minute rest breaks between bouts (for a total exercise time of 30 minutes). After four months of exercise, a maximal exercise test measures her maximal capacity at 70 watts (or 420 kiloponds or approximately 5 METs). She has no adverse response to the exercise program and finds that she has less fatigue during her daily activities. She also reports increased strength in her hip and thigh muscles; and she notes less difficulty in climbing stairs, improved endurance while walking, and less difficulty getting into and out of the bathtub.

Example 3

Upper Limb Ergometer Exercise Testing

You are evaluating a 42-year-old insulin-dependent diabetic with a history of coronary artery disease, hypertension, and a recent below-knee amputation due to peripheral vascular disease. You question the safety of the patient's participation in rehabilitation—especially because of the exertion required for prosthetic training.

You need an appropriate exercise test. For obvious reasons, a treadmill test is ruled out, and the patient would find it difficult to use a bicycle ergometer with only one lower limb. Upper limb ergometry is the exercise test of choice—not only is it convenient, but when the patient begins to use the preparatory prosthesis, the upper limbs will bear much of the stress.

Prior to testing, you measure resting blood pressure, heart rate, and ECG in both the supine and sitting positions. The results show no abnormalities. As the patient is very deconditioned, the exercise test begins at 10 watts, with 10-watt increases every 3 minutes. Table 5.4 summarizes the results.

Although the ECG shows 2 millimeters of ST segment depression, indicative of myocardial ischemia, at the 40-watt stage, the patient denies angina. At the third stage, however, with the heart rate at 124 and the RPE at 14 ("moderately hard"—Borg 1973), the ECG shows neither ST segment depression nor dysrhythmia.

These findings suggest that the patient can safely exercise up to a heart rate of approximately 120 beats per minute and a rating of perceived exertion of "moderately hard." The silent ischemia noted during higher levels of the exercise test, however, is worrisome. For safety reasons, you have the patient wear a heart monitor during therapy, and have the therapist keep the activity level at a heart rate of 120 beats per minute or less.

Table 5.3 Bicycle Ergometer Exercise Testing Results

Stage	Blood pressure	Heart rate	ECG response	RPE
10 watts	110/70	92	Normal	11
20 watts	122/66	106	Normal	12
30 watts	132/64	122	Normal	16
40 watts	144/60	144	Normal	19
50 watts	152/56	156	Normal	20
60 watts	Unable due to fatigue			

Table 5.4 Upper Limb Ergometer Exercise Testing Results

Stage	Blood pressure	Heart rate	ECG response	RPE
10 watts	132/94	98	Normal	11
20 watts	142/90	110	Normal	13
30 watts	150/84	124	Normal	14
40 watts	168/72	146	2 mm ST segment depression	

A Holter monitor, worn during the first 24 hours after the start of therapy, reveals no ECG abnormalities (ST segment depression or dysrhythmia). The monitor also confirms that the patient is able to keep the heart rate at the desired and safe level. With these precautions, the patient safely and successfully completes the rehabilitation program.

EXAMPLE 4
WHEELCHAIR ERGOMETER EXERCISE TESTING

A 44-year-old construction worker falls two floors, sustains a fracture of T12, and becomes paraplegic. After completion of the acute rehabilitation program, he wants to join a wheelchair basketball team. The patient smokes cigarettes and has hypercholesterolemia, and his father had an acute myocardial infarction at age 52. To determine the safety of his participation in any regular exercise, you recommend a wheelchair ergometry test. Table 5.5 shows the results of the exercise test.

The test concludes at the completion of the 100-watt stage due to fatigue. The ECG reveals neither dysrhythmia nor ST segment abnormality. The exercise test is normal. You tell your patient that there is no contraindication for participation in the wheelchair basketball program, and encourage him to join the team after starting a wheelchair aerobic exercise program. The initial exercise is 50 watts, with an exercise heart rate of 120 (74% of his maximal heart rate) and a rating of perceived exertion of 14. You also strongly encourage him to stop smoking!

NEUROMUSCULAR TESTING PROTOCOLS

Assessment of neuromuscular function can be divided into the evaluation of muscle strength and, in special circumstances, the evaluation of muscle endurance or power. Although muscular strength is commonly assessed, muscular endurance and power are rarely assessed—primarily only in research studies. The most common way to assess muscle strength in the clinical setting is with **manual muscle testing** (McPeak 1996). Manual muscle testing, however, is quite subjective and sometimes is not sufficiently accurate to be clinically useful. Clinicians instead need an objective, quantitative assessment of muscular strength that will enable them to assess the effectiveness of a patient's therapeutic program.

All normal activities entail static, concentric, or eccentric muscle contractions. A **static contraction** occurs when there is no movement of the joint(s) that the muscle crosses, but the contraction stabilizes the joint. A **dynamic contraction** occurs with movement of the joint(s) that the muscles crosses. If the muscle shortens during this dynamic contraction, the contraction is **concentric.** If the muscle lengthens during contraction, the contraction is **eccentric.** Muscles may also contract **isokinetically** using special isokinetic testing equipment—the limb is attached to an arm on the isokinetic dynamometer, which can be set at any predetermined angular velocity (such as 60 degrees per second) to assess the strength of the muscle at that specific angular velocity. Isokinetic dynamometers can also be used to measure muscular power. This may be an important factor to measure, as elderly individuals may have a greater loss in muscular power than in muscular strength (Yanagiya et al. 2004). Also muscular power (the ability of the muscle to perform work at a certain rate) is important in the performance of activities of daily living (Bean et al. 2002). Unlike static and dynamic muscular contractions, isokinetic contraction is not performed during normal daily activities.

In all assessments of muscular strength, in order to prevent injury as well as to enhance reliability of the measurements, you should provide clear instructions concerning the evaluation procedure. Have your patient practice with the device before the test, both to warm up and to be certain that she fully understands how to perform the test and that the testing procedure will not cause pain. Pain during the warm-up procedure usually indicates that the individual is not performing the effort correctly and needs further instruction. Stabilization of the patient's body is also important—not only for safety reasons (to minimize the risk of injury), but also to prevent her from using substitution patterns that would result in erroneous measurements of her strength.

There are no universally accepted protocols for evaluating muscle strength. Following are some suggested

Table 5.5 Wheelchair Ergometer Exercise Testing Results

Stage	Blood pressure	Heart rate	ECG response	RPE
25 watts	112/84	92	Normal	12
50 watts	120/78	120	Normal	14
75 watts	134/72	142	Normal	17
100 watts	142/66	166	Normal	20

guidelines. In all methods, take care to avoid injury during testing. With reasonable care, injury can be very rare, and when it does occur, it will be a minor strain.

Assessing Static Strength

Static muscle strength is usually assessed with special dynamometers (e.g., the Cybex, Kin-Com, or Biodex dynamometers for static assessment), cable tensiometry (Andres et al. 1986; Clarke 1952; Clarke 1973; Clarke and Clarke 1984), or loadcell dynamometry (Mundale 1970), which can measure either the force or the **torque** (force times the length of the lever arm) generated during muscular contraction. After properly positioning your patient on the dynamometer and setting the joint at the desired angle, be careful to instruct her in the test procedure. In assessments of static strength, the joint which the muscle crosses should not move during the muscular contraction. At first, have your subject practice with the dynamometer, performing several submaximal muscular contractions; then gradually build up to one or two maximal contractions. After she rests for a short time, she should perform three or four maximal effort contractions of the muscle (usually for 3 to 5 seconds each) with timed rest intervals between efforts.

The rest periods you prescribe depend upon whom you are evaluating. In disabled individuals, we have found 1-minute rest breaks between maximal effort trials to be reasonable. The maximal force or torque generated during these efforts is defined as the **static strength** of the muscle.

Assessing Dynamic Isotonic Strength and Power

The term *isotonic* is actually a misnomer. Isotonic means "equal tension," but its use in strength testing means that the individual is lifting a specific amount of weight. The most common ways to define isotonic strength are

- the determination of the amount of weight that the individual can lift only once through full range of motion with proper mechanics (the one-repetition maximum, or 1 RM), or
- the amount of weight the subject can successfully lift 10 times, but not more, through full range of motion with proper mechanics (the ten-repetition maximum, or 10 RM).

These determinations require spotting or the use of special frames (such as a weight frame) to protect the individual in case the weight slips or in case he cannot successfully lift the weight. As with all strength testing, always provide proper instruction, warm-up, and stabilization for safety, validity, and reliability.

Assessing Dynamic Isokinetic Strength

Special equipment such as the Cybex, Kin-Com, or Biodex dynamometers can assess isokinetic muscle strength. The manufacturers provide specific suggestions for the use of each device. These machines are rather sophisticated and are quite expensive. All isokinetic dynamometers are now computer-controlled, and allow the operator to set the maximum angular velocity at which the arm of the dynamometer moves as well as the range of motion to be tested (figure 5.6). These devices also have mechanisms that continuously measure the torque that the individual is exerting as well as the range of motion through which he is being tested and the time to perform the test. For the dynamometer to measure maximal torque, have your patient try to move the dynamometer arm as fast and forcefully as possible throughout the range of motion you're testing. Because the dynamometer arm has a braking mechanism, and will move only as fast as the angular velocity you set, it

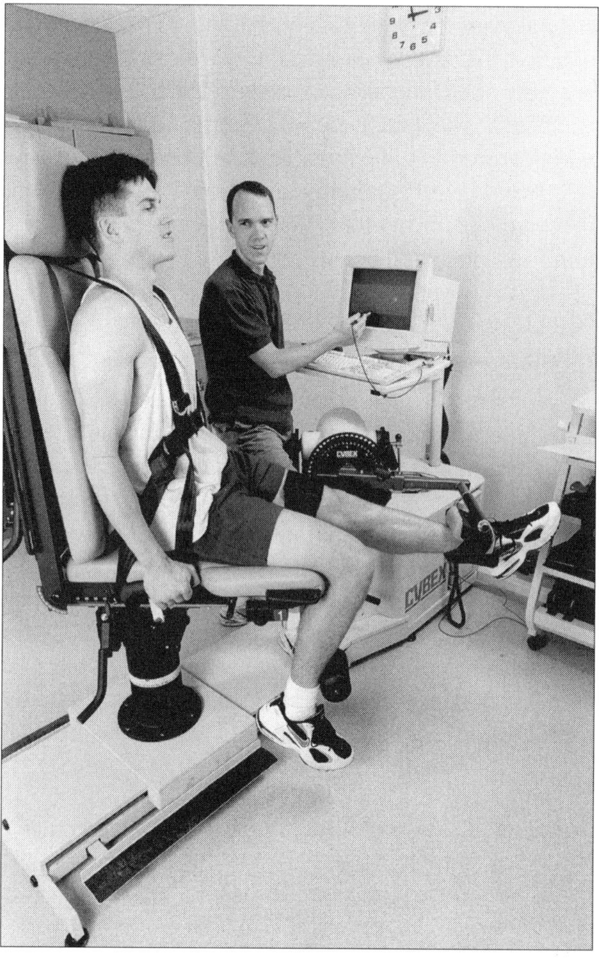

Figure 5.6 A patient on an isokinetic dynamometer warming up prior to a maximal assessment of isokinetic quadriceps femoris strength.

will appear to your patient that the dynamometer is resisting his effort. By moving his arm or leg as fast and forcefully as possible, your patient will generate maximal torque at the predetermined angular velocity. The dynamometer measures and stores in the computer the torque generated throughout the range of motion that was tested.

Ordinarily, straps will stabilize your subject on the dynamometer's chair or bench. Place the fulcrum of the lever arm in the plane of the center of rotation of the joint you're testing. Pass the arm of the dynamometer through the full range of motion to be tested (this allows the dynamometer's computer to measure the weight of the limb throughout the range of motion to be tested). Set the angular velocity for the test (in most cases, between 60 and 300 degrees per second). Instruct your subject in the testing procedure. Have him warm up by moving the arm of the dynamometer gently, gradually increasing the force till he performs one or two full efforts. He should rest for a specified period of time, usually 1 minute. During the test, he extends and flexes the joint through a full range of motion, with maximal muscular effort, for a specified number of contractions—often between three and six maximal efforts. Identify the maximal torque generated by the muscle during the test as the strength of the muscle at the specific angular velocity tested. The isokinetic dynamometer can also measure the power of the muscle at the specific angular velocity being tested. In some situations, especially in clinical research, you might choose to test the muscle at several angular velocities to determine peak torque as well as muscular power.

ASSESSMENT OF ENDURANCE

Although often tested for research purposes, endurance is rarely assessed in the clinical setting. One can assess endurance statically, dynamically, or isokinetically.

STATIC ENDURANCE

You can assess either absolute or relative static endurance. **Absolute endurance** is defined in terms of a specified workload, while relative endurance is defined in terms of a specific percentage of the individual's maximal capacity (see page 60).

Consider the maximum time during which an individual can statically contract a muscle at a certain specified level of effort. If that level of effort is set at 100 newton-meters, then absolute endurance for that person is the time during which she can contract the muscle statically at 100 newton-meters of torque. If the level of effort is defined as 40% of maximum static torque (or any other specific percentage between 0 and 100% of maximal effort), then the subject's relative endurance is determined as the time during which she can contract the muscle statically at that specific relative level of torque.

DYNAMIC ENDURANCE

As with static endurance, you can assess either absolute or relative dynamic endurance. To assess **absolute dynamic endurance,** you would have the individual lift a certain amount of weight with a specific technique (such as knee extension using a table specifically designed to assess knee extension) through full range of motion at a specific cadence (such as one complete lifting motion every 2 seconds), until he is no longer able to successfully lift the weight. You would define the number of successful repetitions as the absolute dynamic endurance for lifting that specific amount of weight. To assess **relative dynamic endurance,** first determine the subject's 1 RM for the test to be performed. Then have him lift a certain percentage of the 1 RM through full range of motion at a specific cadence until he is no longer able to successfully lift the weight. The number of successful repetitions would be the relative endurance for the specific relative amount of weight lifted.

ISOKINETIC ENDURANCE

Although they do not measure absolute or relative endurance, several useful endurance tests employ isokinetic dynamometers (Davies 1987).

- **The 50% decrement test.** The individual performs maximal effort muscle contractions at a specific angular velocity until the peak torque fails to reach 50% of the initial peak torque for a predetermined number of repetitions (usually 2-5 consecutive reps). The number of repetitions successfully performed is used as a measure of endurance.
- **The predetermined time bout endurance test.** The individual performs as many maximal repetitions as possible at a predetermined angular velocity for a predetermined period of time. Measure endurance either as the total number of repetitions performed or as the total work performed by the muscle during the activity (as calculated by the device's computer).
- **The predetermined repetitions bout endurance test** (Davies 1987). The individual performs a predetermined number of repetitions at a predetermined angular velocity. The dynamometer's computer tallies the total amount of work performed by the muscle during the contractions; use the total work performed as a measure of endurance.
- **The 50-repetition decrement test.** The individual performs 50 consecutive maximal effort isokinetic contractions at a predetermined angular velocity. Compare the average torque generated during the last three contractions with that of the first three contractions; use the percent decrement as a measure of endurance.

Examples of Neuromuscular Testing in Physically Disabled Individuals

Below are a few examples of neuromuscular assessments in patients with physical disabilities. Such assessments usually aim either to guide the care of patients or to assess the effectiveness of a therapeutic exercise program.

Example 1

Evaluating the Effect of Strength Training on Strength, Endurance, and Work Capacity in Post-Polio Individuals

Many post-polio individuals complain of fatigue and pain (Halstead and Rossi 1985, 1987). Some are quite weak, with reduced work capacity and a deficit in strength recovery after activity (Agre and Rodriquez 1990). Reduced endurance is also a common problem (Berlly et al. 1991). Several researchers have shown that strengthening exercise can improve muscle strength in post-polio individuals (Agre et al. 1996; Einarsson and Grimby 1987; Feldman and Soskolne 1987; Fillyaw et al. 1991), but until recently, no one had tested whether the improved strength would increase the work capacity or absolute endurance time of muscle.

To investigate this question, we first assessed static strength of the quadriceps muscles of seven post-polio subjects, with the knee positioned 60 degrees from full extension. After permitting the subjects to rest for 5 minutes after the assessment, we gave them static endurance tests at 40% of maximal strength to the point of failure, recording the endurance time in seconds. (We verbally encouraged the subjects to perform this activity as long as possible.) We calculated the static tension time index (or "work capacity") as the product of the endurance time in seconds and the torque (40% of maximal strength) (Agre et al. 1997).

Following a 12-week home exercise program, we reassessed the subjects in the laboratory for strength, endurance, and work capacity, using the same absolute torque as was performed initially (i.e., not 40% of the new strength, but 40% of the previous strength). Table 5.6 gives pre- and postexercise program data.

The exercise program clearly led to significant increases in muscle strength, absolute endurance time, and work capacity—confirming that muscle-strengthening exercise can not only increase strength in post-polio individuals, but also increase work capacity and absolute endurance of the muscle. These findings may have important implications for individuals with weakness due to other neuromuscular diseases or disorders.

Example 2

Evaluating the Effect of Strength Training in an Elderly Man With Degenerative Joint Disease of the Knee

A 70-year-old man is referred to the rehabilitation clinic by his orthopedic surgeon for assessment. He has a history of severe left knee pain due to arthritis. The surgeon is contemplating total knee arthroplasty, but refers the patient to you because the patient wants to try a nonsurgical approach before considering surgery. You find that the patient has severe weakness and atrophy of the left thigh musculature, the strength being barely above antigravity. He keeps the left knee fully extended while he walks (to keep from falling due to the weakness). You believe that a strengthening exercise program might be very beneficial (as will be the use of a cane to decompress the knee). Frontera and colleagues (1988) reported that, in men aged 60 to 72, strength training significantly increased muscle strength as well as hypertrophy of the exercised muscles. You have your patient follow the same exercise program.

In the Frontera study, participants exercised three days per week for 12 weeks, performing three sets of exercise of the knee extensor and flexor muscles, with eight repetitions in each set. They used weights that were 80% of their 1 repetition maximum (1 RM). The 1 RM was measured each week. By the end of the exercise program, the 1 RM increased by over 100% in the knee extensor muscles and 200% in the knee flexors. Dynamic isokinetic assessment showed increases in the knee extensor and flexor strength of 10% and 18%, respectively. Muscle biopsies obtained before and after the program revealed increases in muscle fiber area of the vastus lateralis of over 25%.

After following the described exercise program for three months, the patient is much stronger (with strength increases similar to those found in the research study, as measured with a dynamometer

Table 5.6 Neuromuscular Variables Before and After the Exercise Program (mean ± SD)

Variable	Before	After	Percent change
Strength (N · m)	98 ± 63	134 ± 65	+36%
Endurance (holding time in seconds)	142 ± 46	172 ± 50	+21%
Work capacity (N · m · sec)	6090 ± 2280	7200 ± 2240	+18%

just as in the research study). He also reports that the knee pain has significantly improved: he has minimal difficulty and almost no pain with ambulation, and his gait pattern on physical examination is much improved (because of increased strength as well as use of the cane).

EXAMPLE 3

ASSESSING THE EFFECT OF A WORK HARDENING PROGRAM ON THE FUNCTIONAL LIFTING CAPABILITIES OF AN INJURED WORKER

A 40-year-old heavy manual laborer injured his lower back while lifting a 100-pound box—his third back injury within the past year that has resulted in time off from work. He has undergone several evaluations by other clinicians, but with no specific findings. Radiographs show some evidence of degenerative joint disease and degenerative disc disease. The MRI shows disc bulging at L4-L5 and L5-S1. Analgesics, muscle relaxants, rest, hot packs, and massage did not resolve the problem after six weeks. The patient came to you, a specialist in physical medicine and rehabilitation, for further assessment.

The patient's neurological examination is normal. Through manual muscle testing you observe weak trunk and lower limb musculature, which you believe to be secondary to deconditioning from the past six weeks of inactivity in addition to the inactivity associated with his previous injuries and their treatment. You order physical therapy and have the patient start an active therapeutic exercise program including strength training. After two weeks, the physical therapist reports that the patient has made improvement in strength but is not yet ready to return to his usual work activity. You prescribe a work hardening program, at the completion of which you order a functional capacity evaluation. The physical capacity evaluation assesses a number of factors, including the patient's 1 RM lifting strength to lift from floor to waist height, waist to shoulder height, and shoulder height to overhead. The physical therapist notes that the patient puts forth good effort during this assessment, and believes that the functional capacity accurately reflects the patient's capabilities for work. You advise the patient about his specific capacities for lifting so that he can return to gainful employment and perform his lifting tasks within these guidelines. With this specific information, based upon the functional capacity assessment, the patient successfully returns to work without recurrent injury.

OTHER FUNCTIONAL TESTS

In addition to the tests already described, there are some simple tests that can be performed in the clinical setting that can help to assess the disabled individual's functional capacity. These tests require no expensive or sophisticated equipment. These tests include the Get Up and Go Test (Piva et al. 2004), the Up and Go Test (Podsiadlo et al. 1991), the 6-Minute Walk Test (Kervio et al. 2003), and the Chair and Bed Rise Performance Time (Alexander et al. 2000).

To perform the Get Up and Go Test the subject sits on a standard-height chair with arm rests in front of a 20-meter unobstructed hallway (Piva et al. 2004). The finish line is marked with a strip of tape 15.2 meters away from the front of the chair. Subjects are instructed to sit in the chair with their backs touching the back of the chair. On the command "go," subjects are to stand and then walk as fast as possible through the finish line. A stopwatch is used to measure the time from the command "go" until the subject crosses the finish line. Subjects are to use comfortable footwear; subjects who use canes while walking are permitted to use them during the test. The Get Up and Go Test has been reported to be reliable, and the minimum detectable change has been reported to be adequate for clinical usage (Piva et al. 2004).

The Up and Go Test is a test of basic functional mobility for frail elderly individuals (Podsiadlo et al. 1991). To perform this test the subject sits in a standard arm chair. Upon the command of "go," the subject rises from the chair, walks a distance of 3 meters, turns, walks back to the chair, and then sits down again. A stopwatch is used to measure the time from the command "go" until the subject is again seated in the chair. If the subject uses assistive devices for ambulation, then those devices are used during the test. This test has been widely used with adults and has been determined to be a reliable and valid index of functional mobility (Podsiadlo et al. 1991; DeBolt and McCubbin 2004).

The 6-Minute Walk Test can be performed in an 18-meter corridor free of all obstacles (Kervio et al. 2003). Subjects are asked to walk back and forth at a regular pace, covering as great a distance as possible. Rest stops are allowed if needed by the subject. Standardized encouragement is given every 30 seconds. The time remaining is called every 2 minutes. The total distance covered in meters is measured. This test was found to be reliable after two familiarization attempts were performed, as a learning effect was noted during the first two trials (Kervio et al. 2003).

In a series of tasks composing the Chair and Bed Rise Performance Test, the rise task varied according to the height of the head of the bed (HOB), chair seat height, and use of hands (Alexander et al. 2000). Bed rise tasks included supine to sit-to-edge, sit up in bed with use of hands, and sit up in bed without use of hands, all performed from a bed where the HOB could be adjusted to 0-, 30-, and 45-degree elevations; roll to side-lying, then rise (HOB 0 degrees); and supine to stand (HOB 0 degrees). Chair seat heights could be adjusted according to the percent of the distance between the floor and the knee (%FK). Chair tasks included rises (1) with hands and then without hands at 140%, 120%, 100%, and 80% FK; (2) from a reclining (105% at chair back) and tilting (seat tilted 10 degrees posteriorly) chair (100% FK); and (3) from an 80% FK seat height with a 4-inch cushion added, with and then without hands. Each task was scored as successful or not and, if successful, as the time to complete the task. The total number of tasks successfully completed can also be determined (called the total task score). Test-retest reliability was found to be generally good, with most simple kappa values ranging from 0.6 to 1.0 for rise ability and intraclass correlation coefficients of log-transformed performance times ranging from 0.6 to 0.9.

SUMMARY

Physical activity is a crucial component of healthy lifestyles. Before beginning exercise programs, subjects should be screened for relevant health factors in order to

- optimize the results from an exercise program,
- allow for the development of a sensible and effective exercise prescription, and
- determine safety of participation in an exercise program or exercise testing. There are five general indications for clinical cardiopulmonary testing:

1. The predischarge status after an acute cardiac event
2. The postdischarge status after a cardiac event
3. The medical diagnosis
4. The disease severity and prognosis
5. The patient's functional status

There are three general indications for neuromuscular testing:

1. It helps assess an individual's abilities to function.
2. It aids in the design of a patient's therapeutic exercise program.
3. It can be used to assess the effectiveness of the therapeutic exercise program.

Although there are several ways to assess cardiopulmonary and neuromuscular function, there is no specific set of tests for individuals with physical disabilities. You must simply choose those tests that will be most useful in your patient's particular clinical situation. This chapter has provided several examples that demonstrated how this testing can be helpful in caring for patients with physical disabilities.

CHAPTER 6

A Behavioral Approach to Prescribing Physical Activity for Health and Fitness

Gregory W. Heath, DHSc, MPH

Regular physical activity increases physical working capacity, decreases body fat, increases lean body tissue and bone density, and lowers rates of coronary heart disease (CHD), diabetes mellitus, hypertension, and cancer (Lee et al. 1991; Paffenbarger et al. 1978; Sidney et al. 1977; Smith et al. 1976; Tipton 1991; U.S. Department of Health and Human Services [USDHHS] 1996). It is also associated with greater longevity. Regular physical activity and exercise can also enhance quality of life, improve capacity for work and recreation, and alter the rate of decline in functional status (Shephard 1993).

Both health and fitness should result from exercise prescriptions, where **health** is defined as physical and emotional well-being (not merely the absence of disease), and **physical fitness** is something that people possess or achieve such as aerobic power, muscular endurance, muscular strength, body composition, and flexibility (Caspersen et al. 1985; USDHHS 2000). Exercise rehabilitation programs must take account of physiologic, anatomic, and behavioral factors to ensure a safe, effective, and enjoyable exercise experience for the participant.

Preliminary Factors Important for Exercise Prescription

We can discuss physical activity in terms of health benefits and fitness benefits—not a true dichotomy of benefits, but a useful approach for outlining the outcome-specific nature of the exercise prescription and for providing the rationale for individualized approaches to physical activity recommendations.

Health Benefits of Physical Activity

Physical activity has been defined as any bodily movement produced by skeletal muscles that results in caloric expenditure (Caspersen et al. 1985). Since caloric expenditure enhances weight loss or weight maintenance, physical activity is important in the prevention and management of obesity, CHD, and diabetes mellitus. Healthy People 2010 Physical Activity and Fitness Objective 22.2 highlights the need for every person to engage in regular, preferably daily, physical activity (USDHHS 2000). Current research suggests that light to moderate physical activity for at least 30 minutes per day significantly raises the level of caloric expenditure and confers important health benefits. For example, physical activity equivalent to a sustained walk for 30 minutes per day uses about 1050 kcal per week. Epidemiologic studies suggest that a weekly expenditure of 1000 kcal could have significant individual and public health benefits for CHD prevention, especially among those who are currently inactive.

According to the American College of Sports Medicine (ACSM) and the Centers for Disease Control and Prevention (CDC), the scientific evidence clearly demonstrates that regular, moderate-intensity physical activity provides substantial health benefits (Pate et al. 1995). After an extensive review of the physiologic, epidemiologic, and clinical evidence, the expert panel formulated the following recommendation:

> Every U.S. adult should accumulate 30 minutes or more of moderate-intensity physical activity on most, preferably all, days of the week.

Because intermittent activity confers substantial benefits, people can accumulate the recommended 30 minutes of activity in shorter bouts of 8 to 10 minutes spaced throughout the day. This is not the optimal amount of physical activity for health, of course, but rather a minimum standard to which people can add in order to obtain even more beneficial effects. For someone undergoing comprehensive exercise rehabilitation, the additional effects might be improved cardiorespiratory fitness, muscle endurance, muscle strength, flexibility, and enhanced body composition.

In 2002, the Institute of Medicine (IOM) issued a report addressing the dietary reference intakes for macronutrients (e.g., energy, carbohydrate, fiber, fat, cholesterol, protein) (see www.nap.edu/books/0309085373.html). Within the report the IOM panel acknowledged the importance of regular physical activity for health promotion. They also concurred with the ACSM/CDC statement that moderately intense activity is beneficial. However, the panel further recommended the doubling of the daily 30-minute goal, maintaining that 60 minutes per day of moderate physical activity is necessary to maintain a healthy weight. They further emphasized that this additional volume of physical activity provides further health benefits beyond that of weight maintenance. Similar conclusions about the additional benefits of activity beyond the 30 minutes of daily moderate activity were identified by the ACSM/CDC and the Surgeon General's report on physical activity and health. As Bassuk and Manson have so keenly underscored, "Although the IOM is to be commended for highlighting the importance of physical activity as part of a healthy lifestyle, its recommendation fails to balance the issue of efficacy with feasibility and safety considerations, all of which are crucial in achieving a public health goal." Although the 30-minute recommendation is considered an appropriate starting point in the rehabilitation setting, it is clear that appropriate tailoring of the physical activity prescription is necessary in addressing the health and restorative needs of the individual client.

Fitness Benefits of Physical Activity

Cardiorespiratory endurance, muscular strength, muscular endurance, flexibility, and body composition are the health-related components of physical fitness (Pate et al. 1995).

Regular vigorous physical activity helps achieve and maintain higher levels of cardiorespiratory fitness than light to moderate physical activity. As outlined in Healthy People (HP) 2010, **cardiorespiratory fitness** or **aerobic capacity** describes the body's ability to perform high-intensity activity for a prolonged period of time without undue physical stress or fatigue (Caspersen et al. 1985). Having higher levels of cardiorespiratory fitness helps people carry out their daily occupational tasks and leisure pursuits more easily and with greater efficiency. Vigorous physical activities that help to achieve and maintain cardiorespiratory fitness can also contribute substantially to caloric expenditure, and probably provide more protection against CHD than do less vigorous activities. Vigorous physical activities include very brisk walking, jogging/running, swimming laps, cycling, fast dancing, skating, jumping rope, and selective competitive sports (soccer, basketball, volleyball). Individuals can achieve higher levels of cardiorespiratory fitness

Health-Related Components of Physical Fitness

- Cardiorespiratory endurance
- Muscular strength
- Muscular endurance
- Flexibility
- Body composition

by increasing the frequency, duration, or intensity of activities beyond the minimum recommendation of 20 minutes per occasion, three times per week, at ≥50% of aerobic capacity (ACSM 1998).

Muscular strength is the maximal amount of force generated by a muscle or muscle group, while muscle endurance is the ability of a muscle or muscle group to do prolonged exercise. Muscle strength and endurance are accepted components of health-related fitness (Braith et al. 1989). Strength and endurance greatly affect one's ability to perform the tasks of daily living without undue physical stress and fatigue. Regular use of skeletal muscles helps to improve and maintain strength and endurance. Engaging in regular physical activity, such as weight training or the regular lifting and carrying of heavy objects, appears to be a sufficient stimulus to maintain necessary muscle strength and endurance for most activities of daily living (Barry and Eathorne 1994).

Musculoskeletal flexibility describes the range of motion in a joint or sequence of joints. Those with greater flexibility may have a lower risk of future back injury (Cady et al. 1979). Older adults with better joint flexibility may be able to drive an automobile more safely than less flexible individuals (West Virginia University 1988). Joint movement through the full range of motion helps to improve and maintain flexibility. Stretching exercises can help to maintain a level of flexibility that supports quality activities of daily living, as can a variety of physical activities that require one to stoop, bend, crouch, and reach.

The maintenance of an acceptable ratio of fat to lean body weight is another desired component of health-related fitness. Overweight occurs when individuals expend fewer calories than they consume (Passmore 1971). Data from weight-loss programs focused on diet alone have not been encouraging. Since physical activity burns calories, increases the proportion of lean to fat body mass (lean tissue burns more calories per unit weight than fat tissue), and raises the metabolic rate, a combination of both caloric control and increased physical activity is important for attaining and maintaining a healthy body weight. In a recent consensus report, the International Alliance for the Study of Obesity (IASO) stated that the current guideline for adults of 30 minutes of moderate-intensity physical activity on most days of the week, preferably daily, "is of importance for limiting health risks for a number of chronic diseases including coronary heart disease and diabetes." However, the IASO also emphasized that for preventing weight gain or regain, this guideline is likely to be insufficient for many individuals in the current environment. They concluded that to prevent weight gain or regain in formerly obese individuals requires 60 to 90 minutes of daily moderate activity or lesser amounts of vigorous-intensity activity (Saris et al. 2003).

Determinants of and Barriers to Participation in Regular Physical Activity

When designing any exercise prescription, be sure to consider physiological, behavioral, and psychological variables related to participation in physical activity (Sallis and Hovell 1990). **Self-efficacy**—a construct from social cognitive theory characterized by a person's confidence to exercise under a number of circumstances—is positively associated with greater participation in physical activity, as is **social support** from family and friends. Incorporating some mechanism of social support within the exercise prescription appears to be an important strategy for enhancing compliance.

Significant barriers to participation in physical activity are injury and a lack of time. You can minimize these barriers by encouraging people to include physical activity as part of their lifestyle, integrating not only planned exercise but also transportation and occupational and household activity into their daily routines (e.g., always choose a parking space far from the door, and use stairs rather than elevators). Emphasizing low- to moderate-intensity physical activities, which are more likely to be continued than high-intensity activities and less likely to cause injury or undue discomfort, will increase the rate of patient adherence (Pollock 1988).

A number of physical and social environmental factors can affect physical activity behavior (Sallis et al. 1992). Family and friends can be role models, provide encouragement, or be companions during physical activity. The environment often presents significant barriers to participation in physical activity (e.g., a lack of bicycle and walking paths away from vehicular traffic, inclement weather, and unsafe neighborhoods) (Sallis et al. 1989).

Barriers to Assessment and Counseling for Exercise

Because physicians, therapists, nurses, and clinical exercise scientists have unique access to persons undergoing rehabilitation, they have many opportunities for physical activity assessment and counseling (Harris et al. 1989). Physicians generally believe exercise is important, but indicate that they are not well prepared to provide counseling in that area (Wells et al. 1989). The primary barriers to routine assessment and counseling about exercise in rehabilitation settings are time, reimbursement, perceived effectiveness, and a lack of training in behavioral counseling techniques. A number of programs have attempted to improve the physical activity counseling skills among primary care physicians;

results have been small but generally positive, with from 7% to 10% of inactive patients starting to be physically active (Calfas et al. 1996; Logsdon et al. 1989).

Results from the Activity Counseling TRIAL (Activity Counseling Trial Research Group 2002), and the recent work of Hirvensalo et al. (2003), have demonstrated the effectiveness of provider-based counseling for physical activity among women and older adults, respectively. A number of professional organizations, including the American Heart Association, the American Academy of Pediatrics, and the President's Council on Physical Fitness and Sports, have recommended routine physical activity counseling for people of all ages (American Academy of Pediatrics 1994; American Heart Association 2003; President's Council on Physical Fitness and Sports 1993). Although The U.S. Preventive Services Task Force has acknowledged that physical activity counseling in the primary care setting can be effective in some specific situations, their most recent conclusion is that the evidence is insufficient to generally support the effectiveness of counseling (Eden et al. 2002). Rehabilitation professionals historically have studied exercise therapy and reconditioning methods as part of their training. Yet they often have targeted this information only at specific conditions, with little regard for promoting overall health and for changing their clients' long-term daily behavior. Regardless of their reasons for a clinical visit, patients typically have not responded well to general exercise advice. Often they comply well during the acute rehabilitation phase of therapy, but following a period of "restoration" they begin to discontinue their exercises and eventually fail to maintain the reconditioning effects of their rehabilitation. This pattern is consistently observed in a number of conditions, including orthopedic, cardiac, pulmonary, and stroke rehabilitation.

We must begin to emphasize behavioral-based assessment and counseling approaches, adapting them to the rehabilitation setting and to maintenance of rehabilitation outcomes. As rehabilitation professionals, we have access to patients in multiple settings: hospitals, clinics, nursing homes, athletic departments, community health sites, and rehabilitation centers. Because of this great opportunity, we must expand our roles as providers of preventive care through physical activity and exercise.

Risk Assessment

You can approach exercise prescription in at least three different ways:

1. A program-based level that consists primarily of supervised exercise training (King et al. 1991)
2. Exercise counseling and prescription followed by a self-monitored exercise program (Kriska et al. 1986)
3. Community-based exercise programming that is self-directed and self-monitored (Young et al. 1996)

An excellent review of principles and practices for physical activity assessment and counseling in the clinical setting has recently been published (Estabrooks et al. 2003).

Participants in any kind of exercise program should complete a brief medical history and risk factor questionnaire (see "Medical History and Clearance: Essential Elements") (Hassman et al. 1992).

A questionnaire provides important information regarding potential limitations and restrictions for activity programs. Always encourage clients to consult their personal physicians if they have any questions about their medical status.

After gathering an appropriate medical history, give potential participants a **preprogram evaluation** to document baseline measures of flexibility, cardiorespiratory endurance, strength, and body composition (e.g., at minimum the measurement of height and weight for the calculation of body mass index). These measures not only will help you prescribe an appropriate physical activity level but will also encourage your clients by enabling them to measure their progress. To find more information on patient assessment, please see "Read More About It" (p. 77), and refer again to chapter 5 of this book.

Evaluation measures need not be sophisticated. You can assess flexibility with sit-and-reach tests, both on the floor and in a chair (Shephard et al. 1990). Goniometers can help determine limitations in joint flexibility and mobility. Observations of gait and movement from a seated to standing position provide insight into sensory impairment, impaired equilibrium, or orthostatic hypotension. You can measure strength by simple tests of grip strength combined with modified push-ups and sit-ups. Field tests such as a walking-speed test for 12 minutes or the chair-step test (ACSM 1991) can assess cardiorespiratory endurance, as can submaximal bicycle testing with pulse palpation and blood pressure measurements. These cardiorespiratory tests are intended to be functional evaluations at submaximal levels. For appropriately screened individuals they are relatively safe and effective, while providing data for exercise prescription and physical activity education.

If potential participants have documented CHD, diabetes mellitus, or known risk factors for these diseases, recommend them for diagnostic exercise tolerance testing as well as functional assessment. Chapter 5 deals with such testing in detail. The testing and evaluation should be directed by a physician trained in diagnostic exercise testing. Typical exercise tolerance

Medical History and Clearance: Essential Elements

Medical history

- Cardiovascular disease
- Degenerative joint disease
- Hypertension
- Back syndrome
- Obstructive or restrictive lung disease
- Hypothyroidism
- Diabetes mellitus
- Dizziness
- Ataxia

Risk Factors

- Family history of CAD
- Cigarette smoking
- Physical inactivity
- Obesity
- Hypertension (blood pressure >140/190)
- Elevated blood lipids (cholesterol ≥240 mg/dL or low-density lipoprotein cholesterol ≥130 mg/dL)

Medications

- Beta blockers
- Calcium channel blockers
- Other antianginal medications
- Digitalis preparations
- Antihypertensives
- Nonsteroidal anti-inflammatory analgesics
- Bronchodilators
- Thyroid replacement
- Hypoglycemic

Read More About It

Vivian Heyward's *Advanced Fitness Assessment and Exercise Prescription, Fourth Edition,* published by Human Kinetics, Champaign, Illinois, in 2002, is an excellent resource on patient assessment.

Promoting Physical Activity: A Guide for Community Action (USDHHS 1999) provides guidelines for working with community physical activity promotion advocates.

testing includes graded treadmill exercise testing with continuous electrocardiographic (ECG) monitoring and simultaneous measurement of heart rate and blood pressure. Exercise tolerance testing often involves a symptom-limited testing protocol that provides an estimation of $\dot{V}O_2$max. The modified Balke and modified Bruce protocols, in which the speed and grade are initially at less than 2.5 METs with gradual increases in workload of 1 to 2 METs every 2 to 3 minutes, are examples of appropriate testing protocols (ACSM 1998).

An alternative to treadmill testing is bicycle ergometry. The principles of ECG, heart-rate, and blood pressure monitoring are the same. The most common reason for employing the bike is medical contraindications for use of the treadmill, including the presence of osteoarthritis or an artificial limb, an unstable gait, or severe obesity. The major disadvantage of using the bike for symptom-limited testing is localized muscle fatigue in the legs that sometimes interferes with the participant's ability to achieve heart rates high enough to be of diagnostic value.

In community-based, self-directed programs, medical clearance is left to the judgment of the individual participant. Any campaign promoting physical activity should provide precautions and recommendations for moderate and vigorous physical activity (King et al. 1995). These messages should list steps for participants to follow before beginning a regular moderate-to-vigorous physical activity program, including

1. awareness of pre-existing medical problems (i.e., CHD, arthritis, osteoporosis, or diabetes mellitus),
2. consultation, before starting a program, with a physician or other appropriate health professional if any of the above-mentioned problems are suspected,
3. appropriate modes of activity and tips on different types of activities,
4. principles of training intensity and general guidelines as to rating of perceived exertion (RPE) and training heart rate (THR),
5. progression of activity, with principles of starting slowly and gradually increasing activity time and intensity,
6. principles of monitoring symptoms of excessive fatigue, and
7. making exercise fun and enjoyable.

General Exercise Prescription Guidelines

Exercise prescriptions include five factors that warrant definition:

- **Mode of activity.** Most people who want to participate in regular exercise programming have no significant limitations. But some, especially older persons, have one or more chronic conditions that may necessitate changing the mode of physical activity. Degenerative joint disease, including osteoarthritis, is common among older people. The mode of exercise must accommodate these participants, usually by emphasizing minimal or non-weightbearing activities such as cycling, swimming, and chair and floor exercises. For participants with difficulty in joint mobility of the knees and hips, movement down and up from the floor may initially be contraindicated. Generally, most people will be able to engage in moderate walking activities. Individualization of the mode of activity is important, including variation of activity as well as adjustments for participant bias and preference. Prescribe calisthenics cautiously for individuals suffering from degenerative joint changes, appropriately modifying the stretching and strengthening exercises (see chapter 11). Table 6.1 lists guidelines for prescribing activities for selected chronic conditions.
- **Frequency.** The Surgeon General's most recent recommendations call for more frequent cardiorespiratory endurance and flexibility activities (5-7 days per week) than previous recommendations. Greater frequency provides for greater flexibility and more ready maintenance of endurance capacity. It also enhances compliance and increases the probability that people will assimilate physical activity into their daily routines. Strength-related activities should be done at least twice a week.
- **Duration.** An appropriate goal for most adults is 20 to 40 minutes of endurance activity per session. However, because of physiologic and pathophysiologic limitations, shorter exercise sessions of 10 to 15 minutes repeated two or three times throughout the day may be necessary for some participants. If aging-related limitations require a decrease in intensity of activities, older adults can increase the duration of the activities, preferably approaching one hour in order to derive optimal benefits. If one of the health-related goals of the client/patient is the prevention of weight gain, then the recent recommendations of the IOM may be appropriate. Thus recommending 60 minutes or more of daily moderate intensity activity may be necessary to assist clients/patients in adequately addressing energy balance.
- **Intensity.** Because of the common medical and physiologic limitations among individuals in rehabilitation settings, intensity of activity is of critical importance. For those with a history of CHD, or who are at high risk for CHD, base the exercise prescription on the results of a recent (within three months) ECG-monitored exercise evaluation. You can use the formula of Karvonen to calculate appropriate target heart rates and MET levels, adjusted for symptoms or ECG changes noted in the exercise test (see "Use of Karvonen's Formula for the Calculation of Training Heart Rate" p. 81) (Pollock 1988). "Young-old" (≤75 years) individuals usually can have peak work capacities of 7 METs or greater, whereas the "old-old" (>75 years) frequently have peak levels that do not exceed 4 METs. Unfortunately, the medical and physical activity statuses of participants can vary considerably, making it difficult to generalize workload prescriptions. After assessing an individual's work capacity, you can use MET levels to calculate appropriate exercise intensities. Ratings of perceived exertion (RPE) are quite helpful in regulating intensity. An RPE level of 12 to 15 (on a scale of 6-20) is adequate for most conditioning activities. When people are well oriented to this method, it becomes a very useful self-monitoring mechanism for regulating intensity of exercise.
- **Progression of activity.** A gradual approach to increasing activity levels is best. After beginning an exercise program, most people require from four to six weeks to progress from a low- to moderate-intensity conditioning level. Another four to six weeks is often necessary to achieve an appropriate maintenance level or to progress to a more vigorous conditioning level. Individual variability in fitness and adaptation to the exercise usually dictates the appropriate progression of activity. Once someone achieves a maintenance level of fitness, varying the regimen may enhance compliance. One way to achieve variety is to alter the duration component by interchanging continuous and intermittent activities. Above all, emphasize enjoyment and purpose of the activity sessions needed for maintenance.

Theories and Models Used in Physical Activity Promotion

Historically, health professionals have observed the following sequence in prescribing exercise: assessing the individual (usually with cardiorespiratory fitness measures); formulating the exercise prescription; and counseling the patient regarding exercise mode (usually large muscle activity), frequency (3-5 sessions

Table 6.1 Modification of the Exercise Prescription: Selected Conditions

Condition	Recommended modification
Degenerative joint disease	Non-weightbearing activities such as stationary cycling, water exercises, and chair exercises. Emphasis placed on interval activity. Low-resistance, low-repetition strength training.
Coronary artery disease (CAD)	Physician oversight. Symptom-limited activities. Moderate-level endurance activities preferred (i.e., walking, slow cycling), although at physician's discretion more vigorous activities can be prescribed. Low-resistance, higher-repetition strength training.
Diabetes mellitus	Daily, moderate-endurance activities. Low-resistance, higher-repetition strength training. Flexibility exercises. Monitoring of symptoms and caloric intake. In the presence of obesity, non-weightbearing exercises.
Dizziness, ataxia	Chair exercises may be preferred. Low-resistance, low-repetition strength training. Moderate flexibility activities with minimal movement from supine or prone to standing positions.
Back syndrome	Moderate-endurance activities (i.e., walking, cycling, chair exercises). Modified flexibility exercises. Low-resistance, low-repetition strength training. Modified abdominal strengthening activities. Water activities.
Osteoporosis	Weightbearing activities with intermittent bouts of activity spaced throughout the day. Low-resistance, low-repetition strength training. Chair-level flexibility activities.
Chronic obstructive lung disease	Moderate-level endurance using an interval or intermittent approach to exercise bouts. Low-resistance, low-repetition strength training. Modified flexibility and stretching exercises.
Orthostatic hypotension	Minimize movements from standing to supine and supine to standing. Sustained moderate-endurance activities with short rest intervals. Emphasize activities that minimize the changing of body positions.
Hypertension	Emphasize dynamic large muscle endurance activities; minimize isometric work and focus on low-resistance, low-repetition isotonic strength training.

Reprinted, by permission, from American College of Sports Medicine, 1998, *Resource manual* (Baltimore: Williams & Wilkins), 518.

per week), duration (20-30 minutes per session), and intensity (assigned target heart rate based on the exercise assessment) (ACSM 1998). Often the clinicians review the plans along with the patients and then send the patients on their way. Some professionals schedule follow-up visits for reassessment and revision of the exercise prescription, while others follow up only via telephone. Most researchers who have evaluated this traditional approach to exercise prescription have noted poor long-term compliance, and therefore few long-term benefits (Dishman 1991).

Recent Theories and Models

Exercise scientists have developed a number of theories and models of human behavior for use in exercise counseling and interventions (USDHHS 1996) (table 6.2). The approaches of different models vary in their applicability to promoting physical activity: some are intended primarily as guides to understanding behavior, not designing counseling protocols; others were constructed specifically with a view toward developing intervention protocols.

The **health belief model** suggests that health-related behavior depends on a person's perception of four critical areas:

1. The severity of a potential illness
2. The person's susceptibility to that illness
3. The benefits of taking a preventive action
4. The barriers to taking that action (Rosenstock 1990)

The model incorporates cues to action as important elements in eliciting or maintaining patterns of behavior, and includes the construct of self-efficacy, or a person's confidence in his/her ability to successfully perform an action, perhaps allowing the model to better account for habitual behaviors, such as physical activity.

The **relapse prevention model** can help new exercisers anticipate problems with adhering to their programs. Factors that contribute to relapse include negative emotional or physiologic states, limited coping skills, social pressures, interpersonal conflicts, limited social support, low motivation, high-risk situations, and stress. Principles of relapse prevention include identifying situations containing high risk for relapse (e.g., changes in season) and developing appropriate solutions (e.g., finding a place to walk inside during the winter). It is thought that if exercisers understand that a lapse is not as serious as a relapse, which comprises repeated lapses and requires a more specific strategy to

Table 6.2 Summary of Theories and Models Used in Physical Activity Promotion

Theory/model	Level	Key concepts
Health belief model	Individual	Perceived susceptibility Perceived severity Perceived benefits Perceived barriers Cues to action Self-efficacy
Relapse prevention	Individual	Skills training Cognitive reframing Lifestyle rebalancing
Social cognitive theory	Interpersonal	Reciprocal determinism Behavioral capability Self-efficacy Outcome expectations Observational learning Reinforcement
Theory of planned behavior	Interpersonal	Attitude toward behavior Outcome expectations Value of outcome expectations Subjective norm Beliefs of others Motive to comply with others Perceived behavioral control
Social support	Interpersonal	Instrumental support Informational support Emotional support Appraisal support
Ecological perspective	Environmental	Multiple levels of influence Intrapersonal Interpersonal Institutional Community Public policy
Transtheoretical model	Individual	Precontemplation Contemplation Preparation Action Maintenance

Source: U.S. Department of Health and Human Services 1995.

overcome, their adherence will improve (Marlatt and George 1990).

The **theory of reasoned action** states that individual performance of a given behavior is primarily determined by a person's intention to perform that behavior. This intention is determined by two major factors: the person's attitude toward the behavior and the influence of the person's social environment or subjective norm (i.e., beliefs about what other people think the person should do, as well as the person's motivation to comply with the opinions of others) (Ajzen and Fishbein 1980). The **theory of planned behavior** adds to the theory of reasoned action the concept of perceived control over the opportunities, resources, and skills necessary to perform a behavior (Ajzen 1988). Ajzen's concept of **perceived behavioral control** is similar to Bandura's concept of self-efficacy, i.e., that perceived control over the opportunities, resources, and skills necessary to perform a behavior is critical to the process of changing the behavior (Bandura 1977a).

Social learning theory, later renamed social cognitive theory, proposes that behavior change is affected by environmental influences, personal factors, and attributes of the behavior itself (Bandura 1977b; Bandura 1986). And each factor affects the other two. Self-efficacy is a central tenet of social cognitive theory. People

USE OF KARVONEN'S FORMULA FOR THE CALCULATION OF TRAINING HEART RATE

Mrs. Kim is a 45-year-old Korean American who comes to you for a physical activity prescription. She currently is not taking any medicines, has no history of cardiovascular disease, has no known cardiovascular risk factors, and reports being in good health. She is 5′ 4″ and weighs 135 pounds, with resting blood pressure of 116/82. She played intercollegiate soccer and has subsequently participated in adult senior soccer leagues. Approximately 12 weeks ago she injured her right knee during a soccer match. The injury was precipitated by a quick turn to the inside, pivoting off of the right foot, but with no physical contact with another player. She underwent an MRI evaluation and arthroscopic surgery to remove the distal horn of the lateral meniscus of the right knee. She returns today after six weeks of successful physical therapy, to begin a cardiorespiratory reconditioning program.

As measured using a treadmill, Mrs. Kim's $\dot{V}O_2max$ is 2.8 L/min or 45 ml O_2/kg/min, with maximal heart rate of 179 beats/minute. Her seated resting heart rate was 74 beats/minute. You set her initial exercise prescription at an intensity of 0.6 to 0.8 of $\dot{V}O_2max$ (see Pollock 1988 for Karvonen's formula).

Training heart rate = (Maximum heart rate – Resting heart rate)(0.6 to 0.8) + Resting heart rate

Training heart rate = (179 beats/min – 74 beats/min)(0.6 to 0.8) + 74 beats/min

Training heart rate = (105 beats/min)(0.6 to 0.8) + 74 beats/min = 137 to 158 beats/min

must believe in their ability to perform the behavior, and must perceive an incentive to do so. Additionally, they must value the consequences that they believe will occur as a result of the behavior. Benefits may be immediate (e.g., feeling energized following physical activity) or long-term (e.g., improving cardiovascular health as a result of physical activity). But because these expected outcomes are filtered through a person's expectations of being able to perform the behavior in the first place, self-efficacy is believed to be the single most important characteristic that determines a person's behavior change. To increase self-efficacy in a client, provide clear instructions, provide the opportunity for skill development or training, and see that someone models the desired behavior. To be effective, models must evoke trust, admiration, and respect from the observer; they must not, however, present a level of behavior that the observer is unable to visualize attaining for himself or herself.

Social support for physical activity can be instrumental, as in giving a nondriver a ride to an exercise class; informational, as in telling someone about a walking program in the neighborhood; emotional, as in calling to see how someone is faring with a new walking program; or **appraising**, as in providing feedback and reinforcement in the learning of a new skill. Sources of support for physical activity include family members, friends, neighbors, coworkers, and exercise program leaders and participants. A number of investigators have further explored social support strategies in promoting physical activity using social influence theories such as self-presentation theory, which draws on the strength of people's own perception of their cultural and social identity (King et al. 2002).

A criticism of most models of behavior change is that they emphasize individual processes and pay little attention to sociocultural and physical environmental influences on behavior (McLeroy et al. 1988). Recently, interest has developed in increasing participation in physical activity through **ecological approaches** (Stokols 1992) that place creation of supportive environments on a par with the development of personal skills and the reorientation of health services. Examples of such environmental supports are bike paths, parks, and incentives to encourage walking or bicycling to work. An underlying theme of ecological perspectives is that the most effective interventions simultaneously influence multiple levels and multiple settings (e.g., schools, work sites, etc.).

The **transtheoretical model of behavior change** (Prochaska and DiClemente 1984) integrates an ecological approach with other theories and models of health behavior. In this model, which is demonstrably effective in changing physical activity behaviors (Calfas et al. 1996), behavior change consists of a five-stage process related to a person's readiness to change:

1. Precontemplation
2. Contemplation
3. Preparation
4. Action
5. Maintenance

People progress through these stages at varying rates, often moving back and forth along the continuum a number of times before attaining the goal of maintenance; the stages of change are more spiral or cyclical than linear. In this model, people use different processes of change as they move from one stage to another. Efficient self-change thus depends on doing the right thing (processes) at the right time (stages). According to this theory, tailoring interventions to match a person's readiness or stage of change is essential. For example, for people who are not yet contemplating becoming more active, encouraging a step-by-step movement along the continuum of change may be more effective than encouraging them to move directly into action (Marcus et al. 1992).

PACE—A Behavioral Approach to Physical Activity Counseling

In cooperation with the CDC, investigators from San Diego State University developed the Patient-centered Assessment and Counseling for Exercise (PACE) materials for use especially by primary care providers in targeting apparently clinically healthy adults (Calfas et al. 2002). A number of clinicians have evaluated the materials for both acceptability and effectiveness (Long et al. 1996). The PACE protocols assume that a single counseling approach is not appropriate for all patients. Using the stages-of-change model, the PACE counseling protocols classify patients according to their readiness to become physically active and encourage coupling the counseling approach to the patient's stage (figure 6.1). The theory is that people make behavioral changes progressively and have different counseling needs at each stage. The PACE protocols (figures 6.2-6.5) distill the five original stages of change into three functional stages: precontemplators, contemplators, and actives. Each of these stages has a corresponding counseling protocol.

The score patients receive on the assessment form ("What Is Your PACE Score?", figure 6.2) determines the stage they are in. **Precontemplators** are patients who have not been in nor are currently active in an exercise program and have no interest in doing so. A score of 1 means the patient is a precontemplator, and you may use the "Getting Out of Your Chair" form (figure 6.3) as a guide in counseling him. Your goal is to get such people to consider becoming more physically active. The counseling protocol for this stage requires patients to identify potential benefits of physical activity (e.g., recovery of strength following injury or surgery), thus moving them to the point of realizing that being active is desirable. Patients identify two main reasons why they are inactive and two strategies to overcome these barriers. This sets the stage for you to suggest activities and approaches to overcome any obstacles. Success among these patients is measured by their desire to consider becoming more physically active.

Contemplators (PACE score 2-4) are patients who, although they do little or no regular physical activity, are interested in becoming more active, but usually do not have the knowledge, skills, or the right kind of encouragement. Use "Planning the First Step" (figure 6.4) to counsel them, helping these patients draw up a specific plan to begin an exercise program. Begin with praise for their desire to become more physically active. Ask patients to list at least two benefits they hope to gain from their activity program and to draft a sample activity plan that they will review with you. Have them list the types of activities they enjoy doing and where and when they plan to do them. To elicit social support, ask patients to identify a family member, friend, or coworker who will support their new activity plan. Patients should be as specific as possible in their plans. If necessary you should adjust the exercise plan because of the patient's clinical and health status. The result is a plan that is both realistic and potentially beneficial. The patient agrees to the plan for a specified time period and signs an agreement; signing a contract is an effective behavioral modification technique (Marcus et al. 1994). Contemplators will require more of your time than either precontemplators or actives. It is helpful to provide these patients with additional educational materials and to arrange occasions for them to see people modeling the prescribed exercise behaviors.

Actives (PACE score of 5-8) are already participating in regular physical activity at any level of intensity. These are usually patients who, following their initial rehabilitation sessions, carry the principles of these sessions into lifetime physical activities. Use "Keeping the Pace" (figure 6.5) to counsel these patients, encouraging them to maintain an active lifestyle. Do this by developing strategies to prevent relapse and by encouraging a return to activity after unavoidable time off (e.g., illness, work demands). Counseling these patients also begins with praise for current activities. Ask them to list at least three benefits they receive from their current activity program. Review the program, drawing attention to potential problem areas (e.g., overuse or underexercising). Occasional lapses are expected: challenge these patients to list potential barriers they may need to overcome in the future in order to maintain their programs. Focus on building self-efficacy (i.e., patients' confidence to maintain their programs in the face of certain barriers, such as weather, travel, etc.). Both you and your patient should sign the exercise plan and make a commitment to review and revise it as necessary.

To obtain the PACE forms contact the SDSU Foundation and the San Diego Center for Health Interventions, 5500 Campanile Dr., San Diego, CA 92182-4701.

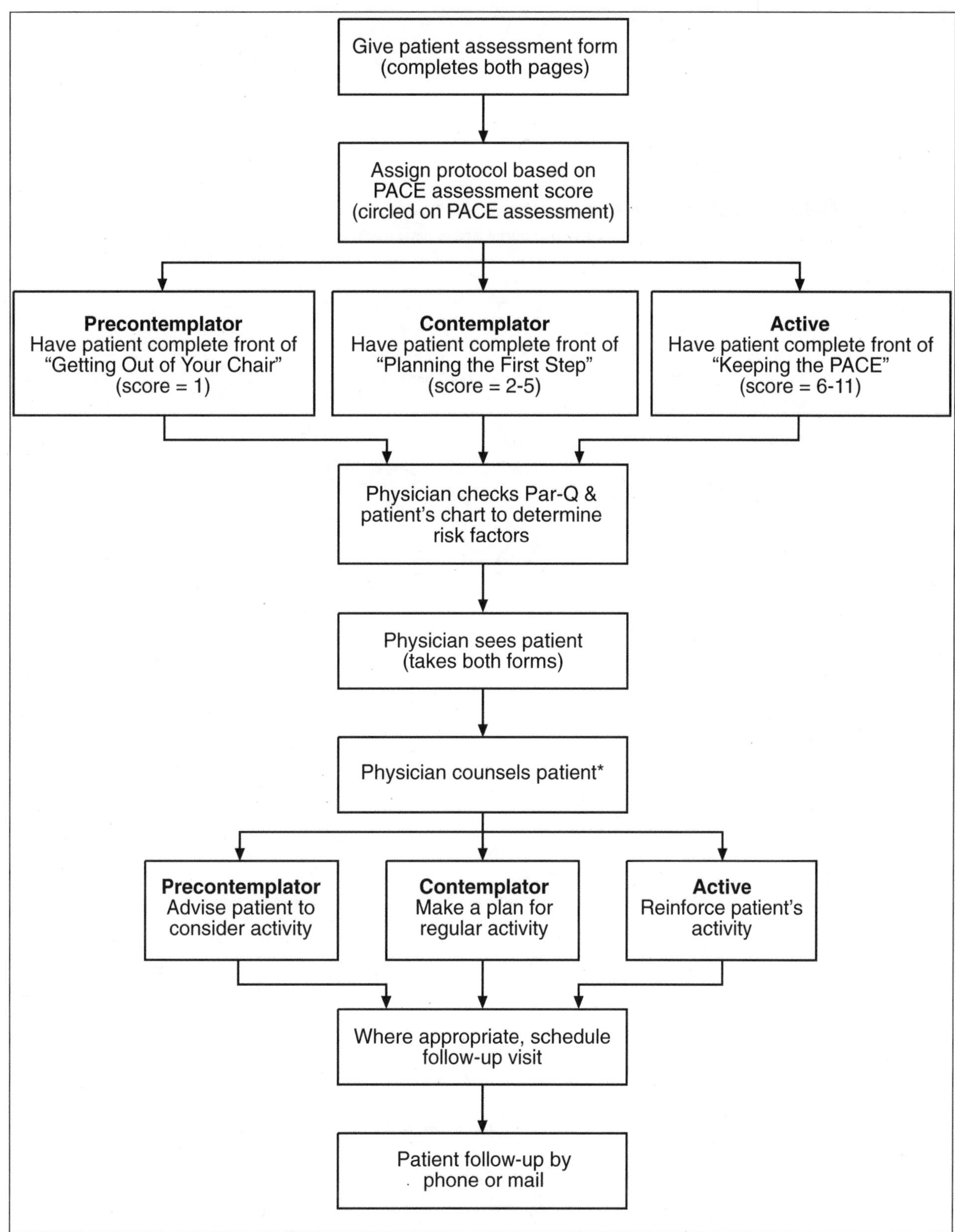

Figure 6.1 PACE assessment and counseling flow chart.

*Physician may emphasize importance of physical activity and refer patient to other health care professionals in the office for counseling.

Permission to reprint from the PACE Manual (Patient-centered Assessment and Counseling for Exercise and Nutrition) granted by the SDSU Foundation and the San Diego Center for Health Intervention.

PATIENT'S NAME DATE

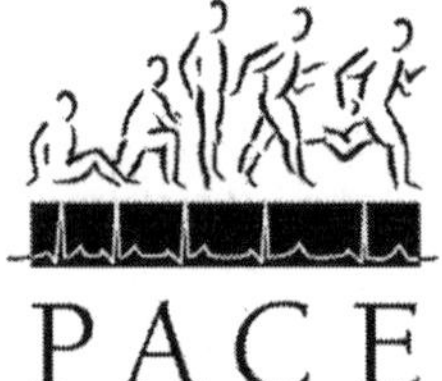

What is Your PACE Score?

This form will help your health care provider understand your level of physical activity. Please read the entire form and then choose the ONE number below that best describes your current level of physical activity or your readiness to do more physical activity. Do not include activities you do as part of your job.

"Vigorous" exercise includes activities like jogging, running, fast cycling, aerobics classes, swimming laps, singles tennis, and racquetball. Any activity that makes you work *as hard as jogging* and *lasts 20 minutes* at a time should be counted. These types of activities usually increase your heart rate, and make you sweat, and you get out of breath. (*Do not count weight lifting.*) *Regular vigorous exercise* is done for at least 20 minutes at a time and at least 3 days a week.

"Moderate" exercise includes activities like brisk walking, gardening, slow cycling, dancing, doubles tennis, or hard work around the house. Any activity that makes you work as hard as brisk walking and that lasts at least 10 minutes at a time should be counted. *Regular moderate exercise* is done at least 30 minutes a day and at least 5 days a week.

CURRENT PHYSICAL ACTIVITY STATUS

Circle one number only.

1. I don't do regular vigorous or moderate exercise now, and I don't intend to start in the next 6 months.
2. I don't do regular vigorous or moderate exercise now, but I have been thinking of starting in the
   next 6 months.
3. I'm trying to start doing vigorous or moderate exercise, but I don't do it regularly.
4. I'm doing vigorous exercise less than 3 times per week (or) moderate exercise less than 5 times per week.
5. I've been doing 30 minutes a day of moderate exercise 5 or more days per week for the last 1-5 months.
6. I've been doing 30 minutes a day of moderate exercise 5 or more days per week for the last 6 months or more.
7. I've been doing vigorous exercise 3 or more days per week for the last 1-5 months.
8. I've been doing vigorous exercise 3 or more days per week for the last 6 months or more.

Please complete other side.

(continued)

Figure 6.2

Permission to reprint from the PACE Manual (Patient-centered Assessment and Counseling for Exercise and Nutrition) granted by the SDSU Foundation and the San Diego Center for Health Intervention.

Physical Activity Readiness Questionnaire - PAR-Q (revised 2002)

PAR-Q & YOU

(A Questionnaire for People Aged 15 to 69)

Regular physical activity is fun and healthy, and increasingly more people are starting to become more active every day. Being more active is very safe for most people. However, some people should check with their doctor before they start becoming much more physically active.

If you are planning to become much more physically active than you are now, start by answering the seven questions in the box below. If you are between the ages of 15 and 69, the PAR-Q will tell you if you should check with your doctor before you start. If you are over 69 years of age, and you are not used to being very active, check with your doctor.

Common sense is your best guide when you answer these questions. Please read the questions carefully and answer each one honestly: check YES or NO.

YES	NO	
☐	☐	**1. Has your doctor ever said that you have a heart condition and that you should only do physical activity recommended by a doctor?**
☐	☐	**2. Do you feel pain in your chest when you do physical activity?**
☐	☐	**3. In the past month, have you had chest pain when you were not doing physical activity?**
☐	☐	**4. Do you lose your balance because of dizziness or do you ever lose consciousness?**
☐	☐	**5. Do you have a bone or joint problem (for example, back, knee or hip) that could be made worse by a change in your physical activity?**
☐	☐	**6. Is your doctor currently prescribing drugs (for example, water pills) for your blood pressure or heart condition?**
☐	☐	**7. Do you know of any other reason why you should not do physical activity?**

If you answered

YES to one or more questions

Talk with your doctor by phone or in person BEFORE you start becoming much more physically active or BEFORE you have a fitness appraisal. Tell your doctor about the PAR-Q and which questions you answered YES.

- You may be able to do any activity you want — as long as you start slowly and build up gradually. Or, you may need to restrict your activities to those which are safe for you. Talk with your doctor about the kinds of activities you wish to participate in and follow his/her advice.
- Find out which community programs are safe and helpful for you.

NO to all questions

If you answered NO honestly to all PAR-Q questions, you can be reasonably sure that you can:

- start becoming much more physically active – begin slowly and build up gradually. This is the safest and easiest way to go.
- take part in a fitness appraisal – this is an excellent way to determine your basic fitness so that you can plan the best way for you to live actively. It is also highly recommended that you have your blood pressure evaluated. If your reading is over 144/94, talk with your doctor before you start becoming much more physically active.

DELAY BECOMING MUCH MORE ACTIVE:

- if you are not feeling well because of a temporary illness such as a cold or a fever – wait until you feel better; or
- if you are or may be pregnant – talk to your doctor before you start becoming more active.

PLEASE NOTE: If your health changes so that you then answer YES to any of the above questions, tell your fitness or health professional. Ask whether you should change your physical activity plan.

Informed Use of the PAR-Q: The Canadian Society for Exercise Physiology, Health Canada, and their agents assume no liability for persons who undertake physical activity, and if in doubt after completing this questionnaire, consult your doctor prior to physical activity.

No changes permitted. You are encouraged to photocopy the PAR-Q but only if you use the entire form.

NOTE: If the PAR-Q is being given to a person before he or she participates in a physical activity program or a fitness appraisal, this section may be used for legal or administrative purposes.

"I have read, understood and completed this questionnaire. Any questions I had were answered to my full satisfaction."

NAME ______________________

SIGNATURE ______________________ DATE ______________________

SIGNATURE OF PARENT or GUARDIAN (for participants under the age of majority) ______________________ WITNESS ______________________

Note: This physical activity clearance is valid for a maximum of 12 months from the date it is completed and becomes invalid if your condition changes so that you would answer YES to any of the seven questions.

 Supported by: Health Canada Santé Canada

continued on other side...

Figure 6.2 *(continued)*

Reprinted from the 2002 revised version of the Physical Activity Readiness Questionnaire (PAR-Q & You). PAR-Q & You is a copyrighted pre-exercise screen owned by the Canadian Society for Exercise Physiology. www.csep.ca/pdfs/par-q.pdf

PATIENT'S NAME DATE

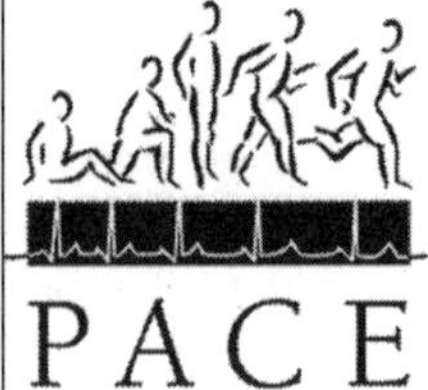

Getting Out of Your Chair

Assessment Score = 1

On your PACE Assessment you said you do not intend to start regular physical activity in the next 6 months. That is fine, because everyone makes changes at his or her own speed.

However, PACE and your health care provider want to make sure you know about the many important benefits of physical activity.

Think About the Benefits of Physical Activity. Please list up to 10 benefits of physical activity. You may have heard these on the news, read about them, or heard about them from friends. Think about benefits you get right away and in the future.

1. ______________________ 6. ______________________
2. ______________________ 7. ______________________
3. ______________________ 8. ______________________
4. ______________________ 9. ______________________
5. ______________________ 10. ______________________

If you listed 10 benefits, that's great. You are well informed. But did you know there are many more benefits? Turn this page over to see a much longer list of the benefits you can get by being physically active.

What are 4 more benefits that are important to you but you did not know about before? List them here.

1. ______________________ 3. ______________________
2. ______________________ 4. ______________________

Because of all these benefits, doctors now realize that being physically active is one of the most important things you can do for your health. We understand that you are not ready to increase your physical activity now, but please think about how these benefits could help you.

Good News About Moderate Physical Activity. Did you know you can enjoy many of these benefits without working up a heavy sweat? The recommendations for physical activity have changed. The new recommendations can be done by everybody, because they emphasize moderate amounts of physical activity on a daily basis. Brisk walking, bicycling, pushing a baby carriage and digging in the garden are all moderate activities. Being active can be an enjoyable part of your day, instead of a chore. Here is the current physical activity recommendation:

> *"Every adult should accumulate 30 minutes or more of moderate-intensity physical activity on most, preferably all, days of the week. An example of moderate intensity physical activity is a brisk walk."*

This means you don't even have to do all 30 minutes at once. You do not have to wear special clothes, use special equipment or spend a lot of money to get the benefits of physical activity.

PROVIDER'S USE ONLY:

○ As your health care provider, I strongly encourage you to plan to be more physically active. I may ask you at your next visit if you are ready to begin.

Based on your medical status and health history, the most important benefits of physical activity for you are:

____
Provider's Signature

(continued)

Figure 6.3

Permission to reprint from the PACE Manual (Patient-centered Assessment and Counseling for Exercise and Nutrition) granted by the SDSU Foundation and the San Diego Center for Health Intervention.

Your physician strongly encourages you to think about the benefits you could get from physical activity.

Most people can improve their health a great deal by taking a walk for 30 minutes a few times every week. If you want information on how to start doing more physical activity, ask your doctor.

Hundreds of research studies show physical activity has dozens of health benefits. It improves many systems of the body and reduces risks for important mental and physical illnesses. Here are some of the benefits of being physically active.

BENEFITS OF PHYSICAL ACTIVITY

Benefits you can get right away

- Reduces blood sugar levels
- Increases metabolic rate after workout
- Improves mental health
- Increases self-esteem and self-concept
- Increases well-being
- Increases quality of life
- Reduces depression
- Reduces anger
- Reduces anxiety
- Helps cope with stress
- Improves vitality and "energy"
- Improves sleep
- Aids relaxation
- Can help quit smoking
- Can help stick with dietary changes
- Builds muscle tissue
- Improves pain tolerance
- Improves some hormonal functions
- Improves blood flow to the brain
- May enhance cognitive functioning
- May aid recovery from substance abuse
- Burns calories

Benefits you get over the long run

- Increases life expectancy. Active people live up to 2 years longer.
- Improves overall quality of life
- Reduces heart attacks by about 50%
- Reduces strokes
- Reduces blood pressure
- Reduces risk of becoming hypertensive
- Reduces triglycerides (fats in the blood)
- Increases HDL (good) cholesterol
- Reduces risk of colon cancer
- Possibly reduces risk of breast cancer
- Possibly reduces risk of prostate cancer
- Improves functioning of immune system
- Reduces risk of becoming diabetic
- Controls body weight
- Helps weight loss
- Promotes loss of body fat
- Promotes loss of dangerous abdominal fat
- Necessary for maintaining weight loss
- Prevents depression
- Prevents anxiety
- Improves immune system
- Makes heart stronger
- Reduces blood clotting
- Can reduce falls in the elderly
- Reduces risk of osteoporosis
- Improves functioning in arthritis patients

Figure 6.3 *(continued)*

Permission to reprint from the PACE Manual (Patient-centered Assessment and Counseling for Exercise and Nutrition) granted by the SDSU Foundation and the San Diego Center for Health Intervention.

PATIENT'S NAME ____________ DATE ________

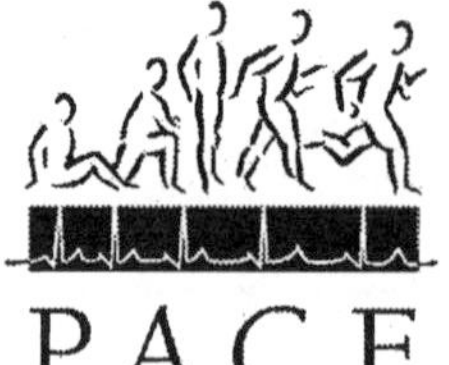

Planning the First Step

Assessment Score = 2-4

Congratulations. On your PACE Assessment you said you are ready to increase your physical activity. You are taking a big step toward improving your physical and mental health. This form can help you start an activity program you can stick with.

What are the two main benefits you hope to get from being active? Writing them down here will help you keep them in mind.

1. ____________________ 2. ____________________

Work up to these physical activity guidelines (see example activities on back).

- Do moderate physical activity for 30 to 60 minutes on 5 to 7 days a week.
- Do vigorous physical activity for 20 to 40 minutes on 3 to 5 days a week.
- Most inactive people should start with moderate activities.

MAKE A PHYSICAL ACTIVITY PLAN

Choose an activity or two. Do you enjoy it? Can you afford the supplies, equipment, facilities, or classes? Are there family or friends to do this activity with you? Can you do it year-round? Consider a back-up activity.

Type of Activity: ____________________

Where will you do your activity? Can you do this activity at home or in your neighborhood? Do you have to go to a gym, a park, or a health club?

Place for Activity: ____________________

What is the most realistic time for you to do this activity? Do you have to reschedule other activities? Start slowly and work up to this goal.

Days and Times for Activity: ____________________

How long do you plan to do your activity each time? You should build up time gradually over several weeks. Start with 5-10 minutes and build up to 30-60 minutes of moderate activity or 20-40 minutes of vigorous activity.

Length of Activity: ____________________

Who can support you or help with your new activity program? It is ideal for someone to work out with you. You may want to ask someone to encourage you or help you to be active.

Who will help you and how? ____________________

PROVIDER'S USE ONLY:

Based on your health status, your doctor recommends you do the following to improve your health:

- ❍ Before you increase your physical activity, you need to have an exercise tolerance test.*
- ❍ You could benefit greatly by starting a program of regular walking or other moderate activity.
- ❍ If you want to do vigorous activities like jogging, you need to have an exercise tolerance test.*
- ❍ You appear to be able to do either moderate or vigorous physical activities.

*Call this office for an appointment or referral.

SUGGESTED PROGRAM (FITT)

Frequency	F______	times per week
Intensity	I ______	moderate______ vigorous activity
Type	T______	type of physical activity
Time	T______	minutes per session (Work up to___minutes in___weeks.)

I agree to try out this physical activity plan from ________ to ________

____
Patient's Signature

____
Provider's Signature

(continued)

Figure 6.4

Permission to reprint from the PACE Manual (Patient-centered Assessment and Counseling for Exercise and Nutrition) granted by the SDSU Foundation and the San Diego Center for Health Intervention.

EXAMPLES OF ACTIVITIES

Moderate Intensity

Walking (at home, to work, on lunch break)
Gardening (must be regular)
Hiking
Slow cycling
Folk, square, or popular dancing
Ice and roller skating
Doubles tennis
Pushing a baby carriage

Vigorous Intensity

Jogging
Aerobic dance
Basketball
Fast cycling
Cross-country skiing
Swimming laps
Singles tennis and racquet sports
Soccer

HOW TO GET PAST YOUR ROADBLOCKS

Roadblock	How To Get Past It
❍ I do not have the time	We're talking about only three 30-minute sessions each week. Could you do without three TV shows each week?
❍ I do not enjoy exercise	Do not "exercise." Start a hobby or way of playing that gets you moving.
❍ I am usually too tired for exercise	Tell yourself, "This activity will give me more energy." This is what most people find.
❍ The weather is too bad	There are many activities you can do in your own home, in any weather. Ask your friends for ideas.
❍ Exercise is boring	Listening to music during your activity keeps your mind occupied. Walking, biking, or running can take you past lots of interesting scenery. Do activity with a friend.
❍ I get sore when I exercise	Slight muscle soreness after physical activity is common when you are just starting. It should go away in 2-3 days. You can avoid this by building up gradually.

ACTIVITY LOG

Use this Activity Log to keep track of your physical activity. Write down how long you do your activity as well as positive feelings and experiences. Note any roadblocks that discourage you from doing your activity and do something about them. When this log is full, make one of your own.

DATE	ACTIVITY	MINUTES	FEELING/COMMENTS

How confident are you that you can do regular physical activity for the next 3 months?

❍ Not at all confident ❍ Somewhat confident ❍ Very confident

Figure 6.4 *(continued)*

Permission to reprint from the PACE Manual (Patient-centered Assessment and Counseling for Exercise and Nutrition) granted by the SDSU Foundation and the San Diego Center for Health Intervention.

PATIENT'S NAME DATE

PACE

Keeping the PACE

Assessment Score = 5-8

Congratulations. You are doing regular physical activity. You have a right to feel proud that you are doing something very positive for yourself. Sometimes you lose sight of the health and mental health benefits you are getting from physical activity.

What motivates you to stay active?

1. ______ 2. ______ 3. ______

REVIEW YOUR PROGRAM

By reviewing the activities you are doing now, you can see if any changes need to be made in your plan. The goal is to improve your chances of staying active.

What *type(s)* of activity do you usually do? ______

How many *times a week?* ______

How long each time? ______

Who *helps* you or does activity with you? ______

Have you had any *injuries?* ______

What parts of your activity plan are you *most satisfied* with? ______

What parts of your activity plan are you *least satisfied* with? ______

What *changes* could you make in your activity plan to make it more enjoyable, convenient, or safe? ______

GETTING BACK ON TRACK

Most people who are regularly active have stopped at one time or another in the past. Sometimes they stop for a few weeks. Sometimes it is years before they start being active again. Planning ahead by answering these questions now can help you get past roadblocks later.

If you have stopped regular activity in the past, what caused you to stop? ______

What could you have done differently that would have helped you stay active or what helped you get back on track quickly? ______

KEEPING THE PACE

How confident are you that you can do regular physical activity for the next 3 months?

○ Not at all confident ○ Somewhat confident ○ Very confident

PROVIDER'S USE ONLY:

SUMMARY OF CURRENT PROGRAM (FITT)	MAJOR CVD RISK FACTORS
Frequency F ______ times per week	○ Smoking ○ Physical Inactivity
Intensity I ______ moderate ______ vigorous activity	○ Hypertension ○ Positive Family History
Type T ______ type of physical activity	○ Elevated Lipids ○ Obesity
Time T ______ minutes per session	
Provider's Signature	

(continued)

Figure 6.5

TIPS FOR KEEPING THE PACE

Injury to muscle, joints and bones may be the *most common* cause of stopping activity. The best way to prevent injury is to avoid over-exercise. Do not do an activity that is too vigorous for you. If you are overdoing it, slow down. If you feel pain during physical activity, stop and take a rest. The *most serious* risk of physical activity is heart trouble, but it is *rare*. If you feel pain in your chest, immediately stop the activity and consult a physician.

The PACE recommendation of 30 to 60 minutes of moderate activity 5-7 days a week or 20 to 40 minutes of vigorous activity 3 to 5 days a week provides maximum benefit at low levels of risk. Exercise scientists also suggest warming up before your main activity and cooling down and stretching after your activity to lower your risk of injury. Warming up and cooling down can be slow versions of your activity, like slow walking. Gently, stretch the muscles you use during the activity. Hold each stretch 5-10 seconds and don't bounce.

There are times when you may stop your regular activity. This may be due to more demands on your time at home or work, travel, house guests, or illness. Interruptions are normal and expected. *The key is starting your regular activity again as soon as possible.*

HOW TO GET BACK ON TRACK

- Remind yourself it is OK to have a pause in your activity once in a while. Don't be hard on yourself. Feeling guilty will make it more difficult to get back on track.
- You may need some extra help to get going again. Ask family and friends to help and encourage you.
- Ask someone to be active with you.
- It may be helpful to tell everybody you know that you are restarting your activity.
- Use an Activity Log to keep track of your activity again.
- Give yourself small rewards each time you go out and do your activity. Make a chart for your refrigerator. Use stickers or gold stars to keep track of your activity. Put change in a jar as a reward. Praising yourself is an effective reward ("I did it and I'm proud of myself!")
- For variety try new activities.
- Do whatever worked for you in the past to restart physical activity.

LOOK AHEAD FOR YOUR ROADBLOCKS

What situation is most likely to make you stop being active? ______________________________

____

What can you do about this roadblock to prevent it or prepare for it? ______________________

____

What is the best way for you to get back on track if you stop? ____________________________

____

Figure 6.5 *(continued)*

Permission to reprint from the PACE Manual (Patient-centered Assessment and Counseling for Exercise and Nutrition) granted by the SDSU Foundation and the San Diego Center for Health Intervention.

SUMMARY

Within the past decade, physical activity has emerged as a key element in preventing and managing chronic conditions. Although for decades clinicians have appreciated the role of exercise in rehabilitation medicine, recent findings regarding the mode, frequency, duration, and intensity of physical activity have modified exercise prescription practices. An important part of these modifications has been a clearer separation of the results of exercise into those related to health and those related to fitness. Most importantly, new behavioral approaches to physical activity assessment and counseling have led to documented improvements in compliance.

Behavioral theories and models of health behavior have been reexamined in light of physical activity and exercise. A set of behavioral principles and guidelines now exists to help health providers guide patients into lifelong patterns of increased levels of physical activity and improved exercise compliance. The PACE materials provide an integrated behavioral approach to exercise prescription that takes into account the providers' limited time and expertise in counseling patients about physical activity, the patients' needs and behavioral readiness for increased physical activity, and the appropriate desired outcomes for health and fitness.

Further refinement of the PACE and other protocols will be necessary for its use in rehabilitation medicine, dictated by the spectrum of patients seen. The more we learn about exercise in specific populations, the more we will be able to refine our prescriptions in terms of mode, frequency, duration, and intensity of exercise for specific classes of people. Combining more refined prescriptions with more effective behavioral paradigms will yield enhanced compliance on the part of previously unmotivated people. The net result will be healthier and more functional patients.

ACKNOWLEDGMENTS

I would like to acknowledge my colleagues at CDC and those at San Diego State University who so profoundly influenced my thinking about "exercise prescription" and health behavior change. I trust that this chapter reflects a bit of their wisdom. Thanks to Dr. Walter Frontera for providing me with the opportunity to pen a few of the animated points from my original Boston presentation. And, finally, thank you to the editorial staff at Human Kinetics for persevering with me on this.

CHAPTER 7

EXERCISE AND THE PREVENTION OF CHRONIC DISABLING ILLNESS

Carlos J. Crespo, DrPH, MS, FACSM; and Edith M. Williams, MS

This chapter discusses the effects of physical activity or exercise in the primary prevention of selected chronic diseases. Being physically active has been associated with lower rates of coronary heart disease (CHD), stroke, certain cancers, type 2 diabetes, osteoporosis, osteoarthritis, and some mental conditions. Table 7.1 shows that about 400,000 deaths per year in the United States are premature due to physical inactivity and poor diet. Epidemiological data have shown that physical inactivity increases the incidence of at least 17 unhealthy conditions, almost all of which are chronic diseases or considered risk factors for chronic diseases (Booth et al. 2000; Chen 2001; Mokdad et al. 2004). While secondary and tertiary prevention approaches were largely unsuccessful in reversing the epidemic emergence of modern chronic diseases in the latter part of the 20th century, primary prevention strategies, which attack the environmental roots of these conditions, are proving to be more effective. The challenge is to differentiate among the independent effects that an active lifestyle, physical fitness, and heredity may have on the occurrence of chronic diseases (Bouchard 1993).

DEFINITIONS

Exercise or exercise training is a planned, structured, and repetitive bodily movement done to improve or maintain one or more components of physical fitness. Physical activity refers to any bodily movement, produced by contraction of skeletal muscle, that substantially increases energy expenditure (Caspersen et al. 1985; Nieman 1996). Thus, exercise is a form of physical activity. Physical activity can be occupational, or can involve housework, leisure activities, transportation (e.g., bicycling), entertainment (e.g., dancing), and, of course, sports. This chapter will use the terms "physical activity" and "exercise" interchangeably.

Physical fitness, defined as a set of attributes that relate to the ability to perform physical activity, can be health-related or skill-related. Health-related fitness has an independent effect on health. Skill-related physical fitness may predispose people to continue or to increase their level of physical activity. Even when skill-related endeavors have no direct health component, they can provide additional psychological confidence that leads people to engage in activities that do improve their health.

Participation in sports or work-related activities requires both health- and skill-related components of physical fitness. Prevention of chronic disease through exercise requires not only that people be physically active but also that they train and improve certain health- and skill-related components of physical fitness.

Table 7.1 Major Causes of Yearly Preventable Deaths in the United States

Cause	Estimated annual deaths	Percentage of total deaths
Tobacco	435,000	18.1
Physical inactivity/diet	400,000	16.6
Alcohol	85,000	3.5
Microbial agents	75,000	8
Toxic agents	55,000	6
Firearms	29,000	4
Sexual behavior	20,000	2
Motor vehicles	43,000	2
Illicit use of drugs	17,000	<2

Source: Mokdad et al. 2004.

Physical Activity and Fitness

Improvements in one or more fitness components can help prevent chronic diseases. Maintaining a healthy body weight or improving cardiorespiratory and muscular endurance can help prevent CHD, type 2 diabetes, osteoporosis, and other chronic diseases. The numerous health benefits of regular exercise depend on the type, intensity, and volume of activity pursued by the individual. These benefits include reduction of low-density lipoproteins (LDL) and increase in high-density lipoprotein (HDL); improvement of glucose metabolism; improved strength, self-esteem, and body image; and reduction of the occurrence of back injuries (Macera et al. 2003; Sothern et al. 1999; Stear 2003).

Earlier longitudinal studies of the relationship between physical activity and chronic disease compared occupations with higher energy expenditure to those with lower energy expenditure (Morris et al. 1966) and found that physical activity protects against heart disease. Later studies found that leisure-time physical activity offers more protection against heart disease than work activities (Haskell 1995; U.S. Department of Health and Human Services [USDHHS] 1996), probably because physical activity has been engineered out of most people's occupations. Unfortunately, data from the National Health Interview Survey and the Third National Health and Nutrition Examination Survey showed that more than half of American adults engage in little or no leisure-time physical activity (Crespo et al. 1996; USDHHS 1996). More recently, the Behavioral Risk Factor Surveillance System (BRFSS) included measures of leisure-time physical activity and new lifestyle activity questions. Even with a more complete measure of physical activity than used previously, findings indicate that the majority of U.S. adults are not physically active at levels that can promote health (Centers for Disease Control and Prevention [CDC] 2003, Aug 15). In addition, the Youth Media Campaign Longitudinal Study (YMCLS), conducted by the CDC, showed that 61.5% of children aged 9 to 13 years do not participate in any organized physical activity during their nonschool hours and that 22.6% do not engage in any free-time physical activity (CDC 2003, Aug 22). It is clear that America is experiencing a virtual epidemic of inactivity.

Simultaneous measurements of physical activity and physical fitness may be useful in epidemiologic studies of habitual physical activity and chronic disease. For example, physical activity and physical fitness correlate significantly and independently with different coronary heart disease risk factors in men and women.

Measuring physical fitness and participation in physical activity among members of different churches in Rhode Island, Eaton et al. (1995) found that physical fitness was more related to systolic and diastolic blood pressure, body mass index, and HDL cholesterol than was physical activity. Multiple regression analysis of physical fitness, physical activity, and their interaction suggested that lack of physical fitness correlates strongly with CHD risk factors. Other studies have found physical fitness to be improved by heavy or vigorous physical activity but not by light to moderate physical activity (Knapik et al. 1993).

In summary, both exercise training and general physical activity can improve physical fitness. The physiological and metabolic changes from improved physical fitness are very likely to produce substantial benefits in the prevention of certain chronic diseases. Physical activity, especially if it is vigorous, plays a crucial role in the maintenance and improvement of acceptable levels of physical fitness.

Physical Activity and Health

Katzmarzyk and colleagues (2000) estimated the health care costs in Canada attributable to physical inactivity in 1999 to be about $2.1 billion. This amount represented 2.5% of the total health care costs that year (calculated at $86.0 billion). The estimated total cost attributable to physical inactivity represented 25.5% of the cost of treating CAD, stroke, hypertension, colon cancer, breast cancer, type 2 diabetes, and osteoporosis that year. The highest costs attributable to physical inactivity were associated with CAD ($891 million), osteoporosis ($352 million), stroke ($345 million), and hypertension ($314 million).

Additionally, there were 207,408 deaths from all causes among Canadian adults in 1995, of which 35.8% were due to the main diseases known to be associated with physical inactivity, specifically CAD, stroke, colon cancer, breast cancer, and type 2 diabetes (Katzmarzyk et al. 2000). A similar figure was reported for the United States in 1995 ($24 billion or 2.4% of the U.S. health care expenditures) (Colditz 1999).

Katzmarzyk et al. (2000) hypothesized that if physical inactivity were completely eliminated in Canada, life expectancy could theoretically increase and 33% of deaths from CAD, colon cancer, and type 2 diabetes could hypothetically be prevented. Similarly, it has been estimated that about one-third of the deaths from CAD, colon cancer, and diabetes in the United States are attributable to inactivity. After recalculation of the direct health care costs attributable to physical inactivity with a reduction of 10% in the prevalence of inactivity (56% vs. 62%), which yielded a cost of $1.97 billion, it was concluded that a 10% reduction would result in savings of about $150 million per year in direct health care expenditures (Colditz 1999; Katzmarzyk et al. 2000).

These estimates do not even take into account the additional risks that inactivity poses for people with stroke, osteoporosis, and depression; nor does it address the issue of quality of life for these and other classes of people. Abundant literature shows the benefits to overall health and quality of life from even moderate amounts of physical activity.

Figure 7.1 compares years of healthy life and life expectancy among the major race/ethnic groups in the United States. Years of healthy life are at least 11 years less than total life expectancy. The difference between total life expectancy and years of healthy life is greater among blacks and Hispanics (around 14 years) than among whites or all races combined (around 12 years). The average American life expectancy had increased to 77.3 years by 2002 (Arias 2003, 2004); yet figure 7.2 shows that the prevalence of high levels of physical activity decrease as the population becomes older (Barnes and Schoenborn 2003). The ability to be independent, functional, and to perform activities of daily living is closely related to being physically active later in life.

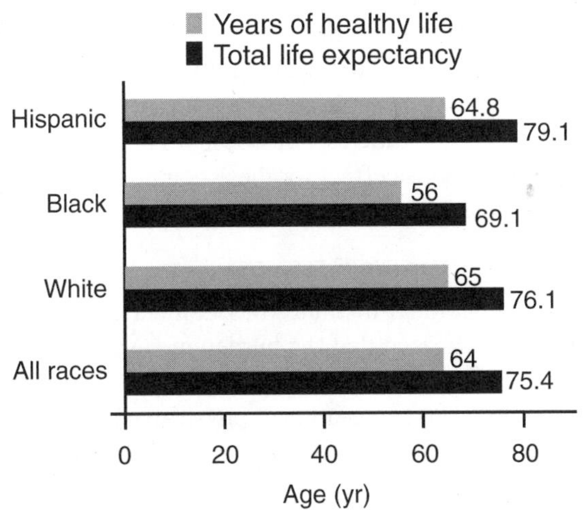

Figure 7.1 Total life expectancy and years of healthy life: United States, 1990.

Source: Erickson, Wilson, and Shannon 1995.

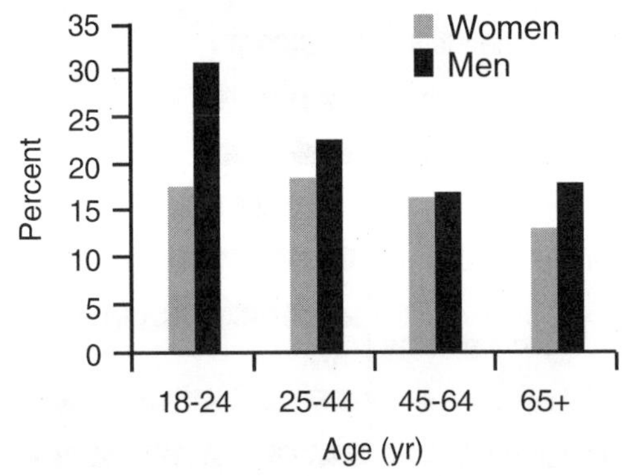

Figure 7.2 Percent of adults achieving high activity levels: United States, 2000.

Note: High activity level is defined as being very active during usual daily activities and engaged in regular leisure-time physical activity.

Source: Barnes and Schoenborn 2003.

Recently, attention has shifted to children, who are displaying increasing rates of childhood obesity and juvenile diabetes. There is evidence that, in this population, activities of a moderate intensity enhance overall health and play a role in preventing chronic disease in at-risk youth (Sothern et al. 1999). Some chronic conditions can severely limit participation in major or outdoor activities for both adults and children. Figures 7.3 and 7.4 show that heart, respiratory, and musculoskeletal problems are primary culprits in limiting physical activities. Table 7.2 shows the top causes of death in the general population as well as in population subgroups. The remainder of this chapter examines the effect of physical activity, exercise training, or physical fitness in the primary prevention of selected chronic diseases shown in table 7.2 and figures 7.3 and 7.4.

Physical Activity and Prevention of Heart Disease

Heart disease, sometimes referred to as cardiovascular disease (CVD), is a general name for more than 20 different diseases of the heart and its vessels. Coronary heart disease (CHD), the number one cause of death

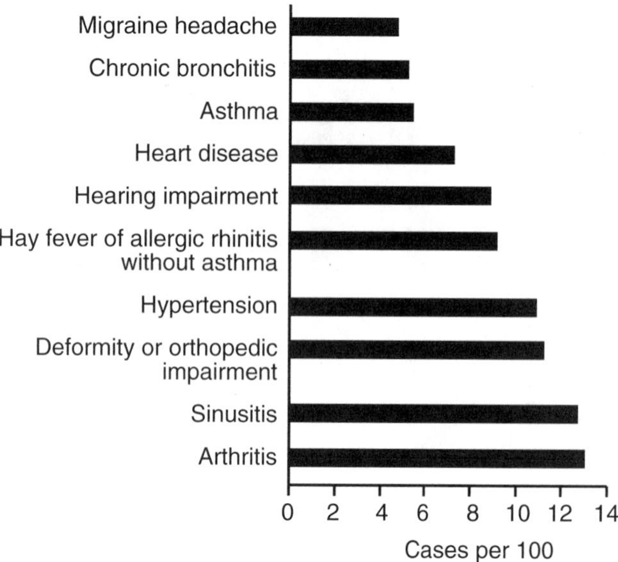

Figure 7.3 Top 10 chronic conditions with highest prevalence in rank order: United States, 1995.

Source: Adams, Hendershot, and Marano 1999.

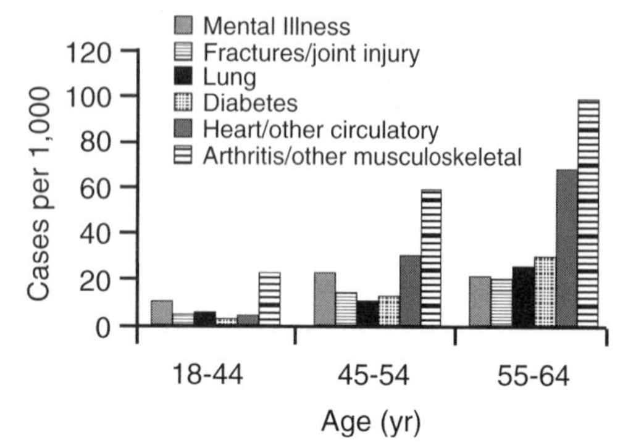

Figure 7.4 Selected chronic conditions causing limitation of activity among working-age adults by age: United States, 2000-2002.

Source: National Center for Health Statistics 2004.

in the United States for both men and women of all racial backgrounds, is one of the most prevalent forms of heart disease and of chronic disease. It is also one of the chronic diseases that causes very high levels of limitation in major or outside activity (see figure 7.4) (National Center for Health Statistics 2004).

Physical Activity and Cardiovascular Disease in General

Physical inactivity is a major independent risk factor for heart disease (NIH 1996; USDHHS 1996). The evidence that physical activity protects against CHD is dramatic, with a clear dose-response effect between physical activity and lower incidence of heart disease. A number of longitudinal, cross-sectional, clinical trials and case-control studies strongly suggest a cause-effect relationship (Blair et al. 1995; Blair et al. 1996; Leon 1991; McBride et al. 1992; USDHHS 1996).

Postmortem studies have shown that death from CHD is twice as common, and occurs at an earlier age, in men who perform light occupational tasks as in those who do heavy work. Physically active men have significantly larger coronary artery luminal areas, less frequent complete or nearly complete coronary occlusions, and less ischemic myocardial damage than less active workers (Leon and Norstrom 1995).

To be effective in preventing coronary heart disease, exercise must be habitual, maintained, and current. Engaging in school athletics does not protect against heart disease later in life, and there is convincing evidence that coronary atherosclerosis originates in adolescence, if not earlier. The general public recommendation to accumulate 30 min of daily physical activity on most, but preferably all, days of the week was recently modified by the National Academy of Science Institute of Medicine to at least 60 min of cumulative daily physical activity in order to maximize cardiovascular health (McKechnie and Mosca 2003). However, critics of the new recommendation argue that this recommendation is so impractical that some people have rejected it. Since epidemiologic data suggest that even 30 min per day of brisk walking can reduce cardiovascular disease risk across gender, public health efforts to promote moderate increases in physical activity may provide the optimal balance between efficacy and feasibility in our largely sedentary society (Bassuk and Manson 2003). Because it is associated with a decrease in CHD, physical activity is today's best buy in public health, especially when one considers the relatively small investment of time, effort, and money that moderate-intensity physical activity requires. Physical activity also provides indirect benefits by reducing other risk factors such as hypertension, hyperlipidemia, diabetes, and obesity. There appears to be a dose-response effect for these conditions (Haskell 1995; Morris 1994).

Some Landmark Studies

At a 1995 National Institutes of Health conference, an expert panel agreed that the burden of CVD and other chronic diseases rests most heavily on the least active (NIH 1996). This association of physical inactivity with CVD is independent of blood pressure, smoking, and blood lipid levels. Many studies have observed that physical activity has a negative association with body fat and a positive association with HDL. Moderately intense physical activity, that need be neither vigorous nor in a structured program, apparently provides the

Table 7.2 Age-Adjusted Death Rates From Selected Chronic Conditions by Race and Gender: United States, 2002

	Age-adjusted rates per 100,000 population				
Cause of death	**All persons**	**Male**	**Female**	**Whites**	**Blacks**
Major cardiovascular diseases	240.8	297.4	197.2	236.7	308.4
Ischemic heart disease	170.8	220.4	133.6	169.8	203.0
Malignant neoplasm	193.5	238.9	163.1	191.7	238.8
Trachea, bronchus, lung	54.9	73.2	41.6	55.3	61.9
Colon, rectum, and anus	19.7	23.7	16.7	19.2	26.8
Prostate†	27.9	27.9	–	25.7	62.0
Breast‡	25.6	–	25.6	25.0	34.0
Cerebrovascular disease	56.2	56.5	55.2	54.2	76.3
Chronic lower respiratory diseases	43.5	53.5	37.4	45.4	24.0
Diabetes mellitus	25.4	28.6	23.0	23.1	49.5
Suicide	10.9	18.4	4.2	12.0	5.3
HIV	4.9	7.4	2.5	2.6	22.5

† Rate for male population only.

‡ Rate for female population only.

Source: National Center for Health Statistics, 2004, *Health, United States, 2004 With Chartbook on Trends in the Health of Americans*. Hyattsville, MD: National Center for Health Statistics.

majority of the preventive benefits of physical activity (Haennel and Lemire 2002). The greatest difference in risk is between those people who do almost nothing and those who regularly perform a moderate amount of exercise. A much smaller risk differential is observed between moderately active and the most active individuals (Bijnen et al. 1996; Haskell 1995; Lakka and Salonen 1993; NIH 1996).

A meta-analysis by Berlin and Colditz (1990) showed that the negative correlation between exercise and CVD is generally stronger when one compares high-activity groups with sedentary groups rather than with moderately active groups.

Physical activity protects both men and women from CVD. Folsom et al. (1997) examined the relationship between physical activity and the incidence of CHD in middle-aged women and men from the Atherosclerosis Risk in Community Study (ARIC), tracking a biracial sample of middle-aged adults over a 4- to 7-year period. The study included 7852 women and 6188 men aged 45 to 64 years who were free of CHD at baseline, and recorded participation in sports, leisure pursuits, and two indexes of work-related physical activity. After adjustment for age, race, ARIC field center, education level, cigarette smoking, alcohol, and (in women) hormone replacement therapy (HRT), the sports and leisure indexes were inversely related to both CHD and total mortality. Physical activity during work was not associated with a protective role against CHD. The findings also confirmed that physical activity can be effective in preventing CHD among women.

Postmenopausal women can lower their risk of nonfatal myocardial infarction (MI) by being more physically active. Lamaitre et al. (1995) compared women who had sustained a nonfatal myocardial infarction (n = 268) to a random sample of women ($n = 925$) enrolled in the same health maintenance organization (HMO), matched by age and calendar year between 1986 and 1991. Women who engaged in modest leisure-time energy expenditures, equivalent to 30 to 45 min of walking three times a week, had approximately 50% fewer MIs (Manson et al. 2002).

MECHANISMS OF HEART DISEASE PREVENTION AND EXERCISE

The biological mechanisms through which physical activity mediates its positive effects appear to be the following:

1. Reduction in severity of coronary atherosclerosis both directly and through favorable effects on other major coronary risk factors (body composition, blood pressure, HDLs, insulin sensitivity, and glucose tolerance)
2. Reduction in myocardial oxygen demands at rest and during submaximal physical effort, evidenced

by decreased heart rate and systolic blood pressure (SBP)

3. Increased myocardial oxygen supply through lengthening of diastole, slowed heart rate, and/or increased vascularization
4. Reduction in risk of coronary thrombosis by decreased platelet adhesiveness and aggregability and by promotion of fibrinolysis
5. Reduced myocardial vulnerability to lethal ventricular arrhythmias in the presence of advanced coronary atherosclerosis, even during heavy physical exertion (Leon and Norstrom 1995; USDHHS 1996)

Previous studies have shown that physical activity exerts an independent effect in the prevention of CHD. However, physical activity indirectly ameliorates other coronary risk factors, leading to decreased hypertension, more favorable body composition, more favorable blood lipid profile (including lowered levels of plasma triglycerides and their lipoprotein carriers), and improvements in cell insulin sensitivity and glucose tolerance (Andersen and Haraldsdottir 1995; Bijnen et al. 1996; Leon 1991; McKechnie and Mosca 2003).

Exercise in the Prevention of Hypertensive Disease

New guidelines for hypertension prevention and management suggest that even individuals with a systolic blood pressure (SBP) of 120 to 139 mmHg or a diastolic blood pressure (DBP) of 80 to 89 mmHg should be considered as pre-hypertensive and require health-promoting lifestyle modifications to prevent CVD. Recommendations include engaging in regular aerobic physical activity, such as brisk walking, at least 30 min per day on most days of the week (Chobanian et al. 2003). Cross-sectional data from the civilian noninstitutionalized population of the United States show a substantial reduction in the prevalence of hypertension among those who are active most days of the week, as compared with those who engage in no leisure-time physical activity (Crespo and Roccella 1997).

Studies on Blood Pressure and Exercise

Several longitudinal studies have confirmed the trend of higher hypertension among those less physically active. Paffenbarger and colleagues (1983) studied approximately 15,000 Harvard University alumni and found that those who were inactive had a 35% greater risk of developing hypertension than their more active counterparts. In a study of approximately 6000 men and women, Blair et al. (1984) observed that people with low fitness levels were 1.52 (95% CI, 1.08-2.15) times as likely to develop hypertension as those with high fitness levels.

Folsom et al. (1990) reported on the longitudinal effect of physical activity among more than 41,000 women, ages 55 to 69 years. After a two-year follow-up, incidence of physician-diagnosed hypertension was inversely associated with physical activity; however, after adjustment for body mass index, waist-to-hip ratio, cigarette smoking, and age, this association disappeared. The consistent pattern among these studies is the association of physical *in*activity with higher risks of developing hypertension. Unfortunately, no longitudinal study has tested the protective role of physical activity in minority populations, who consistently exhibit a disproportionate risk of developing and dying from hypertension.

In a study aimed at finding out whether regular physical activity can reduce the risk of hypertension in both men and women, and in subjects with and without overweight, Hu et al. (2004) prospectively followed 8302 Finnish men and 9139 women aged 25 to 64 years without a history of antihypertensive drug use, coronary heart disease, stroke, or heart failure. They examined both single and joint associations of physical activity and body mass index with the risk of hypertension. Multivariate-adjusted hazards ratios of hypertension associated with light, moderate, and high physical activity were 1.00, 0.63, and 0.59 in men ($p < .001$) and 1.00, 0.82, and 0.71 in women ($p = .005$), respectively. This association persisted both in subjects who were overweight and in those who were not. Multivariate-adjusted hazards ratios of hypertension based at different levels of body mass index (<25, 25-29.9, and ≥30) were 1.00, 1.18, and 1.66 for men ($p < .001$) and 1.00, 1.24, and 1.32 for women ($p = .007$), respectively. This study indicates that regular physical activity and weight control can reduce the risk of hypertension. The protective effect of physical activity was observed in both sexes regardless of obesity.

According to the American College of Sports Medicine's position, it has been firmly established that individuals who engage in some form of physical activity, either by lifestyle or by occupation, are likely to live longer and healthier lives. The college cites research showing that even moderate caloric expenditure from physical activity has a significant impact on life span. The college also states that a physically active person who possesses such factors as hypertension, diabetes, and even a smoking habit can derive significant gains from incorporating regular physical activity into his or her daily activities. Regular physical activity is also likely to help modify a number of risk factors. Additionally, regular exercise is associated with reduction in blood pressure, improved glucose regulation, promotion of better lipid profiles, and stronger/denser bones (American College of Sports Medicine [ACSM] 2002).

Confounding Factors

The effect of exercise on blood pressure can be confounded by changes in body composition and improvements in psychosocial behaviors. Comparing a sedentary population with 571 men and 430 women who had enrolled in a vigorous fitness program, Sedgwick and colleagues (1993) examined the effect of physical fitness on blood pressure and lipid profile over a period of 4 years. They observed almost no direct effect of exercise on either blood pressure or lipids, except for a weak correlation among the women. Almost all the positive effects could be explained by changes in body composition.

Exercise and Mechanisms of Reducing Blood Pressure

The mechanisms by which physical activity lowers blood pressure are complicated (ACSM 1993). There is consensus that physical activity not only is effective in treating hypertension, but also provides significant benefits in preventing hypertension. Some researchers believe that, in addition to its effect on body weight, chronic exercise training attenuates sympathetic nervous system activity, which in turn may decrease the activity of the renin-angiotensin system, reset baroreceptors, or promote arterial vasodilation. Another hypothesis involves the effect of exercise on insulin sensitivity and circulating insulin levels: if exercise reduces insulin or prevents hyperinsulinemia, the kidneys presumably would reduce insulin-mediated sodium reabsorption (USDHHS 1996).

Ishikawa-Takata et al. (2003) examined the dose-response relationship between exercise training and blood pressure, using an 8-week exercise intervention involving 207 untreated subjects with stage 1 or 2 essential hypertension. Subjects were divided into five groups based on the duration and frequency/week of exercise (sedentary control, 30-60 min/week, 61-90 min/week, 91-120 min/week, and >120 min/week). Systolic and diastolic blood pressure at rest did not change in the sedentary control group. Significant reductions in both resting systolic and diastolic blood pressure were observed in all four exercise groups. The magnitude of reductions in systolic blood pressure was greater in the 61 to 90 min/week group compared with the 30 to 60 min/week group. The authors did not observe any obvious relationships between exercise frequency per week and magnitude of blood pressure decreases with exercise training. This study provides evidence that in previously sedentary hypertensive subjects, clinically significant decreases in blood pressure can be achieved with relatively modest increases in physical activity above sedentary levels, and that the volume of exercise required to reduce blood pressure may be relatively small and reasonably attainable by a sedentary hypertensive population.

The proposed mechanism by which exercise is cardioprotective involves reduction in endothelin-1 (ET-1). ET-1, which is produced by vascular endothelial cells, has potent constrictor and proliferative activity in vascular smooth muscle cells and therefore has been implicated in regulation of vascular tonus and progression of atherosclerosis. Maeda et al. hypothesized that plasma ET-1 concentration increases with age, even in healthy adults, and that lifestyle modification (i.e., exercise) can reduce plasma ET-1 concentration in previously sedentary older adults. They measured plasma ET-1 concentration in healthy young women (21-28 years old), healthy middle-aged women (31-47 years old), and healthy older women (61-69 years old). The plasma level of ET-1 significantly increased with aging (1.02 ± 0.08, 1.33 ± 0.11, and 2.90 ± 0.20 pg/ml in young, middle-aged, and older women, respectively), indicating that plasma ET-1 concentration was markedly higher in healthy older women than in healthy young or middle-aged women (by 3- and 2-fold, respectively). In healthy older women, Maeda and colleagues also measured plasma ET-1 concentration after three months of aerobic exercise (cycling on a leg ergometer at 80% of ventilatory threshold for 30 min, 5 days/week). They observed that regular exercise significantly decreased plasma ET-1 concentration in the healthy older women (2.22 ± 0.16 pg/ml, $p < 0.01$) and also significantly reduced their blood pressure. This study suggests that regular aerobic-endurance exercise reduces plasma ET-1 concentration in older women, and this reduction in plasma ET-1 concentration may have beneficial effects on the cardiovascular system in terms of progression of hypertension or atherosclerosis (or both) by endogenous ET-1.

Exercise and the Prevention of Stroke

Stroke is the third leading cause of death in the United States (see table 7.2) and one of the most disabling diseases affecting working Americans. Major risk factors for ischemic stroke include cigarette smoking and high blood pressure, while for hemorrhagic stroke high blood pressure seems to be the predominant risk factor. Figure 7.5 shows the steady decline in the percent of deaths due to stroke ("cerebrovascular accidents") in the United States since 1972. We can attribute part of this decline to decreases in the number of persons with high blood pressure, and, perhaps, to the reduction in

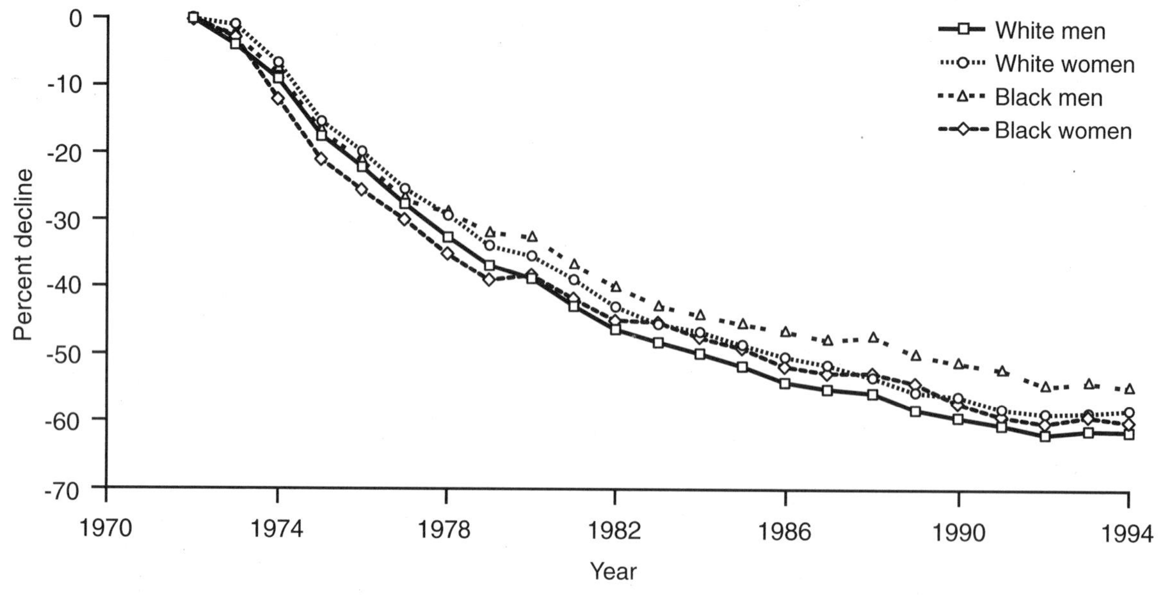

Figure 7.5 Percent decline in age-adjusted mortality rates for stroke by sex and race: United States, 1972-1994.
Source: U.S. National Vital Statistics, 1972-1994: CDC, NCHS.

cigarette smoking that has occurred during the same period. Stroke mortality among persons younger than 75 years of age continues to be higher among racial/ethnic minorities when compared with non-Hispanic whites (CDC 2005).

Kiely and colleagues (1994) prospectively examined the effect of physical activity on the risk of stroke for participants in the Framingham Study. They performed two separate analyses involving 1897 men and 2299 women with mean ages of around 49 years, and again when the cohorts were around 63 years of age (1361 men and 1862 women), calculating a physical activity index for leisure-time and occupational physical activities. The authors concluded that increased levels of physical activity offer a unique independent protective effect in men. It is possible that the women, the majority of whom were housewives, underestimated the level of physical activity associated with their housework and related activities.

Investigators found an inverse association for all strokes and subtypes in a longitudinal study of older Japanese men (ages 55-68 years) from the Honolulu Heart Program (Abbot et al. 1994), particularly in nonsmoking men. Among smokers, however, physical activity did not appear to reduce the risk of thromboembolic stroke. The incidence of hemorrhagic stroke was three- to fourfold greater among inactive older men than among their active counterparts. Wannamethee and Shaper reported in 1992 that moderate-intensity exercise, such as frequent walking and recreational activity, or weekly sporting activity, reduces the risk of stroke and heart attacks in men both with and without preexisting ischemic heart disease. More vigorous activity did not confer any further protection. Lindsted et al. (1991) assessed mortality due to stroke in Seventh Day Adventists. Based on a baseline assessment of physical activity in 1960, the authors observed a nonlinear "U-shape" association between physical activity and risk of stroke. This nonlinear association was based on classifications of low, moderate, and high activity levels, where the lowest risk was observed among those in the moderate category and higher risk was observed in the low and high activity categories. At the very least, these studies suggest in aggregate that moderate-intensity physical activity may confer a primary preventive effect against strokes; and that high-intensity physical activity appears to offer little or no more benefit than moderate activity (or perhaps even can be harmful, according to the Linsted paper).

Whether physical activity reduces stroke risk remains controversial. Lee et al. (2003) recently conducted a meta-analysis to examine the overall association between physical activity or cardiorespiratory fitness and stroke incidence or mortality. They found that there was a reduction in stroke risk for active or fit individuals compared with inactive or unfit persons in cohort and case-control studies and in the two study types combined. For cohort studies, highly active individuals had a 25% lower risk of stroke incidence or mortality (RR = 0.75; 95% CI, 0.69-0.82) compared with low-active individuals. For case-control studies, highly active individuals had a 64% lower risk of stroke incidence (RR = 0.36; 95% CI, 0.25-0.52) than their low-active counterparts. When cohort and case-control studies were combined, highly active individuals had a 27% lower risk of stroke incidence or mortality (RR = 0.73; 95% CI, 0.67-0.79) than did low-active individuals. Lee and associates observed similar results in moderately active individuals compared with inactive persons (RRs were 0.83 for cohort, 0.52 for case control, and 0.80 for the two study types combined). Additionally, moderately and highly active individuals had lower risk of both ischemic and hemorrhagic strokes than low-active individuals.

Another recent investigation yielded similar findings. Kurl et al. (2003) examined the relationship of cardiorespiratory fitness, as indicated by maximum oxygen consumption ($\dot{V}O_2max$), with subsequent incidence of stroke, using a population-based cohort study with an average follow-up of 11 years from Kuopio and surrounding communities of eastern Finland. The relative risk for any stroke in unfit men ($\dot{V}O_2max$ <25.2 mL/kg per minute) was 3.2 (95% CI, 1.71-6.12; $p < .001$; $p < .001$ for the trend across the quartiles) and for ischemic stroke was 3.50 (95% CI, 1.66-7.41; $p = .001$; $p < .001$ for trend across the quartiles) as compared with that for fit men ($\dot{V}O_2max$ >35.3 mL/kg per minute), after age and examination year were adjusted for. The associations remained statistically significant after further adjustment for smoking, alcohol consumption, socioeconomic status, energy expenditure of physical activity, prevalent CHD, diabetes, SBP, and serum LDL-C level for any stroke or ischemic stroke. Low cardiorespiratory fitness was comparable with other modifiable risk factors such as SBP, obesity, alcohol consumption, smoking, and serum LDL-C level as a risk factor for stroke.

Exercise and Some Emerging Risk Factors for Heart Disease

A reduction in plasma fibrinogen is one mechanism through which physical activity may protect against CHD. Several studies have associated fibrinogen with increased risk of heart disease. In 1993, Lakka and Salonen reported the effect of conditioning leisure-time physical activity and cardiorespiratory fitness on plasma fibrinogen concentration in smokers and nonsmokers from the Kuopio Ischemic Heart Disease Risk Factor Study. Plasma fibrinogen was lower among men whose activity intensity averaged more than 4 METs than among men with less intensive physical activity. Durations of the most intensive activities, such as jogging and skiing, were inversely associated with plasma fibrinogen, as was maximal oxygen uptake. The effect was even more pronounced among smokers. These findings suggest that moderate-intensity physical activity is sufficient, but vigorous physical activity is more effective, in reducing fibrinogen, and that physical activity vigorous enough to elevate maximal oxygen uptake has the strongest effect in decreasing plasma fibrinogen. The researchers found no relationship, however, between weekly sessions of vigorous exercise and plasma fibrinogen.

Exercise can also prevent heart disease by inducing adaptations of myocardial blood vessels, such as the development of new capillaries and coronary arterioles (Laughlin 1994; Leon and Norstrom 1995). Niebauer and Cooke (1996) suggested that exercise is associated positively with nitric oxide and prostacyclin, and eventually with reducing the generation of superoxide anions, adherence of monocytes, aggregation of platelets, and proliferation of vascular smooth muscle.

Exercise and Prevention of Peripheral Artery Disease

Peripheral artery disease, characterized by the inability of the circulatory system to deliver oxygenated blood to the limbs, limits activity by decreasing the total cross-sectional area of vascular flow. Housley et al. (1993) examined the protective effects of physical activity on peripheral arterial disease in 1592 men and women, ages 55 to 74 years, from the Edinburgh Artery Study in Scotland. The authors queried the subjects about their participation in moderate and strenuous physical activity between the ages of 35 and 45, and compared those histories to physical activity habits at time of the survey. Decreasing levels of the ankle brachial pressure index (proxy measure of physical activity level) were associated with increased severity of peripheral artery disease. Multiple regression analysis showed that the association of increased ankle brachial pressure index with exercise was most noticeable in men who had at some time in their lives smoked. In men and women who had never smoked, there was no significant association between leisure-time physical activity and the change in mean ankle brachial pressure index after correcting for the other risk factors. Thus, among men who had smoked, leisure-time physical activity seems to exert a protective effect against the development of peripheral artery disease later in life.

Exercise and Prevention of Type 2 Diabetes

One of the most important modifiable risk factors for primary prevention of type 2 (non-insulin-dependent) diabetes is physical inactivity. Most of the direct effect of physical activity in preventing type 2 diabetes occurs because exercise normalizes blood glucose by decreasing insulin resistance and improving insulin sensitivity (Sato et al. 2003). Examining the effect of exercise on glucose tolerance and insulin sensitivity, Heath et al. (1983) found that active individuals had better insulin and glucose profiles than their inactive counterparts. Several studies have shown that exercise training can improve insulin action or decrease insulin resistance, especially among persons at high risk for diabetes or those with hyperinsulinemia.

Significant Studies

Considerable evidence supports the independent effect of physical inactivity in the development of type 2 diabetes. Cross-sectional, longitudinal, and retrospective studies have consistently shown that physically active individuals are less likely to develop diabetes than physically inactive people. Groups of people who migrated to societies with more sedentary lifestyles displayed higher prevalences of type 2 diabetes than their ethnic counterparts who remained in their native lands (Hara et al. 1983; Kawate et al. 1979; Ravussin et al. 1994). Similar findings were observed among urban and rural residents (Cruz-Vidal et al. 1979; Taylor et al. 1983). In a case-control study, Kaye and colleagues (1991) found that women who reported high levels of physical activity were half as likely to develop type 2 diabetes as were women in the same age range with low levels of physical activity. Moderately active women also enjoyed the protective effect of physical activity, but to a lesser extent.

Manson et al. (1991) reported a protective effect against type 2 diabetes among female nurses who reported being vigorously active one or more times per week, as compared to less active female nurses. However, since the assessment of activity in this study consisted of only one question about participation in vigorous physical activity, the authors could say nothing about moderate physical activity. Similar findings were observed with male physicians (Manson et al. 1992).

In another prospective study, Helmrich and colleagues (1994) expanded their assessment of leisure-time physical activity to include walking, stair climbing, and participation in sports. They observed an inverse correlation between physical activity and incidence of type 2 diabetes; the reduced likelihood of type 2 diabetes was more clearly manifested among men with a high body mass index (BMI), a history of high blood pressure, or a parental history of diabetes. For every 500 kilocalories per week of leisure-time physical activity, the authors reported a 6% reduction in the risk of developing type 2 diabetes. Furthermore, among this group of male college graduates, the protective effect of physical activity was greater among those who participated in vigorous sports than among those who obtained their physical activity mostly from climbing stairs or walking.

In these three prospective studies, two (those involving men) found a dose-response relationship. Although female nurses who participated one or more times per week in vigorous physical activity had a significantly reduced likelihood of developing type 2 diabetes, the Manson study failed to show a dose-response relationship.

Recent randomized clinical trials have also demonstrated that lifestyle change can significantly reduce the risk of type 2 diabetes in individuals with impaired glucose tolerance. The Finnish Diabetes Prevention Study and the Diabetes Prevention Program in the United States, in particular, have shown that modest weight change and achievable physical activity goals can translate into significant risk reduction for developing diabetes (Ryan and Diabetes Prevention Program Research Group 2003).

Most Effective Physical Activities for Diabetes Prevention

What type of physical activity is most effective for preventing type 2 diabetes? Aerobic activities, such as brisk walking, biking, swimming, or other activities that use large muscle mass, are probably best for the general public because of their demonstrated benefits in decreasing both type 2 diabetes and cardiovascular risk factors. This recommendation, however, is based on epidemiological data that examined the specific benefits of aerobic physical activities or cardiorespiratory fitness on primary prevention of type 2 diabetes. Strength training, as part of an overall exercise training program that includes aerobic activity, can also provide acute benefits to improve glucose tolerance and insulin sensitivity in individuals with both normal and abnormal glucose tolerance (Kriska 1997; Smutok et al. 1994). However, some recent studies have shown that intense exercise provokes the release of insulin-counterregulatory hormones such as glucagons and catecholamines, which ultimately cause a reduction in the insulin action. Intense exercise has been characterized as exercise that results in $\dot{V}O_2$max of about 50% (plus heart rate of about 120/min for those in their 50s or younger and about 100/min for those in their 60s and 70s), and the recommended type is aerobic exercise, which uses muscles throughout the whole body (e.g., jogging, gymnastic exercise, stationary bicycle exercise, and swimming).

Continued physical training improves the reduced peripheral tissue sensitivity to insulin associated with impaired glucose tolerance and type 2 diabetes, along with regularization of abnormal lipid metabolism (Sato et al. 2003). Therefore, moderate- or low-intensity exercise is recommended. Low- and moderate-intensity physical activities are also easier to incorporate into people's lifestyles, are less likely to result in injury, and (if the population is mostly sedentary) are more likely to be maintained for life (Kriska 2003). It is not certain if lower-intensity activities will help prevent type 2 diabetes in women, since no dose-response relationship has been observed in women. But given the dose-response data for men, one can assume that low to moderate levels of activity will at least provide some protection.

Another benefit of regular physical activity is its effect on body composition. National cross-sectional data indicate that over 60% of people with type 2 diabetes are obese at the time of diagnosis (Diabetes Data Group 1995). Obesity and (probably more importantly) central fat distribution seem to be additional primary risk factors for development of type 2 diabetes. Because increased adiposity in the abdominal (as opposed to the peripheral) area boosts the likelihood that individuals will develop insulin resistance, it is strongly involved in the pathogenesis of type 2 diabetes. Numerous studies have demonstrated the ability of exercise to affect body weight. Physical activity appears to prevent type 2 diabetes, not only by decreasing adiposity; it also acutely affects insulin resistance and glucose tolerance. Much of the effect of physical activity appears to be due to the metabolic adaptation of skeletal muscle, suggesting that exercise training helps prevent type 2 diabetes by increasing sensitivity to insulin. More specifically, it appears that physical activity is more likely to improve abnormal glucose tolerance when the abnormality is caused primarily by insulin resistance than when it is caused by deficient amounts of circulating insulin (Kriska 1997).

Nevertheless, because the effect of exercise that is manifested in improved insulin sensitivity decreases within 3 days after exercise and is not even apparent after 1 week, a continued regimen is necessary (Sato et al. 2003).

EXERCISE AND PRIMARY PREVENTION OF CANCER

Cancer, from which deaths are increasing every year (Peters et al. 1998), is the second leading cause of death in the United States and is also responsible for many days spent in hospital care (Lee 1995). Although the etiologic factors are highly variable, certain cancers are associated with certain behaviors or lifestyles, usually identified through epidemiological studies and not because we have discovered any plausible mechanisms of action. Of course everyone is aware that lung cancer is directly associated with the cancer-causing agents found in cigarettes. Other behaviors associated with different cancers include excess alcohol consumption, diet, and physical inactivity.

According to the American Cancer Society's Web site, a third of all cancer deaths can be attributed to poor diet and physical inactivity (American Cancer Society 2004). Epidemiological evidence has revealed an inverse relationship between increased physical activity and decreased incidence or mortality rates (or both) for various cancers. Physically active people have been shown to have a decreased rate of all-cancer mortality, and the incidence of certain cancers is decreased in more active people when compared with their sedentary peers. This relationship appears strongest for colon cancer and female estrogen-dependent cancers of the breast, ovary, and endometrium (Kiningham 1998; Woods 1998). While some epidemiological studies have controlled for numerous confounding variables such as smoking, body mass index, and percent body fat, it is still difficult to determine whether physical activity affects cancer risk independent of an improved lifestyle and other potential confounding factors (Friedenreich and Orenstein 2002; Woods 1998).

ANTI-CANCER BENEFITS OF EXERCISE

Our immune systems largely regulate our susceptibility to cancer. We have evidence that engaging in moderately intense physical activity can enhance our immune capabilities (Nieman and Nehlsen-Cannarella 1992; Nieman et al. 1995). On the other hand, higher-intensity physical activities, such as running a marathon, appear to suppress the immune system. There seems to be a threshold in the duration and intensity of physical activity that determines whether it will enhance or compromise the immune system.

Some proposed mechanisms by which physical activity decreases cancer risk include decreased lifetime exposure to estrogen or other hormones, reduced body fat, enhanced gut motility, improved anti-oxidant defenses, and stimulation of anti-tumor immune defenses (Woods 1998).

An expert group, convened by the International Agency for Research on Cancer of the World Health Organization, concluded that limiting weight gain during adult life, thereby avoiding overweight and obesity, reduces the risk of various cancers. They considered that excess body weight and physical inactivity account for approximately a quarter to one-third of cancers of the colon, breast, endometrium, kidney, and esophagus. Their claims suggest that adiposity and physical inactivity are the most important avoidable causes of these cancers (Vaino et al. 2002). On the basis of existing evidence, some public health organizations have issued physical activity guidelines for cancer prevention, recommending at least 30 min of moderate- to vigorous-intensity physical activity on 5 or more days per week (Friedenreich and Orenstein 2002).

SIGNIFICANT STUDIES

Physical activity has been inversely associated with cancer mortality in a number of studies. Wannamethee and colleagues reported in 1993 on the relationship between resting heart rate, usual physical activity, and cancer mortality in 7735 men from the British Regional Heart Study. Men were followed for approximately 9.5 years and classified into three physical activity categories. Resting heart rate provided the basis for five categories: <60 bpm, 60 to 69 bpm, 70 to 79 bpm, 80 to 89 bpm, and >90 bpm. Lower resting heart rates were correlated with higher levels of physical activity and with lower cancer mortality rates.

Steenland et al. (1995) reported an inverse association between pulse and cancer mortality in the general population. The data for this study came from the National Health and Nutrition Survey I Follow-Up conducted in the early 1970s and then repeated in 1987. The authors found a modest positive trend between heart rate (highest quartile compared to lowest quartile) and all cancers for men, but not for women. They observed no significant effect for nonrecreational physical activity. The authors caution that lack of participation in nonrecreational physical activity may be an artifact of an existing condition that limits physical activity.

Current research certainly does not justify claims that physical activity can affect all kinds of cancer mortality; however, the observed inverse correlation between low resting heart rates and cancer mortality could be an indicator of a general inverse association between physical fitness and cancer. We need more data.

COLON CANCER

Earlier studies examining the association between physical activity and cancer of the intestinal tract combined data for colon and rectal cancers. We know now that the effect of exercise on colon cancer may be different from that on rectal cancer (USDHHS 1996). The presence of adenomatous polyps in the colon and rectum are believed to be precursors of colorectal cancers. Sandler and colleagues (1995) reported that the risk of developing colorectal adenomatous polyps was inversely associated with physical activity.

Most of the research on physical activity and colon cancer has focused on occupational physical activity, with the majority of studies showing that this type of activity plays a protective role against developing colon cancer. Of the 18 studies described in the Surgeon General's report in 1996 (USDHHS 1996), 14 showed a statistically significant inverse relationship between occupational physical activity and the risk of colon cancer. More recently Kiningham (1998) reviewed 36 studies of men and 21 studies of women, and concluded that physically active men appear to have about half the colon cancer risk of sedentary men. The relationship between women's physical activity and colon cancer was less clear than that observed in men. Many of the studies reviewed included few women with high or moderately high levels of physical activity, so the statistical power to distinguish a difference between activity groups was low. Nevertheless, the bulk of the data suggested a trend toward decreased risk with increased activity in both men and women.

SIGNIFICANT STUDIES

Some researchers have done more carefully designed assessments of leisure-time physical activity or total physical activity in longitudinal or retrospective studies. Most studies show inverse relationships between physical activity and colon cancer.

A case-control Swedish study of 163 men and 189 women, who had been diagnosed with colon cancer, along with 512 matched controls, obtained from a computerized registry of the population of Stockholm County, examined the relationships of occupational and leisure-time physical activity with incidence of colon cancer. Cases were obtained from various hospitals in Stockholm County and from the regional cancer registry. The researchers assessed dietary intake of fiber, fat, protein, browned meat surface, and total energy (Gerhardsson et al. 1990), and stratified participants by levels of leisure-time and occupational physical activity. After adjusting for age, body mass index, and diet, the authors observed a higher incidence of colon cancer in the lower than in the higher physical activity group. There was, in fact, a dose-response relationship between increased levels of physical activity and lower risk of colon cancer.

Giovannucci and colleagues (1995) evaluated data from 47,723 men aged 40 to 75 years, recording weekly participation in leisure-time physical activity and risk of cancer. The investigators used a recreational physical activity index to stratify individuals into quintiles, from least active to most active. This study was unique in that the investigators were able to control for history of endoscopic screening or any diagnosis of polyp, as well as dietary components. Not only did the most active quintile have the lowest incidence of colon cancer, but there was also an inverse dose-response relationship between physical activity and incidence of colon cancer.

CONCLUSIONS ABOUT EXERCISE AND COLON CANCER

Substantial evidence shows that physical activity, after adjusting for family history; for dietary intake of fat, fiber, and total energy; and in some instances for presence of polyps, is inversely related to colon cancer. It is impossible to determine the most beneficial kind of physical activity, since researchers have not designed their projects for that purpose. Studies on occupational physical activity, despite their crudeness, do suggest that occupations with higher energy expenditure enjoy a protective benefit against the development of colon cancer.

In studies of leisure-time physical activity, the protective effect seems to occur among those engaged in higher levels of physical activity. Besides the direct effects that physical activity has on the immune system, the following mechanisms may partially explain the indirect benefits of exercise in preventing of colon cancer:

1. **Shortened intestinal transit time**—most likely because higher-intensity exercises increase peristaltic movement.
2. **Decreased body fat**—abdominal obesity and high-fat diets are risk factors for colon cancer.
3. **Secretion of F-series prostaglandins**—these have been associated with increased gut motility and decreased rates of colonic cell division.
4. **Reduced hyperinsulinemia**—insulin is a growth factor for colonic mucosal cells; and any factor that increases insulin levels may increase colon cancer risk (Kiningham 1998).

Suggestions for Future Research

Given that cancer is a complex disease with multiple etiologic factors, we have yet to solve the problem of controlling for multiple factors (e.g., diet, environmental carcinogens, and socioeconomic status) that are important in evaluating the evidence of a protective effect of physical activity against colon cancer.

Longitudinal studies would benefit from multiple assessments of physical activity throughout individuals' lives. Additionally, the complexities in both the etiology and the development of colon cancer call for careful analyses of intakes of dietary fiber, alcohol, tobacco smoke, fat, and total energy, and also for controls relating to family histories of adenomatous polyps and colon cancer. Few, if any, studies to date have properly assessed all of these confounding factors.

Endometrial Cancer

The etiology and pathogenesis of endometriosis are not well understood, and prevalence estimates vary according to the study population, making it difficult to determine risk factors for the disease (Holt and Weiss 2000). However, environmental and behavioral factors that can potentially influence endogenous factors are of particular interest in prevention of this disease. Regular exercise, which is associated with reduced cumulative exposure to menstrual flow, decreased ovarian stimulation, and estradiol production, is one such factor (Warren and Perlroth 2001).

Prior studies of the association between endometriosis and physical activity have yielded mixed results. A population-based, cross-sectional survey in a Norwegian county found no association, while two case-control studies in the United States reported a decreased endometriosis risk associated with strenuous exercise for at least 3 hours per week (Cramer et al. 1986; Moen and Schei 1997; Signorello et al. 1997). More recently, Dhillon and Holt (2003) evaluated the risk of endometriomas associated with physical activity, both in the recent past and during adolescence and early adulthood. They found that women who reported frequent, high-intensity activity during the 2 years prior to the reference date had a 76% reduced endometrioma risk compared with women who engaged in no high-intensity activity (Dhillon and Holt 2003). The reduction in risk for women who reported such activity at ages 12 to 21 years was nonsignificant, and activities of lower intensity, frequency, and duration were not associated with a woman's risk of endometrioma. While study findings suggest a reduced endometrioma risk associated with regular, high-intensity physical activity during adulthood, there is a need to investigate whether the potential benefits of vigorous and consistent physical activity extend to other affected sites and types of this disease.

Breast Cancer

More women are diagnosed with breast cancer every year than with any other cancer. It is true that effective treatment, early detection, and modification of risk factors have decreased mortality rates due to breast cancer in recent years, yet breast cancer is still the leading cancer killer after lung cancer. Epidemiological data have suggested that obesity, fat intake, nulliparity, and full-term pregnancy after age 35 are possible risk factors.

Significant Studies

Frisch et al. (1985) described an independent and inverse correlation between physical activity and breast cancer. They contacted more than 5300 alumnae from 10 colleges or universities who attended their respective institutions between the years of 1925 and 1981. About half of these women were former athletes, who were matched by a random sample of nonathletes from the same schools. Nonathletes were 86% more likely to develop breast cancer than their athlete counterparts, even after controlling for traditional risk factors.

Some research, however, has found a positive relationship between physical activity and breast cancer. Dorgan and colleagues (1994) found that women in the highest quartile of physical activity were more likely to develop breast cancer than women in the lowest quartile. The researchers followed more than 2300 women in the Framingham Heart Study for approximately 30 years, finally observing that physically active women had 1.6 times the breast cancer risk of those in the least active quartile. This study had the advantage of periodic examinations and adjustments for several confounding factors. However, lack of additional assessments of physical activity after 1954 may not accurately describe secular trends in physical activity among women during these years.

More recently, Chen et al. (1997) found that leisure-time physical activity either during adolescence or in adulthood played no protective role against breast cancer. For this study the investigators selected 747 women aged 21 to 45 years from the Seattle-Puget Sound Surveillance, Epidemiology, and End Results registry who had developed breast cancer and matched them with 961 women from the same area who were free from cancer and otherwise healthy. Leisure-time physical activity was assessed for the two-year period immediately prior to the time of diagnosis, and for the period when the participants had been between the ages of 12 and 21 years. Breast cancer was associated with neither frequency of participation in physical activity, nor hours per week engaged in physical activity, nor METs per week, whether before diagnosis or during adolescent years.

Other retrospective case-control studies have observed a protective role of exercise against breast cancer. Apter (1996) examined 537 women aged 50 to 64 years and matched them with 492 randomly selected women. This time Apter found that, compared to women who reported no exercise, there was a slightly decreased risk of breast cancer in women who exercised more than 1.5 hours per week in the 2 years before the diagnosis of breast cancer. There was no association between the risk of breast cancer and intensity of exercise at ages 12 to 21 years.

Bernstein et al. (1994) studied 545 women aged 40 years or younger who had been diagnosed with breast cancer, and compared them with a control group of 545 healthy women from the same neighborhood matched according to age, race, and parity history. The investigators recorded the hours per week each woman engaged in leisure-time physical activity after reaching menarche, and classified the women into five categories of physical activity. Women who spent 3.8 hours per week of leisure-time physical activity were less likely (OR = 0.42, 95% CI, 0.27-0.64) to develop cancer than women who engaged in no leisure-time physical activity (all other known risk factors being controlled). There was a dose-response relationship, with higher weekly amounts of physical activity related to lower risks of developing breast cancer. The authors concluded that participation in physical activity after menarche is protective against breast cancer.

Mezzetti et al. (1998) examined the effects of diet and physical exercise on breast cancer risks in 2569 Italian women aged 23 to 74 years. The experimenters stratified women by menopausal status (pre- and post), age, education, body mass index, and alcohol intake. Physical exercise included self-reported intensity of activity at work and during leisure time. Women with low levels of physical exercise had 50% higher risk of developing breast cancer than women who were highly active. The protective effect of physical exercise was stronger among post- than among premenopausal women. In women less than 45 years old, Gammon and colleagues (1998) found that physical activity had no protective role against breast cancer. These women reported the intensity and frequency of physical activity during three different time periods that were relevant to two possible biological mechanisms. The authors did not observe a reduced risk of breast cancer among young women with increased recreational physical activity in adolescence, in young adulthood, or during the year prior to interviews.

Findings from longitudinal, case-control, and retrospective studies had been reported as inconclusive concerning the effect of physical activity in preventing breast cancer (Lee 1995; USDHHS 1996). Major problems in some of these earlier epidemiologic studies include crude and incomplete measurements of physical activity and inadequate control for potential confounding factors (Friedenreich and Rohan 1995). Designs of these studies also failed to accurately account for the duration, frequency, and intensity of the physical activity, making it very difficult at present to suggest what type, duration, frequency, or intensity is more protective against breast cancer. More recently, the International Agency on Cancer Research (IARC) concluded that there is consistent evidence to suggest that physical activity is protective against breast cancer (IARC 2002). Other more recent reviews confirm the fact that exercise does confer significant protective effect against breast cancer (Hoffman-Goetz 2003; Lee 2003; McTiernan 2003).

The existence of protective effects is certainly biologically plausible. Exercise can modify production and metabolism of estrogen and progesterone, which are known to affect the development of breast cancer. Other possible mechanisms could involve the effect of physical activity on menstrual cycle, body fat, and fat distribution.

A study of lifetime physical activity and breast cancer in both pre- and postmenopausal women showed that strenuous leisure-time physical activity was protective. The protective effects appeared to be strongest among postmenopausal women who were consistently active throughout their lifetime. The unique aspect of this study is that physical activity data were collected for various time periods, including adolescence, allowing the investigators to examine the important question of when in a woman's life exercise was most beneficial (Dorn et al. 2003). Bernstein et al. (1987) studied the effects of moderate-intensity physical activity on the menstrual cycle and found that adolescent girls who engaged in moderate physical activity had a threefold increase in the likelihood of an anovulatory menstrual cycle. Expenditure of more than 750 kcal of energy per week was associated with menstrual cycles that averaged 2.4 days shorter than those of less physically active girls (Bernstein et al. 1987). These results suggest that moderate physical activity during adolescence might also reduce breast cancer risk by delaying menarche, reducing the number of ovulatory cycles, and thereby reducing a woman's cumulative exposure to ovarian hormones (Kiningham 1998). The inverse relationship between physical activity and obesity in older women suggests the possibility that the protective role is associated with age at menopause (Friedenreich and Rohan 1995).

As part of the Women's Health Initiative cohort study, McTiernan and colleagues (2003) prospectively examined the association between current and past recreational physical activity and incidence of breast cancer in postmenopausal women. Compared with less active women, women who engaged in regular strenuous activity at age 35 years were shown to have a 14% decreased risk of breast cancer, and similar findings were observed for strenuous physical activity at ages 18 years and 50 years (McTiernan et al. 2003). Women who engaged in the equivalent of 1.25 to 2.5 hours per week of brisk walking had an 18% decreased risk of breast cancer compared with inactive women, and a slightly greater reduction in risk was observed for women who engaged in the equivalent of 10 hours or more per week of brisk walking. These data add to literature that suggests an association between increased physical activity and reduced risk for breast cancer in postmenopausal women. Unlike other studies, results from the Women's Health Initiative cohort study also suggest that longer duration of physical activity provides the most benefit and that such activity need not be strenuous (McTiernan et al. 2003).

Conclusions About Exercise and Breast Cancer

More often than not, researchers have reported positive correlations between exercise and lower rates of breast cancer. Differences in methodological design may be responsible for some of the earlier inconsistent results. At present, the preponderance of the evidence suggests that physical activity is protective against breast cancer (IARC 2002). Exercise early and later in life may alter the ages of menarche and menopause, respectively, both of which may in turn affect breast cancer rates (Dorn et al. 2003). Other possible mechanisms of action include reductions in endogenous steroid exposure, alterations in menstrual cycle patterns, increased energy expenditure, reduction in body weight, changes in insulin-like and other growth factors, and enhancement of natural immune mechanisms (Hoffman-Goetz et al. 1998; Rockhill et al. 1998).

Prostate Cancer

Physicians diagnose approximately 165,000 new cases of prostate cancer each year, making it the most frequently diagnosed cancer among men. The prevalence of this cancer varies considerably from one racial group to another; blacks in the United States have one of the highest, if not the highest, rates of prostate cancer in the world. Treatment for this disease can be very disabling. The relationship between physical activity and prostate cancer remains inconclusive (Friedenreich and Thune 2001).

Significant Studies

At the time of the publication of the Surgeon General's report, only 10 epidemiologic studies of cardiorespiratory fitness, leisure-time activity, or total physical activity were reviewed (USDHHS 1996). Of these, only five showed a benefit of physical activity for reducing risk of prostate cancer. A comprehensive review of the literature by Thune and Furberg (2001) examined the relationship between physical activity and dose response in 28 studies and showed that men who expended between 1000 and 3000 kcal per week in exercise at most had a 70% reduction in risk. The data from three studies, however, showed a significant increase in risk among physically active men. Few studies have indicated a significant negative association with increased physical activity increasing the risk. Research examining the relationship between occupational physical activity and prostate cancer has shown no significant association in either direction. Lee and colleagues (1992) reported on the incidence of prostate cancer in a longitudinal cohort of 17,719 men aged 30 to 79 years. They observed a protective effect for men whose age was 70 years or more and who expended 4000 kcal or more per week, compared to men who expended less than 1000 kcal per week. For younger men, however, there was no significant association between exercise level and the risk of prostate cancer.

Between 1971 and 1989 Oliveira et al. (1996) studied the association between cardiorespiratory fitness and prostate cancer in nearly 13,000 men from the Aerobics Institute in Dallas. These men, aged 20 to 80 years, underwent a preventive medical examination that included an exercise treadmill test to estimate cardiorespiratory fitness, and at different intervals provided (via questionnaires) information on physical activity and prostate cancer. Stratifying the subjects by quartile of cardiorespiratory fitness and controlling for age, body mass index, and smoking habits, the investigators observed a protective effect of cardiorespiratory fitness among participants who were younger than 60 years. Participation in physical activity (self-reported via questionnaire) was also inversely associated with prostate cancer in all participants. Those who spent 3000 kcal/week on exercise had lower risk (RR = 0.37, 95% CI, 0.14-0.98) of developing prostate cancer than those who spent less than 1000 kcal/week. More recently, after reviewing more than 36 epidemiological studies, Lee (2003) concluded that the relationship between physical activity and prostate cancer risk is inconclusive. The median relative risk across all studies comparing the most with the least active men is 0.9—which reflects almost similar rates for the two groups. Friedenreich et al. (2004) found no protective effect of total lifetime physical activity on prostate cancer using a large case-control study.

Conclusions About Exercise and Prostate Cancer

Kiningham (1998) speculated that exercise could exert a suppressive effect on prostate cancer development by decreasing testosterone levels. Men with prostate cancer have higher levels of endogenous testosterone than men without the cancer, and aerobically trained men are reported to have lower testosterone levels than sedentary men (Kiningham 1998; Westerlind 2003). However, the relationship between physical activity and sex hormone levels has not been studied as extensively in men as in women. It is also possible that exercise alters the metabolism of fat in a way that decreases its potential association with certain types of malignancies, but this relationship has not been proven. Thus, although there is biological plausibility for a protective effect of physical activity, the current evidence does not consistently support the hypothesis that physical activity protects against prostate cancer (Lee 2003). We need more studies with better assessment of possible confounding factors such as smoking, sexual practices, alcohol consumption, measurements of circulating hormones, cardiorespiratory fitness, body composition, and improved physical activity.

Physical Activity and Testicular Cancer

Data for testicular cancer is as inconsistent as has been the case for prostate cancer. Some studies have shown an increased risk among physically active men, while other studies indicate a protective effect. In the review of the literature by Thune and Furberg (2001), of the five papers published that examined dose-response relationships, three studies showed a graded inverse dose-response relationship.

One of the hypotheses postulated is that athletes display lower levels of circulating testosterone than nonathletes, and the role of testosterone in relation to testicular cancer has guided the research toward the assumption that physical activity might protect against the development of testicular cancer. Testicular injury or trauma, on the other hand, may be a risk factor for testicular cancer (Thune and Furberg 2001). These hypotheses are relatively untested and deserve more research.

Physical Activity and the Prevention of Osteoporosis and Falls

Osteoporosis is characterized by decreased bone mass and structural deterioration of the bone tissue, leading to bone fragility and increased susceptibility to fractures. It occurs most often among postmenopausal white women. It is estimated that 10 million U.S. adults are estimated to have osteoporosis and almost 34 million more are estimated to have low bone mass, placing them at increased risk for osteoporosis. Moreover, nearly 1.5 million fractures are reported each year among people aged 45 years and older.

Risk factors for osteoporosis in the United States are many, the greatest being gender and age, that is, being an older woman. More general risk factors are advanced age, early menopause, premenopausal removal of the ovaries, being Caucasian, being of Asian ethnicity, use of steroids, prolonged bed rest, menstrual irregularity, anorexia nervosa, and family history. Decreased risk is found with high-intensity exercise, African American ethnicity, being overweight, use of estrogen, and dietary calcium intake (Snelling et al. 2001). We need more research on the apparently deleterious effects of alcohol intake, cigarette smoking, use of thiazide diuretics, and excess caffeine intake and on the apparent benefits of fluoridated water and participation in moderate-intensity physical activity (USDHHS 1991).

Exercise and Osteoporosis

It is well established that bones adapt to the stresses imposed upon them through exercise training, heavy lifting, occupational work, or even housework (Hertel and Trahiotis 2001). The effect of exercise in the primary prevention of osteoporosis is not as well documented as its effect in the treatment of osteoporosis, partially because it is difficult and costly to design studies for this purpose. Nevertheless, several investigators (Conroy et al. 1993; Grimston et al. 1993; Kirchner et al. 1996; Nichols et al. 1994; Rubin et al. 1993) have found that children who engaged in weight-bearing or high-impact sports had greater bone density than children involved in swimming or low-impact sports. This observation has significance for public health, since achieving peak bone mass during physical maturity can affect development of osteoporosis later in life (Janz 2002). It is troubling that children are more inactive now than they were in previous generations, and that girls engage in less physical activity than boys (Andersen et al. 1998; USDHHS 1996). In fact, women of all ages are less physically active (especially in vigorous activity) than men (Crespo et al. 1996).

For exercise to produce long-term protection against age-related bone loss, it must be maintained for life. For example, Dalsky et al. (1988) had women exercise between 70% and 90% of their $\dot{V}O_2$max three times per week for 50 to 60 min. At the end of the study, lumbar bone mineral content increased 6%; yet after little more than a year of no exercise, the lumbar bone mineral content fell by 5%.

Lifetime physical activity is related to bone mineral density, but not to the incidence of osteoporotic fractures. In a long-term study, Greendale et al. (1995) measured bone mineral density of 1014 women and 689 men. Exercise habits were calculated beginning in the teenage years, at around 30 years of age, again at around 50 years, and finally at approximately 73 years of age. Bone mineral density in the hip was greater in the current and lifelong recreational exercisers than in those who engaged in mild or no exercise. Yet the authors found no protective effect of exercise against osteoporotic fractures in older men and women.

Exercise and the Prevention of Falls

Physical activity may help prevent falls and fractures among older persons. One component of physical fitness is balance, which has a favorable impact on the prevention of falls (Province et al. 1995). Improved muscle strength certainly can reduce the risk of falls and fractures, and the decline in muscle strength in older persons is correlated with a loss of balance and subsequently with an increased rate of falls (Carter et al. 2001; Judge et al. 1994). It also appears that increased strength of the muscles that produce ankle dorsiflexion can protect against falls (Lord et al. 1991).

Both endurance exercise and strength training exercise have potential benefits in preventing osteoporosis, falls, and fractures. Strength training reduces muscle weakness associated with loss of balance and increased falls; moreover, weight-bearing endurance training can help maintain bone mineral density and overall cardiorespiratory fitness (Henderson et al. 1998).

Exercise in the Prevention of Arthritis

Arthritis is one of the most prevalent chronic diseases. Osteoarthritis, the most common form of arthritis, is characterized by degeneration of cartilage and new growth of bone around the joint. In older persons, arthritis is responsible for more days of limited activity than any other disease, and it is the most cited reason for disability (see figure 7.6). More than 60% of women over the age of 75 report that they have arthritis (Collins 1997).

Running and other sports activities have not been associated with osteoarthritis in people who have not had joint injuries. The primary risk factors for osteoarthritis include joint trauma, obesity, and repetitive joint usage. Obesity can have a causal role in osteoarthritis of the knee. In longitudinal studies, obesity predicts the development of knee osteoarthritis in both men and women. Occupations that require excessive use of specific joints (e.g., bending the knees) are associated with knee osteoarthritis, while farming has been associated with hip osteoarthritis (Nieman 1996).

Because joint trauma is one of the strongest predictors of osteoarthritis, it is difficult to determine whether contact sports or regular noncontact exercise is more effective in preventing osteoarthritis. Cross-sectional and cohort studies suggest that people involved in

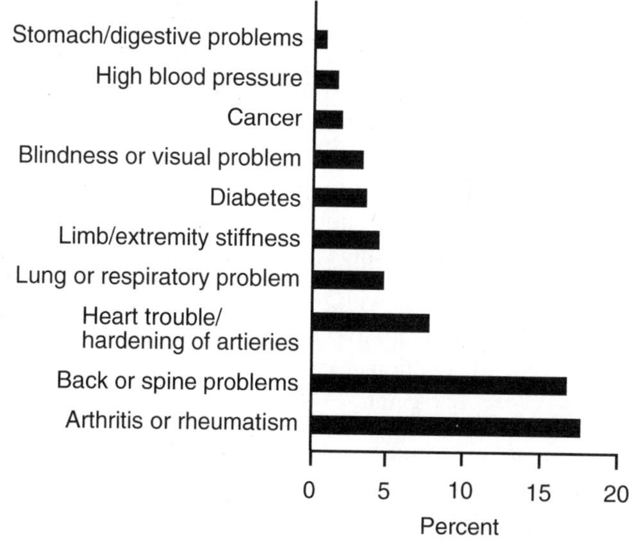

Figure 7.6 Percentage of persons aged 18+ reporting selected conditions as the main cause of the disability in the United States, 1999.

Source: Centers for Disease Control and Prevention 2001.

recreational running over long periods of time have no higher risk of developing osteoarthritis of the knee or the hip than people who engage in no leisure-time physical activity (Lane 1995; Panush et al. 1995). Competitive athletes who train at higher intensities, or compete in sports where specific joints are used excessively, carry the same risk of developing osteoarthritis as people whose occupations require repetitive use of certain joints. Lane et al. (1987) reported that long-distance runners aged 50 to 72 years had less physical disability and greater functional capacity than average members of the community. These runners sought medical services less often, weighed less, and experienced less musculoskeletal disability as they got older. Fries (1994) found that older persons who engaged in vigorous running had a slower development of disability than the general population. This association, however, was more likely to be due to a higher fitness level than to the postponement of the development of osteoarthritis.

Some level of physical activity is necessary to preserve joint function. There is no conclusive evidence that physical activity either causes or prevents osteoarthritis. Injuries sustained in competitive or contact sports, however, can have a comparable effect to that of joint trauma, and thus increase the risk of osteoarthritis.

Exercise in the Prevention of Low Back Pain

Low back pain is one of the most prevalent conditions in the United States. Between 60 and 80% of U.S. adults have reported back pain at some time during their lives, and close to 50% reported having that pain within a given year (Lahad et al. 1994). Figure 7.6 shows that back or spine problems are among the most commonly cited reasons for disability among people aged 18 years or older in the United States, right after arthritis or rheumatism. Low back pain is usually temporary, however, and fewer than 10% of people suffering from low back pain become chronic sufferers (Collins 1997).

The most commonly cited prevention interventions in the literature are

- back flexion, back extension, and general fitness exercises;
- patient education on back mechanics and ergonomic techniques to prevent injury; and
- mechanical back supports (corsets).

Lahad et al. (1994) described three mechanisms by which exercise can prevent low back pain. First, exercise can strengthen the back muscles and increase trunk flexibility, preventing injury and decreasing its severity. Second, exercise can increase blood supply to the spine muscles and joints and to intervertebral disks, minimizing the risk of injury and enhancing the body's natural healing and repair mechanisms. Third, exercise can improve mood and the perception of pain (Casazza et al. 1998). Most of the studies reviewed by Lahad et al. (1994) reported that both exercise of trunk muscles and aerobic exercise were effective and mildly protective against future back pain. Exercise also helps prevent lower back pain by combating obesity, thereby reducing abdominal fat and its disproportionate strain in the lower back.

In summary, exercise, either in the form of aerobic exercise or strengthening of the trunk muscles, appears to be mildly protective against development of low back pain in asymptomatic individuals.

Physical Activity and Primary Prevention of Obesity

Overweight and obesity are increasing in prevalence, and this has created a significant public health burden (Jakicic 2002). Americans are more overweight now than they have ever been (Kuczmarski et al. 1994). Whereas from 1976 to 1980 about 25% of Americans were overweight, by 1988 to 1994 the figure was approximately 33%. Using the new guidelines released by the National Obesity Education Initiative, almost two-thirds (65.1%) of the U.S. adult population is overweight (BMI ≥25) (Hedley et al. 2004; National Obesity Education Initiative 1998). Currently about a quarter of the population does not engage in leisure-time physical activity, an estimate that has changed little since 1985 (Crespo et al. 1996, 2000; CDC 2003, Aug 15, 2004). Reductions in other forms of physical activity can partially explain the increase in overweight. Both obese children and obese adults are less active than normal-weight people. Early studies had shown that obese children spent 40% less time engaging in physical activity than children who were not overweight. Furthermore, on average, obese men walk about 3.7 miles per day (in the course of normal activities) compared to 6.0 miles for those of normal weight; and obese women walk approximately 2.0 miles per day compared to 4.9 miles for normal-weight women (Bullen et al. 1964; Chirico and Stunkard 1960). More recent studies have shown that physical inactivity is one of the strongest risk factors for obesity (Kruger et al. 2002).

Although there is plenty of literature about exercise in the treatment of obesity, only limited research has dealt with physical activity in the primary prevention of obesity. This section addresses physical activity within the context of the prevention of excess weight, rather than the treatment of obesity. The energy expenditure that takes place during physical activity has the potential to affect energy balance, which can in turn affect body weight regulation. There is also some evidence that physical activity can minimize weight gain, and it appears that the activity needs to be moderate to vigorous in intensity to significantly affect body weight. Additionally, it appears that improvements in fitness are associated with reductions in risk of weight gain. Physical activity is also associated with improved maintenance of weight loss (Jakicic 2002).

AMBIGUITY OF THE EVIDENCE

In spite of the studies mentioned, few data exist to unequivocally suggest that physically active people are less likely to become obese than inactive people, that is, that exercise prevents obesity. Cross-sectional studies reveal an inverse relationship (Andersen et al. 1998; Crespo and Wright 1995; DiPietro 1995), and physically active populations exhibit a lower prevalence of obesity than their physically inactive counterparts. Yet the evidence cannot accurately answer whether people are obese because they exercise less, or they exercise less because they are obese.

Ching et al. (1996) analyzed data from the Health Professionals Follow-Up Study, to examine if physical activity or watching TV has independent effects on becoming overweight. Between 1988 and 1990, close to 18,000 men between the ages of 40 to 75 years had provided follow-up information. After adjusting for age and smoking status, the investigators found that more active men (highest quintile) were less likely to become overweight than men in the other four quintiles. Men in the higher third and fourth quintiles were also less likely to become overweight than those in the lowest (first) quintile of physical activity. Time spent watching TV was positively associated with overweight status. Thus, independent of TV watching, physical activity (either strenuous or moderate) conferred protective effects against becoming overweight in this sample of men, especially among those in the highest quintile of physical activity.

Children who spend more time in physical activity during physical education do not necessarily have less adipose tissue than children who engage in less physical activity. Recently, a number of school-based interventions directed at either increasing physical activity or decreasing sedentary behaviors (or both) have shown positive results (Steinbeck 2001). Moore et al. (1995) studied a subset of the Framingham Children's study and found that children with activity counts greater than the median gained fewer millimeters of tricep skinfold thickness over 12 months. In addition, the leaner children who were in the low-activity group were less likely to increase fatness than were the heavier children in the same group (Moore et al. 1995). Sallis and colleagues (1997) evaluated a health-related physical education program for fourth and fifth grade students, designed to increase the amount of physical activity in which children engage during their physical education period and also outside of school. In a quasi-experimental design, seven schools were randomly assigned to one of three conditions. The groups included (1) physical education classes led by an exercise specialist, (2) physical education led by a teacher, and (3) a control group that participated in the usual type of physical education for these seven schools. After 2 years of follow-up, the amount of time spent in physical activity increased significantly in the intervention groups compared to the control group, along with significant improvement in abdominal strength and endurance, and in cardiorespiratory endurance. However, the intervention and control groups did not differ significantly in skinfold measurements or in participation in physical activities outside of school.

Even when physically active people continue to engage in high-intensity physical activity throughout their lives, exercise appears unable to prevent weight gain associated with aging. Dr. Paul T. Williams (1997) studied nearly 8000 runners aged 18 years and older, monitoring them longitudinally and obtaining distance run per week through a questionnaire. This National Runners' Health Study classified the runners into five categories based on distance run in a given week: <16 km, 16 to 32 km, 32 to 48 km, 48 to 64 km, and >64 km. Williams observed that the rate of weight gain through middle age was the same in both shorter-distance and longer-distance runners, and concluded that physical activity guidelines either (1) should recommend substantial increases in activity over time or (2) should use age-adjusted overweight standards. More to the point was the inability of a constant level of physical activity to prevent the age-related weight gain.

More recently the Institute of Medicine has recommended 60 min of physical activity daily for optimal health (Institute of Medicine 2002). This new 1-hour-a-day total activity is higher than the amounts recommended in the Surgeon General's report and supported by the CDC and the ACSM. This recommendation stems from studies of how much energy is expended on average each day by individuals who maintain a healthy weight. The physical activity is expected to be cumulative, and is inclusive of both low-intensity activities of daily life and more vigorous exercise like swimming and cycling.

SUGGESTIONS FOR FURTHER RESEARCH

We need more studies that can assess body weight, fat mass, sedentary activities, and physical activity prospectively in men and women, and in boys and girls of different social classes. Obesity is a complex condition that responds to multiple cues from the environment and also has a genetic component that is not completely clear. The effects of culture, education, occupation, gender, marital status, and neighborhood safety are all key elements in the implementation of a physically active lifestyle. In addition, although minimal public health recommendations can affect health outcomes, additional research is needed to identify the optimal dose of physical activity to prevent weight gain and improve long-term weight loss (Jakicic 2002).

PHYSICAL ACTIVITY AND PSYCHOLOGICAL WELL-BEING

Some mental conditions are chronic, with complex etiologies. Exercise has been shown to improve psychological well-being and to reduce fatigue and stress. Patients who exercise have also shown improvements in depressive symptoms and sleep disorders (Butler et al. 1998). Itself a physical stressor, exercise raises blood pressure, perspiration, heart rate, blood sugars, body temperature, and oxygen supply and stimulates the release of catecholamines. These changes in turn produce acute alterations in moods and mental states. Whether these acute physiological changes of physical activity are responsible for a preventive effect of exercise in maintaining good mental health over time is still unclear. Also, the type of physical activity people engage in seems to affect their moods differently. Recreational or leisure-time physical activities seem to exert a better mood profile, or sense of well-being, than occupational or household activities.

SIGNIFICANT STUDIES

Longitudinal studies have found a negative association between hours per week or calories per week engaged in physical activity and risk of being diagnosed with depression later in life. People who engaged in 3 or more hours of sports or play per week at baseline were nearly 25% less likely to be diagnosed with depression than those engaging in sports or play less than 1 hour a week. A similar level of protection occurred among those who reported spending 2500 kcal per week in physical activity when compared to those who spent less than 1000 kcal a week (Paffenbarger et al. 1994).

Camacho et al. (1991) found involvement in active sports, swimming or walking, daily exercise, and gardening to be negatively associated with depressive symptoms among men and women aged 20 years or more in a population study in Alameda County, California. The researchers collected baseline data in 1965 and data on depressive symptoms in 1974, and classified participants into three levels of physical activity: low, moderate, and high. Compared to those in the high-activity groups, low-activity men and women had higher risks of showing symptoms of depression. The moderately active groups did not differ significantly from the highly active groups of men and women. An interesting aspect of these studies (Camacho et al. 1991; Paffenbarger et al. 1994) was the negative dose-response relationship between physical activity and depression.

Weyerer (1992) published a rather short-term longitudinal study, with baseline assessments in 1975-1979 and follow-ups during 1980-1984. Based on one question that assessed frequency of physical activity, he classified individuals into regular, occasional, or no exercise groups. A psychiatric interview among participants, who were 16 years of age or older at baseline, provided the basis for the depression variable. Physical activity showed no statistically significant relationship with depression in men or women.

More recently, a population-based study in Finland explored the association between physical exercise frequency and a number of measures of psychological well-being in 1856 women and 1547 men of the Finnish cardiovascular risk factor survey. In addition to answering questions about their exercise habits and perceived health and fitness, the participants completed the Beck Depression Inventory, the State-Trait Anger Scale, the Cynical Distrust Scale, and the Sense of Coherence inventory. Hassmen and colleagues (2000) found that individuals who exercised at least two to three times a week experienced significantly less depression, anger, cynical distrust, and stress than those exercising less frequently or not at all. Those who exercised at least twice per week also reported higher levels of sense of coherence and stronger feelings of social integration than their less frequently exercising counterparts (Hassmen et al. 2000).

GAPS IN OUR KNOWLEDGE

At present we do not have enough evidence to suggest a threshold that must be crossed in the intensity, the frequency, or the duration of physical activity to prevent chronic mental disorders. We know of acute changes in physiological responses to exercise that may exert a protective benefit against acute mood changes. We also have evidence that in endurance athletes too much strenuous exercise in one bout leads to mood disturbances that may contribute to adverse mental health. Thus, for the general population, too strenuous a physical activity regimen may have a deleterious effect on mental health (USDHHS 1996). Anecdotal evidence abounds that, after a hard day of work and mental tension, one of the best remedies is a "time-out" 30-min jog. We need more research to better understand the biological mechanisms that may link such episodic but regular bouts of exercise with improved mental health.

SUMMARY

Physical activity and physical fitness appear to be effective in preventing many chronic diseases. More importantly, the chronic diseases that produce the largest limitations in physical activity are also those most amenable to prevention through physical activity.

Moderate-intensity physical activity can prevent or delay coronary heart disease. The risk of inactivity is more common among women and the oldest population than among men. Several chronic diseases are more prevalent among older individuals, and while the mechanisms by which physical activity can ameliorate these diseases are usually not clear, the existence of positive effects from exercise is often well established. Exercise can help prevent hypertension by improving insulin sensitivity and the sensitivity of baroreceptors, but we need more research to identify clear thresholds and types of physical activity for prevention of hypertension in special populations. The indirect effect of exercise on fibrinogens, body composition, and blood flow dynamics are also emerging issues of interest.

Exercise is clearly beneficial in the prevention of type 2 diabetes. Besides its effect on body weight, physical activity helps improve insulin sensitivity and reduce insulin resistance.

The causes of cancer are many and complex. The bulk of research has shown exercise to be protective against colon cancer, breast cancer, and prostate cancer (the leading cancer killers, along with lung cancer). Moreover, all cancer mortality appears inversely associated with lower heart rates, a physical fitness indicator (Lee 1995).

Research on the effect of exercise in preventing bone loss, osteoporosis, fractures, and falls shows that endurance and muscular strength exercises seem to be beneficial in protecting or improving bone health at any age. Participation in physical activity early in life diminishes the risk of osteoporosis later in life. Osteoarthritis, the most common form of arthritis, is not associated with increased participation in physical activity. Improved balance and muscular strength exercise (especially in the lower extremities) may provide additional protective benefit against falls among the elderly.

Although body weight strongly tends to increase with age, lifetime physical activity may help to prevent the excess weight gain observed with aging. Exercise is not a risk factor for low back pain and may be more likely to help prevent low back pain than to cause it. Physically active persons appear less likely to suffer from depression and acute anxiety; we need more research to understand the effect of exercise on other psychological disorders.

In summary: to prevent the onset of many chronic diseases, people can benefit by participating in moderate-intensity physical activity for at least 30 min most days of the week, and also by regularly engaging in muscular strength, flexibility, and endurance exercise.

PART III

Exercise in the Rehabilitation of Specific Diseases and Conditions

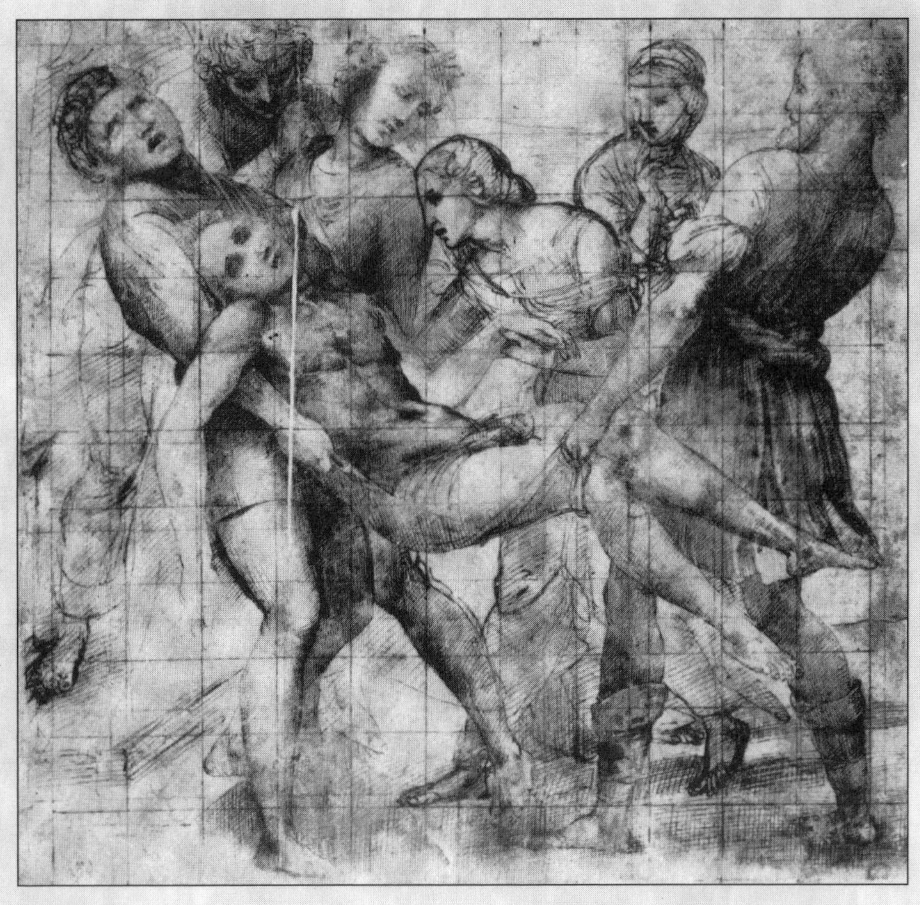

From Vatican Museum.

CHAPTER 8

HEART DISEASES

Ruy S. Moraes, MD, ScD; and Jorge P. Ribeiro, MD, ScD

CASE STUDY

A businessman had an uncomplicated inferior myocardial infarction in July 1988, at the age of 47. Before the myocardial infarction, he was sedentary and he smoked 30 cigarettes per day. His fasting plasma LDL cholesterol level was 180 mg/dL, there was poorly controlled arterial hypertension, and his body mass index was 32 kg/m^2. An echocardiogram demonstrated left ventricular hypertrophy, with inferior akinesis and global ejection fraction of 63%. An exercise tolerance test limited by fatigue at 4 METs demonstrated 2 mm downsloping ST segment depression on the electrocardiogram, compatible with myocardial ischemia at a rate-pressure product of 24,000. He was discharged from hospital on 100 mg daily of both atenolol and aspirin.

Two weeks after discharge from the hospital, the patient entered a comprehensive cardiac rehabilitation program that included a low-fat diet, smoking cessation, and exercise training five times per week. Over the 15 years that followed, the patient attended more than 80% of the scheduled exercise sessions. He was able to quit smoking, his plasma fasting LDL cholesterol declined to 73 mg/dL on sinvastatin 20 mg daily, his blood pressure was adequately controlled on enalapril 10 mg daily, and his body mass index was reduced to 25 kg/m^2. A maximal exercise tolerance test performed in 2003 demonstrated a functional capacity of 12 METs limited by fatigue, with 1 mm ST segment depression at a rate-pressure product of 30,000. An echocardiogram demonstrated normal left ventricular wall thickness, inferior hypokinesis, and a global ejection fraction of 69%.

In the United States, cardiovascular disease causes half of all deaths as well as a great deal of suffering and disability. Coronary artery disease alone is responsible for 1.6 million myocardial infarctions per year, of which 500,000 result in death before hospitalization. Of those patients who are admitted to the hospital with myocardial infarction, 15% die during hospitalization and another 10% die within a year. The mortality rate from coronary artery disease has declined dramatically since 1965, mainly due to widespread efforts to reduce risk factors (Manson et al. 1992). Exercise training has played an important role in the whole spectrum of cardiac disease prevention, including primary, secondary, and tertiary prevention (Smith et al. 1995).

The World Health Organization defines cardiac rehabilitation as the sum of activities required to ensure cardiac patients the best possible physical, mental, and social conditions so that they may, by their own efforts, regain a normal place in the community and lead an active, productive life (World Health Organization Expert Committee 1964). Thus, cardiac rehabilitation implies a multidisciplinary approach to cardiovascular disease that has exercise training as the cornerstone but also involves psychological, behavioral, and vocational support (Thompson et al. 1996). This chapter covers the rationale for and basic principles of physical exercise in cardiac rehabilitation.

RESPONSES AND ADAPTATIONS OF CARDIAC PATIENTS TO EXERCISE

Chapters 3, 4, and 5 described both the physiological responses to a single exercise session and the physiological adaptations to chronic exercise training for healthy individuals. The pathophysiology of exercise in heart disease, as well as the potential risks and benefits of exercise, may differ according to specific clinical conditions.

Coronary Artery Disease

Angina or left ventricular dysfunction may limit maximal functional capacity in patients with coronary artery disease. As is true in healthy individuals, exercise programs for these patients lead to improved exercise capacity as well as lower heart rate, systolic blood pressure, and plasma catecholamines response to a submaximal intensity (Redwood et al. 1972). After a training program, lower myocardial oxygen uptake occurs at a certain submaximal intensity, and these patients are able to tolerate higher exercise intensities before experiencing angina or manifestations of myocardial ischemia. Figure 8.1 compares the effects of exercise training to those of beta-blockers or coronary revascularization in coronary patients with angina pectoris. For most patients with inducible ischemia, the main effect of exercise training is a reduction in oxygen demand by the heart. However, as also shown in figure 8.1, long-term programs that include high training intensities or dietary interventions may improve myocardial blood flow (Froelicher et al. 1984; Hagberg 1991; Ribeiro et al. 1984; Schuler et al. 1988; Schuler et al. 1992), which may be related to regression of coronary artery disease (Hambrecht et al. 1993) or improved endothelial function (Shephard and Balady 1999; Laughlin et al. 1996). In selected groups of patients with left ventricular dysfunction and myocardial ischemia, there is even evidence of collateral coronary formation (Belardinelli et al. 1998).

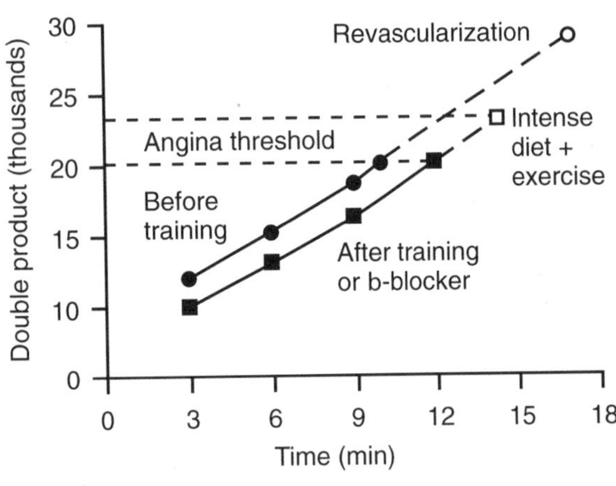

Figure 8.1 Response of the double product (heart rate × systolic blood pressure) to an exercise test, with increments in power every 3 minutes, in a patient with exercise-induced angina pectoris before (●) and after (■) interventions. After commonly used exercise conditioning or β-blockers (—■), the patient is able to tolerate a higher exercise intensity before angina appears. The onset of angina (angina threshold) occurs at the same double product compared to before intervention. After coronary revascularization with angioplasty or surgery (--O) the patient is able to tolerate a higher exercise intensity without angina due to improvement in myocardial blood flow. After prolonged and intense physical training with dietary intervention (--□), the patient is able to tolerate a higher exercise intensity due to both reduction in myocardial oxygen uptake and improvement in myocardial blood flow.

Arterial Hypertension

During incremental dynamic exercise, patients with established systemic hypertension present higher systolic and diastolic blood pressures for a given level of oxygen uptake as compared with normal individuals (Lund-Johansen 1967; Sannerstedt 1966). Although some have proposed exercise testing as a means of detecting individuals at risk of hypertension, there is little clinical evidence to support this concept (Liao et al. 1987). Blood pressure may be reduced for several hours after exercise. Some studies have suggested that exercise training programs may contribute to the reduction of blood pressure in patients with hypertension. Despite the fact that some controlled clinical trials had difficulty isolating the effects of exercise training when co-interventions (e.g., reduction in body weight) were accounted for and 24-hour ambulatory blood pressure devices were used (Blumenthal et al. 2000; Moreira et al. 1999), a recent meta-analysis of 54 randomized, controlled trials indicates that aerobic exercise training may result in a mean reduction of 3.8 mmHg in systolic blood pressure and 2.6 mmHg in diastolic blood pressure (Whelton et al. 2002). There is also some evidence that the response of systolic blood pressure to aerobic exercise training is determined in part by genetic factors (Rice et al. 2002).

Important increments in both systolic and diastolic pressure occur during exercise with static components such as weightlifting. Although some have argued that hypertensive patients should avoid static exercise, a recent meta-analysis of 11 randomized trials demonstrated that strength training may result in mean reduction of 2 to 3 mmHg in systolic blood pressure and 2 to 4 mmHg in diastolic blood pressure (Kelley and Kelley 2000).

Left Ventricular Dysfunction

Patients with congestive heart failure due to systolic dysfunction may present a marked limitation of exercise capacity. In symptomatic patients, functional capacity is usually less than 50% of normal for their ages, while in asymptomatic patients exercise capacity may be 60% to 70% of that predicted for their ages (Liang et al. 1992). Hemodynamic responses to exercise parallel this reduction in functional capacity, with inappropriate chronotropic (Colucci et al. 1989) and inotropic response (Weber et al. 1982), as well as reduced blood flow to exercising muscles (Arnold et al. 1990). The ventilatory response to exercise may also be abnormal, with increased ventilatory drive, increased respiratory dead space, and increased cost of breathing (Ribeiro et al. 1987; Sovijarvi et al. 1992). Skeletal muscle abnormalities in these patients include early lactate release, decreased mitochondrial size, reduced oxidative enzymes, type II fiber atrophy, altered muscle metabolic responses, and ventilatory muscle weakness (Drexler et al. 1992; Hughes et al. 1999; Mancini et al. 1992; Meyer et al. 2001; Minotti et al. 1991; Sullivan et al. 1990). In these patients, physical training improves submaximal as well as maximal exercise performance (figure 8.2) (Sullivan et al. 1989). The magnitude of the improvement in functional capacity is similar to and additional to that obtained by pharmacologic therapy (Ribeiro et al. 1985). However, some heart failure patients, particularly those with reduced cardiac output response to exercise, may not improve functional capacity with exercise training (Wilson et al. 1996). Physical training also induces partial reversal of autonomic (Rovena et al. 2003) and skeletal muscle abnormalities (Coats et al. 1992), as well as improvement in endothelial function (Hambrecht et al. 1998); and, in patients with heart failure and inspiratory muscle weakness, specific programs directed to inspiratory muscle training result in clinically significant improvement in functional capacity and quality of life (Chiappa et al. 2003).

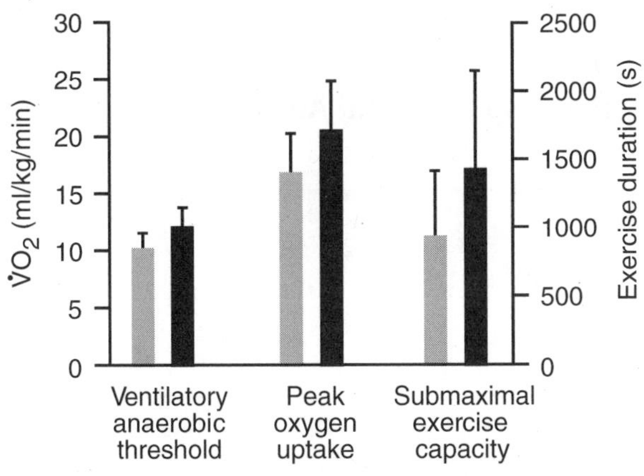

Figure 8.2 Mean ± standard deviation values for the ventilation anaerobic threshold and peak oxygen uptake (both in ml · kg^{-1} · min^{-1}) during incremental tests, and exercise duration (in seconds) on submaximal, constant load protocols measured before (■) and after (■) 16 to 24 weeks of training in 12 patients with chronic heart failure. Maximal and submaximal exercise capacity increased significantly in these patients.

Adapted, by permission, from M.J. Sullivan, M.B. Higginbotham, and F.R. Cobb, 1989, "Exercise training in patients with chronic heart failure delays ventilatory anaerobic threshold and improves submaximal performance," *Circulation* 79: 326-327.

VALVULAR HEART DISEASE

Hemodynamic responses to exercise are quite different in patients with the most common presentations of valvular heart disease. In severe aortic stenosis, the reduction of peripheral vascular resistance during dynamic exercise may result in syncope (Atwood et al. 1988). Because diastolic duration and regurgitation volume decrease during exercise in patients with aortic regurgitation, these patients tolerate exercise well (Weber et al. 1986). In mitral stenosis, this same reduction in diastolic duration impairs left ventricular filling and may reduce cardiac output and increase pulmonary pressure. In mild to moderate mitral regurgitation, cardiac output is maintained during exercise. There is little information on the effects of exercise training in patients with valvular heart disease. Exercise training is useful for improvement in exercise capacity and recovery oxygen uptake kinetics after percutaneous balloon mitral valvuloplasty for mitral stenosis (Douard et al. 1997; Lim et al. 1998). In general, patients with mild to moderate valvular heart disease and a near normal hemodynamic response to exercise may participate in training programs with the benefit of maintaining exercise capacity (Cheitlin et al. 1994). However, patients with severe valvular heart disease should exercise under close supervision.

CARDIAC ARRHYTHMIA

Atrial fibrillation, the most frequent arrhythmia, may affect exercise performance but does not impair the beneficial effects of exercise training (Vanhees et al. 2000). Activation of the sympathetic nervous system may contribute to development of ventricular arrhythmias during exercise, and cardiac patients have a higher risk for sudden death during vigorous exercise than healthy individuals. Chronic exercise training, however, can reduce resting and submaximal exercise plasma catecholamine concentrations, enhance heart rate variability, and increase vagal tone; and long-term training may result in intrinsic adaptations in sinus automaticity and atrioventircular conduction (Stein et al. 2002). After myocardial infarction, patients submitted to cardiac rehabilitation present a reduction of QT dispersion on the electrocardiogram, a finding usually associated with the reduction of malignant arrhythmias (Kalapura et al. 2003).

All these adaptations may potentially benefit patients with ventricular arrhythmias (Malfatto et al. 1996). Indeed, a study in dogs with experimentally induced myocardial infarction demonstrated that exercise conditioning increased the ventricular fibrillation threshold through an increase in vagal and a decrease in sympathetic tone (Billman et al. 1984). Clinical studies have also suggested that cardiac rehabilitation may reduce the incidence of ventricular arrhythmias (Hertzeanu et al. 1993; Mager et al. 2000). Despite these favorable observations, patients with complex ventricular arrhythmias, including those with implantable cardioverter-defibrillators, should exercise under close supervision including those with implantable cardioverter-defibrillators (Vanhees et al. 2001).

Effect of Cardiovascular Drugs on Exercise Responses and Adaptations

In order to document inducible myocardial ischemia, exercise testing should be conducted without any drugs that interfere with the responses of heart rate and blood pressure to exercise. When evaluating patients before they start a formal training program, however, patients should be tested on their usual medications. Table 8.1 describes the effects of frequently used cardioactive drugs on cardiovascular responses and adaptations to exercise. To improve compliance, ask your patients before each exercise session if they have taken their appropriate medications.

Evaluation of Cardiac Patients

Although in the past most patients referred for cardiac rehabilitation were at low risk for cardiac events, today many high-risk patients participate in exercise programs. You need adequate risk stratification and objective measurement of exercise capacity in order to plan individualized programs.

Risk Stratification

Before starting any outpatient exercise program, perform an exercise tolerance test to establish the patient's limits of functional capacity, maximum heart rate, and maximum systolic blood pressure; to look for signs of ischemia or ventricular dysfunction; and to check for arrhythmias. This information permits you to stratify risk for complications during exercise (see "Risk Assessment in Cardiac Rehabilitation," page 121) and prescribe the optimum exercise intensity. While annual reevaluations are sufficient for low-risk patients, you probably should test moderate- to high-risk patients every six months. Reevaluate patients after any change in clinical status suggesting cardiovascular deterioration, or after any new intervention (e.g., a change in medication or the use of revascularization procedures), to determine if exercise is still safe. As appropriate, prescribe a new exercise intensity.

Evaluation of Exercise Capacity

Physicians traditionally have assessed exercise capacity in cardiac patients by subjectively evaluating symptoms resulting from ordinary physical activity. Such information permits use of a categorical scale such as one proposed by the Criteria Committee of the New York Heart Association (1964). Although useful in clinical practice because of its simplicity, this classification system has poor reproducibility, and does not reflect the entire continuum of exercise capacities (Goldman et al. 1981). One can improve the estimate of exercise

Table 8.1 Effects of Commonly Used Drugs on the Responses and Adaptations to Exercise

	Responses		Adaptations
Drug	**Heart rate**	**Blood pressure**	**Functional capacity**
β-blockers	–	–	– + in angina
Arterial vasodilators	0/+	–	0
Calcium antagonists			
Dihydropiridines	0/+	–	0 + in angina
Diltiazem/Verapamil	–	–	0 + in angina
Digitalis	–	0	+ in heart failure
Diuretics	0	–	0
Angiotensin converting inhibitors	0	–	+ in heart failure
Antiarrhythmic agents	0/–	0	0

0 = no significant effect; – = reduction; + = increase.

RISK ASSESSMENT IN CARDIAC REHABILITATION

Low-risk patients

- New York Heart Association (NYHA) class 1 or 2
- Exercise capacity >6 METs
- Absence of heart failure
- Absence of signs of ischemia at rest or during an exercise test intensity ≤6 METs
- Appropriate rise in systolic blood pressure during exercise
- Absence of sequential ectopic ventricular contractions
- Capacity to self-monitor exercise intensity

Moderate- to high-risk patients

- Two or more myocardial infarctions
- NYHA class 3 or greater
- Exercise capacity <6 METs
- ST depression ≥4mm or angina during exercise
- Fall in systolic blood pressure during exercise
- Previous episode of primary cardiac arrest
- Ventricular tachycardia during exercise <6 METs
- Unable to self-monitor exercise intensity
- Any life-threatening clinical problem

Adapted, by permission, from G. Fletcher et al., 1995, "Exercise standards. A statement for health professionals from the American Heart Association," *Circulation* 91:602-603.

capacity by questioning patients about their performance on daily activities with known metabolic costs (Lee et al. 1988), but still with significant misclassification. Estimation of exercise capacity from the total duration on a specific exercise protocol may correlate well with measured maximal oxygen uptake (Franciosa 1984), but oxygen uptake kinetics may differ in patients with heart disease, making the estimation of the metabolic cost of exercise inaccurate (Roberts et al. 1984). Another inexpensive method for estimating submaximal exercise capacity is a self-paced walking protocol that measures the distance achieved by the patient in six minutes (Guyatt et al. 1985).

Cardiopulmonary exercise testing, with measurement of expired gases and determination of anaerobic threshold and peak oxygen uptake, allows objective evaluation of functional capacity and of the effect of medical interventions. It also helps define the prognosis in cardiac patients whose main limitations are not due to myocardial ischemia (Mancini et al. 1991; Ribeiro et al. 1985; Weber et al. 1982). Results from cardiopulmonary exercise testing may also reveal whether exertional dyspnea is secondary mainly to pulmonary or mainly to cardiac disease (American Thoracic Society/American College of Chest Physicians 2003). For patients who are limited by myocardial ischemia, standard exercise testing is appropriate for the assessment of exercise capacity (Fleg et al. 2000).

INDICATIONS FOR CARDIAC REHABILITATION

Cardiac rehabilitation originally was developed for patients recovering from myocardial infarction. For many years, myocardial infarction was managed with several weeks of bed rest, in the belief that it was necessary for complete healing of the myocardium. Because prolonged bed rest may result in loss of muscular mass, bone reabsorption, anemia, thromboembolic events, pulmonary infections, cardiovascular deconditioning, postural hypotension, and tachycardia, survivors were so physically and emotionally limited that returning to normal life was a significant challenge. In recent decades, the concept of early ambulation after myocardial infarction has been well established. Furthermore, early coronary recanalization, risk stratification, and intervention for those at higher risk have gotten most patients out of bed on the second day of hospitalization and discharged from the hospital after five to seven days. Higher-risk patients, however, may still endure prolonged bed rest and its consequences.

Indications for Cardiac Rehabilitation

- Abnormal exercise test indicating ischemia
- Post-myocardial infarction patients
- Stable angina
- Coronary artery bypass surgery
- Post-percutaneous transluminal coronary angioplasty
- Compensated congestive heart failure
- Cardiomyopathy
- Post-heart transplantation
- After other cardiac surgery
- Patients with pacemaker or automatic implantable cardioverter-defibrillator
- Peripheral vascular disease
- High risk cardiovascular disease ineligible for surgical intervention
- Sudden cardiac death syndrome
- End-stage renal disease
- At risk for coronary artery disease

Adapted from American College of Sports Medicine 1995b.

Contraindications for Cardiac Rehabilitation

- Unstable angina
- Resting SBP >200 mmHg or DBP >110 mmHg
- Orthostatic blood pressure drop of >20 mmHg with symptoms
- Critical aortic stenosis
- Acute systemic illness or fever
- Uncontrolled arrhythmias
- Resting heart rate >120 beats/min
- Uncompensated heart failure
- Third-degree AV block (without pacemaker)
- Active pericarditis or myocarditis
- Recent embolism
- Thrombophlebitis
- Resting ST segment displacement >2 mm
- Uncontrolled diabetes
- Severe orthopedic problems
- Other metabolic problems

Adapted from American College of Sports Medicine 1995b.

Traditionally, physicians recommended cardiac rehabilitation after myocardial infarction to restore patients' functional capacity and to allow them an active life. Today, the degree of functional impairment after myocardial infarction depends more on the degree of left ventricular dysfunction and the presence of residual ischemia than on the effects of prolonged bed rest. Although functional capacity on hospital discharge is normal in many cases, regular exercise training promotes important metabolic and cardiovascular adaptations that positively affect secondary prevention. Thus, cardiac rehabilitation is suitable for a great variety of clinical conditions, as listed above in "Indications for Cardiac Rehabilitation."

Contraindications for Cardiac Rehabilitation

Contraindications for starting or maintaining an exercise program are listed in the box above. Before each exercise session, ask your patient about the appearance of new symptoms and for any change in the presentation of their symptoms. Give close attention to changes in the pattern of angina for patients with coronary artery disease, and to weight gain in patients with left ventricular dysfunction. Always measure blood pressure and heart rate. Whenever there is doubt about the safety of performing an exercise session, notify the patient's clinician.

Exercise Prescription for the Cardiac Patient

Encourage cardiac patients to exercise during hospitalization and to maintain active lifestyles after discharge. Inpatient and outpatient programs present different characteristics.

Inpatient Rehabilitation

For patients recovering from myocardial infarction, exercise during hospitalization helps prevent the deconditioning effects of bed rest and prepare the patients to face the demands of daily physical activities after discharge. For most patients, these daily tasks demand less than 4 METs (1 MET = 3.5 $ml \cdot kg^{-1} \cdot min^{-1}$ = the average oxygen uptake while sitting). In uncomplicated cases, you can encourage patients during the first 48 hours of hospitalization to perform arm and leg range-of-motion movements, self-care activities, and low-resistance exercises (figure 8.3).

The posture during these activities should progress from lying to sitting to standing, according to the patient's capacity. Supervision during this period is done by nurses, physical or occupational therapists, or exercise physiologists—all with special training (Pashkow et al. 1988). On the third day after discharge from coronary care unit, patients should start walking for short periods of time, with close monitoring of heart rate, of blood pressure while standing, and, if necessary, of EKG. The exercise heart rate should not exceed 20 beats per minute above resting heart rate, and systolic blood pressure should not exceed 20 mmHg above resting levels. In the beginning, total exercise duration should be around 20 minutes, twice a day, distributed in intermittent bouts lasting 3 to 5 minutes, with rest periods of 1 to 2 minutes between bouts. We recommend that you first increase exercise duration (10-15 minutes of continuous activity), and then raised intensity. During exercise, have the staff watch carefully for symptoms of myocardial ischemia, pulmonary congestion, or a drop in blood pressure. If any of these occurs, interrupt the session and reevaluate the patient before restarting exercise (American College of Sports Medicine 1995b).

OUTPATIENT PROGRAMS

After you have stratified them according to risk, you can offer cardiac patients a variety of outpatient exercise programs.

TYPE OF EXERCISE

Most exercise training in cardiovascular rehabilitation aims to enhance the response of a dysfunctional heart to all kinds of stress—i.e., to diminish the cardiovascular response for a given level of challenge. Aerobic exercise is more efficient in this matter than anaerobic, and is the first choice for cardiac rehabilitation. Most studies using aerobic exercise to control angina in coronary patients have found significant reductions of symptoms (Hagberg 1991; Redwood et al. 1972; Ribeiro et al. 1984).

It is important that predominantly aerobic exercises fulfill the following criteria: low-intensity start, smooth progression; low rate of musculoskeletal injury; and ease of performance and of monitoring. The most popular aerobic exercises are walking and stationary cycling, whose results differ little for most patients. But note that walking demands much more effort for overweight patients than for lean patients—it raises heart rate and blood pressure quickly and imposes a considerable

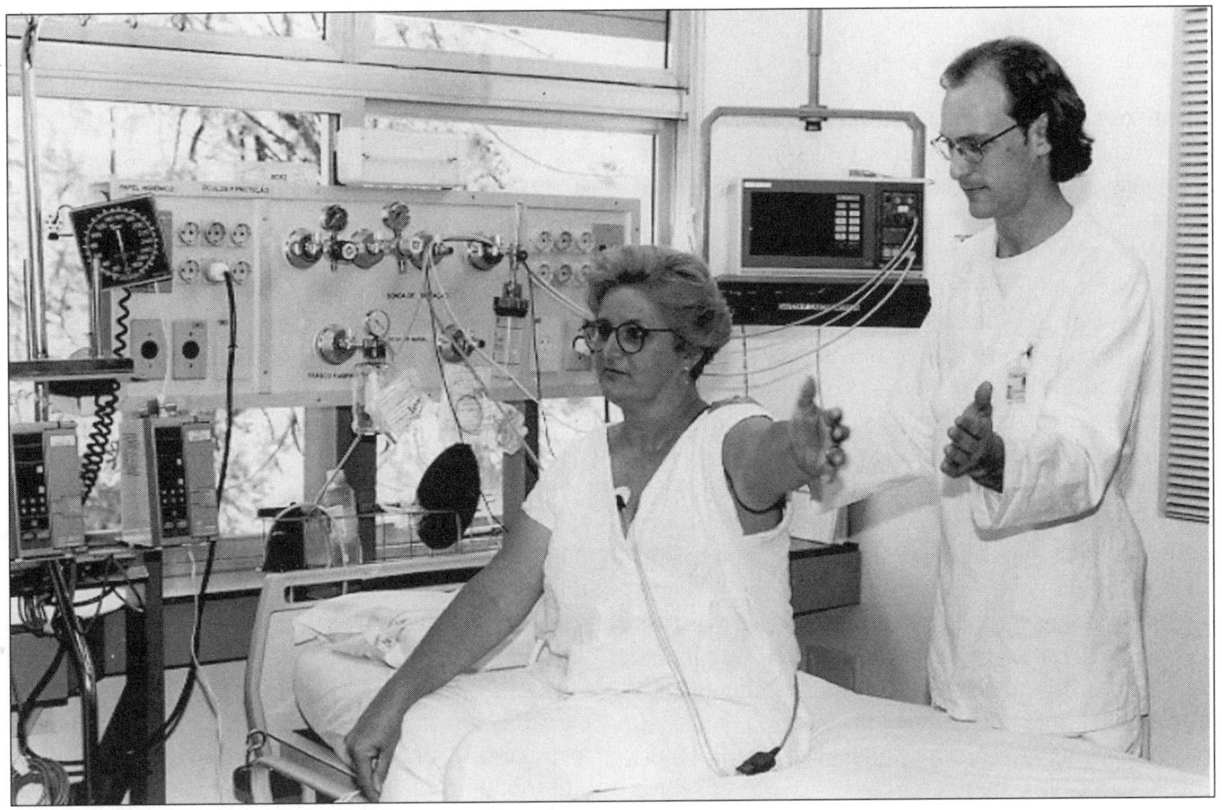

Figure 8.3 Post-myocardial infarction patient performing arm range-of-motion movements under supervision in the intensive care unit.

Courtesy of COFIR – Hospital Moinhos de Vento.

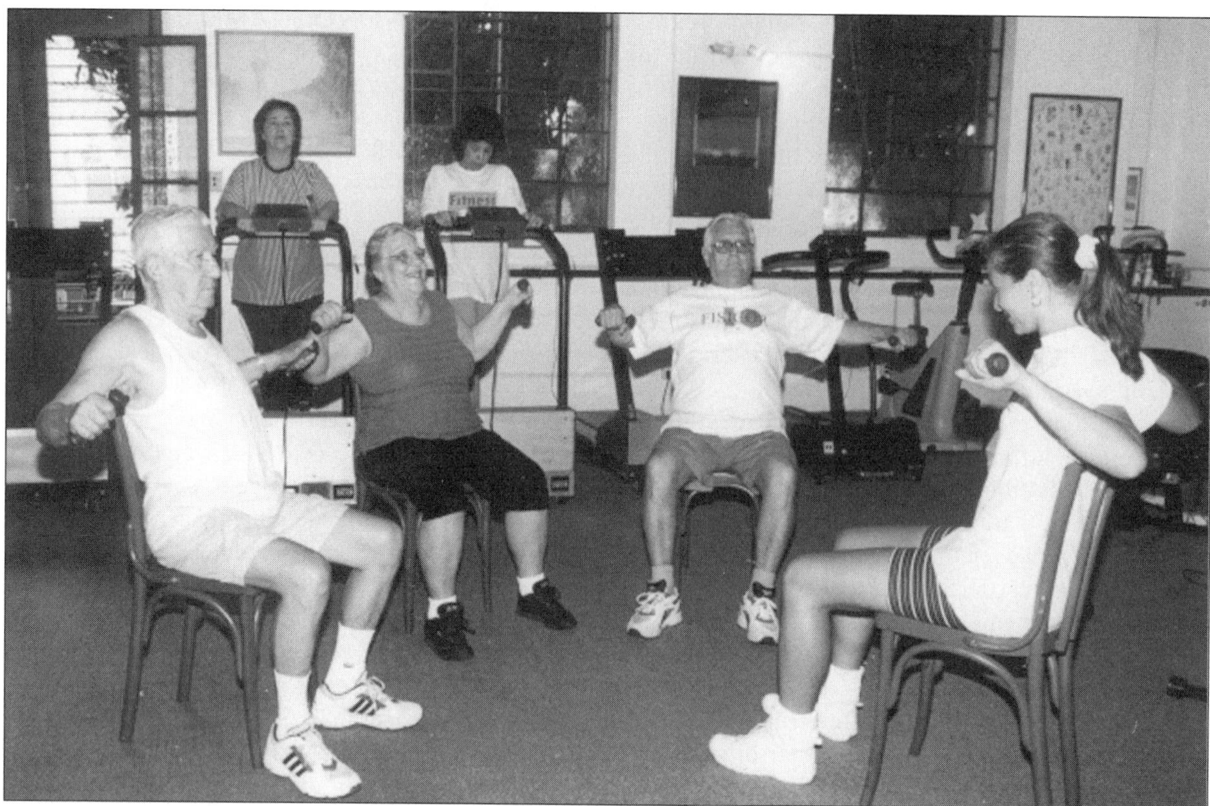

Figure 8.4 Low intensity resistive training in an outpatient cardiac rehabilitation program.
Courtesy of FISICOR – Cardiac Rehabilitation Center.

amount of stress on the musculoskeletal system. Most overweight patients find cycling to be both safer and more enjoyable than walking as they start an exercise program.

Patients who use their arms in the workplace will require upper-body exercise before returning to work after a myocardial infarction. Compared to dynamic exercise, heavy weightlifting and isometric exercise elicit marked and fast elevations in systolic and diastolic blood pressure, less elevation in heart rate, and increased diastolic coronary perfusion, resulting in potentially less myocardial ischemia (Bertagnoli et al. 1990). Therefore, resistive exercise can be safe and useful with proper medical supervision and cardiovascular monitoring (Ghilarducci et al. 1989) (figure 8.4). Low-intensity resistive training may be performed as early as two to eight weeks after myocardial infarction or cardiac surgery (i.e., 0.5- to 4.0-kg hand weights, dumbbells, and elastics). More intense strength training should wait until the patient is aerobically well trained (Verrill 1998, Verrill et al. 1992).

Duration and Frequency

To increase aerobic capacity, exercise should last a minimum of 20 minutes, always beginning with a warm-up period and finishing with a cool-down. Considering that some of the beneficial effects of exercise are short lived, patients should exercise for at least 30 minutes, almost every day, with one or two days of rest every week to avoid osteomuscular injuries. The best results in terms of both weight loss and functional capacity occur with a caloric expenditure of about 800 to 1,000 calories/week, which implies 40- to 60-minute sessions three to five times a week. Some studies have demonstrated that burning 2,200 calories/week can induce plaque reduction. To reach this goal, patients must be highly motivated, exercising intensely for 60 minutes five to six times a week. Patients with very low functional capacity, who experience fatigue after a few minutes of exercise, will benefit from short periods of exercise many times a day (DeBusk et al. 1990).

Target Exercise Intensity

The safety of exercise training for cardiac patients depends mostly on the prescribed intensity. On the basis of information obtained from an exercise tolerance test or from a cardiopulmonary exercise test (American Thoracic Society/American College of Chest Physicians 2003), you can calculate a safe exercise intensity range in several ways. "Range of Exercise Intensities for

Range of Exercise Intensities for Cardiac Rehabilitation

- Workload corresponding to 50% to 80% of $\dot{V}O_2max$
- 70% to 85% of maximal heart rate (HRmax)
- 50% to 75% of heart rate reserve plus heart rate at rest (HRrest)

  ([HRmax – HRrest] × 50%) + HRrest

  ([HRmax – HRrest] × 75%) + HRrest

- Rating of perceived exertion 12 to 16 on the Borg scale
- Exercise intensity corresponding to the anaerobic threshold
- 10 bpm below the point that abnormal responses occur in the exercise test

Cardiac Rehabilitation" lists common methods for estimating target exercise intensity. The "rating of perceived exertion" on that list refers to the patient's perception of the difficulty of each level of exercise according to the Borg RPE Scale (Borg 1998; figure 8.5).

Researchers recently have explored the lower as well as the higher limits of exercise prescription. On one hand, studies have demonstrated that post-myocardial infarction patients may improve functional capacity after training programs that require less than 45% of maximal oxygen uptake (Blumenthal et al. 1988) or as low as 20 beats per minute above resting heart rate (Gobel et al. 1991). These low-intensity programs may result in higher compliance (Lee et al. 1996). On the other hand, selected patients who participated in high-intensity exercise programs (70% to 90% of maximal oxygen uptake) for over a year improved left ventricular function and significantly reduced exercise-induced myocardial ischemia at higher myocardial oxygen uptake (Hagberg 1991). Take special care with patients recovering from large anterior Q-wave myocardial infarctions, with left ventricular dysfunction, as they may experience adverse ventricular remodeling over time with early mobilization and exercise training (Jugdutt et al. 1988; Kubo et al. 2004).

6	No exertion at all
7	Extremely light
8	
9	Very light
10	
11	Light
12	
13	Somewhat hard
14	
15	Hard (heavy)
16	
17	Very hard
18	
19	Extremely hard
20	Maximal exertion

Borg RPE scale

Figure 8.5 The Borg ratings of exertion scale.

Reprinted, by permission, from G. Borg, 1998, *Borg's perceived exertion and pain scales* (Champaign, IL: Human Kinetics), 47.

During the first training sessions, keep exercise intensity in the lower end of the calculated range of intensities. This will permit patients to feel comfortable and confident, and to be free of muscle pains after the sessions. As appropriate for a given patient's cardiovascular and muscular responses, you can gradually and safely increase workload and exercise intensity toward the higher end of the calculated range.

Pulse irregularity makes it difficult to use heart rate to prescribe exercise intensity for patients with atrial fibrillation; instead, use maximal exercise capacity and rate of perceived exertion in setting exercise intensity for these patients (Mertens and Kavanagh 1996). When the patient presents abnormal responses during exercise testing (see "Abnormal Exercise Responses During Stress Testing" heart rate during exercise training should be 10 beats below the heart rate related to the abnormalities.

During the first weeks after coronary artery bypass surgery, patients are still recovering from the surgical trauma, with pain from the thoracotomy and in the leg from which the saphenous vein was removed. For this

Abnormal Exercise Responses During Stress Testing

- Progressive angina, dyspnea, paleness
- ST depression
- Drop in systolic blood pressure
- Systolic blood pressure >240 mmHg
- Diastolic blood pressure >110 mmHg
- Left ventricular dysfunction
- Complex ventricular arrhythmias
- EKG abnormalities

reason, exercise training in this period usually is prescribed without a previous exercise test. During exercise sessions, keep heart rate around 20 beats per minute above resting heart rate and prescribe only low-level aerobic activity. Complete thoracotomy healing takes around 45 to 60 days, so upper body exercises in this period can include no resistance. Because of pain and fear, many patients avoid even moving their arms freely when they walk. It is very important that you respect their limitations in this period and provide whatever physical support is needed to prevent falls. After four to eight weeks, most patients can perform an exercise test for formal exercise prescription. Exercise training in this phase is exactly the same as it is for post-myocardial infarction patients. The preference is for aerobic exercises that rapidly increase maximal oxygen consumption. Strength training in these patients is useful to improve muscle strength, especially in the upper body, but has a smaller impact on maximal oxygen consumption (Wosornu et al. 1996).

Supervision

Outpatient exercise training programs for cardiac patients have different levels of supervision, depending on the time after the index event and the risk for developing cardiac complications during exercise (which is related to the severity of the underlying disease). This supervision can be as strict as continuous electrocardiographic monitoring during sessions, for those patients considered as high risk, right after hospital discharge or no supervision at all for very low-risk patients 12 weeks following a myocardial infarction (see "Risk Assessment in Cardiac Rehabilitation," page 121).

Electrocardiographic monitoring may be appropriate during the first 6 to 12 sessions, gradually reduced to once a week, once a month, or only during symptoms, according to each patient's needs. Individuals at high risk for cardiac complications during exercise, or unable to self-regulate activity levels, may need longer periods of continuous electrocardiographic monitoring. After this intensely monitored phase, patients may enter a gymnasium- or community-based program that offers controlled exercise in an enjoyable environment (figure 8.6). This is the ideal setting to promote self-confidence and risk factor control. Patients have the opportunity to exchange experiences with each other, and group activities help them to increase exercise adherence. Gymnasium staff usually include registered nurses, physical therapists, exercise physiologists, and physical educators, all trained in current basic and advanced cardiac life support. Supervising physicians must be available for emergency response and consultation, but

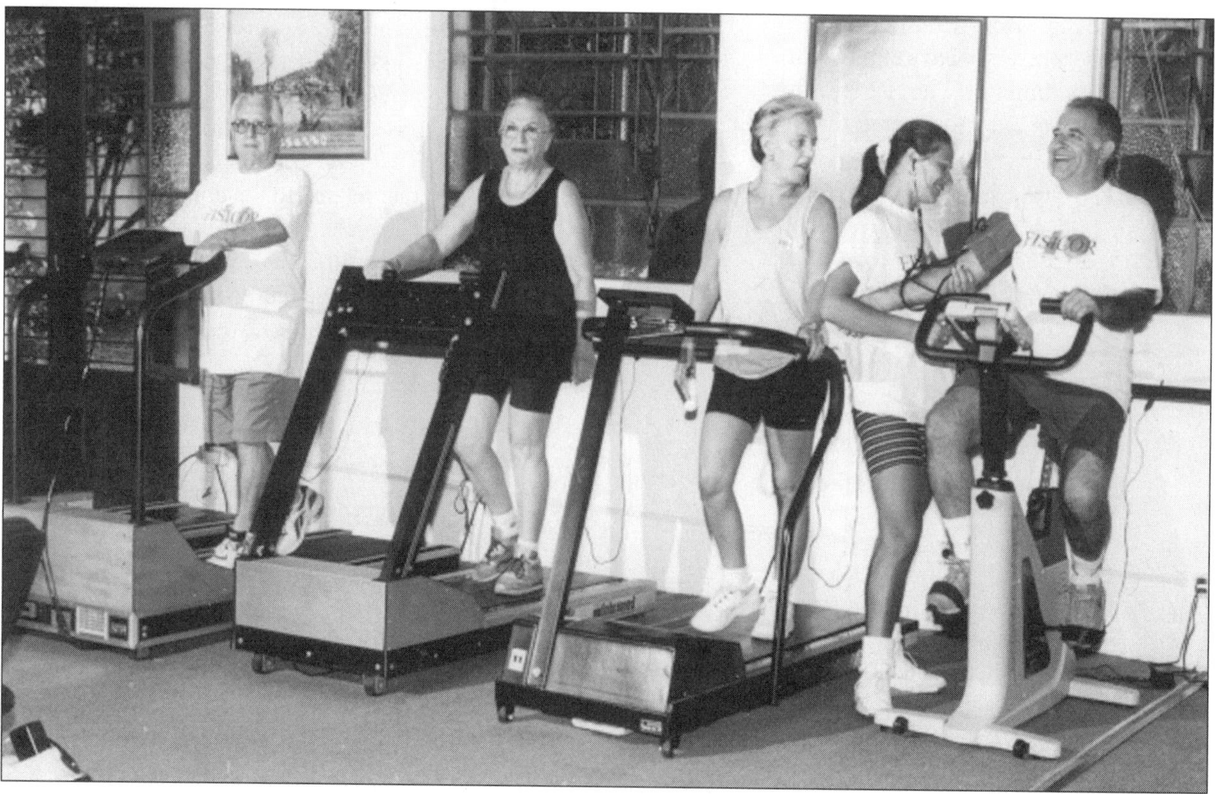

Figure 8.6 Community-based cardiac rehabilitation program that offers a controlled and enjoyable environment.
Courtesy of FISICOR – Cardiac Rehabilitation Center.

need not be present in the gym. (Vongvanich et al. 1996). Staff-to-patient ratio can be from 1:1 to 1:4 in continuously monitored programs during the first 12 weeks, and from 1:10 to 1:20 for group supervised programs (Haskell 1978). For low-risk patients, home exercise rehabilitation is an alternative to supervised group programs. Different monitoring and communication techniques—e.g., regular phone contacts, mail, fax, video recording, Internet, and transtelephonic electrocardiographic monitoring (Balas et al. 1997)—are safe, inexpensive, and convenient for some patients (DeBusk et al. 1985). Finally, exercise training without supervision is acceptable for low-risk patients who are able to prudently control their own exercise intensity.

SAFETY

Heart disease, vigorous exercise, and death have long been associated with each other in the popular mind. Since exercise increases myocardial oxygen consumption, it may be deleterious to a compromised heart. In recent years, scientists have extensively investigated the impact of exercise on the heart, learning that this potentially harmful activity actually can be effective in treating heart disease. According to the cardiac arrest rate reported in the United States for cardiac patients in exercise rehabilitation programs, the average risk is 1 cardiac arrest for 59,142 patient-hours of exercise training. Risk may increase when untrained patients perform intense levels of exercise, like jogging; it tends to decrease with activities like walking, cycling, or treadmill walking with continuous electrocardiographic monitoring (Fletcher et al. 1995). Probably because of close exercise supervision, the successful resuscitation rate for cardiac arrest in rehabilitation programs is around 85% (Haskell 1978; Van Camp and Peterson 1986).

OUTCOMES OF CARDIAC REHABILITATION PROGRAMS

Over the past decades, considerable amount of information has accumulated on the outcomes of cardiac rehabilitation programs.

MORTALITY

Most randomized trials on the effects of exercise training in patients with coronary disease were not powered to show statistically significant effects on mortality. However, meta-analysis of trials conducted before the nineties found that post-myocardial infarction patients enrolled in cardiac rehabilitation programs had lower rates both of overall mortality and of cardiovascular death, but no differences in the incidence of recurrent myocardial infarction. (O'Connor et al. 1989; Oldridge et al. 1988). A recent meta-analysis that included trials conducted in the last decade, with patients under modern clinical care, analyzed the impact of cardiac rehabilitation not only on post-myocardial infarction patients but also on those submitted to coronary artery bypass grafting and percutaneous transluminal coronary angioplasty, as well as patients with angina. Compared to usual care, exercise-based cardiac rehabilitation promoted a reduction of 20% in all-cause mortality and of 26% in cardiac mortality. No difference was observed when exercise was complemented with educational and psychological co-interventions (Taylor et al. 2004). For patients with heart failure, recent meta-analyses indicate that exercise training is associated with a 29% to 35% reduction in mortality (ExTraMATCH Collaborative 2004; Smart and Marwik 2004).

FUNCTIONAL CAPACITY

Patients enrolled in an exercise program for eight weeks may expect an increase in maximum oxygen consumption of about 30%, depending on their previous functional capacity. Patients with lower functional capacity benefit the most. After coronary artery bypass surgery, patients experience a spontaneous and gradual increase in functional capacity over 48 months (Weiner et al. 1981); exercise training significantly improves this response, allowing earlier return to work (Fletcher et al. 1988). When compared to percutaneous transluminal angioplasty, exercise training results in superior event-free survival and exercise capacity, notably due to reduced hospitalizations and repeat revascularizations (Hambrecht et al. 2004). In a training study, the greatest improvement in functional capacity occurred in patients who recovered from myocardial infarction and subsequently had coronary artery bypass surgery; those with the lowest ejection fractions had the greatest increase in exercise capacity (Shiran et al. 1997). Heart failure patients may expect a 17% improvement in peak oxygen uptake when submitted to aerobic training and a 9% improvement when strength training is the only intervention (Smart and Marwick 2004).

RISK FACTOR MODIFICATIONS

Secondary prevention of coronary artery disease—a well-established intervention based on risk factor modification—increases survival, improves quality of life, and reduces both the incidence of subsequent myocardial infarction and the need for interventional procedures. However, it is difficult to implement lifestyle changes for risk modification (Smith et al. 1995). Because of its multidisciplinary approach, cardiac rehabilitation is the ideal setting in which to promote the necessary behavior changes (Gordon and Haskell 1997). As a sole intervention, exercise conditioning can positively affect some of the most important known risk factors (Blair et al. 1993). Exercise increases high-density lipoproteins and decreases both low-density lipoproteins and triglycerides, with small changes in total cholesterol (Lavie and Milani 1996b; Tran and Weltman 1985). In obese patients, these benefits are even greater when associated with weight loss (Lavie and Milani 1996a). Obesity is a risk factor for coronary artery disease (Donahue et al. 1987) and adversely influences other risk factors. Exercise alone cannot always affect weight loss—dietary interventions are usually mandatory. Increases in the level of physical activity improve insulin sensitivity, sometimes preventing non-insulin-dependent diabetes mellitus (Helmrich et al. 1991). Intense endurance training in older people enhances fibrinolysis, possibly reducing the risk of acute thrombosis (Stratton et al. 1991). Although exercise is frequently recommended as a nonpharmacologic treatment for hypertension (Kelley and Kelley 2000; Whelton et al. 2002), there is still controversy about its effectiveness in nonobese patients (Blumenthal et al. 2000); in obese patients, exercise may promote weight loss, which is related to reductions in blood pressure (Schotte and Stunkard 1990). In sum, risk factor modification may be one of the main benefits of cardiac rehabilitation.

VOCATIONAL STATUS

Reemployment after an acute cardiac event depends on factors such as age, educational status, severity of the underlying disease, functional capacity, physician's advice, and the patient's perception of health. An exercise tolerance test after a myocardial infarction is one of the key steps in helping patients return to work. It provides information about the severity of the underlying disease and the functional capacity, and helps patients improve their perception of health. Three weeks after an uncomplicated myocardial infarction, patients may have a functional capacity of more than 7 METs, which meets the physical requirements of most white-collar jobs. For these patients, early return to work does not increase the incidence of recurrent cardiac events (Dennis et al. 1988). For high-risk patients with low functional capacity, exercise training seems to help them return to work faster (Hertzeanu et al. 1993). Manual laborers also may require lower and upper body conditioning before resuming their usual professional activities.

PSYCHOSOCIAL BENEFITS

Acute cardiovascular events strongly affect people's emotional lives. After a myocardial infarction, about 70% of patients report fatigue or lack of energy and are concerned about issues like physical health, return to work, sex life, engaging in physical activities, and the possibility of living an enjoyable life in all aspects (Doerfler et al. 1997). Around 15% to 20% of patients develop signs of depression, which increases the risk of future cardiac events (Carney et al. 1987). Cardiac rehabilitation has been very successful in improving the psychosocial aspects of patients' lives after a major cardiac event. Patients who participate in cardiac rehabilitation programs report improvement in well-being, health, and functional abilities. They also consume fewer tranquilizers and are less depressed when compared to patients not enrolled in cardiac rehabilitation (Denollet and Brutsaert 1995; Lavie and Milani 1997; Milani et al. 1996). These positive effects are not yet fully explained. There is evidence that persons with a low level of activity are at increased risk of developing depression (Camacho et al. 1991), and that intense physical training can improve depression scores (Beniamini et al. 1997). Since cardiac rehabilitation improves fitness and provides an objective assessment of functional capacity, it may create more confidence in patients as they prepare for the usual challenge of daily activities (Dafoe and Huston 1997).

COST EFFECTIVENESS

Since economic resources for health assistance are increasingly more scarce, economic evaluation of health services has become an important issue in modern medicine. To calculate the real cost of an intervention, one must consider health-related improvements in quality of life in addition to reductions in morbidity and mortality. Quality of life is a function not only of physical health, but of the complex interactions among the physical, psychological, and social domains of health (Pashkow et al. 1995; Testa and Simonson 1996). Patients with the same health status may perceive their realities in very distinct ways, having vastly different levels of satisfaction with their lives (Mayou and Bryant 1993).

Investigators have evaluated the costs of cardiac rehabilitation mainly as a secondary prevention measure after acute myocardial infarction. Together with an estimated reduction in mortality of 25% (O'Connor et al. 1989; Oldridge et al. 1988), cardiac rehabilitation reduces costs by lowering the incidence of rehospitalization and of emergency visits (Bondestam et al. 1995; Oldridge et al. 1993). Cardiac rehabilitation after acute myocardial infarction is estimated to cost only US$2,130 per year of life saved, using health care costs of 1985 (Ades et al. 1992); and US$4,950.00 per year of life saved using 1995 figures (Ades et al. 1997; NIH Consensus 1996). Compared to other interventions after acute myocardial infarction—such as coronary artery revascularization, thrombolytic reperfusion, β-adrenergic blocker therapy, angiotensin converting enzyme inhibitor therapy, lipid lowering therapy, and anti-platelet therapy—only smoking cessation programs are more cost-effective.

SUMMARY

Cardiac rehabilitation is a safe, cost-effective intervention that increases functional capacity, usually improves psychosocial status, and may reduce working disability in a variety of cardiac diseases. Patients with lower functional capacity benefit the most. In the many clinical presentations of coronary artery disease, exercise training may reduce mortality and improve risk factor profile. Finally, exercise programs for selected patients with coronary artery disease may reduce the progression and even improve the regression of coronary atherosclerosis.

CHAPTER 9

RESPIRATORY DISEASE

Bartolome R. Celli, MD

CASE STUDY

A 63-year-old woman, S.W., smoked one pack of cigarettes per day from age 17 to age 59. She had begun to experience dyspnea at age 57, and was diagnosed with chronic obstructive pulmonary disease (COPD) at age 59. Although she stopped smoking, her dyspnea continued to progress (at first appearing only with moderate efforts). Over the past year, however, she had become unable to walk up one flight of stairs, and the dyspnea occurred during activities of daily living (washing, bathing, and dressing). She began to limit her exercise, and used a nephew's wheelchair when she went out. She began to use low-flow oxygen at age 62.

A routine chest roentgenogram revealed a right upper lobe nodule measuring 2 centimeters, which had not appeared in an X ray two years earlier. Computerized tomography confirmed the nodule. There were no mediastinal nodes. The same scan confirmed severe hyperinflation, and demonstrated the presence of inhomogeneous changes more prominent in the upper lobes.

Laboratory exams were within normal limits, including cardiac echocardiogram. Physiologic evaluation showed severe airflow obstruction, with a forced vital capacity of 2.05 L and a forced expiratory volume in one second (FEV1) of 0.52 L after bronchodilators. The residual volume determined by plethysmography showed severe air trapping with a value 260% of predicted. S.W.'s six-minute walking distance was 120 meters, and maximal oxygen uptake in a progressive cardiopulmonary exercise test was 11 ml · kg^{-1} · min^{-1}. The working diagnosis was that of neoplasm, very likely malignant, in the right upper lobe.

By conventional criteria S.W. was inoperable, because her FEV1 was very low (26% of predicted). Nevertheless, we explained to her that we could remove the nodule using recently developed lung volume reduction surgery. Even though she understood that poor functional capacity (as expressed by the six-minute walking test) generally predicts poor outcome with this procedure, she wanted to be aggressive and was willing to "do anything" to qualify for the procedure.

We began her on an intense pulmonary rehabilitation program that included lower-extremity exercise at 70% of the determined $\dot{V}O_2$max and upper-extremity unsupported exercise. To aid in the postoperative period, we instructed her in deep-breathing exercises and in assisted cough. S.W. began the program with daily sessions as an inpatient, completing it with three weeks of outpatient training for a total of 20 sessions. Retesting revealed less dyspnea with exercise, and she was able to walk 285 meters over six minutes. Her peak oxygen uptake had risen to 13 ml · kg^{-1} · min^{-1}.

S.W.'s lung volume reduction surgery, which included resection of the nodule, revealed adenocarcinoma of the lung. She recovered in the acute ward of St. Elizabeth's Medical Center for eight days, and was discharged to a rehabilitation facility to continue the program while a small persistent leak (drained with a Heimlich tube) closed. After the leak closed on the 16th day after surgery, S.W. went home. After eight months, the mass has not recurred.

S.W. is still dyspneic, but no longer uses the wheelchair. She has not required hospitalization, and her oxygen requirements have decreased 0.5 liter per minute. She walks daily, and her last six-minute walking distance was 268 meters.

Commentary: This case documents the extreme limitations characteristic of patients with severe COPD. It also shows the frequent association between COPD and lung cancer, as both share cigarette smoking as a common risk factor. More importantly, it shows how pulmonary rehabilitation that includes exercise training can significantly improve certain outcomes. S.W. was well-prepared and confident as she faced surgery. She was also able to walk longer and experience less dyspnea at a higher functional level. It is also possible that the educational components of her pulmonary rehabilitation (especially those that helped her control her breathing) helped improve her postoperative recovery.

Patients with chronic respiratory diseases decrease their overall physical activity, because any form of exercise often results in worsening dyspnea. The progressive deconditioning associated with inactivity initiates a vicious cycle in which dyspnea increases at ever lower physical demands. With time, the patients adopt a breathing pattern (usually fast and shallow) that is detrimental to overall gas exchange, thus worsening their symptoms. Physical reconditioning is a broad therapeutic concept that unfortunately has been equated with simple lower extremity exercise training. This chapter addresses the concept of respiratory muscle training and resting. It reviews current knowledge about reconditioning in broad terms, critically analyzing the effects and roles of leg and arm training, and giving practical recommendations. It also reviews the concept of breathing retraining in its broad definition.

The data on which our current knowledge of reconditioning is based have been obtained from patients with intrinsic lung disease such as emphysema, bronchitis, bronchiectasis, cystic fibrosis, and acute respiratory failure. Very little is known about reconditioning in patients with pure pump failure, such as those with degenerative neuromuscular diseases. There is every reason to believe that, in these patients, physical exercise may worsen rather than improve their overall function and sensation of well-being. On the other hand, pure breathing retraining, such as slow deep breathing, could have a more universal application as long as extra loads are not placed on already weakened and dysfunctional respiratory muscles. As will be reviewed in this chapter, patients with symptomatic "pump failure" may benefit more from ventilatory assistance and resting than from further training.

With these exceptions in mind, this chapter reviews the general principles of physical reconditioning and, specifically, lower and upper extremity training.

PHYSICAL RECONDITIONING

Physical reconditioning is the most important factor in rehabilitating patients with symptomatic respiratory disease. An understanding of the principles and components of exercise conditioning is necessary for anyone who wants to incorporate them in the treatment of such patients.

GENERAL PRINCIPLES

The short- and long-term effects of systematic exercise conditioning have been the subject of extensive investigation. In normal individuals, participation in a well-designed exercise training program results in several objective changes:

- There is increased maximal oxygen uptake primarily due to increases in blood volume, hemoglobin, and heart stroke volume with improvement in peripheral utilization of oxygen.
- With specific training, there is increase in muscular strength and endurance primarily resulting from enlargement of muscle fibers and improved blood and energy supply to the targeted muscle groups.
- Muscle coordination improves.
- Body composition changes, with increased muscle mass and loss of adipose tissue.
- The individual's sense of well-being improves.

In patients with obstructed airflow, participation in a similar program will result in different outcomes depending on the severity of the obstruction. Patients with mild to moderate disease usually respond similarly to healthy individuals; patients with severe obstruction will increase exercise endurance and improve their sensation of well-being with little if any increase in maximal oxygen uptake. Several recent studies have shown improvement in outcomes different from simple exercise performance. They include improved muscle enzyme content, less dyspnea at a similar work level, and decreased production of lactic acid at isowork. Although an initial training effect has been shown, there has been no systematic investigation regarding the effect of maintenance programs on any of the outcomes, including exercise performance.

Chronic obstructive pulmonary disease decreases tolerance to exercise. The most important factors thought to contribute to this limitation of exercise are

- alterations in pulmonary mechanics,
- abnormal gas exchange,
- dysfunction of the respiratory muscles,
- alterations in cardiac performance,
- malnutrition, and
- development of dyspnea.

Although less well characterized, other factors deserve to be mentioned: smoking, abnormal peripheral muscle function, and polycythemia. While the most severely affected patients cannot reach exercise levels where training effects are thought to occur (above anaerobic threshold), a large body of evidence supports exercise training as a beneficial therapeutic tool in helping these patients achieve their full potential.

PHYSIOLOGIC ADAPTATION TO TRAINING

In order to prescribe exercise for patients with severe pulmonary problems, we must understand several principles of exercise training:

1. Specificity of training
2. Intensity, frequency, and duration of the exercise load, and
3. Detraining effect

SPECIFICITY OF TRAINING

This principle states that the training effect is specific to the type of training, and the training of muscles or muscle groups is beneficial only to the trained muscle.

High-resistance, low-repetition stimulus (e.g., weight lifting) increases muscle strength, whereas low-resistance, high-repetition training increases muscle endurance. Strength training increases myofibrils in certain muscle fibers, whereas endurance training increases the number of capillaries and mitochondrial content in the trained muscles.

The training is specific to the trained muscle. Clausen et al. (1973) trained subjects with their arms and legs and observed that the decreased heart rate observed for arm muscle training could not be transferred to the leg group and vice versa. Davis and Sargeant (1975) showed that if training was completed for one leg, the beneficial effect could not be transferred to exercise involving the untrained leg. More recently Belman and Kendregan (1981) tested eight COPD patients who for six weeks trained only their arms, and seven who trained only their legs. Improvements occurred only in the exercise for which the patients trained. Interestingly, biopsies taken before and after the training program revealed no changes in muscle enzyme content in the trained muscles.

INTENSITY, FREQUENCY, AND DURATION OF THE EXERCISE LOAD

This principle states that the intensity, frequency, and duration of the exercise load profoundly affect the degree of the training effect. Although athletes usually train at maximal or near maximal levels in order to rapidly achieve the desired effects, middle-aged nonathletes may require less intense exercise. Siegel et al. (1970) showed that training sessions of 30 minutes about three times a week for 15 weeks significantly improved maximal oxygen uptake, if heart rate was raised over 80% of predicted maximal rate. In patients with chronic lung disease, research by several authors suggests that the greater the number of sessions and the more intense (as a function of maximal performance), the better the results.

Belman and Kendregan (1981) had patients with chronic lung disease exercise four times per week at 30% of their maximal capabilities, gradually increasing their loads as they could individually tolerate the increases. After six weeks, 9 of the 15 patients significantly improved their endurance times. The relatively low training level (30% of maximal) may help explain why six of the patients failed to increase their endurance times. Niederman et al. (1991), who started their subjects at 50% of maximal cycle ergometer level and increased intensity on a weekly basis, observed endurance improvement in most patients. Other authors have used higher starting exercise levels and have achieved higher endurance (Holle et al. 1988; Mohsenifar et al. 1983; Zack and Palange 1985; ZuWallack et al. 1991).

The most thorough study in this regard is that of Casaburi and colleagues. They studied 19 patients with moderate COPD (mean ± *SD* FEV1 [forced expiratory volume in 1 second] of 1.8 ± 0.53 L), who could achieve anaerobic threshold both before and after randomly assigned, low-intensity (50% of maximal) or high-intensity (80% of maximal) exercise. The high-intensity training program was more effective than the low; and after training there was a drop in ventilatory requirement for exercise that was proportional to the drop in lactate at a given work rate (Casaburi et al. 1991). Similar results were reported by Puente-Maestu in 2000. However, Maltais and colleagues (1997) demonstrated that training targeted at high intensity may be difficult to achieve and that the actual level of exercise intensity achieved while aiming to train at high intensity may be lower than previously thought. It appears that a training effect occurs with an exercise intensity at least 50% of maximal and that the intensity can be increased as tolerated. Yet any exercise is better than none, and good results have been shown even for patients with minimal exercise performance (ZuWallack et al. 1991) and with

Table 9.1 Number of Exercise Sessions in Studies on Exercise Endurance

Author	Sessions	Endurance change
Belman	45	50%
Epstein	19	30%
Make	12	12%

relatively low levels of exercise intensity (Normandin et al. 2002).

The number of exercise sessions required to improve endurance is a matter of debate (Belman and Kendregan 1981; Make and Buckolz 1991). Table 9.1 shows that, in general, increases in observed endurance time are a function of the number of sessions. Since stopping the exercise results in loss of the training effect, the optimal plan should involve an intense training phase and a maintenance phase. Difficulty in implementing the latter results in the frequently observed failure to maintain and preserve the beneficial effects of training, yet no study in any respiratory disease has addressed this important issue.

Detraining Effect

This principle states that the effect achieved by training is lost after the exercise is stopped. Saltin et al. (1968) showed that bed rest in normal subjects resulted in a significant decrease in maximal oxygen uptake within 21 days. When the subjects resumed their exercise programs, it took between 10 and 50 days for the values to return to those seen before resting. Keens et al. (1977) examined ventilatory muscle endurance after training in normal subjects who had undergone ventilatory muscle training. Within one month after they stopped training, the subjects had lost the training effect they had achieved. It seems important to continue to train, but the minimum practical and effective timing of maintenance training remains to be determined.

Patients in our program exercise at 70% of the maximal work achieved in a test day. The work is increased weekly, as tolerated by the patients. We aim to complete 24 sessions, typically in an outpatient setting with three weekly sessions. Hospitalized patients can complete the program more quickly, by performing them on a daily basis. Each session lasts 30 minutes if tolerated by the patient. If the patient cannot tolerate 30 minutes of exercise, the program is begun as tolerated by the patient and no further load is provided until the patient can complete the 30-minute session. When metabolic measurements are not possible, we determine a target work rate by using a Borg visual analog scale of the perception of dyspnea. Refer to Horowitz et al. (1997) for further description of this approach. It is helpful to use dyspnea and not heart rate to set performance targets for patients with lung disease, as breathlessness constitutes their most important complaint.

Lower Extremity Exercise

Several early studies have shown that leg exercise benefits patients with lung disease (Beaumont et al. 1985; Christie 1968; Hughes and Davidson 1983; Moser et al. 1980; Paez et al. 1967).

Studies on Lower Extremity Exercise

Working with 39 dyspneic patients younger than 70 years and not on oxygen, Cockcroft et al. (1981) randomly assigned subjects to a treatment group that spent six weeks in a rehabilitation center where they underwent gradual endurance exercise training and to a control group that received medical care but was given no special advice to exercise. After four months, the control group also was admitted to the rehabilitation center for six weeks. As was true for the treated patients, they were instructed to exercise at home afterward. Both groups were similar at baseline. After rehabilitation, only 2 of the 16 control patients manifested improvement in dyspnea and cough, whereas 16 of 18 patients in the treatment group improved. More importantly, the treated patients showed significant improvement in the 12-minute walk and in peak oxygen uptake when compared with the controls.

Sinclair and Ingram (1980) studied 33 patients with chronic bronchitis and dyspnea. The 17 patients randomly assigned to the treatment group climbed up and down on two 24-cm steps twice daily. The exercise time was increased to tolerance. The patients exercised at home and were evaluated by the treatment team weekly. The control group did not exercise. After six months, there were no changes in the degree of airflow obstruction in either group, nor was there improvement in strength of the quadriceps, the minute ventilation, and heart rate. Yet the trained patients significantly increased their performance in the 12-minute walk test.

More recently, O'Donnell et al. (1993) compared breathlessness, six-minute walking distance, and cycle ergometer work between two age-matched groups of patients with moderate COPD. The group trained in endurance exercise ($n = 23$) significantly reduced their dyspnea scores and increased both distance walked and their cycle ergometry work, when compared to the control group ($n = 13$). This trial is important in that it not only documented increased endurance, but for the first time evaluated the patients' perceptions of dyspnea, the most problematic symptom and the one leading to physical limitation.

Since those initial studies, several randomized trials have documented the beneficial effect of lower extremity

Table 9.2 Selected Controlled Studies of Rehabilitation With Exercise in Patients With COPD

Author	No. patients	Frequency	Course	Results
Cockroft	18 T	Daily	16 weeks	↑12 MW ↑VO_2
	16 C	—	—	No change
Sinclair	17 T	Daily	40 weeks	↑FVC ↑12 MW
	16 C	—	—	No change
O'Donnell	23 T	Daily	8 weeks	↑FVC ↑12 MW ↓Dyspnea
	13 C	—	—	No change
Reardon	10 T	2 × /week	6 weeks	↓Dyspnea
	10 C	—	—	No change
Ries	57 T	Daily	8 weeks	↑Exercise capacity ↓Dyspnea ↑Self-efficacy
	62 C	Daily education	8 weeks	No change
Wijkstra	28 T	Daily at home	12 weeks	↑Exercise capacity ↑Quality of life
	15 C	—	—	No change
Goldstein	45 T	Daily	24 weeks	↑6 MW VO_2 ↓Dyspnea ↓S.O.B.
	44 C	None	24 weeks	No change
Griffiths	198 T	3 × /week	8 weeks	↑Exercise ↓Hospital days
	199 C	None	8 weeks	No effect

T = treated; C = controls; MW = minute walk test; FVC = forced vital capacity; VO_2 = peak oxygen uptake; S.O.B. = shortness of breath.

exercise (Bendstrup et al. 1997; Finnerty et al. 2001; Goldstein et al. 1994; Griffiths et al. 2000; Reardon et al. 1994; Ries et al. 1995; Strijbos et al. 1996; Wedzicha et al. 1998; Wijkstra et al. 1994, 1996). Perhaps most important is the study by Ries et al. (1995), who assigned patients either to an education support group ($n = 62$) or to a similar educational program with the addition of three walking exercises per week for eight weeks ($n = 57$). After 2 months and still at 4, 6, and 12 months the exercise group showed increased exercise endurance, less dyspnea with exercise, less dyspnea with activity of daily living, and an increase (not statistically significant) in survival. This landmark study clearly establishes the benefit of exercise in pulmonary rehabilitation. Table 9.2 summarizes the results of several studies.

Physiologic Changes Resulting From Exercise

The mechanism by which exercise endurance is improved remains a matter of debate. Several studies, including those of Paez et al. (1967) and Mohsenifar et al. (1983), have demonstrated a drop in heart rate at similar work levels, a hallmark of a training effect for the specific exercise. This effect may be related to a decrease in exercise lactate level, as suggested by Woolf and Suero (1969). More recent evidence in support of a training effect is provided by the study of Casaburi and colleagues (1991) and by Puente Maestu et al. (2000), whose COPD patients showed reduced exercise lactic acidosis and ventilation in response to training. The reduction was proportional to the intensity of training: there was a 12% decrease in the lactic acidosis rise in patients trained with the low work rate (50% of maximum), and a 32% decrease in those trained with the high work rate (80% of maximum). Both groups exhibited significant decreases in heart rate after training. Other studies have failed to document either increases in maximum O_2 uptake or decreases in heart rate or lactate. The most important study in this group, by Belman and Kendregan (1981), failed to show a decrease in heart rate at the same workload as represented by the $\dot{V}O_2$. They also observed no change in oxidative enzyme content of muscle after training, as determined through analysis of biopsies. Interestingly, nine of the treated patients improved their exercise endurance. As stated previously, it is possible that this study used too low a training effort, since training was started at 30% of the maximum achieved during their testing. This possibility is supported by two studies by Maltais and colleagues. First they showed that muscle biopsies from the legs of patients with COPD had decreased levels of mitochondrial oxidative enzymes (Maltais et al. 1995); subsequently, they observed significant increases in the mitochondrial enzymes after exercise training (Maltais et al. 1996), as well as delayed onset of the lactase threshold.

The evidence therefore indicates that patients with COPD can be trained to a level that produces physiologic changes consistent with improved muscle performance (figure 9.1).

Can Severely Affected Patients Benefit?

Two studies addressed the issue of whether patients with the most severe COPD can undergo exercise training. It is an important question: many patients with the most severe COPD do not exercise to the intensity required to reach their anaerobic threshold or to train the cardiovascular system.

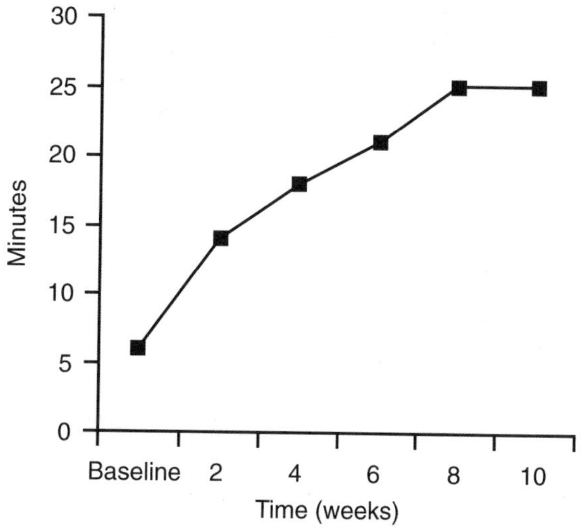

Figure 9.1 Average endurance time that 12 patients with COPD could sustain a submaximal workload targeted at 70% of maximal work measured in a cycle ergometer test. Patients were tested at baseline and at 2-week intervals, training 3 times weekly. Plateau was reached at 8 weeks (24 sessions) of training.

Niederman et al. (1991) studied 33 patients with different degrees of COPD (FEV1 ranging from 0.33 L to 3.82 L). After training, there was no correlation between the degree of obstruction in these patients and their observed improvement—the patients with very low FEV1 were as likely to improve as the patients with high FEV1. Similarly, ZuWallack et al. (1991) evaluated 50 patients with COPD (FEV1 range from 0.38 L to 3.24 L) before and after exercise training. They observed inverse relationships between the level of improvement and the baselines for 12-minute walking distance and for $\dot{V}O_2$. They concluded that patients with poor performance on either the 12-minute walking distance or maximal exercise test are not necessarily poor candidates for an exercise program. These data suggest that any patient capable of undergoing leg exercise endurance training will benefit from a program that includes leg exercise.

Type of Exercise and Testing

Different studies have used different training techniques. Most studies include walking both as a measurement of exercise tolerance and of the training program. The classic 6- or 12-minute walk (the distance walked over 6 or 12 minutes) is very good for patients with moderate to severe COPD but may not be taxing enough for patients with less airflow obstruction (McGavin et al. 1976). However, recent prospective observations by Gerardi et al. (1996) after pulmonary rehabilitation and by Pinto-Plata and coworkers (2004) in our laboratory have demonstrated that the 6 MWD is an excellent predictor of survival in patients with COPD. The latter study compared the predictive power of the 6 MWD with that of the degree of airflow limitation represented by the FEV1 and with the body mass index (BMI). With use of Cox proportional hazard analysis, the 6 MWD was the strongest predictor of mortality. This observation, coupled with the report by Oga and colleagues (2003) that the peak oxygen uptake is also a predictor of mortality, provides evidence of the importance of exercise limitation and its measurement in patients with COPD. In our own studies of stair climbing, we found we could estimate the peak oxygen uptake from the number of steps climbed during a symptom-limited test (Pollock et al. 1993). Several researchers have used a treadmill or steps for testing purposes, even when the training consisted of walking oxygen uptake is higher for stair climbing or treadmill testing than for the more commonly used leg ergometry, presumably because the former uses more body muscles than leg cycling. Leg ergometry is a very popular testing device and has been the training apparatus for most recent studies. It is certainly smaller than the treadmill, and with relatively inexpensive units on the market, it is possible to place several together and train a number of patients simultaneously.

All the studies quoted relied on either inpatient or outpatient hospital training. Little information is available regarding implementation of such programs at home. In a unique report, O'Hara et al. (1984) enrolled 14 patients with moderate COPD (FEV1 = 1.17 ± 0.76 L) in a home exercise program. All patients walked daily while carrying a lightweight backpack (2.6 ± 0.5 kg). Half also did weightlifting and limb-strengthening exercises, including wrist curls, arm curls, partial leg squats, calf raises, and supine dumbbell press. The initial backpack load of 4.3 ± 0.9 kg was increased weekly by 1.2 ± 0.5 kg for six weeks, reaching 10.4 ± 2.6 kg by the last week. The weightlifters performed 10 repetitions three times avoiding dyspnea, breath-holding, and fatigue for a total time of 30 minutes daily. Patients documented their exercises in a diary. Health care personnel visited the patients weekly. After training, all weightlifters had reduced their minute ventilation during bicycle ergometry, when compared with controls. Furthermore, the weight-trained patients showed a 16% increase in exercise endurance. This study suggests that patients can engage in exercise training in the comfort of their homes, with relatively inexpensive programs and no hospital visits. More recent data confirm that supervised home exercise programs achieve the same outcomes as those in hospitals (Wijkstra et al. 1994).

In our pulmonary rehabilitation program we use an electrically braked ergometer for testing and mechanically controlled ergometers for training, on either an outpatient or inpatient basis, depending on the patient's condition. See "Training Method for Leg Exercise" for a practical discussion of how we train our patients. The program may be tailored to each individual and to the available training equipment.

Training Method for Leg Exercise

1. Train at 60% of maximal work capacity (as determined by an exercise test, not necessarily by evaluating heart rate).
2. Increase work every 5th session as tolerated.
3. Monitor dyspnea and heart rate.
4. Increase work after 20-30 minutes of submaximal targeted work.
5. Aim for 24 sessions.

Upper Extremity Exercise

It is unfortunate that most of our knowledge about rehabilitation exercise conditioning derives from programs emphasizing leg training. Performance of many everyday tasks requires not only the hands but also the concerted action of other muscle groups that control upper torso and arm positioning. Some muscles of the upper torso and shoulder girdle serve both respiratory and postural functions. Muscles such as the upper and lower trapezius, latissimus dorsi, serratus anterior, subclavius, and pectoralis minor and major possess both thoracic and extrathoracic anchoring points. They may help position the arms or shoulders or, if given an extrathoracic fulcrum (such as fixing the arms in a supported position), they may exert a pulling force on the ribcage. In patients with chronic airflow obstruction, as severity worsens, the diaphragm loses its capacity to generate force, and the muscles of the rib cage become more important in generating inspiratory pressures (Martinez et al. 1990). When patients perform unsupported arm exercise, some of the shoulder girdle muscles decrease their participation in ventilation; tasks involving complex purposeful arm movements may affect the pattern of ventilation.

Studies on Upper Extremity Exercise

Tangri and Wolf (1973) used a pneumobelt to study breathing patterns in seven patients with COPD while they performed simple activities of daily living such as tying their shoes and brushing their teeth. The patients developed an irregular and rapid pattern of breathing with the arm exercise. After the exercise, the patients breathed faster and deeper, which according to the authors was done to restore the blood gases to normal.

We have explored the ventilatory response to unsupported arm exercise and compared it with the response to leg exercise in patients with severe chronic lung disease (Celli et al. 1986). Arm exercise resulted in dyssynchronous thoracoabdominal excursion that was not due solely to diaphragmatic fatigue. The dyspnea reported by the patients was associated with a dyssynchronous breathing pattern. We concluded that unsupported arm exercise could shift work to the diaphragm and in some way lead to dyssynchrony. To test this hypothesis, we plotted pleural pressure (Ppl) versus gastric pressure (Pg) (measured with gastric and endoesophageal balloons), evaluating the changes as well as the ventilatory responses to unsupported arm exercise. We compared these results with those from leg cycle ergometry in normal subjects and in patients with airflow obstruction (Celli et al. 1988; Criner and Celli 1988) and found increased diaphragmatic pressure excursion with arm exercise. We also found alterations in the pattern of pressure generation, with more contribution by the diaphragm and abdominal muscles of respiration and less contribution by the inspiratory muscles of the rib cage.

Our knowledge of ventilatory response to arm exercise was based on arm cycle ergometry. It is known that at a given workload in normal subjects, arm cranking is more demanding than leg cycling as shown by higher VO_2, VE, heart rate, blood pressure, and lactate production (Bobbert 1960; Davis et al. 1976; Steinberg et al. 1967). At maximal effort however, VO_2, VE, cardiac output, and lactate levels are lower during arm than during leg cycle ergometry (Martin et al. 1991; Reybrouck et al. 1975). Very little is known about the metabolic and ventilatory cost of simple arm elevation. Some recent reports underscore the importance of arm position in ventilation. Banzett et al. (1988) showed that arm bracing increases the capacity to sustain maximal ventilation, when compared to lifting the elbows from the braced position. Others have shown a decrease in the maximum attainable workload, and increases in both oxygen uptake and ventilation, at any given workload when normal subjects exercised with their arms elevated (Dolmage et al. 1993; Maestro et al. 1990). We evaluated the metabolic and respiratory consequence of simple arm elevation in patients with COPD (Martinez et al. 1990). Patients who held their arms in front of them, parallel to the floor, significantly increased both VO_2 and VCO_2, with concomitant increases in heart rate and VE. Evaluating ventilatory muscle recruitment patterns by continuous recording of Pg and Ppl, we observed increased contribution of diaphragmatic and abdominal muscle toward ventilation. The observations suggest that if we train the arms to perform more work, or if we decrease the ventilatory requirement for the same work, we should improve a patient's capacity to perform arm activity.

Results of Upper Extremity Exercise Training

Several studies using both arm and leg training have shown that the addition of arm training results in improved performance that is for the most part task-specific.

Belman and Kendregan (1981) observed a significant increase in arm exercise endurance after exercise training. Lake et al. (1990) had patients engage in arm exercise, leg exercise, or both. There were increases in exercise endurance for arm ergometry in the arm training group, for leg ergometry in the leg training group, and increases in both arm and leg ergometry in the combined group. In addition there was an improved sensation of well-being in the combined group. Ries et al. (1988) compared the effects of two forms of arm exercise—gravity resistance, and modified proprioceptive neuromuscular facilitation—with no arm exercise in a group of 45 patients with COPD who were involved in a comprehensive, multidisciplinary pulmonary rehabilitation program. Even though only 20 patients completed the program, they showed improved performance on tests that were specific for the training, and a decrease in fatigue in all the tests.

A group of cystic fibrosis patients studied by Keens et al. (1977) underwent upper extremity training consisting of swimming and canoeing for 1.5 hours daily. After six weeks, they exhibited increased upper extremity endurance; most importantly, their increase in maximal sustainable ventilatory capacity was similar to that obtained with ventilatory muscle training. This suggests that arm exercise training programs can train ventilatory muscles.

Because simple arm elevation results in significant increases in $\dot{V}O_E$, $\dot{V}O_2$, and VCO_2, we studied 14 patients with COPD before and after eight weeks of three-times-weekly, 20-minute sessions of unsupported arm and leg exercise. Our study was part of a comprehensive rehabilitation program to test whether arm training decreases ventilatory requirement for arm activity. There was a 35% decrease in the rise of $\dot{V}O_2$ and VCO_2 brought about by arm elevation, associated with a significant decrease in $\dot{V}O_E$ (Couser et al. 1993) (figure 9.2). Because the patients also trained their legs, we could not conclude that the improvement was due to the arm exercise. To answer this question, we had patients with COPD undergo either unsupported arm training ($n = 11$) or resistance breathing training ($n = 14$). After 24 sessions, arm endurance increased only for the unsupported arm training group. Interestingly, maximal inspiratory

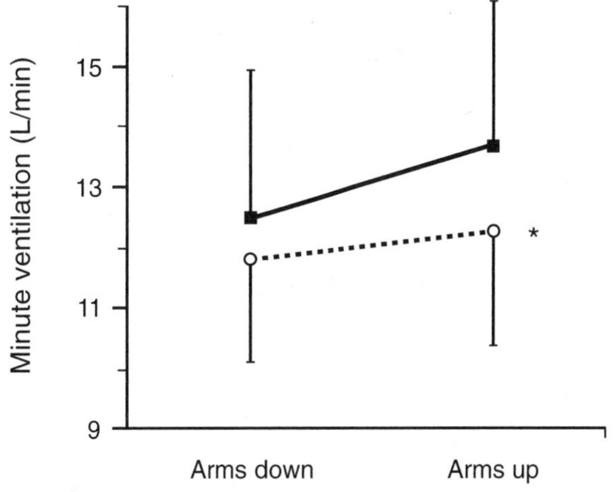

Figure 9.2 Minute ventilation measured with arms down and after 2 minutes of arm elevation before unsupported arm training (■). After 19 sessions of unsupported arm training, the patients manifested a significant decrease in minute ventilation during arm elevation (O). $*p < .05$ using paired t-test.

Reprinted, by permission, from J. Couser et al., 1993, "Pulmonary rehabilitation that include arm exercise," *Chest* 103:37-41.

pressure increased significantly for both groups, indicating that by training the arms, we may induce ventilatory muscle training for those rib cage muscles that hinge on the shoulder girdle (Epstein et al. 1991).

Upper Extremity Rehabilitation Programs

Based on the information available, we include arm exercise in our rehabilitation program. As seen in "Training Method for Supported (Ergometry) Arm Exercise," and "Training Method for Unsupported Arm Exercise" the methods for supported and unsupported exercises vary in their implementation.

Our patients generally perform arm ergometry for 20 minutes per session, starting at 60% of the maximal work (measured in watts) achieved in the exercise test and increasing the work weekly as tolerated. We monitor dyspnea and heart rate. For patients whose limiting symptom is dyspnea at minimal work, we exercise them at 60% of the work that makes them stop. In the most severe patients, the heart rate is unreliable—they may be tachycardic even at rest and may not show any significant increase with exercise. In these patients, dyspnea may be a more reliable index to follow.

In unsupported arm exercise training, patients lift a dowel (750 g) to shoulder level in the same rhythm as their breathing rate. For a total of 30 minutes, they exercise for two minutes then rest for two minutes. We monitor dyspnea and heart rate and we increase the load by 250 grams each week, as tolerated. We aim to complete 24 sessions.

Martinez et al. (1993) compared unsupported arm training with arm ergometry training. Endurance time improved significantly for both groups, but unsupported arm training decreased oxygen uptake at the same workload when compared to arm cranking training. They concluded that arm exercise against gravity may be more effective in training patients for activities that resemble those of daily living.

Table 9.3 summarizes an increasing body of evidence that upper extremity exercise training results in improved performance for arm activities in general and decreases ventilatory requirements for upper extremity activities similar to those in the exercise. The net result is an improvement in the capacity of patients to perform activities of daily living.

Respiratory Muscles and Breathing Training

Leith and Bradley (1976) first demonstrated that, like their skeletal counterparts, the respiratory muscles of normal individuals can be specifically trained to improve their strength or their endurance. Subsequent to that observation, a number of studies have shown that a training response will occur if there is sufficient stimulus. An increase in inspiratory muscle strength (and perhaps endurance) should result in improved respiratory muscle function by decreasing the ratio of the pressure required to breath (PI) and the maximal pressure that the respiratory system can generate (PImax). The PI/PImax ratio, which represents the effort required to complete each breath as a function of the force reserve, is the most important determinant of fatigue in loaded respiratory muscles (Roussos and Macklem 1982). Since patients with COPD have reduced inspiratory muscle strength, considerable efforts have been made to define the role of respiratory muscle training in these patients.

Ventilatory Muscle Strength and Endurance Training

In some cases, training ventilatory muscles is extremely effective. In others, it is of no use or even counterpro-

Training Method for Supported (Ergometry) Arm Exercise

1. Train at 60% of maximal work capacity (as determined by an exercise test, not necessarily by evaluating heart rate).
2. Increase work every 5th session as tolerated.
3. Monitor dyspnea and heart rate.
4. Train for as long as tolerated up to 30 minutes

Training Method for Unsupported Arm Exercise

1. Dowel (weight = 750 grams).
2. Lift to shoulder level for 2 minutes, one repetition for each breath.
3. Rest for 2 minutes.
4. Repeat sequence as tolerated for up to 32 minutes.
5. Monitor dyspnea and heart rate.
6. Increase weight (250 grams) every 5th session as tolerated.

Table 9.3 Controlled Studies of Arm Exercise in Patients With COPD

Author	No. patients	Duration	Course	Type 1	Results
Keens	7 arms	1.5 hr/day	4 wk	Swimming/canoeing	↑VMT (56%)
	4 VMT	15 min/day	4 wk	VMT	↑VME (52%)
	4 control	—	—	VMT	↑VME (22%)
Belman	8 arms	20 min 4 ×/wk	6 wk	Arm ergometry	↑Arm cycle No ↑PFT
	7 legs	20 min 4 ×/wk	6 wk	Cycle ergometry	↑Leg cycle No ↑PFT
Lake	6 arms	1 hr 3 ×/wk	8 wk	Several types	No change in PImax or VME
	6 legs	1 hr 3 ×/wk	8 wk	Walking	No change in PImax or VME
	7 arms and legs	1 hr 3 ×/wk	8 wk	Combined	No change in PImax or VME
Ries	8 gravity resistance arms	15 min/day	6 wk	Low-resistance, high-repetition	↑Arm endurance ↓Dyspnea
	9 neuromuscular facilitation	15 min/day	6 wk	Weight lifts	↑Arm endurance ↓Dyspnea
	11 controls	—	6 wk	Walk	No change
Epstein	13 arms	30 min/day	8 wk	UAE	↓VO_2 and VE for arm elevation ↑PImax
	10 VMT	30 min/day	8 wk	VMT	↑PImax and VME

VMT = ventilatory muscle training; VME = ventilatory muscle endurance; PFT = pulmonary function tests; PImax = maximal inspiratory pressure; UAE = unsupported arm elevation.

ductive. Every clinician should be well aware of when such training is or is not appropriate.

STRENGTH TRAINING

A high-intensity, low-frequency stimulus is needed to train respiratory muscles. Inspiratory muscles are trained by inspiratory maneuvers performed against a closed glottis or shutter.

Several studies have shown an increase in maximal inspiratory pressures when the respiratory muscles have been specifically trained for strength. Lecoq and colleagues studied nine patients (some of whom had COPD) who, after four weeks of training, showed a 50% increase in PImax (Lecoq et al. 1970). Reid and Warren (1984) observed a 53% increase in PImax in six COPD patients after five weeks of training. Both groups noticed a smaller but significant increase in expiratory muscle pressure. Decreasing PI/PImax through respiratory muscle strength training does not appear to be clinically important. Yet respiratory muscle strength often increases as a by-product of endurance training achieved with the use of resistive loads. It is possible that some of the benefits observed after endurance training may relate to the increased strength.

ENDURANCE TRAINING

Endurance is achieved through low-intensity, high-frequency training programs, of which there are three types: flow resistive loading, threshold loading, and voluntary isocapneic hyperpnea.

FLOW RESISTIVE LOADING AND THRESHOLD LOADING

In flow resistive training, the load is created primarily by decreasing the inspiratory breathing hole size—provided that frequency, tidal volume, and inspiratory time are held constant. Although most studies in patients with COPD have shown an improvement in the time that a given respiratory load can be maintained (ventilatory muscle endurance), the results must be interpreted with caution since it has been shown that endurance can be influenced and actually increased with changes in the pattern of breathing. Threshold loading can result in some muscle training, by assuring that at least the inspired pressure is high enough to ensure training, independent of inspiratory flow rate. Although breathing pattern is important (inspiratory time or TI and respiratory rate), it is not as critically important as inspired pressure.

Because many studies have not been controlled, it is difficult to attribute their results to the training. The controlled studies summarized in table 9.4 show an increase in the endurance time during which the ventilatory muscles could tolerate a known load; some show a significant increase in strength (Belman and Shadmehr 1988; Chen et al. 1985; Harver et al. 1989; Larson et al. 1988) and a decrease in dyspnea during the performance of inspiratory load and exercise (Epstein et al. 1991; Falk et al. 1985). In the studies that evaluated systemic exercise performance, there was a minimal increase in walking

Table 9.4 Controlled Trials of Ventilatory Muscle Resistive Training in COPD

Author	No. patients	Type	Frequency	Duration	Results
Pardy	9	RB	2 ×/day	8 wk	↑ET ↑12 MW
	8	PT	3 ×/wk	8 wk	No change
Larson	10	RB	30 min/day	8 wk	↑PImax ↑ET
		30% PImax			↑12 MW
	12	RB	Daily	8 wk	No ↑PI, end time, or 12 MW
		15% PImax		30 min	
Harver	10	RB	15 min 2 ×/day	8 wk	↑PImax
	9	Sham	15 min 2 ×/day	8 wk	No change
Belman	8	RB	Daily	6 wk	↑ET (30 min)
					↑PImax
	9	RB	Daily	6 wk	30 min
Chen	7	RB	Daily	4 wk	↑ET (30 min)
	6	Sham	Daily	4 wk	No change (30 min)
Bjerre	14	RB	45 min/day	6 wk	↑ET, no exercise
	14	Sham	45 min/day	6 wk	No change
Falk	12	RB	Daily	12 mo	↑ET (45 min), no exercise
	15	Sham	Daily	12 mo	No change
Noseda	12	RB	Daily	8 wk	↑ET (30 min) exercise
	13	Breathing	Daily	8 wk	No change
Jones	7	RB	Daily	10 wk	↑Exercise end (30 min)
	6	Sham	Daily	10 wk	↑Exercise end
	8	Exercise	Daily	10 wk	↑Exercise end
Weiner	12	RB and exercise	Daily	3 mo	↑↑Exercise
					↑PImax
	12	Exercise	Daily	3 mo	↑Exercise
	12	Control	None	3 mo	No change
Lisboa	10	RB	Daily	5 wk	No change
		12% PImax			
	10	RB	Daily	5 wk	↑PImax ↑ET
		30% PImax			↓Dyspnea

ET = endurance time for loaded breathing; Exercise end = leg exercise endurance; PImax = maximal inspiratory pressure; RB = resistive breathing; PT = physical therapy.

distance (Jones et al. 1985; Larson et al. 1988; Lisboa et al. 1994; Pardy et al. 1981; Weiner et al. 1992).

Weiner and colleagues assigned 36 COPD patients to one of three groups. Group 1 received specific ventilatory muscle threshold training (VMT) combined with general exercise reconditioning; group 2 received exercise training alone; group 3 received no training. VM training improved VM strength and endurance (as is already known), but patients treated with the combination of exercise and VMT manifested a significant increase in exercise tolerance when compared with those who only exercised (Weiner et al. 1992). In a companion article, the same group reported that asthmatic patients treated with VMT not only increased strength but also showed improvements in asthma symptoms, number of hospitalizations, number of emergency department visits, frequency of school or work absenteeism, and amount of medication consumption (Weiner et al. 1992). Lisboa et al. (1994) have shown that VMT at 30% of PImax seems not only to increase leg ergometry endurance; it also improves baseline dyspnea score and decreases breathlessness with exercise.

It is clear that VMT with resistive breathing results in improved VM strength and endurance. In COPD, however, it is not clear whether this effort results in decreased morbidity or mortality or offers any clinical advantage that makes it worth the effort. In many studies, compliance has been low—with up to 50% of all pulmonary patients failing to complete the programs. On the other hand, if confirmed by others, the studies by Weiner and coworkers (1992) and Lisboa et al. (1994) suggest that this form of treatment for asthmatics should be further explored.

Ventilatory Isocapneic Hyperpnea

This is a training method by which patients maintain high levels of ventilation over time (15 minutes, two or three times daily). The oxygen and carbon dioxide are kept constant in the breathing circuit. In an uncontrolled study, patients with COPD not only increased their maximal sustained ventilatory capacity but also increased arm and leg exercise performance after six weeks of training (Harver et al. 1989). Two controlled studies (table 9.5) also reported increases in maximal sustainable ventilatory capacity (MSVC) in COPD in patients trained for six weeks, but their improvement in exercise endurance was no better than that of the control group (Belman and Mittman 1980; Ries and Moser 1986).

It seems that respiratory muscle training results in increased strength and capacity of the muscles to endure a respiratory load. There is debate as to whether it also results in improved exercise performance or improved performance in activities of daily living. Knowing the respiratory muscle factors that may contribute to ventilatory limitation in COPD, one might logically predict that increases in strength and endurance should help respiratory muscle function. But this is perhaps only important in the capacity of the patients to handle inspiratory loads, for example in acute exacerbations of their disease. It is less likely that ventilatory muscle training will greatly affect systemic exercise performance.

Ventilatory Muscle Training for Intensive Care Patients

Few data exist to justify training the ventilatory muscles of patients in intensive care. It is apparent that as soon as patients are left to breathe on their own (as during any form of weaning), their respiratory muscles are being retrained. We actually use this "training method" whenever we place patients on either T-piece or low synchronized intermittent mandatory ventilation (SIMV), although we don't generally analyze the results as we would for a formal training method. More often, we

Table 9.5 Controlled Trials of Ventilatory Isocapneic Hyperpnea in Patients With COPD

Author	No. patients	Type	Frequency	Duration	Results
Ries	5	VIH	45 min	6 wk	↑MSVC
					↑Exercise
	7	Walking	45 min	6 wk	↑Exercise
Levine	15	VIH	15 min	6 wk	↑MSVC
					↑Exercise
					↑ADLs
	17	IPPB	15 min	6 wk	↑ADLs
					↑Exercise

VIH = ventilatory isocapneic; MSVC = maximal sustainable ventilatory capacity; ADLs = activities of daily living; IPPB = intermittent positive pressure breathing.

think of training in terms of additional external loads in addition to spontaneous respiration.

STUDIES

Few researchers have studied patients recovering from ventilatory failure. Belman and colleagues reported improvement in two patients who had difficulty weaning from mechanical ventilation; after respiratory muscle threshold training, they were able to come off mechanical ventilation (Belman et al. 1981). In a larger but still uncontrolled study, Aldrich et al. (1989) recruited 30 patients who had suffered from stable chronic respiratory failure for at least three weeks, but who had failed repeated weaning attempts. Patients with active infections or unstable cardiovascular, renal, or endocrine problems were excluded, as were those with gross malnutrition (albumin <2.5 g/dL) or neuromuscular disease. Training consisted of intermittently breathing through one inspiratory resistor while either spontaneously breathing or being supported at two to eight breaths per minute with SIMV. The patients' PImax improved from 37 ± 15 to 46 ± 15 cm H_2O while vital capacity increased from 561 ± 325 to 901 ± 480 ml. Of the 30 patients, 12 were weaned after 10 to 46 days of training (40% success). Because the study was uncontrolled and used a selected group of patients, its findings may not apply to most patients recovering from respiratory failure; furthermore, the success rate is little different from those reported in weaning facilities that have not used VMT (Alrich et al. 1989). Before ventilatory muscle training can be recommended as a form of treatment for patients with respiratory failure, more rigorous research is needed.

CAUTION IS NECESSARY

It is important to understand that ventilatory muscle training, especially with resistive or threshold loading, may be deleterious. Breathing at high tension time index with either a PI/PImax or prolonged inspiratory time over the total duration of a respiratory cycle (T_I/T_{TOT}) may induce muscle fatigue (Bellemare and Grassino 1982). Because the muscles of ventilation cannot be rested, as is customary in the training of peripheral muscles in athletes, fatigue may precipitate ventilatory failure in COPD patients. Increased PI is an intrinsic part of VMT, hence it is possible that if an intense enough program is enforced, fatigue may actually be precipitated.

BREATHING RETRAINING

There are other less conventional forms of training that are open to critical review, but that are conceptually solid and may offer new avenues of treatment. The ventilated patient has a high ventilatory drive—patients who failed a ventilator weaning trial manifest higher drive than those patients who successfully weaned.

BIOFEEDBACK

Holliday and Hyers studied 40 patients after at least seven days of mechanical ventilation, weaning them either with conventional methods or with electromyographic feedback training, using the frontalis signal to indicate tension and induce relaxation. They also used surface EMG of the intercostals and diaphragm as indicators of respiratory muscle activity. Compared with the control group, the biofeedback group had fewer mean ventilator days. Their tidal volume and mean inspiratory flow increased significantly when corrected by diaphragmatic EMG amplitude (which was interpreted as improved diaphragmatic efficiency). The authors concluded that breathing retraining resulted in a more efficient breathing pattern, which in turn decreased dyspnea and anxiety and allowed for quicker weaning time in the treated patients (Holliday and Hyers 1990).

To further study some of these factors, we measured the work of breathing (determined by the pressure time integral of the excursions of the continuously recorded Ppl) before and after rehabilitation in 16 patients with COPD. There were no changes in pulmonary functions, but there was a significant decrease in the pressure time index at the exercise isotime after rehabilitation (table 9.6). This drop was due mostly to a decrease in respiratory frequency (Benditt et al. 1990).

Finally, retraining in breathing techniques or pursed-lip breathing that decreases breathing frequency has resulted in increases in tidal volume oxygen saturation and decreases in dyspnea (Roa et al.).

In a previously cited work from our laboratory, analysis of the many factors that may have contributed to improved exercise endurance for upper extremity exercise after upper extremity training indicated that the most striking was a drop in mean inspiratory flow (VT/T_I) at exercise isotime (Epstein et al. 1997). We believe this may represent better coordination of the respiratory muscles.

YOGA

There are other ways to improve ventilatory patterns. Yoga teaches control of posture and voluntary control of breathing, the latter including rapid abdominal maneuvers and/or slow deep breaths with apnea at the end of inspiration and expiration. The breathing rate may be brought down to 6 breaths per minute.

Stanescu et al. (1981) compared breathing patterns of eight well-trained yoga practitioners with eight controls matched for gender, age, and height. The yoga group had a breathing pattern of ample tidal volume and slow

Table 9.6 Work of Breathing, Exercise Endurance, and Maximal Transdiaphragmatic Pressure Before and After Pulmonary Rehabilitation

	Endurance time (sec)	∫ Pesdt (Cm H_2O · min)	Pdimax (Cm H_2O)
Pre-rehab	434	288	48
Post-rehab	512*	219*	52

*$p < .05$

Pdimax = maximal transdiaphragmatic pressure; ∫ Pesdt = work of breathing as estimated by the pressure time index calculated from continuous recording of endoesophageal pressure.

frequency, and a lower ventilatory response to CO_2 rebreathing. The mechanisms of these effects are not clear, but they include habituation to chronic overstimulation of stretch receptors. Since ventilation is automatically controlled by structures in the upper medulla and brain stem, and is voluntarily controlled by the cortex, sustained slow deep breathing may become a "learned" reflex. Whatever the mechanisms, these responses may have practical applications. Tandon (1980) studied the effects of yoga breathing in patients with COPD. The yoga-trained patients controlled dyspnea and improved their exercise tolerance better than the controls.

Postural Changes

Habitual positioning may determine musculoskeletal tone and contraction. Over the last few years, increasing attention has been given to the voluntary inhibition of these musculoskeletal tone and contraction patterns. This focus has been particularly useful for singers. Austin and Pullin (1984) found that proprioceptive musculoskeletal education for better posture improved peak expiratory flow rate, maximal voluntary ventilation, and maximal inspiratory and expiratory pressures in normal subjects. These lessons have not been systematically evaluated in patients with lung disease, but breathing retraining (pursed-lip breathing and diaphragmatic breathing) is a form of therapy that resembles the above-mentioned techniques.

Pursed-Lip Breathing

Pursed-lip breathing (PLB) slows the breathing rate and increases tidal volume. It shifts the recruitment pattern of ventilatory muscles from one that is predominantly diaphragmatic to one that recruits more accessory muscles of the rib cage and abdominal muscles of exhalation (Roa et al. 1991). This shift may contribute to the relief of dyspnea reported by patients when they adopt PLB. Patients on ventilators cannot use pursed-lip breathing techniques. But administration of expiratory retardants or positive-end expiratory pressure improves oxygenation; it also decreases respiratory rate, augments ventilation, and improves the work of breathing in weaning patients. Since pursed-lip breathing (PLB) and positive end expiratory pressure (PEEP) may have similar physiologic effects, the former therapy is often indicated once the latter has been discontinued.

Summary

A critical review of the literature indicates that leg and arm exercise training improve exercise performance and seem to have physiological explanations different from simple dyspnea desensitization. Implementation of such elementary training programs is within the reach of virtually any facility and will result in better quality of life for patients with respiratory disease.

There are more unresolved questions than known facts about training and respiratory muscle function. A wealth of information will be gained if systematic scientific analysis is applied to answer many of the questions we have addressed in this review. It is rewarding to see that widespread interest in applied respiratory physiology has begun to produce results that may benefit the large number of patients suffering from disabling respiratory diseases and for whom there are no other viable therapeutic options.

CHAPTER 10

DIABETES MELLITUS

Edward S. Horton, MD

CASE STUDY

A 52-year-old accountant, J.P., was referred to us for evaluation and treatment of newly diagnosed type 2 diabetes mellitus. He stated that he has been overweight most of his adult life, which he attributes to his sedentary occupation. He has a history of hypertension and hyperlipidemia, which are being treated with a thiazide diuretic and an HMG Co-A reductase inhibitor respectively. He reluctantly admitted to some increasing fatigue, nocturia, and difficulty reading because of blurred vision. He also had noted polyuria, which he attributed to excessive coffee intake. He currently smokes one pack of cigarettes a day and has a 30-year history of smoking. His father had type 2 diabetes and died of a myocardial infarction at age 53.

On physical examination, J.P. was 5 feet 10 inches tall, weighed 235 pounds, and had a sitting blood pressure of 145/92 mmHg. He was obese, with, predominantly, an abdominal distribution of body fat, but otherwise appeared generally well. Fundoscopic examination revealed hard exudates, microaneurysms, and some blot hemorrhages, but no neovascularization. Cardiovascular examination was normal except for moderate hypertension, and carotid and peripheral pulses were normal without bruits. On neurological examination, the ankle jerks were absent and vibration sense was diminished, but touch sensation was normal when tested with a 10-g filament. Laboratory tests revealed a fasting plasma glucose of 260 mg/dL, hemoglobin A1C 9.2%, total cholesterol 220 mg/dL, LDL-cholesterol 105 mg/dL, HDL-cholesterol 32 mg/dL, and triglycerides 400 mg/dL. Urinalysis revealed glucosuria, but no albuminuria or ketone bodies.

We reconfirmed that J.P. does have type 2 diabetes mellitus, as well as inadequately treated hypertension, dsylipidemia, and obesity. In addition, he has moderately severe background retinopathy and has early peripheral neuropathy.

Our treatment goal was to institute a lifestyle modification program to reduce his body weight by 7% to 10% through dietary modification and increased aerobic exercise, to reduce cardiovascular risk factors through smoking cessation, and to treat his hypertension and dyslipidemia more effectively. After an initial three-month trial of appropriate diet and exercise, glycemic control would be reassessed, and oral antidiabetic agents started, if necessary, to achieve control of his hyperglycemia.

To achieve these goals, the thiazide diuretic was replaced by an angiotensin converting enzyme inhibitor (ACEI), and the HMG Co-A reductase inhibitor was continued at the same dose. We referred J.P. to our diabetes management team for basic education and implementation of a calorically restricted diet that provided a daily negative energy balance of 500 to 1,000 kcal and followed the National Cholesterol Education Program Step 1 Guidelines. He was seen by the exercise physiologist who assessed his physical fitness and prescribed a program of moderate-intensity aerobic exercise for 30 to 45 minutes daily for at least 5 days per week. Because of the peripheral neuropathy, appropriate shoes were recommended, and exercises such as cycling, rowing, and swimming were prescribed rather than jogging or running. J.P. also undertook a smoking cessation program and decreased his coffee drinking as part of his lifestyle modification program.

(continued)

(continued)

After three months, J.P. lost 15 pounds and was successfully exercising 5 days a week. His blood pressure was 135/85, fasting glucose was 140 mg/dL, and hemoglobin A1C was 7.8%. Total cholesterol was 215 mg/dL, LDL-cholesterol 100 mg/dL, HDL-cholesterol 38 mg/dL, and triglycerides 300 mg/dL. His symptoms of fatigue, blurred vision, nocturia, and polyuria were much improved, and he had decreased his smoking to one or two cigarettes per day. Because of his substantial progress, we elected to continue the same program and did not start him on an oral antidiabetic agent at that time. This proved to be a good decision, since he continued to improve over the next three months with a further 10-pound weight loss and improvement in his glucose, blood pressure, and lipid levels.

This case illustrates several points about type 2 diabetes mellitus. First, as many as 50% of patients will have evidence of long-term complications when diabetes is first diagnosed. A thorough history and physical examination are required before starting a program of exercise and lifestyle modification. Second, patients with type 2 diabetes frequently have multiple risk factors for cardiovascular disease. In this case, hypertension, dyslipidemia, obesity, and cigarette smoking were all present and had to be addressed in the treatment plan. Third, a program of lifestyle modification to treat the diabetes and comorbidities requires a team approach involving diabetes education, nutrition, exercise physiology, and behavior modification, as well as appropriate medications. Finally, such an approach can be very successful in achieving the goals of treatment and should form the basis on which all other therapies are built. Over time, many patients with type 2 diabetes will require the addition of oral antidiabetic drugs or insulin, but a healthy lifestyle remains a fundamental pillar of the treatment program.

There are approximately 18 million people with diabetes in the United States and 200 million worldwide. Over 90% have type 2 diabetes, and the incidence is increasing rapidly in many populations. Perhaps one-third to one-half of people with type 2 diabetes in the United States are receiving no treatment, because their disease is undiagnosed. In those who are diagnosed, treatment is frequently inadequate, leading to long-term complications that might be prevented. In the United States, diabetes is still the leading cause of new-onset blindness, of chronic renal failure requiring dialysis or kidney transplant, and of nontraumatic lower-extremity amputation. Approximately 60% of mortality in diabetes is due to coronary artery and other heart disease, while 15% results from cerebrovascular disease. The costs of treating diabetes and its complications may exceed 100 billion dollars per year in the United States nearly 15% of the total health care budget. Because of the increased mortality and morbidity associated with diabetes and the high costs of medical care for people with diabetes, it is imperative that physicians become more familiar with diabetes and its treatment. A healthy lifestyle, including increased physical activity and weight reduction, is essential both to prevent and to treat diabetes. This chapter reviews current information about diabetes including the diagnosis, pathophysiology, and classification of its different forms and discusses the role of physical (particularly aerobic) exercise as a key element in its treatment.

WHAT IS DIABETES?

Diabetes mellitus is not a single disease but a group of metabolic disorders characterized by increased fasting and postprandial blood glucose concentrations that result from decreased insulin secretion, decreased insulin action, or both.

Although defects in the regulation of glucose metabolism are considered to be the primary abnormality in diabetes, alterations in lipid and protein metabolism also can occur including hyperlipidemia and a protein catabolic state in inadequately treated patients. The most common symptoms of diabetes are related to chronic **hyperglycemia** and include fatigue, increased thirst and urination (**polydipsia** and **polyuria**), weight loss, increased hunger (**polyphagia**), blurred vision, poor wound healing, and increased susceptibility to infections. Prolonged, severe hyperglycemia may lead to dehydration, mental confusion, and loss of consciousness (**hyperosmolar nonketotic syndrome**) or, when severe insulin deficiency is present, to **diabetic ketoacidosis** and death.

Hypoglycemia may occur in patients treated with insulin or drugs that stimulate insulin secretion. Symptoms of hypoglycemia include those associated with activation of the sympathetic nervous system such as tachycardia, palpitations, perspiration, and sensations of anxiety or hunger. With severe or prolonged hypoglycemia, neuroglucopenia may lead to mental confusion, loss of consciousness, or seizures. Symptoms usually respond rapidly to restoration of normal blood glucose concentrations, but prolonged, untreated hypoglycemia may lead to permanent brain damage.

The major morbidity and mortality of diabetes relate to long-term complications of chronic hyperglycemia.

These include potential loss of vision; chronic renal failure; damage to peripheral nerves leading to loss of sensation, foot ulcers, Charcot joints, and risk of amputation; and damage to the autonomic nervous system causing gastrointestinal, genitourinary, and cardiovascular symptoms, as well as sexual dysfunction. Collectively these have been termed the **microvascular complications** of diabetes, and their development and progression are clearly linked to the degree and duration of hyperglycemia (DCCT 1993; Ohkubo et al. 1995; United Kingdom Prospective Diabetes Study Group 1998).

People with diabetes also have an increased incidence of **macrovascular diseases** including atherosclerotic cardiovascular, peripheral vascular, and cerebrovascular disease. The increased risk of atherosclerosis in diabetes is multifactorial and not well understood. Hyperglycemia may play a role, but diabetes is associated with increases in many of the recognized risk factors for atherosclerosis in nondiabetic individuals: hypertension, hyperlipidemia, obesity, insulin resistance, and alterations in the regulation of thrombosis and fibrinolysis. When adjustments are made for these risk factors, however, the incidence of coronary artery disease is still significantly greater in people with diabetes compared to those without the disease (Kannel 1990; Koskinen et al. 1992). Current research is directed toward understanding the relative roles and mechanisms by which hyperglycemia, hyperinsulinemia, and insulin resistance may contribute to the increased risk of macrovascular disease in diabetes.

Classification of Diabetes

Several pathogenic processes are involved in the development of diabetes ranging from destruction of insulin-producing pancreatic beta cells by autoimmune, toxic, or other mechanisms, to defects in regulation of insulin secretion and action on its target tissues. Insulin deficiency may be "absolute," as in the case of pancreatic beta cell destruction, or "relative," when insulin secretion is present but inadequate to maintain blood glucose within the normal range.

In 1997, an expert committee of the American Diabetes Association revised the **diagnostic criteria** and classification of diabetes. The new classification divides diabetes into four major diagnostic groups, based on etiology (American Diabetes Association 2005).

- In **type 1 diabetes,** destruction of beta cells leads to absolute insulin deficiency. The damage may be immune mediated or idiopathic.
- **Type 2 diabetes,** the most common form of the disease, is characterized by relative insulin deficiency. Patients may range from predominantly insulin resistant, with relative insulin deficiency, to having a predominantly insulin-secretory defect with only mild to moderate insulin resistance.
- A large number of other specific, but generally uncommon, forms of diabetes have been defined, including diabetes associated with genetic defects of beta cell function or insulin action, or with diseases of the endocrine pancreas; diabetes induced by various endocrinopathic drugs or chemicals; diabetes caused by various infections; uncommon forms of immune-mediated diabetes; and other genetic syndromes sometimes associated with diabetes.
- Finally, **gestational diabetes mellitus (GDM)** refers to diabetes that first appears during pregnancy, usually during the second or third trimester. In most cases, glucose tolerance returns to normal after delivery, but women with a history of GDM are at increased future risk of developing type 2 diabetes. Untreated GDM is frequently associated with fetal macrosomia, complicated delivery, and increased neonatal morbidity.

The ADA also modified the diagnostic criteria for diabetes from those previously used, and created a new category of **impaired fasting glucose.** Criteria for diagnosing **impaired glucose tolerance** remained unchanged, however, and are still based on the plasma glucose concentration two hours after a 75-gram oral glucose load. See "Criteria for the Diagnosis of Diabetes Mellitus, Impaired Glucose Tolerance, and Impaired Fasting Glucose."

Pathogenesis of Type 1 and Type 2 Diabetes

The most common cause of type 1 diabetes is autoimmune destruction of the pancreatic beta cells, which can occur rapidly or over many months or years. Markers of the immune process, which often appear before the onset of clinical diabetes, include islet cell autoantibodies, insulin autoantibodies, autoantibodies to glutamic acid decarboxylase, and autoantibodies to the tyrosine phosphatases IA-2 and IA-2B. There are also strong HLA (human leukocyte antigen) associations, with linkage to the DQA and DQB genes. Autoimmune destruction of the beta cells has multiple genetic modulators with both susceptibility and protective alleles, and is also related to environmental factors that are not well understood. Current research seeks to identify and modulate the autoimmune process in susceptible individuals, with the goal of preventing or delaying the onset of clinical diabetes and preserving residual beta cell function in those who have already developed diabetes. Once diabetes is established, treatment with insulin is required

CRITERIA FOR THE DIAGNOSIS OF DIABETES MELLITUS, IMPAIRED GLUCOSE TOLERANCE, AND IMPAIRED FASTING GLUCOSE

Diabetes Mellitus

- Symptoms of diabetes plus casual glucose concentration ≥ 200 mg/dL (11.1 mmol/L). Casual is defined as any time of day without regard to time since last meal. The classic symptoms of diabetes include polyuria, polydipsia, and unexplained weight loss.

or

- Fasting plasma glucose ≥ 126 mg/dL (7.0 mmol/L). Fasting is defined as no caloric intake for at least 8 hours.

or

- Plasma glucose ≥ 200 mg/dL (11.1 mmol/L) 2 hours after the oral ingestion of a glucose load equivalent to 75 g anhydrous glucose dissolved in water in a previously fasting subject (oral glucose tolerance test—OGTT).

In the absence of unequivocal hyperglycemia with acute metabolic decompensation, these criteria should be confirmed on a different day.

Impaired Glucose Tolerance

Plasma glucose ≥140 mg/dL (7.8 mmol/L) and <200 mg/dL (11.1 mmol/L) 2 hours after oral ingestion of a glucose load equivalent to 75 g anhydrous glucose dissolved in water in a previously fasting subject (OGTT).

Impaired Fasting Glucose

Fasting plasma glucose ≥100 mg/dL (5.6 mmol/L) and <126 mg/dL (7.0 mmol/L).

Source: American Diabetes Association 2005.

to maintain blood glucose concentration as close to normal as possible in order to relieve symptoms, restore metabolism, and prevent the development of acute and long-term complications of the disease.

Unlike type 1 diabetes, type 2 diabetes is associated not with beta cell destruction and absolute insulin deficiency, but rather with defects in the regulation of insulin secretion and action. Several factors contribute to development of type 2 diabetes. The disease is strongly familial and polygenic in character. As yet undetermined genetic factors contribute to both insulin resistance and impaired beta cell function.

A number of environmental factors contribute to insulin resistance. The most important of these are obesity (particularly intra-abdominal fat deposition), physical inactivity, and advancing age. Thus, as the population becomes older, fatter, and less physically active, insulin resistance increases and the incidence of type 2 diabetes also increases at a rapid rate. Figure 10.1 illustrates the sequence of events in the development of type 2 diabetes. Since insulin secretion adequately compensates for the insulin resistance before diabetes develops, the body is able to maintain normal fasting and postprandial plasma glucose concentrations. As insulin resistance increases or β-cell function decreases, insulin secretion can no longer fully compensate and impaired glucose tolerance develops. Genetic factors and the presence of increased glucose and/or free fatty acid concentrations may further impair beta cell function leading in turn to further worsening of glucose tolerance and eventually to the development of overt diabetes.

Interventions that reduce insulin resistance, such as weight reduction and increased physical exercise, are the first steps in both the prevention and treatment of type 2 diabetes. A large number of cross-sectional and prospective studies show that regular physical exercise decreases the risk of developing type 2 diabetes (Diabetes Prevention Program Research Group 2002; Helmrich et al. 1991; Kriska et al. 1991; Manson et al. 1991, 1992; Pan et al. 1997; Tuomilehto et al. 2001).

EXERCISE IN TYPE 1 DIABETES

Before the discovery of insulin, diet and exercise were the principal therapies for diabetes. However, the ability

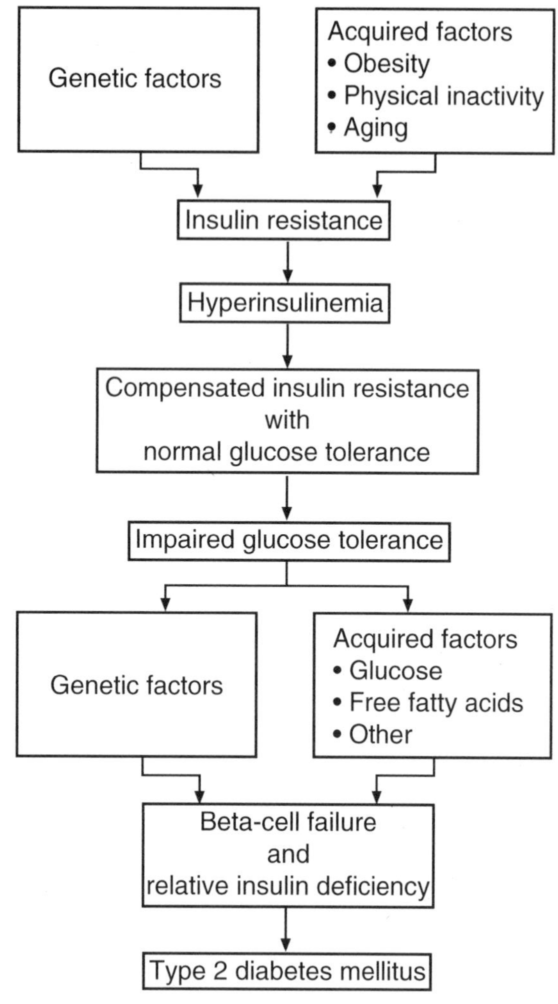

Figure 10.1 Steps in the development of type 2 diabetes mellitus.

Source: Kruszynska and Olefsky 1996.

to exercise was often severely limited in patients with type 1 diabetes because of the associated metabolic abnormalities, including muscle wasting, dehydration, and ketosis. Survival was rarely longer than two to three years. With the advent of insulin therapy in 1921, vigorous exercise became possible for patients with type 1 diabetes, although difficult to manage. Successful therapy of type 1 diabetes depends on a carefully managed interaction among food intake, physical exercise, and insulin administration. Increased knowledge about metabolic regulation in response to acute exercise and physical training, along with development of newer insulin preparations and methods for self-monitoring of blood glucose, now make it possible for people with type 1 diabetes to participate in a wide variety of recreational and competitive sports. Many such individuals have become world-class athletes. However, the appropriate role of physical exercise in the treatment of type 1 diabetes is still somewhat controversial. Some health care professionals instruct all individuals with diabetes to exercise regularly as an integral part of their treatment plan; others merely evaluate and educate patients so they can participate in exercise and sports if they wish to do so. The latter approach has gained favor in recent years. Physicians are realizing that exercise can present both benefits and significant risks to patients with type 1 diabetes and that appropriate advice requires careful evaluation of each patient with regard to his or her personal desires, the types of exercise to be performed, and the relative benefits and risks involved. Most diabetologists now seek to educate those with type 1 diabetes who want to participate in sports or other forms of physical exercise, but they do not recommend exercise for everyone. Educational programs should enable patients to maintain good metabolic control before, during, and after exercise, and to avoid or minimize the various complications of exercise (Horton 1988).

Potential Benefits

Regular physical exercise benefits the health of nearly everyone, including those with diabetes. See "Benefits of Exercise for Patients With Type 1 Diabetes." In addition to acutely lowering blood glucose (Berger et al. 1977; Kemmer et al. 1979) and increasing insulin sensitivity (Bjorntorp et al. 1970; Sato et al. 1984), regular exercise improves several of the recognized risk factors for cardiovascular disease. Serum cholesterol and triglyceride concentrations may decline with physical training, due to decreases in low-density and very low-density lipoproteins (Huttunen et al. 1979; Lipson et al. 1980) and increases in high-density lipoprotein cholesterol (Wood and Haskell 1979). Also, mild to moderate hypertension declines (Horton 1979), resting pulse rate and cardiac work decrease, and physical working capacity usually measured as maximal aerobic capacity ($\dot{V}O_2max$) increases with physical training. Since people with diabetes are at increased risk for developing cardiovascular disease, all of the above effects may provide the rationale for encouraging daily exercise. Psychological benefits of exercise such as an increased sense of well-being, improved self-esteem, and an enhanced quality of life are also important for people with diabetes, who must cope with the anxieties and limitations of living with a chronic disease.

Although exercise can acutely lower blood glucose and increase insulin sensitivity, some studies have failed to demonstrate a beneficial effect of regular exercise on long-term glycemic control in patients with type 1 diabetes (Wallberg-Henriksson et al. 1986; Zinman et al. 1977); others have shown that a program of regular exercise does result in improved glucose control (Marrero et al. 1988; Stratton et al. 1987). The negative results may be attributable to increased food intake that compensates

BENEFITS OF EXERCISE FOR PATIENTS WITH TYPE I DIABETES

1. Lower blood glucose concentrations during and after exercise
2. Improved insulin sensitivity and decreased insulin requirement
3. Improved lipid profile
   - Decreased triglycerides
   - Slightly decreased LDL-cholesterol
   - Increased HDL-cholesterol
4. Improvement in mild-to-moderate hypertension
5. Increased energy expenditure
   - Adjunct to diet for weight reduction
   - Increased fat loss
   - Preservation of lean body mass
6. Cardiovascular conditioning
7. Increased strength and flexibility
8. Improved sense of well-being and quality of life

for the increased energy expenditure of exercise, so that average blood glucose concentrations throughout a 24-hour period may not be altered (Zinman et al. 1977). One should not prescribe exercise programs for patients with type 1 diabetes for the sole purpose of improving long-term glycemic control. It is probably best to initiate an exercise program for such people only if they express desire to participate in sports or to obtain the general health benefits of an exercise program.

RISKS

Exercise presents several risks for patients with type 1 diabetes (see "Risks of Exercise for Patients With Type 1 Diabetes"). Weigh these risks against the potential benefits when advising patients about participation in vigorous physical activity. Hypoglycemia may occur during or after exercise, and superimposing exercise on the insulin-deficient state may lead to rapid increases in blood glucose and the development of ketosis. Even in well-controlled individuals, brief periods of high-intensity exercise may cause hyperglycemia.

In adults, exercise may precipitate angina pectoris, myocardial infarction, cardiac arrhythmias, or sudden death if there is underlying coronary artery disease. Exercise may also worsen several of the long-term complications of diabetes. Physical activity does not appear to affect the development or progression of proliferative retinopathy in patients with type 1 diabetes (Cruickshanks et al. 1995), but individuals who have proliferative retinopathy are at increased risk for developing retinal or vitreous hemorrhages or retinal detachment. Although there is no firm evidence that these complications occur more frequently during or following exercise, it is usually recommended that individuals with proliferative retinopathy should avoid extremely vigorous exercise that increases blood pressure or causes jarring of the head. While vigorous exercise also increases proteinuria (Mogensen and Vittinghu 1975; Viberti et al. 1978), it is probably a

RISKS OF EXERCISE FOR PATIENTS WITH TYPE 1 DIABETES

1. Hypoglycemia
   - Exercise-induced hypoglycemia
   - Late-onset postexercise hypoglycemia
2. Hyperglycemia after very strenuous exercise
3. Hyperglycemia and ketosis in insulin-deficient patients
4. Precipitation or exacerbation of cardiovascular disease
   - Angina pectoris
   - Myocardial infarction
   - Arrhythmias
   - Sudden death
5. Worsening of long-term complications of diabetes
   - Proliferative retinopathy
     a. Vitreous hemorrhage
     b. Retinal detachment
   - Nephropathy
     a. Increased proteinuria
   - Peripheral neuropathy
     a. Soft-tissue and joint injuries
   - Autonomic neuropathy
     a. Decreased cardiovascular response to exercise
     b. Decreased maximum aerobic capacity
     c. Impaired response to dehydration
     d. Postural hypotension
     e. Altered gastrointestinal function

transient hemodynamic response; exercise appears to have no deleterious effect on the progression of renal disease.

Injuries to soft tissues and joints may occur when patients with peripheral neuropathy engage in vigorous exercise. In those with autonomic neuropathy, physical working capacity may significantly decrease (Storstein and Jervell 1979), accompanied by increased resting pulse rate and reduced cardiovascular response to exercise (Hilsted et al. 1979; Kahn et al. 1986; Margonato et al. 1986), lower $\dot{V}O_2max$ (Rubler 1981), and impaired response to dehydration. Gastroparesis, with altered rates of gastric emptying, may affect the absorption of food, fluid, and electrolytes.

Carefully screen adults for long-term complications of diabetes prior to prescribing an exercise program of moderate to vigorous intensity. In addition to a complete history and physical examination, complete a dilated retinal examination to identify proliferative retinopathy; renal function tests, including a screen for microalbuminuria; and a neurological examination for peripheral and autonomic neuropathy. For individuals age 35 or older, an exercise stress test can help screen for undiagnosed ischemic cardiac disease.

However, long-term epidemiological data for children with type 1 diabetes suggest that regular physical activity early in life is not associated with an adverse effect on health; in fact, it may be beneficial (LaPorte et al. 1986).

Management of exercise in patients with type 1 diabetes requires knowledge of the integrated cardiovascular, hormonal, and neural responses that ensure delivery of oxygen and fuel to muscles, to the central nervous system, and to other organ systems, and that remove potentially toxic metabolic end products. Chapters 1 and 2 describe these processes in detail. In brief, metabolic fuels are regulated by a complex system that involves both (1) breakdown of glycogen and triglyceride stores within muscle tissue, and (2) increased delivery of glucose and free fatty acids (FFAs) from the circulation. Blood glucose concentrations are maintained during exercise by increased hepatic glucose output, derived from hepatic glycogenolysis and gluconeogenesis and from the digestion and absorption of ingested carbohydrates. Normally, hepatic glucose output is closely linked to glucose utilization, and blood glucose concentration is maintained within the normal range during exercise. Hypoglycemia is rare and occurs only with extreme, prolonged, and exhausting exercise.

During exercise, circulating FFA concentrations increase through release from adipose tissue triglycerides; exercising muscles and the liver then take up the FFAs and oxidize them for energy. Insulin plays a key role in regulating both glucose and FFA metabolism during exercise. It inhibits hepatic glucose production and stimulates peripheral glucose uptake, thus lowering the blood glucose concentration. It also inhibits lipolysis in adipose tissue, decreasing the release of FFAs, an important energy source for both the muscles and the liver. During exercise, activation of the sympathetic nervous system normally inhibits insulin secretion, decreasing plasma concentrations to a low physiological level and thereby increasing hepatic glucose production and adipose tissue lipolysis. Following the cessation of exercise, there is a transient increase in insulin secretion that reverses the increased rates of hepatic glucose production and lipolysis. Because patients with type 1 diabetes depend on exogenous insulin, they lack this finely tuned system—and regulation of metabolic fuel homeostasis during and after exercise is difficult to achieve. Too much insulin results in hypoglycemia, whereas too little leads to hyperglycemia and ketosis.

In the following sections common problems that patients with type 1 diabetes encounter in response to physical exercise, as well as the strategies used to prevent these problems, are discussed.

Exercise-Induced Hypoglycemia

Whereas changes in blood glucose are very small in normal subjects during exercise, several factors may complicate glucose regulation during and following exercise in patients with type 1 diabetes. Since exercise potentiates the hypoglycemic effect of injected insulin, regular physical activity leads to decreased insulin requirements and increased risk of hypoglycemic reactions. Several studies have confirmed that physical training increases sensitivity to insulin (Horton 1986). Athletes have normal or increased tolerance to oral glucose, in conjunction with low basal and glucose-stimulated insulin responses (Lohmann et al. 1978), and physical inactivity rapidly results in decreased glucose tolerance (Lipman et al. 1972). Both normal subjects and patients with diabetes have a 30% to 35% increase in insulin-stimulated glucose disposal after physical training, when studied by the hyperinsulinemic–euglycemic clamp technique (DeFronzo et al. 1983). This increase in insulin sensitivity correlates well with the training-induced increase in $\dot{V}O_2max$, and is due primarily to increased glucose uptake by muscle, associated with an increase in skeletal muscle GLUT 4 (glucose transporter isoform 4) content (Goodyear et al. 1992).

Acute exercise in untrained subjects leads to increased insulin sensitivity and increased glucose metabolism—which persist for several hours following the exercise (Bogardus et al. 1983). These increases appear to stem from the need to replenish decreased muscle and liver glycogen stores and to increased glucose metabolism in muscle. Unless an individual adjusts the insulin dose, the increased sensitivity to insulin during and after exercise may result in hypoglycemia.

Another problem for people with type 1 diabetes is that plasma insulin concentrations do not respond to exercise in a normal manner, thus upsetting the balance between peripheral glucose utilization and hepatic glucose production. Plasma insulin concentrations do not decrease during exercise; they may even increase because of enhanced insulin absorption from the injection site. This effect of exercise on insulin absorption is most marked with short-acting insulin and when the injection site is in an exercising part of the body (Koivisto and Felig 1978). At rest, soluble human insulin is absorbed more rapidly than porcine insulin, but during exercise this difference disappears, both being absorbed more rapidly than in the resting condition. The increased absorption rate during exercise is not associated with increased cutaneous blood flow but may be due to mechanical stimulation of the injection site (Fernqvist et al. 1986). It is preferable to choose an injection site in a nonexercising part of the body (e.g., the abdominal wall).

Enhanced insulin absorption during exercise is most likely to occur when the injection occurs shortly before the onset of exercise, due to increased absorption of insulin from the subcutaneous tissue. The longer the interval between injection and the onset of exercise, the less significant this effect will be and the less important it is to choose the site of injection to avoid an exercising area. The injection site (such as the thigh, abdomen, or arm) may affect the rate of insulin absorption more than the exercise itself. To avoid this problem, individuals should postpone vigorous exercise for at least 60 to 90 minutes after an insulin injection. Even with this precaution, however, plasma insulin concentrations do not decrease in a normal way during exercise in insulin-treated patients, possibly impairing glucose homeostasis.

The sustained insulin levels during exercise may enhance peripheral glucose uptake and stimulate glucose oxidation by exercising muscle. However, the major effect is an inhibition of hepatic glucose production (Zinman et al. 1977). The high insulin levels inhibit both glycogenolysis and gluconeogenesis. Even though counter-regulatory hormone responses may be normal or even enhanced, blood glucose concentration falls because the hepatic glucose production rate cannot match the rate of peripheral glucose utilization. During mild to moderate exercise of short duration, this decrease may be beneficial, but during more prolonged exercise, hypoglycemia may result.

It is now well recognized that one of the trade-offs for intensive metabolic control is an increased incidence of severe hypoglycemic reactions, many of which are associated with exercise. One possible mechanism for the increased incidence of exercise-induced hypoglycemia in patients on intensive insulin therapy is a subnormal response of epinephrine, growth hormone, and cortisol when blood glucose is lowered to 50 mg/dL (Simonson et al. 1985). Strict control of blood glucose by insulin pump therapy significantly decreases the threshold glucose concentration for epinephrine and growth hormone release and increases the liver's sensitivity to insulin for inhibiting glucose production (Amiel et al. 1987). Thus, intensively treated patients achieve much lower blood glucose concentrations before counter-regulatory mechanisms are activated and hepatic glucose production increases.

Autonomic neuropathy may also contribute to exercise-induced hypoglycemia. Studying patients who experienced frequent hypoglycemic reactions during intensive insulin therapy, White et al. (1983) found that defective autonomic nervous system function was associated with decreased catecholamine responses and inadequate glucose counter-regulation to insulin-induced hypoglycemia. In addition, patients with autonomic neuropathy often do not develop the classic warning signs of hypoglycemia before developing severe neuroglucopenia—further compounding the problem of exercise-induced hypoglycemia.

Strategies to avoid hypoglycemia during prolonged, vigorous exercise include decreasing insulin dosage prior to exercise and eating supplemental carbohydrates before and during exercise. For example, individuals should inject insulin at least 60 minutes before exercise and decrease the dose by 25% to 50%. If blood glucose is less than 100 mg/dL, they should take supplemental carbohydrates prior to and during exercise.

In patients treated with an insulin pump, blood glucose responses following breakfast and in response to exercise are similar to those in normal control subjects, and there is an appropriate 30% decrease in insulin requirement during exercise. Infusing insulin at a constant rate (i.e., when it is not decreased during exercise) can cause symptomatic hypoglycemia, further demonstrating the interaction between insulin and exercise in lowering blood glucose concentration in insulin-treated subjects (Nelson et al. 1982).

Caron and colleagues (1982) studied metabolic responses, in type 1 diabetes and in normal subjects, to 45 minutes of moderate-intensity aerobic exercise performed 30 minutes after breakfast on one day and compared the results to the metabolic responses following breakfast without any exercise on another day. In the controls, exercise rapidly reversed the expected postprandial rise in blood glucose and insulin concentrations, and both returned to fasting levels within 45 minutes. When the normal subjects stopped exercising, there was a moderate rebound in glucose and insulin concentrations that did not exceed those occurring after breakfast alone. Thus, the postbreakfast exercise significantly but transiently lowered blood glucose concentrations in the normal individuals. In the diabetic subjects (treated with subcutaneous insulin), the responses were variable. Blood glucose concentrations improved for most of the subjects, remaining lower after breakfast and even through lunch. Some, however, showed improved glucose levels only during lunch. A few showed no significant improvement at all. Thus, the effect of postprandial exercise on blood glucose concentrations, and the appropriate adjustments in insulin dosage, may vary considerably from person to person. Individuals should experimentally determine their own responses in order to achieve improved glucose control and avoid symptomatic hypoglycemia.

Postexercise Hypoglycemia

Another major problem for people with type 1 diabetes is postexercise hypoglycemia. Many diabetics experience increased insulin sensitivity and have hypoglycemic reactions several hours following exercise, in some cases even the following day. In one study (MacDonald 1987), 16% of 300 young patients with type 1 diabetes who were followed prospectively for two years experienced postexercise, late-onset hypoglycemia—usually occurring at night 6 to 15 hours after the completion of unusually strenuous exercise or play. Although the mechanism of postexercise hypoglycemia is not well understood, it is most likely due to increased glucose uptake and glycogen synthesis in the previously exercised muscle groups, associated with increased insulin sensitivity and activation of glycogen synthase in skeletal muscle (Bogardus et al. 1983). Hepatic glycogen stores also recover following exercise, but at a slower rate than in muscle, so that increased requirements for dietary carbohydrate may persist for up to 24 hours following prolonged, glycogen-depleting exercise. Various strategies have been used to prevent postexercise hypoglycemia—including decreasing pre-exercise doses of intermediate- or short-acting insulin, and taking supplemental feedings after exercise—but no universal guidelines are totally effective. Treatment regimens must be individualized.

Exercise-Induced Hyperglycemia

In contrast to moderate-intensity, sustained exercise (during which blood glucose concentrations remain constant or decrease slightly), short-term, high-intensity exercise at 80% of $\dot{V}O_2$max is normally associated with a transient increase in blood glucose levels (Mitchell et al. 1988). In nondiabetic exercisers, blood glucose peaks 5 to 15 minutes after exercise ends and then gradually returns to the pre-exercise level within 40 to 60 minutes. This glycemic response to intense exercise results from marked stimulation of hepatic glucose production, so that it exceeds the rate of glucose uptake in muscle. This stimulation is associated with activation of the sympathetic nervous system, with a sharp rise in glucose counter-regulatory hormones (particularly epinephrine), and with a suppression of insulin secretion. The energy for muscular contraction comes predominantly from glycolysis and from oxidation of glucose derived from breakdown of muscle glycogen—glucose uptake from the circulation increases only gradually. Hepatic glucose production, on the other hand, is stimulated rapidly by the decrease in portal vein insulin concentration, by an increase in the glucagon-to-insulin ratio, and by the rapid rise in plasma epinephrine. When exercise is stopped, there is a rapid, two- to threefold increase in plasma insulin, which has an inhibitory effect on hepatic glucose production and increases postexercise glucose uptake in muscle. As a result, the transiently elevated blood glucose concentration returns rapidly to normal (Calles et al. 1983).

Because this highly integrated response to brief, high-intensity exercise is abnormal in type 1 diabetes, sustained hyperglycemia may occur. Mitchell and associates (1988) studied the effects of exercise to exhaustion at 80% $\dot{V}O_2$max on glucose and hormone responses, both in diabetics treated with insulin pumps and in normal controls. Blood glucose rose to much higher levels during postexercise recovery in the diabetic subjects than in the normals and remained elevated for the entire two-hour postexercise observation period. Pre-exercise glucose concentration affected the pattern of postexercise hyperglycemia, which was considerably greater when the pre-exercise level was elevated. The most likely mechanism of the sustained hyperglycemic response is intense autonomic nervous system stimulation of hepatic glucose production and the absence of any increase in plasma insulin during postexercise recovery.

Since many sports and recreational activities require relatively short periods of very high-intensity exercise, the sustained hyperglycemic response to this type of exercise may present a problem for people with diabetes. At present there are no clear guidelines for prevention or management of this response, although it is possible that administration of small doses of insulin following exercise may shorten the period of hyperglycemia. Careful self-monitoring of blood glucose levels before, during, and following exercise of different intensities and duration may help individuals to develop strategies that minimize the risks of either hyper- or hypoglycemia.

Exercise-Induced Ketosis

When insulin-dependent individuals exercise in the presence of severe insulin deficiency, hyperglycemia and ketosis can develop. The onset of exercise increases peripheral glucose utilization but also enhances lipolysis and stimulates hepatic glucose production and ketogenesis. The already poor metabolic control rapidly becomes worse, and instead of lowering blood glucose, the exercise results in a rise in blood glucose and the development of ketosis (Berger et al. 1977). The mechanism for the rapid development of ketosis is not altogether clear. Recent studies suggest that there is a defect in peripheral clearance of ketones rather than a marked increase in ketogenesis during exercise in insulin-deprived individuals (Fery et al. 1987). Individuals with type 1 diabetes should check their blood glucose concentration and urine ketones prior to undertaking vigorous physical activity. If they note blood glucose greater than 250 mg/dL and ketones in their urine or blood, they should postpone the exercise and take supplemental insulin to reestablish good metabolic control.

Strategies for Management of Exercise in Type 1 Diabetes

"Suggested Strategies to Avoid Hypo- or Hyperglycemia During and After Exercise" is a helpful reference. Individuals anticipating exercise should plan to start it one to three hours after a meal, when the blood glucose is above 100 mg/dL. If exercise is prolonged and vigorous, they should have frequent carbohydrate snacks during exercise and extra food following the exercise to avoid postexercise hypoglycemia. If exercise is intermittent, of high intensity and short duration, hyperglycemia may be a problem, and small supplemental doses of insulin may be needed during postexercise recovery.

No precise guidelines indicate how much carbohydrate one should eat during prolonged exercise to avoid hypoglycemia. However, one can make some estimate of energy requirements based on the intensity and duration of the physical exercise to be performed. In most situations, a snack containing 15 to 25 g of carbohydrate every 30 minutes during prolonged exercise will maintain normal blood glucose concentration.

Individuals who plan exercise in advance may alter their insulin dosages and schedules to decrease the likelihood of hypoglycemia during or following exercise. Those who take a single dose of intermediate-acting insulin may decrease the dose by 30% to 35% on the morning prior to exercise. Or they may change to a split-dose regimen—taking 2/3 of the usual dose in the morning, and 1/3 before the evening meal if they need supplemental insulin following the exercise. Those who use a combination of intermediate- and short-acting

Suggested Strategies to Avoid Hypo- or Hyperglycemia During and After Exercise

1. Adjustments to the insulin regimen
   - Take insulin at least one hour before exercise. If less than one hour before exercise, inject in a nonexercising part of the body.
   - Decrease the dose of both short- and intermediate-acting insulin before exercise.
   - Alter daily insulin schedule.
2. Meals and supplemental feedings
   - Eat a meal one to three hours before exercise and check to see that blood glucose is in a safe range (100 to 250 mg/dL) before starting exercise.
   - Take carbohydrate snacks or beverages during exercise—at least every 30 minutes if exercise is vigorous and of long duration. Monitor blood glucose during exercise, if necessary, to determine size and frequency of feedings needed to maintain safe glucose levels.
   - Increase food intake for up to 24 hours after exercise (depending on its intensity and duration) to avoid late-onset postexercise hypoglycemia.
3. Self-monitoring of blood glucose and urine ketones
   - Monitor blood glucose before, during, and after exercise to determine the need for and the effect of changes in insulin dosage and feeding schedule.
   - Delay exercise if blood glucose is <100 mg/dL or >250 mg/dL and ketones are present. Use supplemental feedings or insulin to correct glucose and metabolic control before starting exercise.
4. Determination of unique metabolic responses
   - Learn individual glucose responses to different types, intensities, and conditions of exercise.
   - Determine effects of exercise at different times of the day (e.g., morning, afternoon, or evening) and effects of physical training on blood glucose responses.

insulin may decrease the short-acting dosage by 50% or even omit it altogether prior to exercise. They may also decrease the intermediate-acting insulin before exercise and take supplemental doses of short-acting insulin after exercise if needed.

Those using multiple daily injections of short-acting insulin may decrease the dose before exercise by 30% to 50%, adjusting postexercise doses based on glucose monitoring and their personal experience with postexercise hypoglycemia. If they use insulin pumps, they may decrease the basal infusion rate during exercise and decrease or even omit premeal boluses. Although failure to make these adjustments may result in hypoglycemia during exercise (Schiffrin et al. 1984), this has not been a universal experience. In practice, individuals can adjust intra- and postexercise basal infusion rates as well as premeal boluses based on glucose monitoring and personal experience. In advising patients regarding these strategies, always stress the individual nature of the problem—including the need for careful glucose monitoring and for carefully recording their experiences. If their exercise patterns are relatively consistent with respect to the time of day and the intensity/duration of the exercise, your patients can often develop a routine program to avoid hypo- or hyperglycemia during or following exercise. If their exercise is unusual or without a strong pattern, then frequent glucose monitoring will help them make adjustments in insulin dosage and in the frequency and size of supplemental snacks.

Exercise in Type 2 Diabetes

The role of exercise in the management of type 2 diabetes is quite different from that in type 1 diabetes. Approximately 80% of people with type 2 diabetes are obese and insulin resistant, and only about 35% require insulin therapy. Exercise-induced hypoglycemia is uncommon, even in insulin-treated patients, and physicians often prescribe exercise—along with diet and oral antidiabetic agents—to achieve and maintain weight reduction and improve glycemic control. There is abundant evidence that regular physical exercise protects against the development of type 2 diabetes in high-risk populations (Diabetes Prevention Program Research Group 2002; Pan et al. 1997; Tuomilehto et al. 2001). Along with the prevention and treatment of obesity by dietary restriction, increased physical activity is an important component of lifestyle modification for people with impaired glucose tolerance, with a family history of type 2 diabetes, or with other risk factors for its development.

As with type 1 diabetes, exercise presents specific risks and benefits for each patient. While exercise-induced hypoglycemia and acute regulation of blood glucose are less of a problem in type 2 than in type 1 diabetes, the risks of cardiovascular disease and musculoskeletal injuries are generally greater. People with type 2 diabetes develop the same long-term complications as those with type 1 diabetes—including retinopathy, nephropathy, neuropathy, and macrovascular disease—and must be screened for these before starting an exercise program. Proper selection of exercise type, intensity, and duration can avert most of the risks, although for some patients a program of physical exercise may be impractical or contraindicated.

Exercise and Insulin Sensitivity

Bjorntorp and colleagues (1973) first suggested the use of physical exercise to treat the insulin resistance associated with obesity and type 2 diabetes. They observed that physically active middle-aged men had significantly lower fasting insulin concentrations and lower insulin responses to oral glucose than untrained men of the same age and body weight (Bjorntorp et al. 1972). This finding suggested that regular physical activity is associated with increased insulin sensitivity and led them to study the effects of physical training in obese patients with normal glucose tolerance but insulin resistance. After 12 weeks of moderate-intensity aerobic exercise (30-60 minutes, 5 days/week), there was no change in the subjects' blood glucose responses—but insulin levels were significantly lower, both fasting and following glucose administration (Bjorntorp et al. 1970). Subsequently, numerous investigators have used a variety of techniques to demonstrate increased insulin sensitivity and responsiveness in physically trained subjects (Horton 1986). For example, both normal subjects and patients with type 2 diabetes have a 30% to 35% increase in insulin-stimulated glucose disposal after physical training, when studied by the hyperinsulinemic–euglycemic clamp technique (DeFronzo et al. 1983; Sato et al. 1984). This increased insulin sensitivity correlates closely with the training-induced increase in $\dot{V}O_2$max (Rosenthal et al. 1983; Yki-Jarvinen and Koivisto 1983); presumably it is due mainly to increased glucose uptake in skeletal muscle, since no changes have been observed in hepatic glucose production rates. Recently it has also been demonstrated that resistance training improves insulin sensitivity in people with type 2 diabetes without increasing $\dot{V}O_2$max (Ishii et al. 1998).

The increase in insulin sensitivity and responsiveness associated with physical conditioning rapidly disappears when exercise is discontinued. Burstein et al. (1985) found that much of the effect is gone within 60 hours; others have demonstrated that the effect is no longer present after 5 to 7 days without exercise. In a study by Bogardus and colleagues (1984) comparing the effects in type 2 diabetes of a very low-calorie diet with the same diet plus a physical (mainly aerobic) training program, the physically trained group had a significant increase in insulin-stimulated glucose disposal rates; the group treated by diet alone had no change after three months of treatment. The rise in insulin-stimulated glucose disposal in the diet-plus-exercise group was due entirely to increased nonoxidative glucose disposal, presumably reflecting increased glycogen synthesis. Since the glucose clamp procedures were done 5 to 7 days after the last exercise session in this study, these data presumably demonstrate a true effect of physical training rather than a carryover effect from the last bout of exercise.

In more recent studies, Mikines and associates (1988) observed that a single bout of aerobic exercise increased the sensitivity and responsiveness of insulin-stimulated glucose uptake in untrained individuals. The effect lasted at least 2 days, but was not observed after 5 days. In addition, physically trained subjects (as compared with untrained subjects) had increased insulin action 15 hours after their last training session. Five days after the last training session, insulin responsiveness remained elevated compared with that of untrained subjects, suggesting that training engenders a long-term adaptive increase in whole-body responsiveness to insulin (Mikines et al. 1989). Although the mechanism of this increase is not yet known, it may be related to increased capillary density in skeletal muscle, to enhanced oxidative capacity of skeletal muscle, or to other adaptations to training such as elevated skeletal muscle GLUT 4 content (Goodyear et al. 1992).

Despite the increase in insulin-stimulated glucose uptake that can last 5 to 7 days following cessation of exercise in previously trained subjects, patients with type 2 diabetes generally do not have improved fasting blood glucose concentrations during this same period. Some researchers, however, have observed that physical training is associated with lower glycosylated hemoglobin levels (Schneider et al. 1984)—likely the cumulative result of decreased blood glucose concentrations during and after aerobic exercise rather than a specific effect of physical training. Since moderate-intensity aerobic exercise usually lowers blood glucose concentrations toward normal in hyperglycemic patients with type 2 diabetes, and since increased insulin-stimulated glucose disposal persists for many hours following a single bout of exercise (Devlin and Horton 1985), it is likely that regular exercise 4 to 7 days a week may decrease blood glucose and glycohemoglobin concentrations without a significant effect on fasting blood glucose or glucose response to meals. Thus, the net effect of exercise repeated on a regular basis would be to improve long-term blood glucose control in patients with type 2 diabetes.

GUIDELINES FOR EXERCISE IN TYPE 2 DIABETES

Before starting an exercise program, all patients should have a complete history and physical examination—with particular attention to identifying any long-term complications of diabetes that may affect exercise safety or tolerance. Individuals with diabetes are considered to be at high risk for exercise-induced cardiovascular events and should have a stress test if they intend to start a program of moderate or vigorous exercise (American College of Sports Medicine 2000). The test will help identify previously undiagnosed ischemic heart disease and abnormal blood pressure responses to exercise. All individuals also should have a dilated retinal examination to identify proliferative retinopathy, renal function tests (including screening for microalbuminuria), and a neurological examination to determine peripheral or autonomic neuropathy. To avoid significant risks or worsening complications, individuals with abnormalities should engage only in exercises of appropriate type and intensity. In general, an exercise program should consist of moderate-intensity aerobic exercises that can be sustained for 30 minutes or longer and that result in a sustained heart rate of 60% to 70% of the individual's predetermined maximum heart rate. Patients with no proliferative retinopathy or significant hypertension may tolerate some resistance training or high-intensity exercises.

Each exercise session should begin with a warm-up of low-intensity aerobic exercise and stretching for 5 to 10 minutes to prevent musculoskeletal injuries. The moderate- to high-intensity exercise phase should last at least 30 minutes, with longer durations as tolerated by the level of physical conditioning. Patients should monitor their heart rates periodically during exercise, to ensure that they are in the target range. Each exercise session should conclude with a cool-down phase of 5 to 10 minutes to reduce the risk of postexercise cardiovascular and musculoskeletal complications. Activities such as walking, stretching, and slow, rhythmic exercises are appropriate.

To significantly increase cardiovascular fitness, to improve insulin sensitivity and glycemic control, and to lose or maintain reduced body weight, patients should exercise at least three days a week; five to seven days a week is preferable. Individual or group activities are appropriate, and many patients find that variety sustains their interest. For individuals who are new to exercise or who have significant complications of diabetes, supervised exercise programs may be beneficial. Most patients, however, do not require formal supervision once they have completed an initial assessment and established an appropriate exercise program. Although blood glucose regulation during exercise in type 2 diabetes differs from normal in several ways, elevated blood glucose concentrations usually fall toward normal with moderate-intensity exercise. Exercise-induced hypoglycemia is rare. Exceptions may occur in patients taking insulin, sulfonylureas or other oral insulin-secreting agents such as meglitinides or phenylalanine derivatives. Metformin, thiazolidinediones, or α-glucosidase inhibitors are rarely associated with exercise-induced hypoglycemia. Patients treated by diet alone need not use supplemental feedings before, during, or after exercise, except when the exercise is exceptionally vigorous or of long duration. Individuals being treated with sulfonylureas or insulin may need supplemental feedings to prevent hypoglycemia; they may also decrease insulin doses to avoid hypoglycemia.

SUMMARY

The role and management of physical exercise in patients with diabetes mellitus is complex, and is associated with both benefits and significant risks. In type 1 diabetes, the main goal should be to educate patients about regulation of blood glucose during and after exercise by glucose monitoring and appropriate adjustments in food intake and insulin administration. Individuals with type 2 diabetes should employ regular exercise and diet to achieve and maintain weight reduction (in obese patients), to reduce insulin resistance, to improve glycemic control, and to reduce cardiovascular risk factors including hypertension and hyperlipidemia. Those at risk of developing type 2 diabetes should engage in regular exercise as a preventive measure.

Before starting an exercise program, all patients with diabetes should undergo a careful medical evaluation to determine their general state of health, the presence and degree of long-term complications of diabetes, and any limitations or contraindications to exercise. Particular attention should be paid to the cardiovascular system, since people with diabetes have an increased risk of coronary artery disease (which may be asymptomatic). A dilated eye examination to detect proliferative retinopathy, an evaluation of renal function, and a neurological and musculoskeletal examination are important to detect diabetic complications that may be aggravated by exercise.

Exercise programs should be tailored to each individual's goals and medical condition. Patients must become proficient and faithful in self-monitoring—learning through careful experimentation the effects of specific types, intensities, and durations of exercise on their blood glucose. By following these guidelines, most diabetic patients can exercise effectively and safely.

CHAPTER 11

MAJOR INFLAMMATORY AND NON-INFLAMMATORY ARTHRITIDES

Maura Daly Iversen, DPT, SD, MPH; Matthew H. Liang, MD, MPH; and Axel Finckh, MD, MS

CASE STUDY

A 42-year-old nurse, E.M., has had sero-positive erosive rheumatoid arthritis for 3 years. Her rheumatologist initially treated her with Methotrexate and NSAIDs but recently added anti-TNF-alpha therapy because of an insufficient response. E.M. had little functional limitation but increasingly has to arrange her day around the physical demands of her activities. Her occupation requires lifting and a great deal of dexterity of the hands. She complains of occasional shoulder and neck pain, some tenderness and stiffness of her hands, and discomfort in her forefeet that worsens by the end of her shift. E.M.'s general physical examination and vital signs are normal. She has mild synovitis of her wrists and her second through fourth metacarpophalangeal joints (MCPs) with mild ulnar deviation. The elbows are minimally involved. She has a rheumatoid nodule on her left elbow. Her knees have small effusions and fine crepitus. Her MTPs are painful with compression.

What rehabilitation program would you advise? What restrictions to her activities would you recommend?

Rehabilitation program for E.M.: This patient has early, mildly active rheumatoid arthritis (RA). Her rehabilitation program should include active range-of-motion exercises for the involved joints, strength training (both static and dynamic) of low to moderate intensity, and progressive aerobic exercise either in the water or on a bicycle to maximize her endurance and function while reducing stress on her feet. The therapist should address static posture (particularly while standing), ergonomic factors, and adaptive equipment (dynamic and resting wrist splints) and an assessment for orthotics and proper footwear. The educational component of the program should contain a thorough discussion of her disease, information about whole body and joint-specific rest, and information on how to modify her exercise program based on her disease activity.

Arthritis and musculoskeletal disorders are among the most common chronic conditions, affecting approximately 70 million people in the United States (Bolen et al. 2002) and resulting in severe activity limitations. The 100+ forms of these disorders spare neither age nor race, and cause joint pain, deformity, and disability. Some systemic rheumatic conditions can lead to death. Arthritis and musculoskeletal conditions are classified generally as systemic versus nonsystemic and monoarticular versus polyarticular; polyarticular diseases may be subclassified as inflammatory, metabolic, or degenerative (Decker 1983). Table 11.1 lists selected rheumatic diseases, their pathology, and clinical presentation.

All joint diseases may cause a series of events that compound one another—principally joint stiffness, pain and deformity, soft tissue contracture, muscle atrophy, general deconditioning, and diminished function. Patients with inflammatory or non-inflammatory joint disease can have decreased muscle strength and atrophy surrounding the involved joint. Diminished strength may result from inactivity, inflammation of muscles, or inhibition of muscle contraction due to joint swelling or inflammation. Agents used to treat these conditions (e.g., corticosteroids or, rarely, hydroxychloroquine, which can cause myopathy) may compound the reduction in strength (Gerber 1990). It is possible, in the case of osteoarthritis of the knee, that weakness is not the result, but a cause of the disease (Slemenda et al. 1997).

Restricted joint mobility and deformity are common in arthritis. These may result from pain, soft tissue contractures, poor posture, improper positioning, joint capsule thickening, joint effusion, and subluxation of the joints (Semble et al. 1990). Collagen shortens when not periodically stretched (Gerber 1990). Systemic or local inflammatory disease may impair cardiopulmonary function or restrict activity, leading to contracture, muscle atrophy, diminished stamina and endurance, general deconditioning, and diminished function.

Despite concerns, studies of exercise therapy show that exercise maximizes range of motion (Brighton et al. 1993), muscle strength (Ekdahl et al. 1990; Lyngberg et al. 1994), endurance (Ekblom et al. 1975; Harkcom et al. 1985; Minor et al. 1989), proper joint alignment, function (Stenstrom et al. 1996; Semble et al. 1990), and bone density (Aloia et al. 1978) and does not increase arthritis symptoms. However, clinicians continue to prescribe sub-optimal exercise programs or not at all. The reasons in part stem from the belief that exercising patients with inflammatory arthritides could stress the joints and supporting tissues and cause more joint inflammation (Jensen and Lorish 1994). In a survey assessing rheumatologists' opinions about the benefits of exercise and their attitudes toward exercise, about 80% of rheumatologists believed that range-of-motion exercises were useful in managing the symptoms of rheumatoid arthritis, while only 42% believed that aerobic exercises were useful and 52% that strengthening exercises were useful (Iversen et al. 1999).

This chapter reviews major rheumatic conditions and the role of exercise in their management.

Table 11.1 Features of Rheumatic Diseases

Disease	Dominant pathology	Clinical features
Rheumatoid arthritis (RA)	Synovitis	Symmetrical and bilateral joint involvement Joint pain, swelling, stiffness, contracture Muscle weakness and fatigue
Osteoarthritis (OA)	Cartilage degeneration	Weight-bearing joints involved Joint pain Joint malalignment Muscle weakness
Spondylarthropathies	Enthesitis	Axial skeleton, hip, shoulder, knee Reduced spinal flexibility Pain
Systemic lupus erythematosus (SLE)	Systemic inflammation	Diverse and varied organ involvement Fatigue
Polymyositis/dermatomyositis (PM/DM)	Myositis	Proximal weakness Decreased ROM/contracture
Scleroderma	Fibrosis	Skin and visceral organs involved Contracture of soft tissue Respiratory involvement

RHEUMATOID ARTHRITIS

Rheumatoid arthritis (RA) is a chronic, systemic, inflammatory disorder of unknown etiology. The prevalence of RA, about 1% to 2% of the population (Lawrence et al. 1989), increases with age. It affects women twice as often as men, shortens life expectancy about 10 years (Harris 1990), and causes a great deal of suffering.

Rheumatoid disease primarily affects the synovium of diarthrodial joints, resulting in synovitis. It is characterized by exacerbations and remissions. Joint involvement is generally symmetrical. Uncontrolled, rheumatoid synovitis results in progressive, disabling, joint destruction. Extra-articular manifestations of RA may involve the heart, lungs, blood vessels, skin, and nervous system (Harris 1990). Fatigue, which is common, probably results from production of cytokines, deconditioning, depression, and altered biomechanics from affected joints (which require greater energy expenditure for the same activities). All these factors significantly limit a patient's function and restrict independence.

The goals of rehabilitation in the management of RA are to maximize strength, flexibility, endurance, mobility, and to promote independence. A well-designed exercise program is based on the extent of the joint impairments as well as the patient's motivation and adherence to therapy. Psychosocial effects from RA are pervasive and include depression, reduced confidence in the ability to manage the disease, and disruption of personal relationships (Smedstad and Liang 1997; Stenstrom 1994). Depression and reduced self-confidence decrease motivation to perform exercises. Social support for exercise increases the chance that the patient will participate and continue in an exercise program. In fact, positive social support for exercise increases the likelihood of adherence by threefold (Iversen et al. 1999).

JOINT PAIN

Pain is common and disabling in RA. During acute flares, therapeutic cold helps to reduce inflammation and relieve pain; heat is avoided as it may exacerbate the inflammatory process. When the inflammation resolves, patients may apply either heat or cold to relieve symptoms, based on their preference, disease states, and treatment goals (Hayes 1996). Exercise also may help reduce joint pain. Ekdahl et al. (1990) found that circulating endorphin levels increase in proportion to the intensity and frequency of dynamic exercise. These endogenous opiates may be responsible for the decrease in pain experienced with exercise.

JOINT STIFFNESS, SWELLING, AND CONTRACTURES

Rheumatoid arthritis can lead to tightening of the soft tissues, tendons, and joint capsules. Loss of bone and cartilage reduces joint space, structurally restricting joint motion. Patients with early disease should perform range-of-motion and flexibility exercises daily on affected joints to maximize joint function. Two to three repetitions of range-of-motion exercises performed once a day, either independently or with assistance are recommended during acute flares. As inflammation subsides, passive stretching will increase joint range of motion and repetitions of exercise can increase (see chapter 4). Patients may apply heat prior to stretching, as it appears to increase the extensibility of collagen and maximizes the stretching effect (Hicks 1994; Warren et al. 1976).

Research shows that range-of-motion exercises safely and efficiently maximize joint motion in patients with variable disease activity. They do not appear to increase joint damage, joint flares, or swelling over periods from 6 weeks to 48 months (Brighton et al. 1993; Ekblom et al.1975; Lyngberg et al. 1988; Perlman et al. 1990; van den Ende et al. 1996). Table 11.2 summarizes a variety of exercise studies in RA.

WEAKNESS

Strengthening programs enhance muscular strength and contractility, improving the ability to perform activities of daily living. Patients with RA are weaker than their healthy counterparts; those with severe disease have 33% to 55% less strength compared to healthy individuals (Nordesjo et al. 1983). In RA, muscle weakness may result from direct and indirect manifestations of the disease process. Patients with RA exhibit type I and type II muscle fiber atrophy (Semble et al. 1990), which may be related to pathological changes from the disease within the tissue and/or to disuse. Myositis can be subtle in RA; one can check muscle enzymes if it is suspected. If the myositis is not severe, patients may exercise and achieve a training effect (Gerber 1990).

Strengthening programs may be static or dynamic, or a combination. In **static exercises** (also known as isometric exercises), an individual generates muscle force without moving the joint. These exercises help prevent muscle atrophy and cause less inflammation and fewer rises in intra-articular pressure than do other forms of resistive exercise (Hicks 1994). Patients tolerate them well, even during periods of acute joint inflammation (Semble 1995). However, since sustained static exercises may place high demands on cardiac function, they are relatively contraindicated in the presence of ischemic heart disease or congestive heart failure. Patients with these conditions should consult the appropriate specialists.

Dynamic exercises produce muscle fiber lengthening and/or shortening, allowing the joint to move through a range of motion and generate a force. The combination of low resistance and high repetitions enhances endurance;

Table 11.2 Randomized Controlled Trials of Exercise in Rheumatoid Arthritis

Author	Subjects (no.)	Intervention	Result
Ekblom et al. 1975	23 with nonactive disease, Class II-III	6 wk general rehabilitation (1 ×/day) plus: ROM or strength training and aerobic bicycle ergometry, 5 days/wk, 20-40 min/day	The endurance training group decreased walk test time by 14%, increased VO_2 20%, reported less pain; no change in articular indices in either group.
Ekblom 1975	30 with nonactive disease, Class II, III	6-mo follow-up on patients enrolled in study described above	6 patients who exercised ≥4 ×/wk demonstrated sustained benefits.
Wessel and Quinney 1984	32 with stable disease, Class II	7 wk of either static or isokinetic exercise, 3 ×/wk vs. control	No change in knee swelling detectable; exercise pain about 25% greater in static than isokinetic group.
Harkcom et al. 1985	20 with nonactive disease, Class II	12 wk low-intensity bicycle exercise 3 ×/wk at 70% max heart rate, 50 rpm; 4 groups: 15, 25, 35 min, and control group	17/20 completed; all exercisers improved aerobic capacity ($\dot{V}O_2$max); exercise duration (mean increase 3.4 min), symptoms, and pain; only the 35 min group demonstrated statistically significant differences in aerobic capacity.
Minor et al. 1989	40 with variable disease activity	12 wk aerobic walking; aerobic aquatic; aerobic ROM, 3 ×/wk for 60 min	Improved endurance and aerobic capacity in walkers and aquatic groups; anxiety, depression, and physical activity AIMs improved; no difference in joint activity among groups.
Ekdahl et al. 1990	67 with low to moderate disease activity, Class II	6 wk of home exercises and supervised PT visits; 4 groups: dynamic plus 12 PT visits; dynamic plus 4 PT visits; static exercise plus 12 PT; static plus 4 PT visits; patients followed for 3 more mo	62/67 completed; significant increases in strength, endurance, and function; dynamic exercisers increased aerobic capacity by 30%; effects still seen at 3 mo; no significant change in static groups; no joint flares in any group.
Brighton et al. 1993	44 with active disease, Class I	48 mo of hand exercises; reinforcement provided when necessary	Significant increases in grip strength and pincer grip strength in the exercise group.
Baslund et al. 1993	18 with moderate disease activity	8 wk progressive biking, 4-5 ×/wk for 35 min at 80% $\dot{V}O_2$max	Max VO_2 uptake increased 18% trained vs. 6% controls; heart rate at stage 2 and perceived exertion decreased; no change in immune response.

Author	Subjects (no.)	Intervention	Result
Hansen et al. 1993	75 with mixed disease activity, Class I-II	2-year study; 4 groups. Exercised 45 min total (15 min general, 30 min aerobic) 2-3 ×/wk: self-exercisers (SE); SE plus weekly group exercise; SE plus weekly group and PT exercises; and no exercise	65/75 completed; no significant differences between groups; strength increased in all groups; no change in aerobic fitness; no difference in X-ray progression of disease.
Hoenig et al. 1993	57, functional Class II-III	All patients performed exercises twice daily for 10-20 min over 3 mo: (A) hand range-of-motion, (B) hand resistive exercises, (C) hand ROM plus resistive, or (D) none	41/57 completed. Improvements were found in muscle strength and disease activity.
Hakkinen et al. 1994	43, disease activity not stated	10 mo progressive dynamic strength training (2-3 ×/wk at 40%-60% max) vs. regular activity (3-4 ×/wk)	39/43 completed; exercisers increased bilateral dynamic strength 32% and unilateral strength by 49%; ESR decreased and function increased; only slight changes in joints of subjects.
Ekdahl et al. 1994	30 with low to moderate disease activity, Class II; and 20 healthy	6 wk of (1) high-intensity (60 min 2 ×/wk); (2) low-intensity dynamic exercise, (3) control	47/50 completed; initially RA and healthy subjects differed in CRH levels; RA exercisers increased CRH levels (3 pmo/L; $p < .05$) compared to others; significant difference in β-endorphin levels in RA and healthy exercisers.
Hall et al. 1996	148 with Class I, II, III	4 wk; 30 min 2 ×/wk seated immersion, hydrotherapy; land exercise or relaxation	139/148 completed; all patients improved physically and emotionally; 27% decrease in joint tenderness; average knee ROM increased 6.6 degrees in women in hydrotherapy; at 3 mo hydrotherapy group maintained psychological improvements.
Stenstrom et al. 1996	54 with Class I, II disease	2 groups; dynamic exercise or relaxation training, 5 ×/wk for 30 min for 3 mo	48/54 completed; dynamic group improved walking speed (*md diff* = 0.7) and perceived exertion ($p < .05$); relaxation group improved on Nottingham Health Profile, joint tenderness, and lower extremity muscle function.

(continued)

Table 11.2 *(continued)*

Author	Subjects (no.)	Intervention	Result
Rall et al. 1996	30 with well-controlled disease	12-wk program with 4 groups: 8 healthy elders, 8 RA, and 8 young healthy; performed resistance exercises 2 ×/wk at 80% 1 rep max contraction; 6 elderly performed warm-up swimming exercises	Exercisers increased muscle strength compared to controls: RA 57%, young exercisers 44%, elderly exercisers 36%; no change in joint symptoms; RA patients reported improvements in pain and fatigue.
Van den Ende et al. 1996	100 with stable disease	12 wk exercise with 2-wk follow-up; 4 groups: dynamic weight-bearing exercises and bike, ROM and static exercises in group, supervised ROM and static exercises; or home ROM and static exercises	90/100 completed; 17% increase in aerobic capacity and muscle strength, 15% increase in joint mobility in high-intensity group; gain lost after stopping; no damage to joints.
Komatireddy 1997	49 with Class II-III	Progressive resistive circuit exercises for 20 to 30 min at 30-40% of max load >3 ×/wk for 12 wk plus video vs. no exercise	41/49 completed. Improvements seen in joint counts and number painful joints, knee extension HAQ scores, sit-to-stand time. No significant changes in $\dot{V}O_2max$.
Senstrom et al. 1997	54 with RA Class I and II disease and 6 PA	12-mo program; 2 groups: dynamic training or relaxation 5 ×/wk for 3 mo, then 2-3 ×/wk for 9 mo	Improved physical impact (median 1.7 vs. 1.2, $p \leq .05$) and work effects (AIMS2) in dynamic group; relaxation group less pain and emotional reaction.
Bostrom et al. 1998	45 with mild RA	Progressive dynamic shoulder exercises performed 3 ×/wk for 40-60 min at 30% max load for 10 wk vs. static shoulder exercises.	37/45 completed. Both groups reported fewer UE swollen joints and less shoulder-arm pain. Dynamic exercisers showed improvements in physical and overall dimensions in the Sickness Impact Profile.
McMeeken et al. 1999	36 non-active RA	Knee extensor and flexor strengthening 2-3 ×/wk for 45 min at 70% max for 6 wk vs. attention control	35/36 completed. Knee extensor and flexor strength increased significantly. Exercisers reported improvements in pain and function as measured by HAQ and increased TUG time.
Hakkinen et al. 1999	70 with <2 years onset RA	Dynamic whole-body exercises 2 ×/wk for 45 min at 50-60% max load vs. ROM exercises 2 ×/wk for 12 mo	65/70 completed; 22-35% increase in muscle strength in dynamic group vs. 3-24% in ROM group. No significant changes in BMD.

Author	Subjects (no.)	Intervention	Result
van den Ende et al. 2000	64 with active RA, no TKR	Progressive dynamic (3 sets of 8 reps) and static strengthening (70% MVC) plus biking at 60% max HR for 15 min 3 ×/wk plus ROM vs. ROM plus isometrics 5 ×/wk for 1 mo	61/64 completed. Increase in strength, joint mobility, and function with decrease in disease activity.
Westby et al. 2000	30 women with Class I-II on low-dose steroids	Weight-bearing aerobic exercise 3 ×/wk for 45 to 60 min for 12 mo vs. usual activity	21/30 completed. Significant improvements in function and activity levels noted among exercisers. No change in BMD.
Hakkinen et al. 2001	70 with onset of dx <2 years	Dynamic whole-body strengthening 2 ×/wk for 45 min at 50-70% max vs. ROM 2 ×/wk for 24 mo. All encouraged to participate in recreational activities 2 ×/wk .	62/70 completed. Muscle strength disease activity (HAQ) and function improved in both groups but greater improvements seen in dynamic exercisers (19-59% increase in muscle strength). ROM group decreased BMD while dynamic exercisers showed slight improvements in BMD femoral neck (0.51 ± 1.64%) and spine (1.17 ± 5.34%).

Adapted, by permission, from J.E. Hicks, 1994, Exercise in rheumatoid arthritis, *Physical Medicine and Rehabilitation Clinics in North America* 5:708, 717.

higher resistance and low repetitions produce muscle hypertrophy and increase strength. **Isokinetic exercise,** a form of dynamic exercise, is done on machines that control the velocity of joint movement. Since the machines provide resistance proportional to muscle strength at each point in the range, the machine speed controls the muscle torque.

Early studies of strength training in RA focused on the impact of low-intensity training regimens of various duration and frequency. Over the past 20 years, studies have focused on the impact of high-intensity strength training programs to determine whether patients can tolerate increased stresses on the joint and whether their joints will be damaged.

RELEVANT STUDIES

Both static and dynamic strengthening programs improve strength and function in patients with RA. To study the effects of dynamic strength training on knee flexor and extensor muscle force, McMeekan et al. (1999) randomly allocated 36 patients with nonactive RA to either 6 weeks of strengthening exercises, two to three times per week for 45 minutes at 70% maximum voluntary contraction, or to an attention control group. At the end of the trial, patients in the exercise group demonstrated significant improvements in strength as measured with isokinetic torques at speeds of 60 degrees and 120 degrees per second. These patients also demonstrated significant improvements in pain and function as measured by the Health Assessment Questionnaire (HAQ) and increased Timed Up and Go times.

Lyngberg et al. (1994) saw improvements in muscle strength from a 6-week strengthening program with 3 weeks of isokinetic exercise for the right knee extensors, followed by 3 weeks of static knee exercises for the left knee extensors. Using an isokinetic dynamometer, patients performed 48 repetitions of relatively low-intensity exercise (50% of maximal voluntary contraction) at four different angular velocities, three times per week for 15 minutes during the first 3 weeks of the trial. In the subsequent 3 weeks, the subjects trained their left knee extensors using static exercises at 50% of the maximal voluntary contraction at two joint angles, 60 and 90 degrees. They held each contraction for 3 seconds. Nine of the 11 patients with mild to moderate disease activity completed the study, with a mean increase in knee strength of 21% in the isokinetic program. The relatively large increase in strength with this modest exercise program may be attributed to the patients' low baseline level of conditioning. The subjects tolerated the static exercise training about the same as the isokinetic program of similar intensity.

Komatireddy et al. (1997) randomized 49 patients with functional class II and III and a mean duration of illness of 10.5 years to 12 weeks of progressive resistance exercises of 30% to 40% max load 20 to 30 minutes, 3 × per week versus control. The exercise group was instructed in circuit exercise program using light resistance and high repetitions and received a videotape of the exercises to continue the program at home. Muscle strength, joint involvement, physical function, and endurance were assessed at baseline and 12 weeks. During the study period, patients in the exercise group demonstrated significantly increased knee extension strength, reduced number of painful joints, joint count, reduced sit-to-stand time and increased time to anaerobic threshold compared to the control group. Although the intervention group exercised at a relatively low intensity, their function improved and joint symptoms did not worsen. Dynamic exercises even at low intensity appear to enhance functional performance.

To evaluate high-intensity exercise on muscle strength, Rall and colleagues (1996) studied 30 subjects: 8 healthy untrained subjects, 8 untrained subjects with RA, and 14 untrained healthy elderly subjects. The healthy elderly were randomized to dynamic resistance exercise or to the warm-up exercise in a swimming pool. Subjects in the high-intensity resistive exercise group trained all major muscle groups twice a week at 80% of their 1-repetition maximal contraction. After 12 weeks, the subjects with RA had a 57% increase in strength, the young healthy exercisers a 44% increase, and the healthy elderly subjects a 36% increase in strength. Subjects with RA also reported a 21% reduction in joint pain and a 38% decrease in fatigue.

Conclusions About Strength Exercises and Rheumatoid Arthritis

Static and dynamic exercises increase muscle strength in patients with RA over periods of 3 to 12 weeks. Static exercises produce less intra-articular force and place less shear force across joints (leading to less discomfort during exercise), and are appropriate during acute flares to prevent muscle atrophy. Patients with stable disease tolerate dynamic as well as static exercises at moderate to high intensity (50%-70% maximum voluntary contraction), and dynamic exercise leads to greater improvements in muscle strength and function. Isokinetic exercises performed at high speeds, such as a velocity of 180 degrees per second, appear to reduce the discomfort normally associated with dynamic exercise. As most studies of strengthening exercises in RA do not include patients with active or severe disease, one should not generalize the results of these studies to such populations. We recommend that individuals avoid dynamic strengthening exercises during acute flares. Other contraindications to dynamic exercises in RA include the presence of ligamentous laxity, which may increase the risk of ligament rupture during strengthening programs, and the presence of tense popliteal cysts, which could rupture during isokinetic exercise (Hicks 1994).

Fatigue and Endurance

Aerobic exercise can improve immune responses, aerobic capacity, endurance, and function in healthy individuals (Åstrand and Rodahl 1986). Patients with RA have decreased aerobic capacity compared to healthy subjects. With short-term conditioning programs, cardiovascular fitness can be improved by 20%, as measured by $\dot{V}O_2max$ and physical function can increase (Ekblom et al. 1975; van den Ende et al. 1996). Training regimens of 50% to 80% of $\dot{V}O_2max$ appear to be best. Most maximal stress tests for RA patients use a modified Bruce protocol and employ bicycle ergometers to reduce stress on weight-bearing joints. Bicycling, swimming or aquatic exercises, and walking are also appropriate aerobic activities for RA patients' joints (see figure 11.1). The buoyancy of water facilitates exercises that are difficult to perform on land. Warm water also relaxes muscle tension and reduces

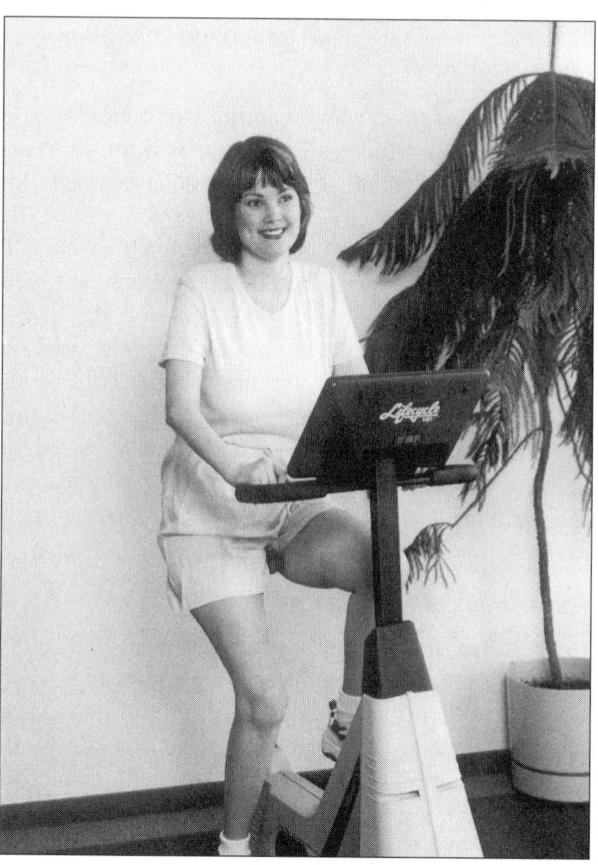

Figure 11.1 Bicycling is a safe and effective approach to exercise that patients can do at home.

pain. The recommended water temperature for patients with arthritis is 37 to 40 degrees Celsius (Gerber and Hicks 1990). There has been little research on aquatic programs for RA patients, although theoretically they are ideal for maximizing range of motion and endurance in such patients.

RELEVANT STUDIES

Baslund and colleagues (1993) evaluated the effects of an 8-week, moderate-intensity bicycle training program on the immune system of 18 patients with moderate RA disease activity. The researchers found a training effect, as measured by maximal O_2 uptake, but no changes in natural killer cell activity, blood mononuclear cells, plasma cytokines, or lymphocyte proliferative responses.

Harkcom et al. (1985) tested 20 patients with nonactive RA at three levels of low-intensity aerobic conditioning for 35, 25, or 15 minutes, performed three times a week over a 12-week period. The 35-minute, low-intensity conditioning program produced statistically significant improvements in aerobic capacity (6.9 $ml \cdot kg^{-1} \cdot min^{-1}$ on average). The 25- and 15-minute programs appeared to improve aerobic capacity, but the results were not statistically significant. A comparison of the three exercise groups to the control group showed an increase in mean aerobic capacity of 6.2 $ml \cdot kg^{-1} \cdot min^{-1}$ and a mean increase in endurance time of 3.4 minutes. All exercisers reported significant decreases in joint pain and swelling compared to the non-exercising controls ($p < .01$). This study demonstrated that a low-intensity conditioning program of as little as 15 minutes' duration, performed three times per week over 3 months, improved aerobic capacity in patients with RA (see figure 11.2).

In a large randomized controlled trial, van den Ende et al. (1996) found improvements in aerobic capacity, muscle strength, and joint mobility with a 12-week program of high-intensity exercise. One hundred patients were allocated to either a high-intensity dynamic program, including weight-bearing exercises and bicycling, in which patients exercised at 70% to 85% of their age-predicted maximal heart rate; a low-intensity group exercise program, consisting of range-of-motion and static strengthening exercises for the trunk and lower extremity; a low-intensity individual range-of-motion and static exercise program, with instructions by a physical therapist; or a written home program of range-of-motion and static exercises.

The high-intensity exercise group met for 1 hour, three times per week; the low-intensity exercise group met for 1 hour, twice a week; the patients receiving individual instruction also performed their exercises twice a week. Patients in the home program were encouraged to exercise twice a week for at least 15 minutes. Following the 12-week program, the high-intensity group demonstrated a 17% increase in aerobic capacity and knee muscle strength and a 15% increase in joint mobility; both low-intensity groups demonstrated a small increase (about 7%) in knee muscle strength. Joint symptoms did not increase in any of the groups and actually decreased among the high-intensity exercisers. Twelve weeks after discontinuation of the program, the improvements in aerobic capacity and joint mobility were no longer present although the gains in 50-foot walk time and muscle strength remained.

Earlier studies examined the benefits of bicycle ergometry (Ekblom et al. 1975; Harkcom et al. 1985). Recent research has focused on alternative forms of aerobic exercise for RA patients. Minor and colleagues (1989) tested how aerobic walking and aquatic programs could improve aerobic capacity in patients with RA. In addition to the improvements in aerobic capacity for both groups, patients reported improvements in mood.

Few studies have evaluated the efficacy of hydrotherapy on physical and psychological outcomes in patients with RA. Hall and colleagues (1996) randomly assigned patients to 4 weeks of hydrotherapy, seated immersion, land exercises, or relaxation training. Each session met twice a week for 30 minutes. All subjects improved both physically and emotionally. Subjects in

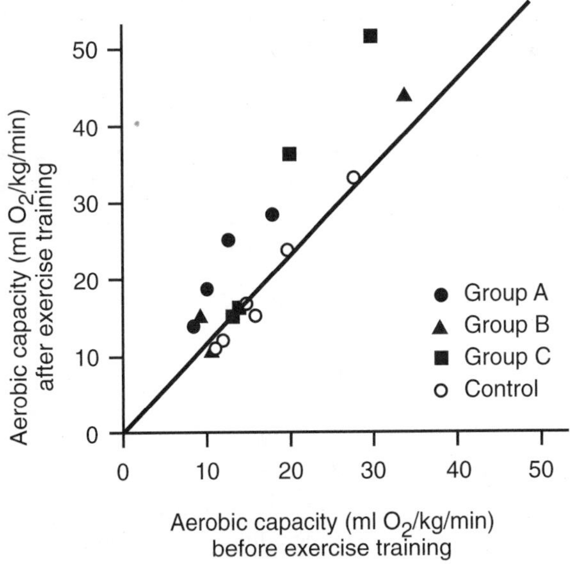

Figure 11.2 Aerobic capacity for each subject before and after exercise training. $p < .05$ for group A. Group A = 14-min final total duration exercise. Group B = 24-min final total duration exercise. Group C = 35-min final total duration exercise.

Adapted from T.M. Harkcom et al., 1985, "Therapeutic value of graded aerobic exercise training in rheumatoid arthritis," *Arthritis and Rheumatism* 28:35. Copyright 1985 John Wiley & Sons, Inc. Adapted with permission of Wiley-Liss, Inc., a subsidiary of John Wiley & Sons, Inc.

the hydrotherapy group reported 27% less joint tenderness than patients in the other groups. Women in the hydrotherapy treatment increased their total combined knee range of motion by 6.6 degrees. At follow-up, hydrotherapy patients maintained their emotional and psychological improvement.

Conclusions About Aerobic Conditioning and Rheumatoid Arthritis

Studies of aerobic conditioning in RA have varied considerably in the frequency, duration, intensity, and mode of exercise tested, and the outcomes measured (physiologic versus self-report). While it is difficult to combine these results in a quantitative manner, the collective data suggest that short-term aerobic exercise programs in which patients exercise at least three times per week can increase aerobic capacity by about 20% and improve both endurance and mood. A significant problem with programs of short duration (6 to 12 weeks), however, is that the benefits are not maintained once the program has ended. Programs of longer duration and intensity produce the greatest aerobic effects. The conflicting results surrounding the impact of aerobic exercise on joint symptoms may reflect the variation in patient selection and sample size and the use of differing measures of disease activity and joint symptoms. Aerobic exercise programs that incorporate weight-bearing exercises, once believed to be harmful, have proven to be well tolerated by patients with stable disease. In our experience, it is very difficult for patients to adhere to these programs over the course of a chronic disease. Programs must be flexible, incorporating a variety of exercise modes that reduce boredom and enable patients to modify their programs based on their joint symptoms. Research is needed to assess the benefits of such programs for patients with varying levels of disease activity, and to determine the intensity required to maintain long-term aerobic effects.

Structural Joint Damage in RA

A common clinical concern is the safety of high impact training on joint integrity in patients with RA. A study by de Jong et al. (2003) examined the effectiveness and safety of a long-term exercise program compared to usual therapy. Patients with RA, some with structural damage in the hip and knee joints, were allocated to either a high-intensity program including classical aerobic and strengthening exercises and impact sporting activities or usual care. Increased joint damage progression was observed in patients who started with more structural damage and longer disease duration as measured by follow-up X-rays. This progression was more apparent in the exercise group, despite the fact that, on average, these patients had markers of less serious disease at baseline, such as less structural joint damage, shorter disease duration, and less medication requirements. This is one of only two controlled studies that examined the safety of exercise by follow-up X-rays of involved joints, and one of only five studies that has looked at X-ray progression as an endpoint (de Jong et al. 2003; Hansen 1993; Nordemar et al. 1981; Stenstrom et al. 1991; Stenstrom 1994). Both controlled studies showed a trend to more progressive joint damage in the exercise intervention groups. These studies suggest caution in prescribing exercise to patients who already have significant joint damage, especially of weight-bearing joints.

Recommendations for Exercise Prescription in RA

In summary, exercise improves function, strength, endurance, and mood in patients with RA. Short-term static and dynamic exercises improve muscle strength from 27% to 57%, with little effect on joint effusion and pain. These exercises may even reduce joint synovitis. Short-term aerobic exercise increases aerobic capacity by 20%. Research is still needed to describe the effects of long-term exercise training on joint structures and its impact on synovitis.

The degree of synovitis, amount of joint destruction and deformity, and the patient's pain tolerance set the parameters for the exercises prescribed. Patients in an acute flare should engage in static strengthening and gentle active range-of-motion exercises and learn about joint protection techniques to minimize trauma to inflamed joints. These patients should not perform resistive exercises, since there is a possibility of tendon rupture. Static exercises, on the other hand, do not require joint movement, yet they generate maximal muscle contractions and improve muscle strength. Static exercises of 6-second duration appear most effective for maximizing strength; individuals should perform them once a day on each muscle group during an acute flare. Table 11.3 summarizes the exercise recommendations.

Patients with RA should perform range-of-motion exercises daily to prevent loss of motion. This is important because joints generally feel more comfortable in a flexed position as flexion relieves pressure and discomfort but may lead to flexion contractures. During a flare, two to three repetitions of active range-of-motion exercises help maximize joint mobility while placing minimal stress on the articular structures. Performing exercises in the evening may reduce early morning stiffness commonly experienced by patients with active disease (Byers 1985). As the inflammation subsides, the exercises can increase to 8 to 10 repetitions a day for each involved joint.

During remissions or relatively inactive disease, patients with RA may undertake a more active exercise program that incorporates active range-of-motion exercises as well as strength and endurance training. Aerobic exercise sessions of as little as 15 minutes'

Table 11.3 Summary of Exercise Recommendations

Disease	Disease status	Recommendation
RA	Acute flare "hot joint"	Active ROM exercises to involved joints: 2 repetitions/joint/day
	Subacute	Active ROM exercises: 8-10 repetitions/joint/day Static exercises: 4 to 6 contractions of 6-second durations Dynamic exercises with light resistance (avoid if joints are unstable, in presence of tense popliteal cysts or internal joint derangement) Aerobic training (15 to 20 min, 3 ×/wk). Cardiac evaluation for men over 35 and women over 45 is recommended. Establish heart rate parameters and use perceived rating of exertion scale (e.g., BORG)
	Stable or inactive	Active ROM and flexibility exercises Static and dynamic strength training (avoid dynamic exercises if joints are unstable or in presence of tense popliteal cysts) Aerobic training 15 to 20 min, 3 ×/wk. Cardiac evaluation for men over 35 and women over 45 is recommended. Establish heart rate parameters and use perceived rating of exertion scale (e.g., Borg).
OA of hip and knee	Mild pain	Active ROM exercises (10 repetitions), 3 to 5 repetitions of flexibility and static exercises (8 to 10 repetitions of 6 second duration). Dynamic exercises especially to quadriceps and hamstrings (8 to 10 repetitions). Low-impact aerobic activities (pool, bicycling) 20 min, 3 ×/wk. Static and dynamic exercises reduce to 5 repetitions, 3 to 5 repetitions of flexibility exercises to maintain muscular balance around joints.
	Moderate pain	Low-impact aerobic exercises (pool, biking) 20 min, 3 ×/wk. Balance activities (BAPS and tilt board), single limb stance. Static and dynamic exercises (no resistance) 3 to 5 repetitions (contraindication: internal joint derangement).
	Severe pain	Low- to no-impact aerobic exercises (pool). *Note:* Advise functional activities to keep moving, use balance and proprioception activities.
	Bone-on-bone	Same as severe but few to no repetitions of dynamic exercises. Patient education very important. *Note:* In patients with ligamentous laxity and malalignment, caution should be taken with prescribing quadriceps strengthening exercises
Hand OA		Active movements, few repetitions, low amount of resistance. Teach home exercises that patient should repeat daily. Aim to maintain the full range of motion of MCP, PIP, and DIP joints.
Spondylarthropathies		Stretching of pectorals, back extensors, hamstrings, psoas, and active ROM exercises (8 to 10 ×/day). Breathing exercises (diaphragmatic and lateral costal expansion) frequently throughout day. Dynamic exercises especially for trunk and hip muscles 5 to 8 repetitions. Aerobic exercises (pool especially helpful in presence of hip involvement) 20 min, 3 ×/wk.
SLE	Active but stable	Active ROM if synovitis present and endurance activities as tolerated.
	Inactive	Dynamic exercises, 8 to 10 repetitions. Aerobic exercises (bicycle, pool, walking), > 20 min, 3 ×/wk.
PM/DM	Active but stable	Use RA guidelines for strengthening as a basis.
	Inactive	Active ROM and static exercises, 8 to 10 repetitions. Dynamic exercises, 8 to 10 repetitions (*Note:* Careful with eccentric exercises, use fewer repetitions). Aerobic exercises as tolerated (20 min, 3 ×/wk).

(continued)

Table 11.3 *(continued)*

Disease	Disease status	Recommendation
Scleroderma		Active ROM exercises (heating of tissue prior to stretching helpful) or use of prolonged stretch Dynamic and static exercises 8 to 10 repetitions Aerobic exercises 20 min, 3 ×/wk

duration, performed three times per week, increased aerobic capacity in patients with RA (Harkcom et al. 1985) without placing undue stress on joints.

Patients should let their pain determine the intensity of the program. Acute pain during exercise indicates a need to modify the program; vague, diffuse pain that resolves in less than 2 hours does not indicate a need for program modification (Hayes 1996). Patients must recognize the signs of an acute flare including redness, inflammation, pain, and stiffness and reduce the frequency and intensity of their exercise with their disease activity. Exercise prescriptions should include the intensity, frequency, and duration at which each exercise should be performed.

Osteoarthritis

Osteoarthritis (OA), also called osteoarthrosis and degenerative joint disease, is the most common form of chronic arthritis. It increases with age and affects nearly 40 million individuals in the United States. Although its exact pathogenesis is unknown, genetic, environmental, and biological determinants are important. **Primary osteoarthritis,** the most common, includes a number of clinical syndromes of specific joints for which there is no etiologic basis. **Secondary osteoarthritis** is osteoarthritis due to underlying factors that accelerate age-related degeneration of cartilage. The factors include inflammatory arthritis (such as RA or spondylarthritis); metabolic diseases (such as hemochromatosis, acromegaly, or diabetes); congenital abnormalities which produce joint surface incongruities, thereby accelerating damage of cartilage; or trauma/sports-related injuries.

Whether primary or secondary, the pathology of OA is in the cartilage, which over time, with variable amounts of inflammation and changes in loading across the joint lead to joint surface destruction. On X-ray the classic appearance includes unequal joint space narrowing, eburnation of the subchondral bone, osteophytes, and subchondral cysts (see figure 11.3). These findings increase in frequency after the age of 50. One of the most impressive features of the epidemiology of OA is the lack of concordance between X-ray pictures and symptoms; roughly 2/3 of patients with radiographic features have few or no symptoms. Patients with early OA experience joint stiffness with progressive cartilage destruction and pain when loading the affected joint. Secondary contractures occur around the involved joint and contiguous joints. These contractures can be biomechanically disadvantageous and increase energy requirements for the patient. The most commonly affected and symptomatic joints are the apophyseal joints of the spine, the distal and proximal interphalangeal joints, the carpometacarpal joint, the first metatarsal phalangeal joint, and the knee, hip, and patellofemoral joints. OA of the axial skeleton and of the large weight-bearing joints has the greatest negative impact on patient mobility and function.

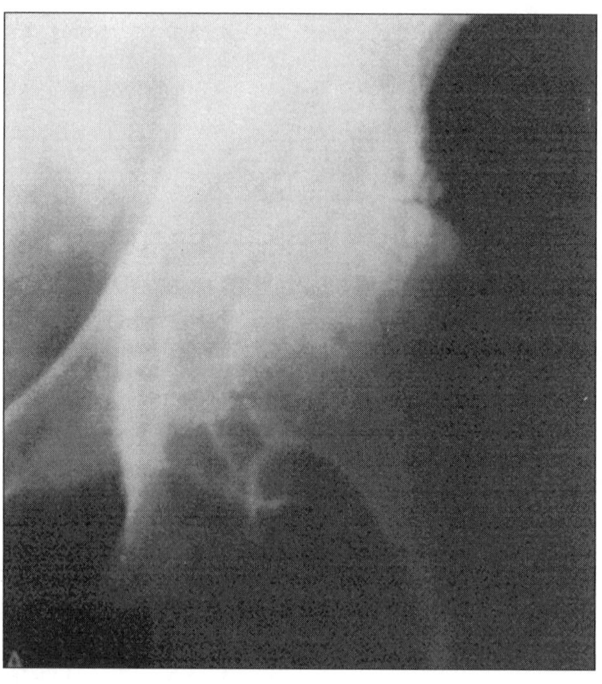

Figure 11.3 Moderately advanced osteoarthritic changes are present, with asymmetric joint space narrowing and superior migration of the femoral head. Eburnation and cystic changes are seen in the subchondral region.

Reprinted, by permission, from W.N. Kelley et al., 1997, *Textbook of rheumatology,* 5th ed. (Philadelphia: W.B. Saunders), 665.

Finger Stiffness/Pain

Osteoarthritis of the fingers causes pain, aching, or stiffness, and an unsightly appearance with gradual loss of ability to grip or hold small objects tightly. With severe deformities, some patients may be unable to grip objects tightly or to make a tight fist. Very often with time the finger pain or stiffness diminishes, probably because the deformities prevent motion.

There has been little study of range-of-motion exercise for OA of the fingers. A trial addressed the effect of joint protection and home exercises on hand function of patients with hand OA. Patients were trained to protect their hand joints in activities of daily living and instructed to perform a 15-minute daily home exercise program: making a fist, flexing the MCP joint while keeping the PIP and DIP stretched, touching the tip of each finger with the tip of the thumb, spreading the fingers as far as possible with the hand lying flat on a table, pushing each finger in the direction of the thumb with the hand lying flat on a table, and touching the fifth MCP joint with the tip of the thumb. Grip strength and hand function improved in the intervention group, but no significant difference was seen in pain or in quality of life (Stamm et al. 2002). In one small trial, yoga and relaxation techniques over a 10-week period diminished pain and tenderness and improved joint motion of finger joints (Garfinkel et al. 1994).

Decreased Proprioception

Proprioceptive changes within the joint contribute to or result from OA. Proprioception is necessary for motor output and provides feedback regarding joint positioning. Changes in proprioception may result from destructive changes in the ligaments, cartilage, capsule, muscle, or tendon that alter joint alignment. Two studies demonstrate that individuals with knee OA have poorer knee proprioception than their healthy older counterparts (Barrett et al. 1991; Sell et al. 1993). Sharma et al. (2003) enrolled 28 adults with unilateral knee OA (Kelgren scale grade 2 or greater) and 29 adults without knee OA in a study to examine the impact of OA on joint proprioception. Proprioception was measured using a computer-driven device consisting of a stepper motor that provided angular motion at 0.3 degrees per second and a precise measurement of angular displacement. Patients were asked to report the threshold at which knee joint deflection was detected. Patients with unilateral knee OA demonstrated worse proprioception than their healthy counterparts. However, a between-knee difference was not found in adults with OA. These data should be interpreted with caution, as cause and effect could not be ascertained. Balance exercises, such as double limb stance activities progressing to single limb stance activities, may help to improve joint proprioception and strength. Activities on unsteady surfaces, such as BAPS boards and tilt/rocker boards, may be incorporated into an exercise routine. It is important to address proprioception in the rehabilitation program, as proprioception does not spontaneously return when pain decreases (Hurley and Scott 1998;Wegener et al. 1997).

Muscle Weakness

It is generally believed that OA causes joint symptoms that reduce activity and contribute to disease-specific muscle atrophy and overall deconditioning (Sharma 2001; Steultjens et al. 2002). However, a study suggested for the first time that muscle weakness may be a cause rather than a result of knee OA (Slemenda et al. 1997). Muscle weakness may alter the biomechanics of the joint and place unequal forces across the joint surface. Joint laxity from muscle inhibition and joint space narrowing distributes the forces across the cartilage surface unequally and can accelerate the process of cartilage degeneration. A subsequent study compared elderly subjects with painful radiographic knee OA to subjects who reported knee pain but had no radiographic evidence of knee OA, and to a group that had neither knee pain nor radiographic evidence of disease. The researcher found that in contrast to subjects with symptomatic OA and radiographic evidence of disease, those with no radiographic evidence of knee OA had less obesity, greater hamstring as well as quadriceps weakness (balanced weakness across the joint may be protective for knee OA), and depression (Brandt et al. 2000).

Patients with advanced radiographic structural changes have the worst deformity, range of motion, quadriceps weakness, and deconditioning (Philbin et al. 1995). Disuse atrophy probably results from ligament stretching, reflex inhibition from pain, capsular contraction, and joint irritation due to pain and effusion. Atrophy of the quadriceps muscle group due to reflex inhibition starts a vicious cycle, increasing force across the damaged cartilage and altering the mechanics of the patellofemoral joint. Malalignment of the patella and abnormal tracking may produce retropatellar pain and chondromalacia patellae. Because muscle weakness and deconditioning accompany OA of the hip and knee, improving both is a goal of rehabilitation. Recent studies have addressed the local factors influencing the genesis and progression of knee OA. These studies focus on the role of joint alignment, ligamentous laxity, and quadriceps and hamstring strength in disease progression. In a systematic review of exercise therapy in knee and hip OA, van Baar et al. (1999) found small to moderate effects on pain, small effects on disability, and moderate effects of exercise on self-reported global assessments. Few investigators have examined the impact of strengthening programs and potential long-term adverse effects on cartilage, or compliance. Table 11.4 summarizes the studies of exercise in individuals with knee OA.

Relevant Studies

For individuals with mild to moderate OA of the knee or hip, a 12-week aerobic exercise program (walking

Table 11.4 Randomized Controlled Trials of Exercise in Knee OA (KOA)

Author	Subject (no.)	Intervention	Result
Minor 1989	80 with KOA 40 with RA	3 groups: aerobic exercise or aerobic aquatics for 30 min at 60-80% max HR 3 ×/wk for 12 wk vs. non-aerobic exercise 3 ×/wk for 12 wk vs. control	Exercisers increased aerobic capacity, increased activity, decreased anxiety and depression. Benefits sustained at 9-mo follow-up. 83% completed 12-wk program and 72% completed follow-up.
Kovar et al. 1992	102 with chronic, stable KOA	8 wk of supervised fitness walking and patient education re: functional status, pain, use of medications vs. routine care	Increased walk distance in exercise group, decreased in control group. Exercisers also reported reduced pain, increased activity, and decreased use of medications.
Borjesson et al. 1996	68 with medial KOA scheduled for surgery	5 wk of physiotherapy 3 ×/wk vs. no treatment	No significant differences in gait, range-of-motion, or isokinetic strength between groups. Patients in PT group increased ability to descend stairs and reported improved mood.
Schilke et al. 1996	20	8 wk isokinetic exercise, 6 sets of 5 max voluntary contractions of knee flexors and extensors vs. control (no Rx)	Significant decrease in pain, stiffness, and AIMS activity and OASI scores. Increased mobility in exercise group. Control group increased right knee flexion and left knee extension.
Bautch et al. 1997	20	12 wk of low-resistance strengthening exercises 3 ×/wk, 3 reps of each exercise increased to 10 reps at 4 wk plus education vs. education only	Exercisers showed decreased pain levels. Education-only group demonstrated better AIMS scores. No change in synovial fluid composition.
Ettinger et al. 1997	439 with X ray evidence of KOA and disability	18-mo program; 3 groups: (a) aerobics, (b) resistive exercise, (c) education; exercise 60 min at 60-80% max HR	365/439 completed. Adherence rate 68% for aerobic group and 70% for strengthening group. Aerobic exercisers showed 10% decrease in disability, 12% less knee pain, improved walk time, stair climbing, and carrying ability compared to controls. Strength group showed 8% decrease in disability and knee pain, improved walk time, stair climbing, and carrying ability compared to controls. No change on X ray in any group.
van Baar et al. 1998	201	Individual exercise program for 12 wk, 1-3 ×/wk for 30 min by a PT, vs. education	Exercisers showed 17% decrease in pain and 19% reduction in disability (effect sizes medium to small, respectively).
Rogind et al. 1998	25 with severe KOA	Outpatient group exercise by PT including general fitness, balance, coordination, flexibility, and strengthening exercises 2 ×/wk for 3 mo vs. control	23/25 completed. 78% adherence. Exercise group increased quadriceps strength by 20%. At 1 year, improved walking speed by 13%, algofunction index decreased 3.8 pts, pain reduced 2 pts. Increase in palpable effusions.

Author	Subject (no.)	Intervention	Result
O'Reilly et al. 1999	191	Daily strengthening exercises for 6 mo, home-based program vs. control	Decrease in WOMAC pain scores by 22.5% and by 6.2% in controls. Significant improvement in VAS pain and 17.4% change in function among exercisers.
Deyle et al. 2000	83	Intervention group: manual therapy to knee, spine, hip, and ankle plus exercise program and home exercise vs. subtherapeutic ultrasound	At 4 and 8 wk significant improvements found in exercisers for 6-min walk time and WOMAC scores. At 8 wk, 6-min walk time improved 13.1% and 55.8% in WOMAC compared to control. Gains still found at 1 year.
Hopman-Rock and Westhoff 2000	103 with hip and knee OA	Comprehensive education and exercise program led by a peer and exercise led by a PT vs. control	Significant improvements in pain, quadriceps strength, knowledge, self-efficacy at post-assessment. Benefits still evident at 6 mo in Rx group.
Fransen et al. 2001	126	3 groups: (a) 8 wk of individualized exercise by PT; (b) small group exercise 1-hr sessions 2 ×/wk for 8 wk supervised by a PT plus home program vs. wait list control	Both PT treatment groups showed significant improvements in pain, physical function, health-related quality of life. Improvement maintained for 2 mo. No difference between PT groups.
Petrella and Bartha 2000	179	Home-based progressive exercise program: simple ROM and resistance exercises utilizing common items in the home	At 2 mo: improvement of measures of activity (self-paced walking, stepping) and activity-related pain.
Penninx et al. 2001	250	- Aerobic exercise program (3 ×/wk walking program for 1 hr) - Resistance exercise program (3 one-hour sessions per week consisting of 9 different exercises)	At 3 mo: both exercise programs reduced the incidence of disability in activities of daily living (self-reported questionnaire).
Baker et al. 2001	46	Home-based progressive strength training program (squats, step-ups, and isotonic exercises of the lower limbs)	At 4 mo: improvements in strength, pain, physical function, and quality of life.
Quilty et al. 2003	87	Nine 30-min PT sessions over 10-wk; PT sessions included 7 quadriceps exercises, postural education, functional exercises, footwear recommendations, and patellar taping; exercises performed at home 10 ×/day vs. usual care	At 5 mo, treatment group showed small decrease in pain and significant improvement in quadriceps strength. No difference at 1 year.

or in water) increased aerobic capacity by almost 20% without exacerbating joint symptoms and decreased pain by almost 10% and morning stiffness by 20 minutes.

Minor and colleagues (1989) studied 80 patients with mild OA of the hip, knee, or ankle for 3 months with three interventions:

1. Stretching and strengthening exercise program (comparison group)
2. Same program with aerobic pool activities
3. Same program with aerobic walking

All patients had supervised range-of-motion and isometric exercises three times a week for an hour. The two aerobic exercise groups also did up to 30 minutes of exercise to increase their heart rates to 60% to 80% of baseline maximum. At 3 months, the researchers assessed 80% of the participants for maximum oxygen uptake as a measure of aerobic capacity, for flexibility, for endurance on a treadmill, for time to walk 50 feet, and health status.

The pool and walking programs increased aerobic capacity 20% and 19%, respectively; the control group had no change. In no case was there exacerbation of joint symptoms in the two aerobic groups. On average, moreover, pain decreased by almost 10% and morning stiffness by 20 minutes in both groups. Physical activity, anxiety, and depression also improved in both aerobic groups significantly more than for the controls (Minor et al. 1989).

Kovar and colleagues (1992) randomly assigned 102 patients with primary knee OA to either

- an 8-week program of lectures, group discussions, and supervised light stretching and strengthening followed by up to 30 minutes of walking or
- routine care and telephone follow-up calls three times a week (control group).

The unblinded investigators evaluated the subjects at baseline and at 8 weeks. Intervention participants had an 18% increase in 6-minute walking test time, compared with a 17% decrease in controls. The intervention group also improved more than controls on measures of physical activities, arthritis pain, and use of medications (Kovar et al. 1992).

Ettinger and his colleagues (1997) studied the effects of exercise in a less controlled setting and randomized 439 community-dwelling subjects 60 years or older, with radiographic knee OA, pain, and physical disability, to

- an aerobic exercise program,
- a resistance exercise program, or
- a health education program.

Overall, patients in the aerobic or resistance exercise groups had modest improvements in pain and disability, and better scores on performance measures and function, than those in the health education group. The effects were smaller than those observed in previous studies; the authors speculated that differences between the three raters might not be apparent since all interventions, even education alone, had previously been shown to be effective. Prior exercise behavior was the strongest predictor of exercise compliance in this sample (Rejeski et al. 1997). A similarly designed study (Penninx et al. 2001) confirmed that aerobic and resistance exercise reduce disability in older adults with knee OA.

Rogind et al. (1998) evaluated the effects of a physical training program on patients with severe OA of the knees. Twenty-five subjects were allocated to a 3-month training program consisting of general fitness exercises, balance and coordination activities, and stretching and lower extremity strengthening plus a home program at an outpatient clinic or allocated to control. Subjects exercised in groups, twice a week. At the 3-month assessment, quadriceps strength had increased 20%, as measured by isokinetic testing. At 1 year, improvements were found in pain (a reduction of 2 points) and in algofunctional index scores (a 3.8 reduction) compared to controls.

Hopman-Rock and Westhoff (2000) randomized 105 patients with hip and knee OA to a 6-week program of health education and exercise or control. The program consisted of weekly sessions of 2 hours' duration. The program began with 1 hour of instruction focused on education and self-management, including a discussion of the pros and cons of exercise and the importance of rest and alternating activity, led by a peer. In the second hour a physical therapist led the exercise program, which consisted of a 15-minute warm-up, followed by static and dynamic strengthening exercises for the hip and knee, and a cool-down. Significant improvements were found for pain, quality of life, quadriceps strength, knowledge, self-efficacy, and physically active lifestyle in the intervention group. The effects were present, but to a lesser degree, at the 6-month assessment.

Petrella and Bartha (2000) found that a progressive exercise program, which included a series of simple range-of-motion and resistance exercises using common household items, in addition to nonsteroidal anti-inflammatory therapy, improved pain and functional performance in knee OA. Baker et al. (2001) evaluated a high-intensity, home-based strength training program (squats, step-ups, and isotonic exercises of the lower limbs) and demonstrated substantial improvements in strength, pain, physical function, and quality of life in persons with knee OA.

Conclusions About Exercise and Osteoarthritis in the Knees and Hips

Aerobic exercise improves endurance and reduces fatigue and has modest effects on muscle strength. With structured exercise (three times/week over 4 months), individuals can improve strength and endurance leading to decreased dependency and pain, and increased functional activity. Some of these benefits continue for up to 8 months after an intense program (Fisher et al. 1991). There is some evidence that exercises focused on proprioception and balance may decrease disability and improve strength. However, more research is needed in this area.

Despite the evidence that symptoms of OA of the hip and knee can be improved with exercise and the fact that exercise is recommended in practice guidelines (American College of Rheumatology 2000), most patients with OA have not had a prescription for exercise. Even when physicians prescribed exercise, only a small percentage of patients exercised in a manner that can achieve a therapeutic effect (Dexter 1992). Certain patients with OA of the hip can exercise at home as effectively as with outpatient hydrotherapy to improve joint mobility and increase muscle strength (Green et al. 1993). Caution needs to be applied in patients with lax or malaligned knees, especially with tibiofemoral OA, in which quadriceps strengthening may exacerbate symptoms and accelerate damage (Sharma et al. 2003).

Patients with mild to moderate knee and hip OA can safely engage in effective aerobic and strengthening exercise without exacerbating joint symptoms. When patients are supervised and compliant, the results are good. No one has studied the long-term and possible adverse effects of such programs. Practical barriers may prevent these modalities from being used more widely.

Gait Problems in Osteoarthritis

Contracture of soft tissues and of tendons surrounding a joint, destruction of joint cartilage, persistent faulty posture, or an imbalance between agonist and antagonist muscle groups may lead to limited joint motion and abnormal gait. Although a flexed position minimizes intra-articular pressure and reduces pain, it leads to flexion contracture. A flexion contracture across the acetabulum toward the lateral margin (Hicks et al. 1993) increases valgus forces at the knee and ankle and causes inefficient gait patterns and increased energy expenditure. Patients describe difficulty and pain when walking or climbing stairs and reduced functional independence. Decreased muscle strength and reduced joint proprioception is also associated with an increased incidence of fall (Wegener et al. 1997).

Evaluations of regimens to correct or prevent contractures are almost nonexistent. In practice, heat followed by passive range-of-motion (ROM) exercises and joint mobilization often can help prevent or at least reduce contractures. Patients also should assume appropriate positions during extended inactivity or sleep, and engage in active ROM exercises to maximize functional range and strength. Patients with knee flexion contractures should not sleep with pillows under the knee. In difficult cases, serial casting or splinting can reduce contracture when followed by maintenance exercises. An exercise program consisting of individualized progressive training including isometric and dynamic exercises for patients with knee OA (Fisher et al. 1997) significantly improved muscle function, functional capacity, walking time by as much as 21%, and reduced self-reported difficulty with walking and pain. Stationary cycling has also demonstrated improvements in walking speed, aerobic capacity, and pain (Mangione et al. 1999).

Loss of joint motion at the hip has functional effects that some clinicians may not appreciate such as impaired ability to sit and may affect personal hygiene and sexual function. Loss of hip range adversely affects the spine and other joints, including the knee and ankle. Preventive posturing, as in prone lying, is important. Repetitive sit-to-stand exercise maintains strength in hip and knee extensors and can be started with standing up from a seat whose level is progressively lowered as the maneuver becomes easier to complete. For patients unable to tolerate full-gravity exercise, the use of water allows exercise with reduced load.

Six patients with severe OA of the hip, who were waiting for total hip arthroplasty, increased hip adduction by 8.3 degrees, increased type I and II fiber cross-sectional area, and increased glycogen levels after passive muscle stretching perpendicular to the direction of the adductor muscle (without hip movement). The subjects stretched with a 20- to 30-kg force applied manually for 30 seconds, rested for 10 seconds, and repeated; sessions lasted 25 minutes and took place 5 days a week for 4 weeks (Leivseth et al. 1989). Recent studies have also demonstrated improved rates of recovery in patients with end-stage hip arthritis following pre-operative and peri-operative exercise programs for total hip arthroplasty (Crowe and Henderson 2003; Wang et al. 2002).

In conclusion, gait problems are common in patients with OA of any of the weight-bearing joints and are a clue to underlying pathology of the soft tissues or the joints themselves. Left untreated, they can cause problems. Clinicians should be attentive to the diagnosis and should design treatments that maximize joint function.

Spondylarthropathies

Spondylarthropathies (SPA) include a group of disorders: ankylosing spondylitis, reactive arthritis, formerly called Reiters disease, psoriatic arthritis, enteropathic arthritis, juvenile onset spondylarthropathy, and undifferentiated spondylarthropathy. The prototypic spondylarthropathy, ankylosing spondylitis (AS), occurs in about 0.1% of the general Caucasian population, predominantly in males. The common finding of these diseases is inflammation of the tendons and ligaments at their insertion into bone, or enthesitis that causes spondylitis, sacroillitis, or arthritis. Stiffness, pain, and restrictions in spinal mobility limit functional abilities. Occasionally skin lesions and aortic valve involvement may be manifest. Over years, SPA leads to variable degrees of restricted mobility of the spine, resulting in loss of functional capacity. In extreme cases of spinal ankylosis, the entire spine may fuse in a flexed position. These patients may also have a rigid thorax associated with kyphosis due to bony ankylosis and osteopenia of the thoracic vertebrae, costovertebral, costotransverse, sternoclavicular, and sternomanubrial joints. This can lead to restricted pulmonary functions but with normal pulmonary compliance, diffusing capacity, and blood gases.

Besides axial spine involvement, peripheral joints may be affected, especially hip, shoulder, or knee. Ankylosing spondylitis is associated with exercise limitation and breathlessness. Carter et al. (1999) have shown that peripheral muscle function is the most important determinant of exercise intolerance in these patients, suggesting that deconditioning is the main factor in the production of the reduced aerobic capacity. Although researchers have focused most exercise therapy studies on AS, there is no reason to believe that the results of such research involving spinal symptoms would not apply to the other SPA. Table 11.5 summarizes the main randomized controlled trials of exercise in SPA.

The goals of exercise prescription are to maximize range of motion, maintain and improve spinal mobility, and maintain a neutral posture. Rehabilitation guidelines for RA are generally appropriate for patients with SPA and peripheral arthritis. Exercises should include passive range-of-motion activity; strengthening of the muscles of the trunk, the back, the abdomen, and the legs; and activity to improve overall fitness. Several forms of exercise for SPA have been shown to be effective: supervised

Table 11.5 Studies of Exercise in AS

Author	Subject (no.)	Study design	Intervention	Result
Sweeney et al. 2002	155	RCT	Home-based exercise intervention (inform. video, exercise chart, booklet, reminder stickers...)	No improvement in function, disease activity, and well-being. Significant improvement in self-efficacy and self-reported levels of exercise.
Van Tubergen et al. 2001	120	RCT	3 wk combined spa-exercise therapy, followed by 37 wk group physical therapy	Significant improved pooled index of change at 4 wk. No significant difference at 40 wk.
Hidding et al. 1993	144	RCT	9 mo group physical therapy vs. individualized home therapy	Intention to treat analysis: group physical therapy proved superior to home therapy in improving thoracolumbar mobility, fitness, and global assessment.
Hidding et al. 1994	68	RCT, continuation of Hidding et al. 1993	18 mo group physical therapy vs. individualized home therapy	Intention to treat analysis: global health and functioning were sustained or even improved further if group physical therapy continued; spinal mobility decreased slightly in both group and home therapy.
Kraag et al. 1990	53	RCT	4 mo home physiotherapy	Intention to treat analysis: significant improvement in finger to floor distance and functional ability but no difference in pain, and Schober test.

individualized exercises, supervised group physiotherapy, and unsupervised home exercises. Rehabilitation is most effective if it is started before significant ankylosis occurs. In a cohort study of patients with AS, exercise was associated with significant improvements in pain, stiffness, and functional disability only in patients who had had AS for less than 15 years (Uhrin 2000).

LIMITED SPINAL MOBILITY

Data indicate short-lived benefits of physiotherapy on pain, stiffness, and spinal mobility from exercises with and without hydrotherapy (or spa therapy) in SPA (Dagfinrud 2001). There is a tendency for additional benefits if the exercises are performed in a supervised group setting as compared to home exercise, and this is most likely due to social support and enhanced compliance.

A 4-month home exercise program combined with patient education was effective in patients with AS (Kraag et al. 1990). Including education about the disease process and its physical management, this program aimed to decrease local and generalized pain, increase spinal mobility and function, improve pulmonary vital capacity, increase muscle strength and endurance, improve exercise compliance, and enhance psychosocial adjustment. Patients in the treatment group showed significant improvements in finger-to-floor distance and functional ability ($p < .001$), but not with pain (100 mm visual analog scale) or lumbar flexion (Schober test). The benefits from the treatment program remained after 8 months (Kraag et al. 1994).

Hidding and colleagues (1993) showed that 9 months of supervised group physical therapy was superior to individualized therapy in improving thoracolumbar mobility and fitness, and significantly improved general health status. Group therapy consisted of 1-hour physical training to improve mobility of the spine and peripheral joints and to strengthen muscles of the trunk and legs, followed by 1 hour of sports such as volleyball or badminton and 1 hour of hydrotherapy. A follow-up study noted sustained global health and function in the treatment group, but slightly decreased spinal mobility in both treatment and control groups over the longer term (Hidding et al. 1994). It's likely that the higher adherence to home exercises among the group therapy patients strengthened the beneficial effects of group therapy.

The concern with short-term physical therapy in SPA is that its benefits may not be sustained after the supervised therapy is discontinued. Self-management is a prerequisite for long-term progress; therefore patients should be encouraged to incorporate exercise as part of their daily routine. Regular recreational exercise and back stretching at home should be strongly encouraged by all therapists. In a prospective longitudinal cohort study, Uhrin et al. (2000) found that unsupervised recreational exercise and back exercises were effective in improving pain, stiffness, and functional disability in patients with AS. However, benefits were seen only when patients performed recreational exercise at least 30 minutes per day (200 minutes/week) and back exercises at least 5 days per week. Table 11.5 summarizes the studies of exercise in AS.

CONCLUSION

Further research is needed to determine the most effective physiotherapy modalities. Few studies were controlled and most were short-term using small numbers of subjects. Nevertheless, the overall clinical impression is that exercise is beneficial for at least the symptoms of stiffness and pain. In practice, exercise programs must be adjusted to the stage of the disease and the patient's problems. In patients with advanced ankylosed spine or an osteoporotic spine, vigorous spinal exercise may cause spinal fractures and is unlikely to improve mobility significantly. Since patient compliance is the key to long-term success, it is important to incorporate stretching and exercise into routine activities. To enhance proper posture, for example, patients may want to read in the prone position or sleep on a hard bed with a low pillow height. Recreational exercises such as swimming, volleyball, or badminton provide carryover of the exercise program. Group exercise therapy can socially reinforce continuing exercise and is less costly than individual programs (Bakker et al. 1994).

SYSTEMIC LUPUS ERYTHEMATOSUS

Systemic lupus erythematosus (SLE) is a multisystem autoimmune disease, characterized by immune hyperactivity, autoantibodies, and immunologically mediated tissue injury. It can affect many organs in the body, most commonly the joints, the skin, and kidneys, but cardiac, pulmonary, neuropsychiatric, gastrointestinal, and hematological involvement also occur. Estimated to afflict 40 or 50 per 100,000 population, lupus is 9 times more prevalent in women (particularly in their reproductive years) than in men, and is 3 to 4 times more prevalent in African-Americans. Advances in management of lupus have improved survival and reduced morbidity. Improved survival makes rehabilitation important, but there are few studies on the efficacy of rehabilitation in the management of patients with SLE.

Exercise strategies for lupus should be individualized. For patients with predominant arthralgias or arthritis, we recommend the rehabilitation techniques used in RA. In patients with avascular necrosis of weight-bearing

Table 11.6 Exercise in SLE

Author	Subject (no.)	Study design	Intervention	Result
Tench et al. 2003	93	RCT	Moderately supervised home exercise program 30-50 min, 3 ×/wk vs. relaxation vs. control	Significant decrease in fatigue. No change in aerobic fitness measures.
Daltroy et al. 1995	34	RCT 2-stage trial	1st stage: moderately supervised 3 mo aerobic exercise; 2nd stage: minimally supervised 3 mo aerobic exercise	Significant improvements found with fatigue but not with other outcomes. Unsupervised home exercise may benefit only a select subgroup of patients.
Robb-Nicholson et al. 1989	23	RCT	Supervised 8 wk anaerobic exercise	Anaerobic capacity ($\dot{V}O_2$max) increased by 19% in contrast to 8% in controls, decreased fatigue.

joints, a complication of lupus, loading of involved joints should be avoided and treated by range-of-motion and isometric exercises (e.g., aquatic exercises) that do not stress affected joints. Patients with muscle weakness caused by myositis or steroid-induced myopathy can be managed with the rehabilitation strategy for polymyositis/dermatomyositis.

Fatigue is a very common complaint (~80%) in patients with both active and inactive disease. It is important to determine whether fatigue is a manifestation of treatable causes such as anemia, depression, cardiopulmonary involvement, or myositis. Most often fatigue results from a number of factors, such as low aerobic exercise capacity (Tench 2002), disease activity, depression, or associated fibromyalgia. For nonspecific fatigue, aerobic exercise training is helpful. Robb-Nicholson et al. (1989) found a significant reduction in fatigue and improved aerobic capacity after an 8-week supervised aerobic program including walking, bicycling, and jogging. Daltroy et al. (1995) tested a minimally supervised home aerobic training program, observing a significant reduction in fatigue, but only smaller statistically nonsignificant improvements in fitness, depression, fatigue and helplessness. These studies suggest that a home aerobic training program can be effective. Tench et al. (2003) randomized 93 lupus patients to a graded exercise therapy, relaxation therapy, or no intervention; after 12 weeks, half of the patients in the exercise group felt "much" or "very much" improved, compared to 22% in the non-exercise groups. Another study (Ramsey-Goldman et al. 2000) compared an aerobic exercise program with a range-of-motion and muscle strengthening exercise program and found no clinically significant differences in outcomes between the two programs. All studies demonstrate that exercise programs consisting of different forms of exercise can be prescribed safely to patients with lupus of mild to moderate severity (see table 11.6). Future research should address how to improve compliance with aerobic training.

Polymyositis/ Dermatomyositis

Polymyositis and dermatomyositis (PM/DM) are rare idiopathic inflammatory disorders of the muscles characterized by proximal muscle weakness of the limbs, reduced muscle endurance, and pain and are sometimes associated with neck and respiratory muscle weakness. Although PM/DM are primarily diseases of skeletal muscles, the skin, heart, lungs, gastrointestinal tract, or joints may be involved. Chronic muscle weakness in this population can be attributed to the effects of the disease on muscle, corticosteroid myopathy, or disuse.

The goal of exercise for patients is to maximize muscle strength. In the presence of synovitis, exercise can help prevent contractures or improve range of motion. With ectopic calcification (most commonly seen in children), maintaining a functional range may be very difficult. Preserving range of motion is particularly important in children and in markedly weakened adults, who can develop contractures rapidly.

Wiesinger et al. (1998) found significant improvements in muscle strength (29.4% in the exercise group) and activities of daily living and no increase in muscle inflammation following 6 weeks of supervised, progressive bicycle exercise and step aerobics. Patients exercised for a total of 1 hour at an intensity of 60% of maximum heart rate twice weekly during the first 2 weeks, and then three times per week for the remaining 4 weeks. A physical therapist supervised the exercise sessions. Alexanderson et al. (1999) demonstrated improved muscle function, walking distance, and general health following a 12-week program of home exercise. Ten of 13 patients with stable, inactive PM/DM completed the study and performed muscle strengthening exercises for the upper and lower extremities, trunk, and neck, as well as mobility and stretching exercises, 15 minutes a day for 5 days a week. The program also included a 15-minute walk 5 days per week. There were no signs of increased disease activity as measured by creatine phosphate kinase (CPK), MRI, or muscle biopsy.

These trials support the use of active exercise in patients with stable, inactive disease. However, patients with acute, active disease are frequently told to avoid strengthening exercises for fear of aggravating muscle inflammation. An earlier case study of a patient with active, stable polymyositis by Hicks et al. (1993) showed that static exercise significantly increased strength without a significant increase post-exercise creatinine phosphate kinase (CPK). Escalante et al. (1993) also found increases in muscle strength without clinically significant rises in serum levels of muscle enzyme with resisted exercise in five patients with active, stable polymyositis. Alexanderson et al. (2000) replicated her study of home exercise in patients with stable inactive disease in a sample of patients with active PM/DM. In this low- to moderate-intensity program, patients with active disease also demonstrated improvements in muscle strength and function, without exacerbation of muscle inflammation. Overall evidence of small nonrandomized trials shows that exercise can improve function in patients with PM/DM; however, more research is needed.

Active exercises in patients with active, stable disease appear to be safe and effective but patients should be monitored for elevation in muscle enzymes or increased muscle pain. Eccentric exercises should be undertaken with caution, as they are associated with greater post-exercise discomfort and muscle damage. The mechanism for this increased pain with eccentric exercise is unknown, but it may be related to mechanical stress. Patients with PM/DM may be at even greater risk of post-exercise discomfort because of their inflammatory disease. They should begin an exercise program with fewer repetitions of eccentric exercises per set, increasing their effort gradually, as tolerated. Although there are no empirical data regarding the benefits of breathing exercises, we recommend them to strengthen respiratory muscles.

SYSTEMIC SCLEROSIS

Systemic sclerosis, also known as scleroderma, is a rare connective tissue disease characterized by fibrosis of the skin and potential involvement of visceral organs such heart, lung, kidney, and gastrointestinal tract. The natural history of the disease evolves from an edematous phase to a sclero-atrophic phase. The progression of the disease varies in pace and the extent of the fibrosis (limited-acral form, diffuse-systemic form). Restrictive lung disease, interstitial fibrosis, and pulmonary hypertension may occur. No controlled studies on rehabilitation have been published in scleroderma; therefore, exercise guidelines rely on expert opinions or experiences from related conditions (Casale et al. 1997).

Skin, muscle, and joint involvement leads to contractures of the fingers and other joints, which are traditionally treated with range-of-motion (ROM) exercises and manual stretching. Other physical techniques have been recommended. These increase the mobility of the joints, reduce the edema and stimulate vascularization and include massage, heat, spa, ultrasound, CO_2 laser, biomechanical stimulation, acupuncture, and transcutaneous electrical nerve stimulation (TENS). However none of these therapies has been formally evaluated. Particular focus should be given to the finger joints and the mandibular joint, as the quality of patients' life depends heavily on the use of their fingers and of their mouth.

Joint pain becomes some patients' major complaint. Some authors have reported good results with topically applied therapies; in particular, TENS, acupuncture and laser therapy have been put forth, but there are no controlled studies. Clinicians often recommend aerobic training for patients with systemic sclerosis aiming to improve patients' long-term autonomy. However, safety is a concern in this clinical setting; in one study one-third of exercising patients developed arrhythmias (Blom-Bulow et al. 1993). These arrhythmias might result from myocardial fibrosis, triggering ventricular tachycardia, a cause of sudden death. Since there are no data regarding safety of aerobic exercise in scleroderma, we recommend only progressive, mild to moderate aerobic exercises.

IMPROVING PATIENT ADHERENCE

As documented earlier, exercise therapy has a role in many rheumatic conditions and yet appears underutilized and frequently underprescribed. Doctors' attitudes and beliefs influence the way in which they present treatments to their patients; they also modify the dynamics of the conversation, directly affecting even whether or not rehabilitation programs are prescribed (Iversen et al. 1999). Information that is personally relevant and delivered by experts can influence attitudes and beliefs. Doctors therefore can affect patients' beliefs and attitudes about exercise, either through reinforcing the use of exercise or by communicating misgivings. The greatest barrier to having a dialogue about exercise promotion is that providers lack confidence in their ability to promote change (Iverson et al. 1985).

Studies show that arthritis patients' adherence to exercise prescriptions is low, in the range of 35% to 60% (Bradley 1989; Deyo 1982; Stenstrom et al. 1997). In specific subgroups the compliance rates may be even lower. Factors associated with nonadherence in arthritis treatment include education, gender, and age; features of the disease (such as disease activity or severity); characteristics of the treatment source (hospital or clinic); and the quality of the doctor-patient interaction (Hicks 1985). For example, the more severe the disease, the more likely patients are to adhere to the treatment regimen. However, more complex treatment regimens are associated with lower adherence rates. Demographic factors and characteristics of the treatment source (hospital-based versus clinic) explain only a small proportion of differences in adherence rates. Beliefs and attitudes, including patients' confidence in their ability to manage the disease, explain a fair amount of the differences seen in adherence with treatments (Gecht et al. 1996). For example, Stenstrom et al. (1997) have shown that high self-confidence and previous participation in exercise strongly predict exercise compliance at 1 year among patients with inflammatory rheumatic diseases.

The clinician needs to consider the patient's physical and psychosocial characteristics, as well as his or her own beliefs regarding the effectiveness of exercise, when designing a rehabilitation program (Iversen et al. 1999). Iversen (1999) and Jensen and Lorish (1994) have demonstrated how patients' and providers' attitudes about the effectiveness of exercise in managing arthritis symptoms can affect patients' intention to exercise as well as their subsequent exercise behavior. Godin (1987) has shown that the pleasantness or unpleasantness associated with exercise is a stronger determinant of intention to exercise than patients' perceptions of the effectiveness of the exercise. This means a clinician should describe the positive attributes of the prescribed program (e.g., warm-water exercises are soothing and relaxing), and the benefits of exercise (e.g., enhanced mood, improved appearance, and increased functional mobility), to enhance adherence.

In chronic arthritides, exercise prescriptions are exercises for life. Patients who are successful in adhering to an exercise regimen are those who modify their program to accommodate the specific features of their disease. To instruct patients properly, you must understand the role of various exercises (dynamic versus static strength training, aerobic exercise, range-of-motion exercises), and when to prescribe each exercise. This information needs to be clear and concise in terms patients can understand. An effective communicator elicits patients' expectations of exercise, their perceived barriers to adhering to the prescription, and their confidence in performing the exercises appropriately. Using this information as a framework, one collaborates with patients in setting goals. It is also important to incorporate exercises into activities of daily living. For example, patients can perform postural exercises in front of the mirror either before or after a shower and range-of-motion exercises

TIPS FOR ENHANCING PATIENT ADHERENCE TO EXERCISE

1. Elicit patients' beliefs and attitudes regarding the benefits of exercise and past experience with exercise.
2. Discuss patients' expectations of exercise.
3. Establish realistic goals. Small, incremental, attainable goals will encourage and promote long-term adherence.
4. Help patient identify and reduce barriers to exercise.
5. Promote the positive attributes of exercise.
6. Provide written instructions and have patient demonstrate exercises.
7. Provide intensity, frequency, and duration of each form of exercise, whether aerobic or strength training.
8. Teach patient to take a radial pulse and give patient an exercise range heart rate (e.g., 60% to 80% age-predicted heart rate).
9. Encourage use of an exercise diary or log.
10. Link patient to community resources (such as the Arthritis Foundation).
11. Incorporate recreational activities.
12. Identify a significant other to support patient's participation in exercise.

at the edge of the bed before going to sleep, to reduce early morning stiffness and discomfort.

Feedback enhances adherence to exercise programs. Providing target heart rates based on age-adjusted predicted heart rate values (ACSM 1995), or targeting levels of perceived exertion (Borg 1982), can be especially useful to ensure that patients achieve aerobic benefits from their exercise programs. Similarly, they can use a log of these results to track progress and exercise-induced symptoms. By encouraging patients to participate in recreational activities and linking them with community resources, you can increase their physical activity while also enhancing their psychological well-being. The Arthritis Foundation has designed exercise programs specifically for patients with arthritis. These programs, such as PACE (People with Arthritis Can Exercise), are taught by certified instructors educated in the principles of exercise as they pertain to individuals with arthritis. Exercise videos are also available through the Arthritis Foundation as an adjunct or alternative to home exercises. For a summary of suggestions for helping patients stick with their exercise programs, see "Tips for Enhancing Patient Adherence to Exercise" (on previous page).

The final step in enhancing compliance is to help patients identify significant others who will support their participation in exercise. Educating the partners along with the patients will reinforce patient learning and increase adherence to the program. This multifaceted approach in the design and implementation of an exercise regimen will enhance patient carryover and safety.

SUMMARY

This chapter discusses the role of exercise therapy in major arthritic disorders, the evidence supporting the use of various exercise modalities, the strengths and limitations of these studies, and new recommendations in the face of uncertainty. Future research areas are suggested. We highlight the importance of prescribing the correct frequency, duration, intensity, and type of exercise, and present techniques to enhance patient adherence to exercise regimens and to help health care providers develop goals of exercise therapy with their patients, based on the patient's disease, status, goals for rehabilitation, and preferences for treatment.

CHAPTER 12

NEUROMUSCULAR DISEASES

David D. Kilmer, MD; and Susan Aitkens, MS

CASE STUDY

A 44-year-old woman with hereditary motor and sensory neuropathy, type I (HMSN), came to us for assessment of rehabilitation needs. She was functionally independent in self-care but reported difficulty with fine motor tasks. Distal weakness in the lower extremities led her to use ankle–foot orthoses for community ambulation, but she noted increasing fatigue as she walked longer distances. Although she used to enjoy walking and gardening, she now spent most of her day sedentary at home.

We carefully assessed her interests, motivations, and her reasons for not exercising, and formulated realistic goals for an exercise prescription. She probably had a component of disuse weakness due to lack of activity, and worked at a higher percentage of her maximal capacity during routine physical activities. An exercise program to build her muscular endurance was the primary focus—so we initially prescribed a 15-minute walking program three days a week, at an intensity requiring fairly hard breathing but maintaining the ability to carry on a conversation. We also encouraged her to garden or perform other enjoyable recreational activity on alternate days, working toward a goal of some physical exertion each day. However, we cautioned her to stop exercising if she noted any increased muscle weakness or pain. Initially testing her lower extremity strength with a hand-held dynamometer in the clinic, we scheduled subsequent tests at one-month intervals to reassure both the patient and ourselves of her progress and to motivate her to continue the program.

At the three-month follow-up, the patient reported that she was able to walk 45 minutes without stopping and noted increased energy to enjoy her garden. She still had to be careful not to perform continuous physical activity for more than one hour, lest she endure excessive soreness and fatigue the following day. Objective strength testing using hand-held dynamometry showed no significant improvement or decrement of isometric force.

Despite advancing knowledge regarding the beneficial effects of habitual physical exercise in the able-bodied population over the last several decades, the role of exercise in the rehabilitation of diseases of the peripheral nervous system remains unclear. The term **neuromuscular diseases (NMDs)** encompasses disorders of the anterior horn cell, peripheral nerve, neuromuscular junction, and skeletal muscle. Each specific disease may respond differently to exercise. However, researchers commonly group NMDs together due to their relative rarity and common clinical issues: progressive muscular weakness, fatigability, and disability. Until recently, clinicians have understood few of the specific structural or biochemical abnormalities distinguishing many conditions, with diseases diagnosed primarily by common clinical characteristics.

This situation is changing. There is now a high level of scientific interest in the molecular basis for a number of diseases of the peripheral nervous system. The ultimate goal is to determine the genes and gene products responsible for normal and abnormal functioning of the motor unit. However, it will be clear from this chapter that we still know little about how diseased muscle responds to physical activity. The basic principles of an adaptive response to muscle overload may not be valid in neuromuscular conditions, and in fact certain types of exercise could be detrimental. This chapter reviews current understanding of the effects of exercise in neuromuscular disease, discusses etiologies for the decline in neuromuscular function in these disorders, and makes reasonable exercise recommendations based upon the limited scientific research available.

Physiologic and Functional Consequences of Neuromuscular Diseases

This discussion highlights diseases at each anatomic level of the peripheral nervous system leading to progressive impairment, disability, and compromised exercise performance. The primary focus is on hereditary diseases, since few exercise studies exist in acquired diseases such as polymyositis (see chapter 11) and Guillain-Barré syndrome. It should be evident that muscle weakness is the common impairment linking each disorder.

Anterior Horn Cell

Amyotrophic lateral sclerosis (ALS) results in degeneration of bulbar and spinal motor neurons, causing progressive, usually rapid, loss of strength both in the limbs and bulbar musculature. It is known to affect maximal oxygen uptake and exercise capacity early in the disease, possibly due to functional skeletal muscle loss as well as deconditioning (Sanjak et al. 1987). ALS subjects may also have a higher oxygen cost for a given level of submaximal exercise (Sanjak et al. 1987). Spasticity and other causes of biomechanical inefficiency are important contributing factors.

Several studies suggest increased muscle fatigability in ALS patients, possibly due to an abnormality distal to the muscle membrane (Sharma et al. 1995; Sharma and Miller 1996). The implications of these findings for exercise performance and rehabilitation are not known.

Other causes of anterior horn cell dysfunction include primarily autosomal recessive **spinal muscular atrophies (SMA)** of childhood and adult onset, resulting in gradual loss of lower motor neuron function. In general, an earlier onset of weakness implies more severe disability, with a higher likelihood of contractures, progressive scoliosis, and restrictive lung disease (Carter et al. 1995a). An exercise program may be appropriate for persons with the later onset forms.

Peripheral Nerve

The most common hereditary neuropathy leading to disability is **hereditary motor and sensory neuropathy, type I (HMSN,** or **Charcot-Marie-Tooth Disease).** The majority of cases are associated with duplication of a gene locus on chromosome 17 involved in peripheral nerve myelination (Murakami et al. 1996). The primary pathology of this autosomal dominant disorder is uniform demyelination of peripheral nerve progressing to axonal degeneration, manifested by weakness and sensory loss primarily in the feet and hands. However, systematic studies demonstrate significant deficits in proximal muscle strength as well, even in mildly affected subjects (Carter et al. 1995b; Lindeman et al. 1994). These deficits correspond with a reduction in functional abilities (Lindeman et al. 1994). It is unclear whether the proximal weakness is a direct result of the neuropathy, or is related to disuse.

In a closely related hereditary disease of the peripheral nerve, termed **hereditary motor and sensory neuropathy, type II,** axonal degeneration is the primary pathology rather than demyelination as in type I. There seems to be less proximal muscular involvement with this disease, with less overall disability. It is not known if exercise responses differ between the forms of hereditary neuropathy.

Neuromuscular Junction

The most common neuromuscular junction disorder is **myasthenia gravis (MG),** caused by antibodies directed against acetylcholine receptors. Characteristic symptoms include fluctuating weakness exacerbated by exercise. Unlike other NMDs considered here, MG may be treatable with anticholinesterase and cytotoxic medications, although in generalized MG there may be persistent muscle weakness. Aerobic and strength characterization studies have not been performed in MG.

Muscle

The muscular dystrophies comprise a heterogeneous group of hereditary diseases exhibiting progressive loss of muscle fibers, resulting in weakness first usually noted in the proximal musculature. The most common dystrophy is **Duchenne muscular dystrophy (DMD),** an X-linked, recessive, rapidly progressive disease of boys causing gait difficulty during childhood, wheelchair dependence in late childhood or early adolescence, and death by the early third decade. **Becker's muscular dystrophy (BMD)** shares a similar pattern of weakness and X-linked inheritance, but typically has a later onset and a much slower rate of progression.

The protein **dystrophin,** which is deficient in DMD, is closely associated with the cell membrane (Bonilla et al. 1988; Hoffman et al. 1987). Although its exact function is not known, dystrophin is probably important in maintaining the cytoskeletal framework of the muscle cell during active muscle contraction (Ervasti and Campbell 1993). When dystrophin is absent (as in DMD), or decreased or altered (as in BMD), the muscle fiber may be predisposed to damage with normal activities (Petrof 2002). The dystrophin-associated glycoproteins or other membrane constituents have been found to be abnormal or absent in most subtypes of **limb-girdle muscular dystrophy syndromes (LGS),** possibly causing disorders of skeletal muscle similar to but less severe than those seen in DMD (Brown 1997). Whether other muscular dystrophies or neuropathic disorders have structural muscle cell membrane defects is not yet known. The genetic defect in **myotonic muscular dystrophy (MMD)** is known to involve the presence of CTG codon repeating sequences on chromosome 19. The abnormal gene then transcribes into a potentially pathogenic RNA, although ramifications at the muscle cellular level are not yet clear (Mankodi and Thornton 2002). Table 12.1 lists the major muscular dystrophies and current knowledge about the deficient or abnormal proteins.

With knowledge of muscle cell membrane abnormalities in at least some dystrophies, it seems plausible that

Table 12.1 Classification of the Major Muscular Dystrophies

Dystrophy	Inheritance	Responsible chromosome	Altered gene product
DYSTROPHIES WITH EXERCISE-TRAINING INVESTIGATIONS			
Duchenne (DMD)	Sex-linked recessive	X	Dystrophin (absent)
Becker's (BMD)	Sex-linked recessive	X	Dystrophin (partial/ abnormal)
Myotonic (MMD)	Autosomal dominant	19	–
Facioscapulohumeral (FSH)	Autosomal dominant	4	–
Limb-girdle 1A-1E (LGS)	Autosomal dominant	Various	–
Limb-girdle 2A-2J (LGS)	Autosomal recessive	Various	Various sarcolemmal proteins
SELECTED DYSTROPHIES WITHOUT EXERCISE-TRAINING INVESTIGATIONS			
Emery-Dreifuss	Sex-linked recessive	X	Emerin
Classic merosin-positive congenial muscular dystrophy (CMD)	Autosomal recessive	–	–
Classic merosin-negative CMD	Autosomal recessive	6	Merosin
Fukuyama CMD	Autosomal recessive	9	–
Walker-Warburg Syndrome CMD	Autosomal recessive	9	–
Scapuloperoneal	Autosomal dominant	12	–
Autosomal dominant distal myopathy	Autosomal dominant	14	–
Autosomal recessive distal myopathy	Autosomal recessive	2	–
Oculopharyngeal	Autosomal dominant	14	–

activities stressing the muscle fiber, such as exercise, might be detrimental for persons with these disorders. Indeed, intense physical exercise results in marked release of creatine kinase in a number of myopathies, implying muscle membrane damage. The lack of dystrophin may weaken the sarcolemma, making muscles more susceptible to injury (Moens et al. 1993; Petrof et al. 1993; Weller et al. 1990). As we gain further knowledge about the function of these cellular proteins, researchers may be able to design scientifically based protocols, using different types of exercise interventions, to determine beneficial and detrimental effects of physical activity on the muscle fiber. Identifying the implications of the specific protein dysfunction will then be possible.

Subjects with DMD and other dystrophies have reduced maximal oxygen uptake during exercise, probably due to loss of functional muscle mass rather than a defect in muscle energy metabolism (Haller et al. 1983; Haller and Lewis 1984; Sockolov et al. 1977). In fact, there is some evidence for an inverse relationship between leg weakness and maximal oxygen uptake (Carroll et al. 1979). However, since muscle strength and endurance may affect daily physical abilities more than cardiorespiratory limitations in NMD, improving maximal oxygen uptake is of limited value (Bar-Or 1996). Progressive loss of muscle fibers with motor weakness is the hallmark of the dystrophies. The primary goals of intervention should be to maintain or reverse loss of muscle strength and function.

CAUSES OF REDUCED NEUROMUSCULAR FUNCTION IN NMD

Progressive muscle weakness from the primary disease is only one cause of the disability resulting from disorders of the peripheral nervous system. In fact, disability may be out of proportion to the severity of muscle involvement. Other factors often play an important role in defining the extent of one's disability, and it is these components that may be primarily amenable to an exercise program.

MUSCLE DISUSE

Disuse of muscle fibers results in reduced myofibril size, decreased fiber cross-sectional area, lower force production, and reduced muscle endurance (Appel 1990; Mujika and Padilla 2000). Although there is no direct evidence linking muscle disuse with disability in persons with NMD, clinical experience, as well as limited studies examining aerobic fitness, suggests that persons with neuromuscular disorders are sedentary and poorly conditioned (McCrory et al. 1998; Wright et al. 1996). Likely explanations include poor physical fitness skills learned during childhood and adolescence, social isolation, concern on the part of health care professionals and physical educators about the potential harm from exercise, and lack of available adapted programs (Kilmer and McDonald 1995). Further evidence comes from the frequent clinical observation that short periods of bed rest, particularly in rapidly progressive disorders such as DMD, result in significant loss of strength and function that may not be reversible (Vignos 1983).

It seems clear that muscle disuse often contributes to the muscular weakness, easy fatigability, and poor endurance seen with NMD. In the nonmetabolic myopathies and neuropathic syndromes, there appear to be no primary defects in muscle oxidative transport or phosphorylation. However, muscle adapts to the absence of stresses, likely resulting in low concentrations of important enzymes in these pathways. Diseased muscle may at least partially respond in the same fashion as intact muscle to progressive overload during aerobic training.

The biomechanical disadvantage in persons with NMD, due to weakness and/or sensory loss, leads to inefficient performance of physical tasks. For example, weakness in the prime movers of a joint forces the musculature to work at a higher percentage of maximal capacity, leading to fatigue (Dolmage and Cafarelli 1991). Recruitment of secondary, less efficient muscles further increases the energy expended to perform a task, fatiguing muscle more rapidly (figure 12.1). It is not surprising that persons with NMDs complain of poor exercise capacity, fatigue, and muscle soreness when they attempt physical tasks. A similar phenomenon is noted in the post-polio population with residual muscle weakness (Borg et al. 1988; Perry et al. 1988). These people often adopt sedentary, inactive lifestyles, increasing the spiral of disability. A key question for researchers and clinicians is the relative contribution of disuse in an individual patient's disability, and potential for reversal without damaging the muscle.

MUSCLE OVERUSE AND ECCENTRIC CONTRACTIONS

NMD patients often say they "pay the price" for physical exertion, reporting residual muscle soreness and fatigue for several days following exercise. Clinicians have long been concerned about potential damaging effects of vigorous exercise (commonly called **overwork weakness**) in NMD patients. This concern is pervasive, despite lack of evidence from systematic studies in NMD subjects showing deleterious effects of exercise. Evidence for overwork weakness is only anecdotal, known from a series of case reports.

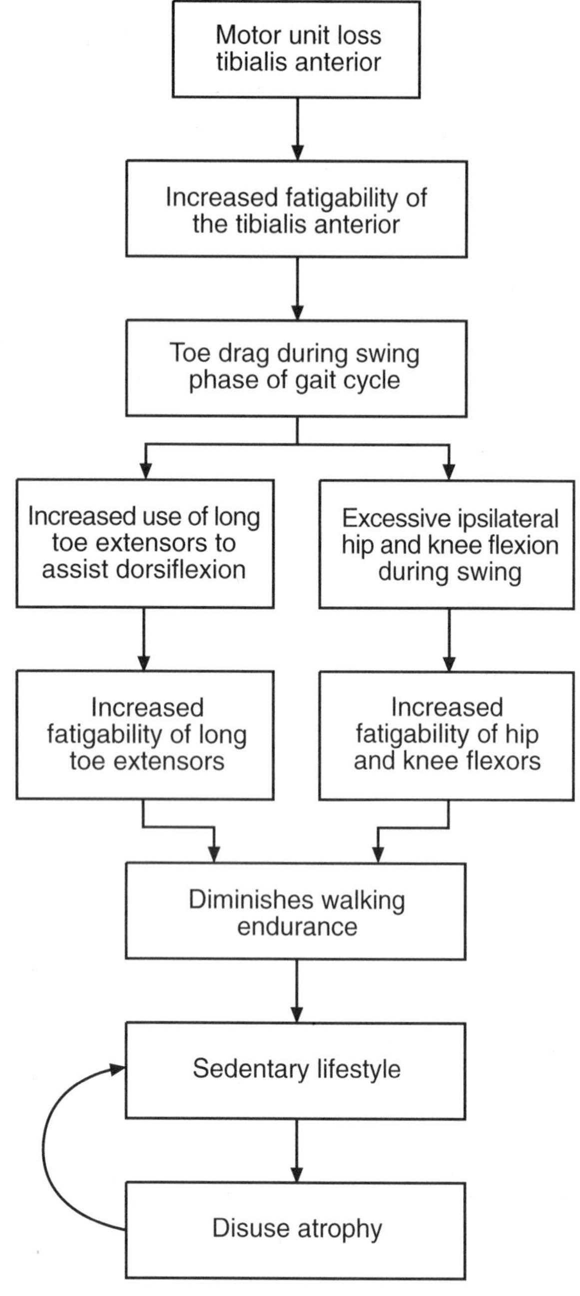

Figure 12.1 An example of the cascade of dysfunction which may occur with weakness in the prime mover of a joint, in this case the tibialis anterior. From Kilmer D.D. 1996. Functional anatomy of skeletal muscle.

An influential case series in the 1950s reported signs of overwork weakness in persons with poliomyelitis during both supervised submaximal resistance exercise and unsupervised community activities (Bennett and Knowlton 1958). In a pathologic study of a person with DMD, the greatest degeneration occurred in muscles undergoing sustained physical activity, suggesting the possibility of overwork weakness (Bonsett 1963). Additional circumstantial evidence exists in a report of persons with **facioscapulohumeral dystrophy (FSH),** demonstrating greater weakness in the dominant limb subjected to heavy loads during work or involved in unsupervised weight lifting (Johnson and Braddom 1971). In another study, right-hand dominant persons with FSH were found to be weaker in the right upper limb compared to the left (Brouwer et al. 1992). However, a natural history profile reports frequent asymmetric upper extremity weakness in FSH (Kilmer et al. 1995).

Recent work involving experimental models of muscle overuse in able-bodied subjects may have relevance for the NMD population. It is well established that a bout of maximal **eccentric (lengthening) contractions** causes damage to muscle fibers and results in transient muscle weakness over a period of weeks (Clarkson et al. 1992; Clarkson and Hubal 2002; Friden and Lieber 1992). This weakness is associated with delayed muscle soreness, changes in resting joint angle, and elevations of creatine kinase. There appears to be high strain on selected individual fibers rather than equal transmittal of load through the entire muscle, possibly disrupting the cytoskeletal framework with myofibrillar damage (Friden and Lieber 1992; Lieber and Friden 1993; Lieber et al. 1996). The actual muscle fiber damage may result from calcium influx through the disrupted sarcolemma, stimulating protease and phospholipase activity within the muscle cell (Armstrong et al. 1991). However, an adaptive response seems to occur, and repeated bouts within several months cause less damage (Clarkson et al. 1992). The mechanism for this repeated-bout effect may involve longitudinal addition of sarcomeres and beneficial inflammatory adaptations (McHugh 2003). It is not known if this adaptive response occurs in diseased skeletal muscle or whether damage is cumulative.

In the primary animal model of DMD, the mdx mouse, there is a similar lack of dystrophin but with a milder phenotypic expression of weakness and muscle necrosis (Cooper 1989). Several studies demonstrate that muscles from mdx mice sustain greater injury than those from control mice after eccentric exercise, resulting in higher levels of intracellular calcium and potential muscle necrosis (Franco and Lansman 1990; Stedman et al. 1991; Turner et al. 1991). Overall, there is strong evidence that dystrophin deficiency reduces the muscle cell's ability to tolerate mechanical stress (Petrof 1998). A similar mechanism may exist in deficiencies of the dystrophin-glycoprotein complex as seen in LGS (Petrof 2002). Jacobs and colleagues (1996) mechanically induced muscle damage in prednisone-treated mice, which sustained less damage than controls. The authors suggest that prednisone protects against mechanically induced damage, possibly by stabilizing the muscle cell membrane. Prednisone is known to help slow the rate of progression in human DMD (Fenichel et al. 1991).

There may be similarities between models of muscle overuse from eccentric muscle contractions and weakness in diseases of the muscle fiber cytoskeletal framework. Indeed, Edwards et al. (1984) proposed that submaximal eccentric contractions, so important in postural muscles during routine activities, may damage diseased muscle over time. This hypothesis is attractive in light of recent findings that, in a number of dystrophies, abnormalities in sarcolemmal structural proteins may increase susceptibility to mechanical damage from routine eccentric contractions (Petrof 2002). Myopathic patients complaining of soreness and weakness on the day after unusual exertion may be manifesting the untoward effects of eccentric muscle contractions. Dystrophic muscle may not repair itself sufficiently to return strength to a baseline level (Jejurikar and Kuzon 2003).

The only way to avoid eccentric contractions in daily life would be to live in a gravity-free environment. However, there is now at least a theoretical rationale to design exercise programs minimizing this type of muscular contraction, made particularly feasible by use of isokinetic dynamometers. In a study of patients with post-polio muscular atrophy, a training technique involving primarily concentric contractions showed beneficial strengthening results with no serological or histological evidence of muscular damage (Spector et al. 1996).

Cardiopulmonary Involvement

When it directly affects the cardiopulmonary system, NMD compromises exercise performance—as certainly occurs in some neuromuscular disorders, particularly DMD (McDonald et al. 1995b), BMD (McDonald et al. 1995a), and MMD (Johnson et al. 1995). In DMD, cardiomyopathy becomes a clinical concern during the adolescent years, along with restrictive lung disease from weakness of the respiratory musculature. At this stage, however, profound extremity and truncal weakness already severely limit exercise capacity. Even during earlier stages of the disease, Sockolov et al. (1977) observed reduced maximal exercise capacity and endurance along with reductions in stroke volume, cardiac output, and peripheral oxygen utilization.

In the slowly progressive disorders, BMD may exhibit disproportionately severe cardiomyopathy as compared with skeletal myopathy (McDonald et al. 1995a), and MMD is associated with well-described cardiac conduction defects (Johnson et al. 1995)—but the extent to which either problem limits exercise performance is not known.

In most other NMDs, deconditioning likely plays a more prominent role in reduced stroke volume and cardiac output than intrinsic cardiac malfunction. While Carroll et al. (1979) demonstrated a wide range of exercise capacities among subjects with various NMDs, there were generally reductions in maximal oxygen uptake. Haller et al. (1983) noted similar ratios between NMD subjects and controls for cardiac output and systemic A-VO_2 difference from rest to maximal exercise, implying normal cardiac function.

Body Weight

That many persons with NMD are overweight, with increased adiposity compared to similar-aged controls (McCrory et al. 1998), probably results from a sedentary lifestyle, poor nutritional choices, and reduced income. Important ramifications of this problem include

- increased muscular demand for movement, causing the muscle to exercise at a higher percentage of its maximal capacity;
- accentuated biomechanical inefficiencies due to altered body habitus; and
- increased atherosclerotic risk factors for ischemic cardiac disease.

Reversing this tendency to become overweight may lead to improved function.

Contractures

A comprehensive review of hereditary NMDs found that, with the exception of DMD, joint contractures were not a significant functional problem until people were forced to rely on wheelchairs (McDonald et al. 1995b). This is not surprising, since contractures are generally a consequence of muscle imbalances, chronic postural adjustments to maintain the ability to stand and take steps, improper positioning, and habitual wheelchair use. This results in more significant weakness and limited exercise capacity (Vignos 1983). In DMD, progression of contractures in the heelcords, hip flexors, and iliotibial bands may allow continued upright standing at the cost of reduced muscle endurance and increased effort during ambulation. In other NMDs, contractures do not limit exercise performance until late in the disease.

Effects of Resistance (Strengthening) Exercise in NMD

The first controlled study of strengthening exercise used a high-resistance regimen in 24 rapidly and slowly progressive NMD patients over a one-year period, reporting strength improvement throughout the first four months of exercise with a subsequent plateau in strength (Vignos and Watkins 1966). The authors determined that, since the degree of improvement was related to the initial strength of the exercised muscle, exercise programs should begin early in the course of disease.

Milner-Brown and Miller (1988) had 16 patients with gradually progressive NMD (6 FSH, 4 MMD, 3 SMA, 1 BMD, 1 LGS, and 1 idiopathic polyneuropathy) perform elbow curls using dumbbells, and knee extensions using ankle weights. They initially used weights that could be lifted a maximum of 12 to 15 times, and completed one set on alternate days—gradually increasing the number of sets, training days, and weight over time to model a high-resistance weight training program. While most patients demonstrated strength gains, those with severely weak muscles (<10% normal strength) generally did not improve. The authors concluded that NMD patients should initiate weight training at the onset of muscle weakness, as the training provides no benefit once muscles have become severely weak.

McCartney et al. (1988) trained 5 subjects with NMD (3 spinal muscular atrophy, 1 LGS, 1 FSH) over a nine-week period, three times per week. The progressive weight training program was based on initial one-repetition maximums (1RM) for single arm curl and double leg press; the contralateral limb served as control for the arm exercise. By the end of the study, the strength of the trained arms increased between 19% and 34%, while the strength of the untrained arms changed between −14% and +25%, demonstrating cross-training effects in some cases. Leg strength increased from 11% to 50%. Muscular endurance also improved considerably. By the end of the training period, the pretraining 1RM could be lifted from 3 to 48 times in the trained limbs, and from 1 to 13 times in the untrained limbs. The authors concluded that strength training may be useful in managing selected NMDs.

In a small study of 9 subjects with MMD, there were modest gains in knee extensor strength with a high-resistance training program (3 × 10 reps at 80% 1RM) three times per week over 12 weeks. Importantly, no changes in quadricep muscle histopathology were noted on biopsy after the training (Tollback et al. 1999) (see table 12.2).

Aitkens and colleagues (1993) studied moderate resistance exercise in 14 control and 27 slowly progressive NMD subjects over a 12-week period, three days per week. They prescribed submaximal exercise, using ankle and wrist weights and a handgrip exerciser (table 12.3). Both groups demonstrated significant increases

Table 12.2 Summary of Strength Training Studies in NMD

Author	Study population and sample size	Duration of training	Training modality	Training protocol	Response(s)
Vignos and Watkins 1966	Various NMD (24)	12 months	Weight training (multiple muscle groups)	Unspecified, but based on 10-repetition maximum (RM)	Strength increased; % increase correlated with initial strength
Milner-Brown and Miller 1988	Various NMD (12)	>12 months (variable)	Weight training (elbow flexion and knee extension)	Initially 1 set of 10 reps based on 15-RM performed on alternate days; gradually increased to a maximum of 5 sets 4 days per week; protocol individualized	Strength increased significantly when the initial degree of strength loss was not severe (<10%)
McCartney et al. 1988	Various NMD (5)	9 weeks	Weight training (arm curl and leg press)	3 days per week; initially 2 sets of 10-12 reps at 40% max; gradually progressed to 3 sets of 10-12 reps (1 set at 50%, 60% and 70% max); contralateral arm control	Strength and muscular endurance increased; considerable intersubject variability Cross-training effect in nonexercised limb

Author	Study Population and Sample Size	Duration of training	Training modality	Training protocol	Response(s)
Aitkens et al. 1993	Slowly progressive NMD (27) and able-bodied controls (14)	12 weeks	Weight training (elbow flexion, knee extension, grip)	See table 12.3	Significant improvement in most strength measures (not grip) in both groups; cross-training effect
Kilmer et al. 1994	Slowly progressive NMD (10) and able-bodied controls (6)	12 weeks	Weight training (elbow flexion, knee extension)	See table 12.4	Results mixed: some increase in leg strength coupled with decrease in arm strength in NMD
Lindeman et al. 1995	MMD (33) and HMSN (29); non-exercise control group	24 weeks	Weight training (knee extension and flexion, hip extension and flexion)	3 days per week; initially 3 sets of 25 reps at 60% 1 RM; progressed to 3 sets of 10 reps at 80% 1 RM	In MMD group, no change in strength In HMSN group, increased strength of knee extensors
Tollback et al. 1999	MMD (9)	12 weeks	Weight training (knee extension)	3 days per week; 3 sets of 10 reps at 80% of 1-RM	Significant increase in 1-RM; no change in histopathology

Table 12.3 Moderate-Resistance Exercise Training Schedule Over 12 Weeks

	Knee extension			Elbow flexion			Hand grip		
Week	Sets	Reps	% max*	Sets	Reps	% max*	Sets	Reps	% max*
1	3	4	30	3	4	10	3	4	100
2	3	6	30	3	6	10	3	4	100
3	3	8	30	3	8	10	3	4	100
4	3	8	30	3	8	10	3	4	100
5	3	4	35	3	4	15	3	4	100
6	3	6	35	3	6	15	3	4	100
7	3	8	35	3	8	15	3	4	100
8	3	8	35	3	8	15	3	4	100
9	3	4	40	3	4	20	3	4	100
10	3	6	40	3	6	20	3	4	100
11	3	8	40	3	8	20	3	4	100
12	3	8	40	3	8	20	3	4	100

*Exercise performed 3 days per week based on one-repetition maximum weight.

Adapted, by permission, from S.A. Aitkens, M.A. McCrory, D.D. Kilmer, and E.M. Bernauer, 1993, "Moderate resistance exercise program: Its effect in slowly progressive neuromuscular disease," *Archives of Physical Medicine and Rehabilitation* 74:711-715.

in most strength measures. Since the strength gains did not significantly differ between the exercised and nonexercised limbs in either group, a cross-training effect was apparent.

The same research group modified the moderate-resistance protocol described above into a high-resistance program with 10 slowly progressive NMD and 6 control subjects, again using elbow flexion and knee extension exercise (Kilmer et al. 1994) (table 12.4). The results of this regimen were less consistent in the NMD group than those of the moderate-resistance study. While most strength parameters showed improvement over the 12-week period, a few indices declined in the NMD group. Finding no benefit of high- versus moderate-resistance protocol, the researchers suggested caution with high-resistance exercise.

The only randomized, controlled trial of strength training in NMD examined 33 subjects with MMD and 29 subjects with HMSN (Lindeman et al. 1995), exercising three times per week over 24 weeks. Initially subjects completed three sets of 25 repetitions at 60% of 1RM, increasing to three sets of 10 reps at 80% of 1RM as the study progressed. In the MMD group, investigators found no deleterious or beneficial effect on strength. This could be related to the significant weakness at baseline in some subjects. In the HMSN group, there was a significant increase in the strength (14%) of the knee extensors, and a nonsignificant increase of 13% for knee flexors. Neither group experienced a change in muscle endurance—but because the endurance test was a timed maximal isometric contraction sustained at 80% of maximal voluntary contraction, and the training was dynamic, this finding is not surprising. The authors also noted that most participants enjoyed the training and intended to continue exercising.

No one has examined the relative contribution of neural factors versus actual muscle fiber hypertrophy in NMD strengthening studies. However, during brief 8- to 12-week protocols, improved recruitment of motor units and efficiency of contraction (neural factors) are probably the primary causes for increases in strength. The cross-training effects described above to the nonexercised limb are consistent with this conclusion.

In summary, it appears there are significant benefits to appropriate strength training in persons with slowly progressive NMD, particularly if they start training before manifesting significant weakness. Limited research suggests that high-resistance is no more beneficial than moderate-resistance exercise. Importantly, there have been no signs of overwork weakness in these systematic investigations.

Table 12.4 High-Resistance Exercise Training Schedule Over 12 Weeks for Knee and Elbow Exercise

Week	Exercise days per week	Sets	Repetitions per set*
1	3	1	10
2	3	2	10
3	3	3	10
4	3	4	10
5	4	4	10
6	4	4	10
7	4	4	10
8	4	4	10
9	4	5	10
10	4	5	10
11	4	5	10
12	4	5	10

*Based on maximum weight lifted 12 times.

Adapted, by permission, from D.D. Kilmer, M.A. McCrory, N.C. Wright, S.A. Aitkens, and E.M. Bernauer, 1994, "The effect of a high resistance exercise program in slowly progressive neuromuscular disease," *Archives of Physical Medicine and Rehabilitation* 75: 560-563.

Effects of Aerobic (Endurance) Exercise in NMD

Because the hallmark of NMD is motor weakness, more investigators have dealt with muscle strengthening than with aerobic capacity. This discussion demonstrates the challenges of aerobic testing in this population and reviews the few studies performed.

Testing Approaches

Since NMD subjects may have difficulty with stability and ambulation, measuring aerobic capacity with graded bicycle ergometry offers significant advantages (i.e., it is stationary and provides support) over treadmill exercise. Additionally, it is possible to start at a very low power output (e.g., 0 to 200 kilopond-meters/min) and increase the exercise intensity in small increments. It is often a challenge to find the "right" protocol for a given subject population: if the protocol is too rapid or aggressive, a weaker subject cannot keep pace; if it is excessively slow-paced, local muscular fatigue (legs) can cause premature termination of the test.

An additional challenge in testing the aerobic capacity of NMD subjects is determining the end point. One end point is a clearly defined $\dot{V}O_2max$ (i.e., the point at which oxygen uptake plateaus in response to an increase in power output). Even in motivated, able-bodied individuals, achieving this objectively definable end point is an arduous task. It is often beyond the physical capacity of NMD subjects, and peak rather than maximal $\dot{V}O_2$ is the end point. Another end point is "volitional fatigue," the voluntary limit beyond which a subject no longer desires to continue the prescribed protocol. This end point is highly dependent on the motivation of the subject, the influence of the person administering the protocol (e.g., verbal encouragement), and established discontinuation criteria.

Typical aerobic testing protocols are continuous, with an increase in power output every 1 to 2 minutes. Most exercise protocols involving NMD subjects do not achieve steady-state oxygen consumption at each progressive workload. In general, poorly conditioned individuals require longer to reach steady state at any given workload—yet it is desirable to achieve steady state if the oxygen cost of a given submaximal exercise level is of interest. This generally requires that each step be longer in duration (e.g., 3-5 minutes).

RESPONSE TO TRAINING

After earlier studies demonstrated reduced aerobic capacity in persons with NMD, several investigators examined the response of individuals with NMD to aerobic exercise training. Florence et al. (1984) tested four control and eight NMD subjects (various slowly progressive or non-progressive disorders) in a 12-week aerobic training program, three days per week. The subjects performed six 5-minute bouts on a bicycle ergometer, with a 2-minute rest period between each bout, at 70% of each individual's previously determined $\dot{V}O_2max$. The $\dot{V}O_2max$ increased significantly in both groups, with the majority of the increase occurring in the first six weeks. After 12 weeks of training, the NMD subjects increased $\dot{V}O_2max$ from 24.2 ± 3.2 to 29.6 ± 3.4 ml · kg^{-1} · min^{-1}, and the control subjects increased from 29.9 ± 1.4 to 35.5 ± 2.0 ml · kg^{-1} · min^{-1}. The two groups responded similarly to the training program when expressed as a percentage of the initial value. Interestingly, the increase in $\dot{V}O_2max$ in the NMD subjects brought their values up to the initial level of the able-bodied control subjects. The authors concluded that persons with a variety of neuromuscular disorders may develop relatively normal adaptations to training, although they cautioned that there may be disease-specific differences.

Wright et al. (1996) studied the effects of a 12-week, home-based aerobic walking program on eight NMD subjects (5 MMD, 2 HMSN, 1 LGS). Training heart rate corresponded to resting heart rate plus 50% to 60% of heart rate reserve (Reserve HR = Max HR – Resting HR). They began with 15-minute exercise periods and increased to 30 minutes three to four days per week. Graded exercise testing to volitional fatigue using a semirecumbent cycle ergometer found significant decreases in sub-maximal heart rate and systolic blood pressure for a given power output following the training period; increases in $\dot{V}O_2max$ were not significant.

In a study including 10 subjects with various chronic myopathic disorders, eight weeks of training three to four times per week, at 70% to 85% of estimated heart rate reserve on the treadmill for 20 to 30 minutes, resulted in improvement in aerobic capacity similar to that in controls. Specifically, a decreased heart rate was noted at the same submaximal workload. The authors reported evidence of improved quality of life based on a self-assessed measure of functional status (Taivassalo et al. 1999).

Although these studies demonstrate modest improvements in function without untoward effects, it is not yet possible to draw firm conclusions about the role of endurance exercise training in diseases of the peripheral nervous system.

EXERCISE RECOMMENDATIONS IN NEUROMUSCULAR DISORDERS

Before prescribing exercise for persons with NMD, be sure to differentiate between physical activity and exercise, terms often used interchangeably. Casperson (1989) defines exercise as a subcategory of physical activity, involving planning, structure, and repetition leading to improved fitness. With NMD, it may be beneficial to prescribe physical activities not clearly defined as exercise. For example, gardening does not meet the strict definition of exercise, but as a physical activity it may be a successful method to gradually improve endurance in a person with limited motivation and resources and easy fatigability. Indeed, low levels of activity such as walking and gardening, although not improving maximal oxygen uptake, may reduce the risk of coronary artery disease in the general population, a condition certainly important in the NMD population as well (Leon and Connett 1991). Unstructured activities are more feasible in this disabled group because of their low levels of employment (Fowler et al. 1997). There are often limited financial resources to join health clubs, purchase equipment, and travel to events.

Based on our understanding of available research, our general recommendations for strengthening programs include focusing on muscles with greater than antigravity strength, emphasizing concentric rather than eccentric muscle contractions, and encouraging moderate- rather than high-resistance weight training.

Exercise Prescription Recommendations

- To improve compliance, consider both a formal exercise program and enjoyable physical activities.
- Include activities with opportunities for social development and personal accomplishment.
- Strengthening programs should emphasize concentric rather than eccentric muscle contractions.
- High-resistance strengthening programs probably have no benefit over moderate-resistance programs.
- Muscles with less than antigravity strength have little capacity to improve: the program should focus on stronger muscles.
- Periodically monitor muscle strength to assess for possible overwork weakness, particularly in unsupervised programs.
- Activity modification should include periods of physical activity alternating with rest.

When available, structured and supervised exercise programs for NMD patients are highly desirable. You can define and ensure the exercise mode, intensity, frequency, and rest periods. In fact, some advocate that NMD patients use only therapist-supervised programs, although others have found beneficial improvements in both strength and endurance measures using home-based programs (Aitkens et al. 1993; Kilmer et al. 1994; Vignos 1983; Wright et al. 1996). If a therapist-supervised program is not available or not practical, and the patient is motivated to perform a home program, it is prudent to follow the patient closely for the first several months using quantitative strength measures to reassure yourself and the patient. The hand-held dynamometer is a quick, inexpensive, and reliable device to measure strength in this population (Kilmer et al. 1997).

Adequate rest is an important component of exercise prescriptions in NMD. Extrapolating from the post-polio population, there is evidence that alternating periods of activity and rest forestall the development of fatigue (Agre and Rodriguez 1991). These same principles should benefit patients with other diseases of the peripheral nervous system.

Do not overlook the potential psychological benefits of exercise. Being involved in a sport, even at a low level, can have tremendous effects on self-esteem. Participating in an exercise program improves energy, reduces weight, and often brings a new sense of independence.

Summary

This chapter highlights the consequences of peripheral nervous system pathology for exercise performance, including the specific neuromuscular defects associated with compromised physical abilities. Disability in NMD is a complex phenomenon, however, and many other factors play an important role, including muscle disuse, cardiopulmonary involvement, excess body weight, and contractures. Muscle overuse is a particular concern in NMD; although no one has conclusively demonstrated the association experimentally, overuse may be related to habitual or sporadic eccentric muscular contractions. As we gain knowledge of the specific gene product abnormalities with each NMD, exercise recommendations may have a more rational scientific basis.

Overcoming the psychological and social barriers that make the NMD population sedentary is a challenge to clinicians working with these patients. Unfortunately, review of the scientific literature does not yet allow us to confidently assure safety and effectiveness for all types of exercise. A prudent and thoughtful exercise prescription takes into account the person's goals, motivations, abilities, limitations, and concerns. A personalized, well-devised physical activity program may currently be the most effective prescription we can give to people with NMD to improve their quality of life, enhance self-image, and provide greater energy for both work and play.

Acknowledgments

This work was supported by Research and Training Grant H133B031118 from the National Institute on Disability and Rehabilitation Research (NIDRR), United States Department of Education.

CHAPTER 13

Spinal Cord Injury

Mark S. Nash, PhD, FACSM

Case Study

The patient is a 46-year-old male who was in excellent health until age 41 when he was involved in a motor vehicle accident and sustained T6 neurologically complete (ASIA A) paraplegia. In the five years since injury he has gained considerable weight and has experienced pain in his shoulders when propelling his wheelchair and performing other activities of daily living. A recent physical examination showed fasting glucose of 156 mg/dL and an HbA1c level of 8.6%. His lipid profile was consistent with an isolated low high-density lipoproteinemia (HDL-C = 29 mg/dL). The patient was placed on metformin 1,000 mg bid. He was further advised to restrict intake of calories and fat and to undergo exercise reconditioning directed toward reduction of shoulder pain and cardiovascular disease risks.

The patient entered a circuit resistance exercise training program incorporating resistance and endurance activities of the upper extremities. He trained for 45 min three times weekly with resistance settings at 50% of his measured 1-repetition maximum for six resistance maneuvers. After 16 weeks of training, his percentage of body fat was significantly reduced. He reported less shoulder pain and an improvement in both activities of daily living and personal independence. As he could now lift himself from his swimming pool without assistance from his daughter, he added two days of swimming to the weekly exercise regimen. After 24 weeks his fasting blood glucose was 128 mg/dL, which mandated tapering of the metformin dose by half. Loss of body fat, reduction of body weight, and lessened shoulder pain improved his health and quality of life.

The human spinal cord is an elaborate network of upper motoneurons that functions as a bidirectional relay between the brain and most motor, sensory, and autonomic targets of the body. Disruption of spinal cord transmission by trauma and disease dissociates central control of most body functions, and undermines the essential reflex interplay between body sensors and their motor and autonomic effectors. As the spinal cord is rarely severed by trauma, most persons surviving spinal cord injury (SCI) experience varying patterns and degrees of motor, sensory, and autonomic dysfunction depending on the specific neural structures affected. The interruption of spinal cord functions by trauma affects 8,000 to 10,000 Americans annually, with an estimated 179,000 persons having survived their initial injury (DeVivo et al. 1993, 2002).

While SCI was described millennia ago as an ailment not to be treated (Hughes 1988) and until 60 years ago was a fairly certain death sentence, advances in field injury stabilization, medical treatment, and rehabilitative care now allow those with SCI to experience relatively normal life spans. Those life spans, however, are filled with unique physical, social, and psychological changes that diminish participation in, and benefits derived from, exercise conditioning (Nash 2002). These limitations are a concern for patients and health care providers alike, as individuals with SCI are usually young and physically active at the time of injury (DeVivo et al. 1992) and thereafter undergo profound physical deconditioning (Noreau et al. 1993; Washburn and Figoni 1998). Physical deconditioning following SCI likely causes or contributes to lifelong medical complications such as accelerated cardiovascular disease risk, insulin resistance, obesity, and metabolic syndrome X (Demirel et al. 1998; Kocina 1997; Nash 1997; Shields 2002), as well as activity limitations (Dallmeijer 1998; Janssen et al. 1994) and accelerated aging (Bauman et al. 1999d; Gerhart et al. 1993).

The need for persons with SCI to adopt habitual exercise as part of a healthy lifestyle has been endorsed by many investigators and health care practitioners. The question of *how* persons with SCI should safely benefit from exercise participation is far more difficult to answer. Most exercise options for those with SCI employ movement generated by muscles located above the level of lesion, forces generated by muscles that are partially spared by injury, or sequenced contractions of paralyzed muscles stimulated by electrical current. Credible evidence shows that exercise of almost any kind performed by those with SCI both enhances physical conditioning and reduces multisystem disease susceptibility. It further suggests that habitual exercise reduces fatigue, pain, weakness, musculoskeletal decline, and incipient neurological deficits that appear as persons age with disability. The prevention of these deficits will allow those with SCI to enjoy fullest health and life satisfaction.

Compared to the situation for persons without disability for whom exercise is readily available and easily accomplished, exercise options available to those with SCI are more limited (Jacobs et al. 2002b) since their acute exercise and training responses are less robust than those of persons without SCI (Davis 1993; Nash et al. 1995) and risks of imprudent activity greater and potentially irreversible. This makes an understanding of exercise opportunities and risks important if exercise undertaken by those with SCI is to provide benefit, not harm. The text that follows addresses common medical problems experienced by persons with SCI, common modes and benefits of exercise conditioning, and risks imposed by unsound exercise recommendations.

Health Consequences of Spinal Cord Injury

Persons with SCI usually live sedentary lives (Dearwater et al. 1986; Washburn and Figoni 1998) and have been classified among the least physically fit of all humans (Dearwater et al. 1986). This fact alone could easily explain their accelerated cardiovascular morbidity and mortality (Bauman and Spungen 2000). In many cases their physical deconditioning results from muscle paralysis sufficient to make voluntary exercise ineffective. In many cases persons with SCI simply adopt a sedentary lifestyle, or fail to identify personnel and equipment that will assist their training. Without regard for the cause of their sedentary lifestyle, nearly one in four healthy young persons with SCI fails to achieve levels of oxygen consumption on an arm exercise test sufficient to perform many essential activities of daily living (Noreau et al. 1993). While those with paraplegia have far greater capacities for activity and more extensive choices for exercise participation than persons with tetraplegia, they are barely more fit (Bostom et al. 1991; Dearwater et al. 1986).

Not unexpectedly, young persons with chronic SCI experience accelerated pathological states and conditions normally associated with physical deconditioning, including dyslipidemias and heart disease (Bauman and Spungen 2000; Bauman et al. 1999d), arterial circulatory insufficiency (Hopman et al. 1998; Nash et al. 1997) and clotting disorders (Green et al. 1992), bone and joint diseases (Segatore 1995a, 1995b), and pain of musculoskeletal and neuropathic origins (Levi et al. 1995; Widerstrom-Noga and Turk 2003). All these conditions, of course, can be caused and exacerbated by inactivity in uninjured persons and persons with SCI. SCI also results in dysfunctions beyond musculoskeletal paralysis that promote inactivity, contributing to the vicious cycle of decline observed in persons with SCI.

Alterations in Cardiac Structure and Function

Individuals with chronic SCI experience various types of circulatory dysregulation depending on the level of their cord lesion (McKinley et al. 1999). When injury occurs above the level of sympathetic outflow at the T1 spinal level, resting hypotension with mean arterial pressures of 70 mmHg is common (King et al. 1994). Low mean arterial pressures challenge the ability of persons with SCI to regulate pressure accompanying orthostatic challenge (Figoni 1984) and further alter cardiac structure and function (Kessler et al. 1986). As size and architecture of the human heart are influenced to a great degree by peripheral circulatory volume and systemic pressures, withdrawal from normal activity levels and altered circulatory dynamics transform the structure of the heart and alter its pumping efficiency (Cooper and Tomanek 1982). For those with tetraplegia, a chronic reduction of cardiac preload and myocardial volume coupled with pressure underloading causes the left ventricle to atrophy (Kessler et al. 1986; Nash et al. 1995). By contrast, long-term survivors of paraplegia are normotensive and have normal left ventricular mass and resting cardiac output but experience a cardiac output composed of elevated resting heart rate and depressed resting stroke volume (Davis 1993; Nash et al. 1991). This lowered stroke volume is attributed to decreased venous return from the immobile lower extremities or frank venous insufficiency of the paralyzed limbs (Hopman et al. 1996).

Vascular Structure and Function

The blood volume and velocity of lower extremity arterial circulation are significantly diminished after SCI, with volume flow of about half to two-thirds that reported in those without paralysis (Nash et al. 1996; Taylor et al. 1993). This circulatory "hypokinesis" (Hjeltnes 1977) results from loss of autonomic control of blood flow as well as diminished regulation of local blood flow by vascular endothelium (Nash et al. 1996). The lowering of volume and velocity contributes to heightened thrombosis susceptibility commonly reported in those with acute and subacute SCI (Green et al. 1992). A contributing factor to thrombosis disposition appears to be a markedly hypofibrinolytic response to venous occlusion of the paralyzed lower extremities (Boudaoud et al. 1997), a poor response likely attributable to low blood flow conditions in the paralyzed lower extremities (Nash et al. 1996) or interruption of adrenergic pathways that regulate fibrinolysis in the intact neuraxis (Winther et al. 1992).

Cardiovascular Disease, Dyslipidemia, and Disease Comorbidities

Epidemiological studies beginning in the early 1980s reported emergence of cardiovascular disease as a major cause of death in persons with SCI (DeVivo et al. 1993; Gerhart et al. 1993). While genitourinary complications accounted for 43% of deaths in the 1940s and 1950s, mortality from these causes was reduced to 10% of cases in the 1980s and 1990s (Gerhart et al. 1993; Whiteneck 1992). Cardiovascular diseases currently represent the most frequent cause of death among persons surviving more than 30 years after injury (46% of deaths) and among persons more than 60 years of age (35% of deaths) (Bauman et al. 1992; Whiteneck 1992).

Decline of cardiovascular function in persons aging with SCI is similar to that experienced by persons who age without SCI, but occurs at an accelerated rate (Bauman et al. 1999). Asymptomatic cardiovascular disease also occurs at earlier ages after SCI (Bauman et al. 1994, 1992), and its symptoms may be masked by interruption of sensory pain fibers that normally convey warnings of cardiac ischemia (Bauman et al. 1994, 1992). Several major risk factors commonly reported in persons with SCI have been linked with their accelerated course of cardiovascular disease; these include dyslipidemia (Bauman and Spungen 1994) and a sedentary lifestyle imposed by muscle paralysis and limited exercise options (Noreau et al. 1993; Washburn and Figoni 1998). The cardiovascular disease risks of individuals without SCI are worsened by hyperinsulinemia (Bauman and Spungen 1994; Karlsson 1999) and elevated percentages of body fat (Maki et al. 1995; Zlotolow et al. 1992), which are common among persons with SCI (Gerhart et al. 1993).

An atherogenic lipid profile is commonly reported in persons with chronic SCI (Bauman et al. 1999a). Elevated total cholesterol (TC), triglyceridemia, and plasma low-density lipoprotein cholesterol (LDL-C) have all been reported in sedentary persons with SCI, although elevated TC is not observed in all cases (Bauman et al. 1999a; Spungen et al. 1995) and LDL-C concentrations tend to show elevation typical of the general population (Bauman et al. 1999a). The most consistent finding of reports on the lipid profiles of persons with SCI is a depressed blood plasma concentration of the cardioprotective high-density lipoprotein cholesterol (HDL-C) (Bauman et al. 1999a; Washburn and Figoni 1999), whose levels are inversely associated with cardiovascular risk (Grundy 1995). More than 40% of persons with SCI have HDL-C levels below the earlier criterion score for high cardiovascular risk (HDL >35 mg/dL). Unfortunately, dyslipidemia is not the sole cardiovascular disease risk common among those with SCI. Truncal obesity (Zlotolow et al. 1992), elevated body mass indices (Maki et al. 1995), physical inactivity (Noreau et al. 1993; Washburn and Figoni 1998), reduced lean body mass (Aksnes et al. 1996; Bauman et al. 1999c), diabetes (Bauman et al. 1999b; Duckworth et al. 1980), metabolic syndrome X (Kuhne et al. 2000), and advancing age (Ragnarsson 1993) all represent additional risks for disease that magnify risk for disease progression.

Insulin Resistance

Insulin resistance occurring in a high percentage of persons with SCI was first reported in 1980 (Duckworth et al. 1980) and has since been confirmed as a risk sustained by those with an SCI (Bauman and Spungen 1994; Karlsson 1999). Almost half the persons with SCI live in a state of carbohydrate intolerance or insulin resistance (Bauman and Spungen 1994; Duckworth et al. 1980). A reason for prevalent insulin resistance in persons with SCI has not been firmly identified, although physical inactivity (Burstein et al. 1996), obesity (Maki et al. 1995; Zlotolow et al. 1992), and sympathetic dysfunction (Karlsson 1999; Karlsson et al. 1995) have all been suggested as possible causes. An association may also exist between abnormal lipid profiles and insulin resistance in those with SCI. Such an association has been identified in persons without SCI having depressed serum HDL-C, as they are also especially prone to insulin resistance (Hashimoto et al. 1995; Jeppesen et al. 1998). This risk profile closely matches that of persons with SCI, in whom isolated low HDL-C and insulin resistance are often comorbid (Bauman and Spungen 2000).

Alterations of Muscle Mass, Fiber Morphology, and Tone

Interruption of spinal transmission alters structural and contractile properties of muscle and limits the ability of totally paralyzed and weakened muscle to sustain intense contractions for extended durations. Most studies of sublesional muscle after SCI in humans demonstrate fibers that are smaller than those above lesion and than those of persons without SCI (Castro et al. 1999a, 2000), have less contractile protein (Castro et al. 1999b), and produce lower peak contractile forces (Levy et al. 1990; Rochester et al. 1995b). These fibers also evolve toward fast phenotypic protein expression (Andersen et al. 1996; Castro et al. 2000), increase fast myosin heavy chain isoforms (Talmadge et al. 2002, 1995), and decrease their resistance to fatigue (Burnham et al. 1997; Shields 2002; Shields et al. 1997). Muscle fiber cross-sectional area declines within one month of SCI (Castro et al. 1999a), while electrical stimulation of muscle paralyzed for more than one year evokes forces only one-seventh to one-third those of subjects without SCI (Rochester et al. 1995a, 1995b).

In addition to altered muscle fiber morphology and contractile properties, muscles below the level of spinal lesion develop hypertonia or atonia depending on the level and type of SCI. Hypertonia is the more common condition, in which exaggerated rate-dependent stretch results in spastic contraction (Priebe et al. 1996). This results from damage to the upper motor neuron alone, in which descending inhibition of reflex response is interrupted by cord injury. Hypertonia in these individuals can be worsened by a number of anoxious stimuli unrelated to muscle stretch, including urinary voiding, venous thrombosis, thermal dysregulation, occult fracture, or infection (McKinley et al. 1999). By contrast, damage to lower motor neurons involving injury below T10 often results in flaccid paralysis, which confers greater muscle and bone atrophy than upper motor neuron lesion, as well as loss of neuromuscular response to administration of alternating electrical currents.

Skeletal Decline After Spinal Cord Injury

Considerable sublesional bone demineralization is expected during the first year after SCI, after which bone density levels continue to slowly decay (Bloomfield et al. 1996). Increased urinary excretion of calcium and hydroxyproline and progressive rarefying of bone are evident on radiographs throughout this period (Garland et al. 1999; Lazo et al. 2001). About one-third to one-half of bone mineral density is lost by one year after injury, with primary losses occurring in the supracondylar femur. During this time bone becomes underhydroxylated and hypocalcific (Uebelhart et al. 1995; Chantraine et al. 1986) with permanently heightened susceptibility to fracture, even accompanying trivial or imperceptible trauma (Ragnarsson and Sell 1981; Vestergaard et al. 1998). Joints suffer similar deterioration and heightened injury susceptibility brought on by cartilage atrophy and joint space deformities (Nash et al. 1994).

Adrenergic Dysregulation After Spinal Cord Injury

Limitations in physical function after SCI are typically explained by profound sensorimotor deficits accompanying cord damage, although tracts of the sympathetic nervous system also descend in the spinal cord within the intermediolateral columns and exit with motor nerves in the thoracolumbar segments. This makes these nerve tracts equally susceptible to disruption, and the targets they control highly vulnerable to dysregulation after injury. As sympathetic autonomic tracts exit the cord at T1-L2 spinal levels, individuals with complete cervical-level injuries often lose all central command over sympathetic nervous functions, while loss of autonomic outflow to the adrenals and their sympathomedullary cell targets is also observed in persons with paraplegia above the T6 spinal level. Injury above the sacral cord segments abolishes central parasympathetic regulation of genitourinary organs (S2-4), which explains the neurogenic bowel and bladder commonly experienced after SCI, as well as erectile dysfunction experienced by males (Brackett et al. 1996). Autonomic dysfunction that results from injury above the thoracolumbar levels of sympathetic nerve outflow is associated with cardiac and circulatory dysfunction (Kessler et al. 1986; Nash et al. 1995), clotting disorders (Green et al. 1992), altered insulin metabolism (Duckworth et al. 1980; Karlsson et al. 1995), resting and exercise immunodysfunction (Campagnolo et al. 2000; Cruse et al. 2000; Nash 2000), orthostatic incompetence (King et al. 1992), osteoporosis and joint deterioration (Minaire 1989), and thermal dysregulation at rest and during exercise (Gass et al. 1988; Hopman et al. 1992b).

A blunted chronotropic response to exercise in persons with tetraplegia is well documented, and usually yields peak heart rate in the mid-120 beat per minute range—similar in magnitude to that of persons without SCI who exercise under conditions of pharmacological adrenergic blockade (Nash et al. 1995). Absence of or meager catecholamine responses to exercise (Schmid et al. 1998a) explain the suppressed heart rate responses to exercise and also the widely variable pressor, fuel, peripheral circulatory, thermal, and work capacity responses after SCI. For those with paraplegia from T2 to T5 (or T6), sparing of sympathetic efferents to the heart with resulting noradrenergic-mediated cardiac acceleration will be observed. A relatively normal response is observed below T5 or T6 (Gass and Camp 1984) as central inhibitory control of the adrenals (normally innervated from T6-T9) is maintained below these levels (Bloomfield et al. 1994). When compared to what occurs in persons exercising after sustaining paraplegia, the combination of diminished muscle mass and adrenergic dysfunction experienced by individuals with tetraplegia roughly halves their peak exercise capacity (Franklin 1985; Jacobs et al. 2002a).

PAIN

Various forms of nociceptive and neuropathic pain trouble most persons with SCI throughout their life span. While a complete discussion of post-SCI pain is beyond the scope of this chapter, the problem of upper extremity musculoskeletal pain is especially relevant to exercise in persons with SCI. Upper limb pain is the most common symptom of physical dysfunction reported by those with SCI (Sie et al. 1992; Subbarao et al. 1995), and the shoulder is the most common site for pain (Escobedo et al. 1997; Pentland and Twomey 1994). Persons with SCI are also highly susceptible to rotator cuff tears, impingement, and resulting shoulder dysfunction (Burnham et al. 1993; Lal 1998). A large cross section of the paralyzed population lives with pain in the shoulders, arms, and wrists, with complaints reported in 35% (Silfverskiold and Waters 1991) to 73% (Subbarao et al. 1995) of persons with chronic paraplegia. These figures cause special concern because onset of pain occurs earlier in persons with SCI than in those without disability, and because pain from muscle and joint overuse worsens with time and advancing age (Gellman et al. 1988).

While a single cause for shoulder pain has not been identified, many studies attribute pain to deterioration and injury resulting from insufficient shoulder strength, range, and muscle endurance (Curtis et al. 1999a; Pentland and Twomey 1994). Pain that accompanies wheelchair locomotion and other wheelchair activities interferes with functional performance including, but not limited to, upper extremity weight bearing for transfers, high-resistance muscular activity in extremes of limb range, wheelchair propulsion up inclines, and frequent overhead activity (Pentland and Twomey 1991, 1994). Wheelchair propulsion and depression transfers cause the most pain and increase the intensity of existing pain more than other daily activities (Taylor et al. 1986). As many as half of persons with SCI experience significant shoulder pain intensified by wheelchair propulsion and body transfers (Nichols et al. 1979), which are critical to activity and health maintenance. Although upper limb pain during transfer activities increases as time following injury lengthens (Gellman et al. 1988), exercises focusing on the posterior shoulder and upper back appear to lessen the pain (Curtis et al. 1999b).

An understanding of upper limb pain is critical if function is to be enhanced by exercise and the progression of incipient disability into newfound dysfunction is to be avoided. Common explanations for shoulder pain involve both generalized weakness and strength imbalances imposed by suboptimal scapular motion (Burnham et al. 1993; Powers et al. 1994), which limit shoulder joint motion and overstress muscles required for dynamic glenohumeral joint stabilization. Because the four joints composing the shoulder complex have the most extensive range of any joint complex, they also have the least stability (Hart et al. 1999). They are thus structurally and functionally ill-suited for locomotory functions needed by those with SCI and are highly susceptible to loading injury, development of intraglenoid capsular pressures during body transfers exceeding flow pressures of capillaries that nourish subchondral bone, and avascular necrosis of the shoulder head (Barber and Gall 1991; Bayley et al. 1987).

EXERCISE FOR PERSONS WITH SPINAL CORD INJURY

Exercise performed by persons without physical disability has been shown to enhance their activity, satisfaction, productivity, and health and also to benefit personal independence. While similar exercise benefits would clearly enhance the lives of those with SCI, the exercise options and benefits from training are often limited by need for special equipment or by the unique responses of persons with SCI to acute exercise and exercise training. Therefore, an appreciation of how physiology is altered by SCI is critical to an understanding of both resting and exercise responses of these individuals. Table 13.1 shows the body systems affected by SCI and how these changes influence exercise performance.

ATYPICAL PHYSIOLOGICAL RESPONSES TO ACUTE EXERCISE STRESS

Damage to the spinal cord dissociates homoeostatic mechanisms whose integration regulates necessary physiological responses to exercise (Hopman et al. 1993a; Sawka et al. 1989). It further disrupts to varying degrees the necessary signal integration among motor, sensory, and autonomic targets and thus profoundly affects acute adjustments to activity and peak exercise capacity (Schneider et al. 1999). These limitations are associated with the level of SCI and are explained by various factors. First, progressively higher levels of injury cause greater loss of mass of muscles necessary to serve as prime movers and stabilizers of trunk position. Thus, arm exercise performed by persons with SCI requires that the arms simultaneously generate propulsive forces and steady the trunk. Second, progressively higher levels of injury are associated with greater adrenergic dysfunction, and at key spinal levels totally dissociate adrenal, cardiac, and sympathetic nervous system regulation from central command. As the adrenergic and noradrenergic systems play key roles in cardiovascular regulation and fuel homeostasis during exercise, their loss decays the cardiovascular and metabolic efficiencies achieved during exercise by persons with SCI compared to those exercising with an intact neuraxis.

A direct relationship exists for those with SCI among level of injury, peak workload attained, and peak oxygen uptake (VO_2peak) reached during arm crank testing. This association serves as the basis for sport classification used during Paralympic and other sport events for persons competing with physical disability (Nash and Horton 2002). Exercise performance after SCI is limited by suboptimal circulatory adjustments (Hjeltnes 1986; Hopman et al. 1992b, 1993b). Individuals with injuries below the level of sympathetic outflow at T6 have significantly lower resting stroke volumes (SV) and higher resting heart rates (HR) than persons without paraplegia (Hopman et al. 1992b; Van Loan et al. 1987). The significant elevation of resting and exercise HR is thought to compensate for a lower cardiac SV imposed by pooling of blood in the lower extremity venous circuits, diminished venous return and cardiac end-diastolic volumes, or frank circulatory insufficiency (Houtman et al. 1999; Hjeltnes 1977).

Table 13.1 Effects of Spinal Cord Paralysis on Key Body Systems and How They Affect Exercise

System	Influence of SCI	Influence of SCI on exercise; influence of exercise on SCI
Cardiovascular	Orthostatic incompetence Diminished infralesional vascular tone Resting and exercise hypotension (tetraplegia) Left ventricular atrophy (tetraplegia)	Suboptimal pressor adjustments Chronic left ventricular volume underloading Venous stasis or pooling Lowered exercise HR and Q (tetraplegia) Exaggerated HR with normal Q (paraplegia)
Pulmonary	Level of injury-dependent reduction of inspiratory volumes Loss of expiratory force Inefficient cough	Diminished abdominothoracic pump and suboptimal gas exchange
Muscle	Loss of active muscle mass Lost or diminished infralesional muscle force Shift toward faster motor units	Postural deficiencies Rapid muscle fatigue Lowered work capacities
Skeletal	Infralesional osteopenia Heterotopic ossification Need for use of the upper limbs for locomotion and most exercise	Heightened fracture susceptibility with minor overuse or trivial injury Overuse injuries Charcot Limitation from pain
Autonomic	Autonomic hyperreflexia and mass effects Reflex crisis hypertension (above T6 level) Neurogenic bowel and bladder Urinary tract infections Thermal dysregulation Immune suppression	Lost or deficient adrenergic stimulation to autonomic targets Exercise-induced immunosuppression
Endocrine	Diminished infralesional autonomic outflow to adrenergic targets Attenuated mobilization of fatty fuels	
Skin	Pressure ulcers Attenuated central → peripheral shunting of blood	Induction of ischemic necrosis requiring chronic rest, skin protection, or surgery Exercise hyperthermia and syncope

Compensatory upregulation of the intact adrenergic system after SCI may also regulate the excessive chronotropic response to work, as higher resting catecholamine levels and exaggerated catecholamine responses to physical work occur in paraplegics with middle thoracic (T5) cord injuries (Bloomfield et al. 1994). These exceed resting and exercise levels of both high-level paraplegics and healthy persons without SCI (Hopman et al. 1992a; Schmid et al. 1998a). Hypersensitivity of the supralesional spinal cord is believed to regulate this adrenergic state and dynamic, which contrasts with the down-regulation of adrenergic functions observed in persons with high thoracic and cervical cord lesions (Hopman et al. 1992a; Schmid et al. 1998b). The exaggerated HR response to endurance exercise in persons with paraplegia (Bloomfield et al. 1994) may limit performance, as they consume higher levels of oxygen to perform at the same work intensity as persons without SCI (Davis and Shephard 1988; Hoffman 1986; Hopman et al. 1992b). As the sympathetic nervous system regulates hemodynamic and metabolic changes during activity, the elevated oxygen consumption and HR response to endurance exercise in paraplegics with injuries below T5 may be due to adrenergic overactivity accompanying their paraplegia (Bloomfield et al. 1994; Schmid et al. 1998a, 1998b).

ENDURANCE AND RESISTANCE TRAINING

For many, recovery from SCI leaves the upper extremities unimpaired or with sufficient strength and endurance to perform arm exercise. For these individuals, various exercise options are available, including arm endurance training and resistance training of the upper extremities. In some cases, this exercise requires specialized equipment, although intense wheelchair locomotion or arm exercise using free weights may promote similar benefits.

ARM ENDURANCE TRAINING

Despite the described physical and homeostatic limitations imposed by SCI, many persons can still undergo and benefit from exercise reconditioning. Summary benefits from various forms of exercise are shown in table 13.2. Those who retain upper extremity function can participate in a wide variety of exercise activities and sports (Curtis et al. 1986; Nash and Horton 2002) and ambulate with the assistance of orthoses and computer-controlled electrical neuroprostheses (Graupe and Kohn 1998; Klose et al. 1997; Triolo et al. 1996). Individuals with upper motor neuron lesions have pedaled cycle ergometers using surface electrical stimulation of selected lower extremity muscle groups delivered under computer control (Glaser 1994; Ragnarsson et al. 1988). Many body organs and tissues respond to exercise despite their decentralized or denervated states; and because many survivors of SCI experience complete sensory loss or significantly diminished nociceptive responses, electrically stimulated muscle contractions can often be utilized without pain.

In most cases SCI leaves the lower limbs either entirely paralyzed or else with insufficient strength, endurance, or motor control to support safe and effective physical training. This explains why most exercise training after SCI employs the upper extremity exercise modes of arm crank ergometry, wheelchair ergometry, and swimming. All of these training modes improve peak oxygen uptake in those with SCI by an average of 15% to 25% (Cowell et al. 1986; Franklin 1985; Gass et al. 1980; Hoffman 1986; Hooker and Wells 1989), with a magnitude of fitness improvement usually inversely proportional to level of spinal lesion. While it is possible for persons with low tetraplegia to train on an arm ergometer, special measures must be taken to affix the hands to the ergometer, and their gains in peak oxygen uptake fail to match those of their counterparts with paraplegia (Yim et al. 1993). Thus, level of injury is a key to predicting outcome from arm endurance training (DiCarlo 1988; Drory et al. 1990).

Guidelines for training after SCI have been published by several authorities (Franklin 1985; Hoffman 1986; Phillips et al. 1998), although limited testing for superiority of training algorithms has been performed. Given, however, that most persons with SCI are sedentary long after injury and the accepted dictum that training benefits are most easily gained in the most deconditioned of individuals, these methods are nonetheless successful in achieving higher levels of fitness. Endurance training recommendations for those with paraplegia do not vary dramatically from advice directed to the general population (Figoni 1997; Lockette and Keyes 1994). The need to attain long-term compliance and avoid disabling injury represent major training goals for those with SCI. Warning is required for assignment of target exercise intensities grounded in typical chronotropic or metabolic standards, as they may promote exaggerated exercise responses or exceed exercise tolerance for those with SCI.

RESISTANCE TRAINING AFTER SPINAL CORD INJURY

Upper extremity weakness, pain, and need for use of upper limbs in performance of many daily activities would seem to identify increased strength of the shoulders, upper back, chest, and arms as essential exercise training goals for those with SCI. As manual wheelchair propulsion causes considerable pain and dysfunction, incorporation of resistance training into the health care plan would appear needed and justified. Surprisingly, however, far less is known about the effects of resistance compared to endurance training in persons with SCI. This might seem counterintuitive, since muscle weakness has been reported to precipitate pain and dysfunction as persons with SCI age with their disability.

Several investigators have studied effects of resistance exercise in persons with paraplegia. In a study of Scandinavian men (most having incomplete low thoracic lesions), a weight training program emphasizing triceps strengthening for crutch walking yielded modest but significant increases in peak exercise capacity accompanied by increased strength of the triceps brachii (Nilsson et al. 1975). Others (Davis and Shephard 1990) have examined effects of arm ergometry in subjects assigned to high intensity (70% of their VO_2peak) or low intensity (40% of their VO_2peak) for 20 or 40 min per session, respectively. Strength gains were limited to subjects assigned high-intensity training and occurred only in the shoulder joint extensor and elbow flexor muscles. Otherwise, no changes in shoulder joint abduction or adduction strengths were reported, and none of the muscles that move or stabilize the scapulothoracic articulation or chest were stronger following training. These results suggest that arm crank exercise is a poor choice for use as a training mode for upper extremity strengthening because it fails to target the muscles most involved in performance of daily activities. Conditioning of five paraplegic and five tetraplegic subjects three times weekly for nine weeks using a hydraulic fitness machine was reported. Exercises performed were chest press and row, shoulder press, and latissimus pull (Cooney and Walker 1986). Significant increases in average arm oxygen consumption and power output were observed, although direct measurement of strength in muscle groups undergoing training was not performed. A recent study showed reduced shoulder pain following a series of shoulder resistance exercises using elastic bands (Curtis et al. 1999b).

As both endurance and resistance exercises benefit those without SCI, the effects of circuit resistance training (CRT) (Gettman et al. 1978) on various attributes of fitness, dyslipidemia, and shoulder pain have been studied in young and middle-aged subjects with paraplegia. The exercise program incorporates periods of low-intensity, high-paced movements interposed within activities performed at a series of resistance training stations. The CRT exercise program adapted for persons with paraplegia consisted of three circuits of six resistance stations encompassing three pairs of agonist/antagonist movements (e.g., overhead press and pull) and three 2-min periods of free wheeling arm cranking performed between resistance maneuvers (see figure 13.1). No true rest periods are allowed during the performance of CRT, with active recovery limited to the time necessary for the subject to propel the wheelchair to the next exercise station. Three weekly sessions were completed, with each session lasting approximately 45 min.

Subjects undergoing 16 weeks of mixed resistance and endurance exercise increased their average peak arm oxygen consumption by 29%, with accompanying upper extremity strength gains of 13% to 40% depending on the site tested (Jacobs et al. 2001). Subjects undergoing CRT lowered their total and LDL cholesterol while increasing their HDL cholesterol by nearly 10% (Nash et al. 2001). Subjects aged over 40 years undergoing the same treatment for 12 weeks experienced significant gains in endurance, strength, and anaerobic power, even though the latter was not specifically targeted by training (personal communication). Shoulder pain present in these subjects before training was assessed by a pain instrument validated in the population and was significantly reduced. In 4 of 10 subjects, pain

Table 13.2 Summary Benefits of Exercise Training After Spinal Cord Injury

Training mode	Established or suggested benefit
Voluntary arm or wheelchair ergometry	Enhanced extremity endurance and exercise tolerance, with benefits improving with descending level of injury. Lipid profiles should be improved with reduction in cardiovascular disease risk. The pressor response to orthostatic repositioning is improved, with benefits favoring lower levels of injury. Many patients report improved feelings of well-being and life satisfaction.
Circuit and resistance training	Improved upper extremity strength, power, and endurance reduce upper extremity pain; improved lipid profile favoring reduced cardiovascular disease risk; and enhanced cardiac function, with reduced resting heart rate and increased stroke volume.
Electrical stimulation of paralyzed muscle	*Individual muscles:* Increased muscle size; increased muscle blood flow, increased muscle endurance through electrical stimulation. Shift toward slower motor units depending upon type of electrical current. *Complex activity:* Increased muscle size and lower limb blood flow; reversal of cardiac atrophy (quadriplegics only); improved endurance and improved feelings of well-being.

was eliminated. This circuit was then replicated by use of elastic bands (Nash et al. 2002) so that access to expensive weightlifting equipment would not impose a limitation to participation in training. Evidence thus supports the health and fitness advantages of CRT over either endurance or resistance exercises alone for persons with paraplegia.

BASIC PRINCIPLES OF ELECTRICALLY STIMULATED MOVEMENT

A dominant feature of SCI is the loss of voluntary motor control below the level of lesion. In many cases, however, electrical current can elicit contraction of paralyzed or weakened muscles and thus provide a stimulus for exercise training. When these contractions are sequenced by a computer microprocessor, they can often generate purposeful movement that can be exploited for exercise.

Use of electrical current to initiate purposeful movement after SCI dates to 1960 when Kantrowitz used surface stimulation to initiate contraction of the quadriceps and gluteus muscles of a T3 paraplegic. Since that time, many forms of electrically stimulated exercise have been applied to use by persons with SCI. These include site-specific stimulation of the lower extremities (Dudley et al. 1999; Greve et al. 1993; Rodgers et al. 1991) and upper extremities (Bryden et al. 2000; Klefbeck et al. 1996; Mulcahey et al. 1997; Scremin et al. 1999), leg cycling (Hooker et al. 1990; Nash et al. 1995; Ragnarsson et al. 1988; Raymond et al. 1999), leg exercise with upper extremity assist (Mutton et al. 1997; Raymond et al. 1999), lower body rowing (Laskin et al. 1993), electrically assisted arm ergometry (Cameron et al. 1998), electrically stimulated standing (Mulcahey et al. 1997; Triolo et al. 1996), and electrically stimulated bipedal ambulation with an orthosis (Phillips et al. 1995;

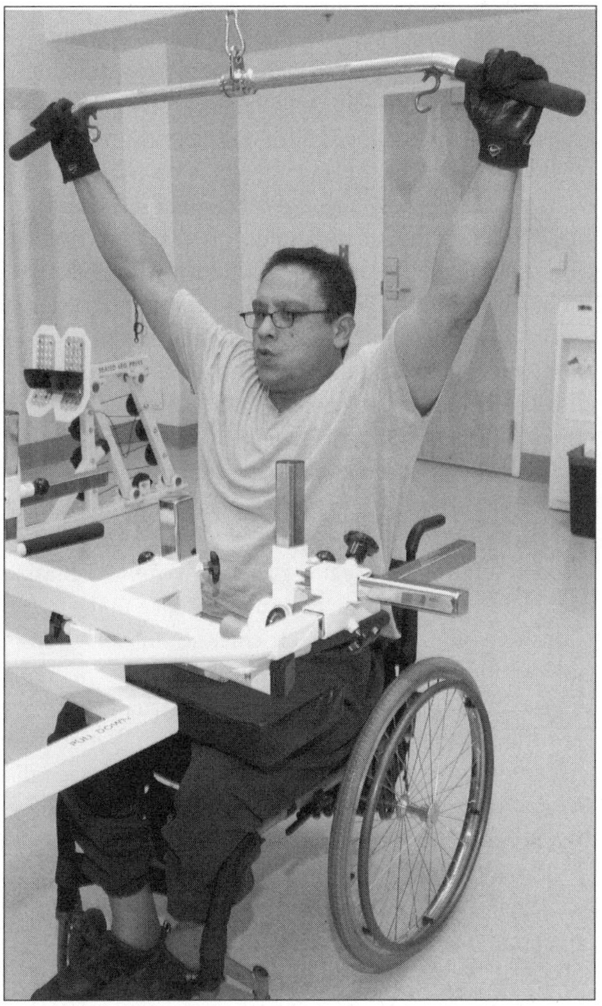

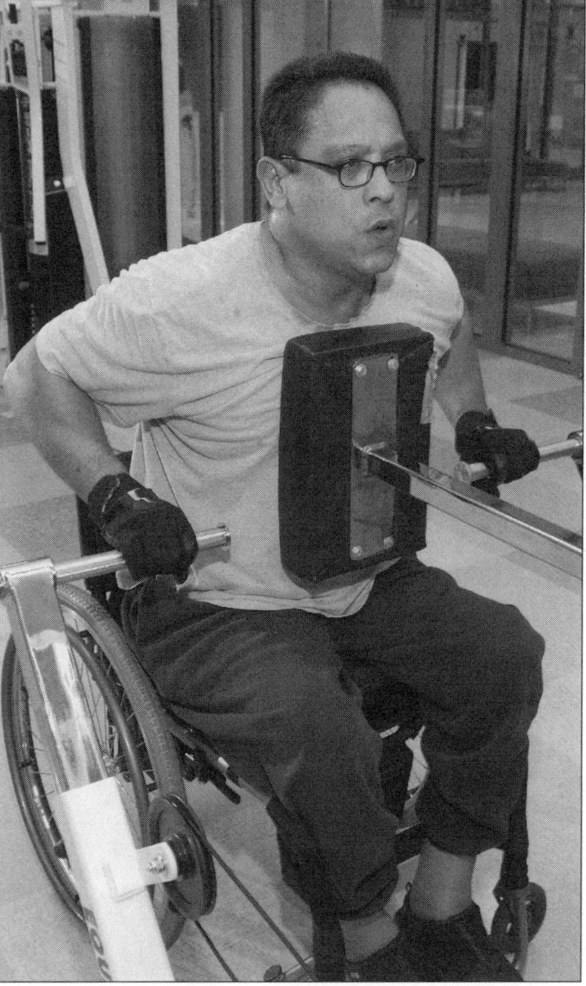

Figure 13.1 Resistance exercises performed by a person with paraplegia to enhance daily function and strengthen muscles that stabilize the shoulder girdle. The bolster positioned on *(a)* the thighs and *(b)* the chest stabilizes the body during execution of the maneuvers.

Courtesy of Robert Camarena, the Miami Project to Cure Paralysis.

Solomonow et al. 1997; Triolo et al. 1996) or without an orthosis (Brissot et al. 2000; Klose et al. 1997). Walking can also be achieved with assistance of a driven gait orthosis as shown in figure 13.2 (Dietz et al. 1997; Field-Fote 2001).

Most forms of electrically stimulated exercise require that the lower motor neuron system remain intact following injury, as muscle activation occurs via indirect electrical stimulation of the intact peripheral nerve and not muscle directly (Phillips 1987). This requirement excludes most individuals having cauda equina or conus medullaris syndromes from use of electrically stimulated exercise. It may also compromise the efficiency of muscle activation in spinal segments that have sustained injury to the anterior horn cells or spinal (Wallnerian) degeneration from injured adjacent spinal areas. Many applications of SCI target muscle strengthening of limb segments whose motor function is partially spared by injury (Triolo et al. 1996), while others use electrical current as a neuroprosthesis for the lower extremities (Graupe and Kohn 1998; Phillips et al. 1995) and upper extremities (Peckham and Creasey 1992; Mulcahey et al. 1997). Qualifications to safely participate in these exercise programs have been described (Graupe 2002; Graupe and Kohn 1998; Klose et al. 1997), while benefits and risks of exercise participation are described in tables 13.2 and 13.3, respectively.

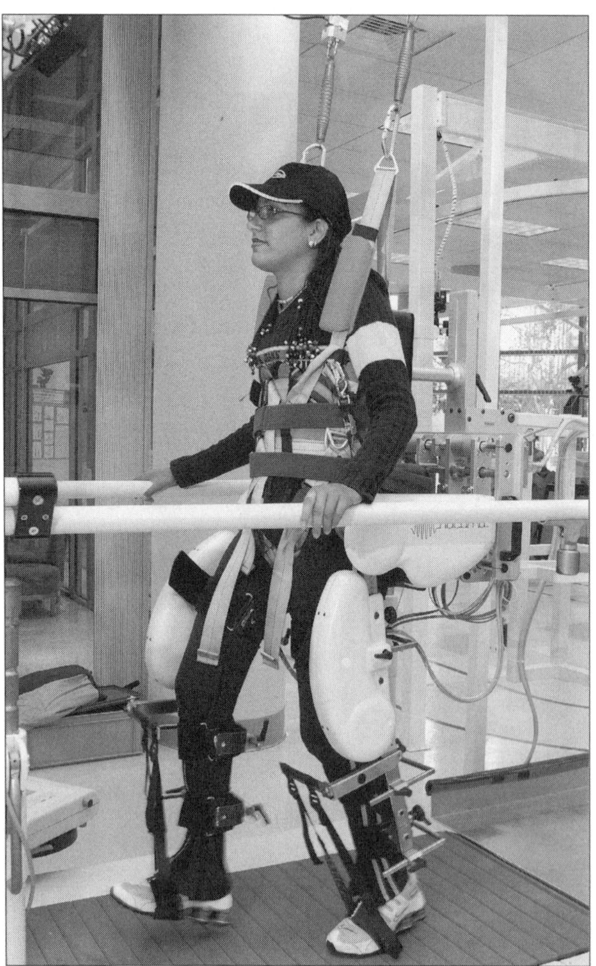

Figure 13.2 A patient with C5 motor-complete tetraplegia undergoes treadmill stepping with assistance from a Lokomat driven gait orthosis.

Courtesy of Robert Camarena, the Miami Project to Cure Paralysis.

Electrically Stimulated Leg Cycling Exercise After Spinal Cord Injury

A cycling motion in the slightly recumbent position is the simplest form of multilimb segmental exercise used by persons with SCI. Pedaling force is initiated by electrically stimulated contractions of the bilateral quadriceps, hamstrings, and gluteus muscles sequenced under computer microprocessor command (Glaser 1994). Pedal cadence and muscle stimulation intensity are controlled by feedback from position sensors integrated within the pedal gear (Petrofsky and Phillips 1984).

Training with electrically stimulated cycling is often preceded by electrically stimulated strengthening of the quadriceps muscles, which is necessary in cases of severe muscle atrophy or diminished muscle endurance (Dudley et al. 1999; Ragnarsson et al. 1988). These factors will generally slow success in training, especially for individuals with long-standing paralysis, low muscle tone, and flexor patterns of spasticity. Notwithstanding poor levels of muscle strength and endurance observed early in most training programs, and despite limited ability to exercise against intense workloads, enhanced levels of fitness (Hooker et al. 1995; Mutton et al. 1997), improved gas exchange kinetics (Barstow et al. 1995, 1996), and increased muscle mass (Scremin et al. 1999) are reported following exercise training using electrically stimulated cycling. For those with neurologically incomplete injuries, gains in lower extremity mass as well as isometric strength and endurance under conditions of voluntary and electrically stimulated exercise are reported (Scremin et al. 1999).

Reversal of the adaptive left ventricular atrophy reported in persons with tetraplegia has also been observed, with near normalization of pretraining cardiac mass (Nash et al. 1991). This adaptation may be caused by significantly improved lower extremity circulation following training (Gerrits et al. 2001; Schmidt-Trucksass et al. 2000), which is also accompanied by a more robust hyperemic response to an occlusion stimulus (Nash et al. 1997, 1996). Attenuation of paralytic osteopenia has been observed by several investigators (BeDell et al. 1996; Mohr et al. 1997) and an increased rate of bone turnover by another (Bloomfield et al. 1996), with sites benefiting from training at the lumbar spine and proximal tibia, not the proximal femur (Mohr et al.

1997). Not all studies have shown a posttraining increase in mineral density for bones located below the level of the lesion (Leeds et al. 1990), but those failing to do so have usually studied subjects with long-standing paralysis that lowers the likelihood of stimulating osteogenesis. Even absent improved bone mineral density, a study examining the appearance of lower extremity joints and joint surfaces using magnetic resonance imaging showed no degenerative changes induced by cycling, and less joint surface necrosis than previously reported in sedentary persons after injury (Nash et al. 1994).

Training using electrically-stimulated muscle contractions has improved body composition by increasing body lean mass and decreasing fat mass (Hjeltnes et al. 1997) and has enhanced whole-body insulin uptake, insulin-stimulated 3-0-methyl glucose transport, and expression of the quadriceps GLUT4 transport protein (Hjeltnes et al. 1998). According to a recent report, this training resulted in improved profiles of insulin resistance (Mohr et al. 2001). When simultaneous upper extremity arm ergometry is combined with electrically stimulated cycling, the acute cardiovascular metabolic responses are more intense, and the gains in fitness are greater than observed with lower extremity cycling alone (Mohr et al. 2001; Mutton et al. 1997).

USE OF AMBULATION NEUROPROSTHESES

Sequenced electrical stimulation has been used as an ambulation neuroprosthesis for those with motor-complete injuries (Graupe 2002; Klose et al. 1997) and as an assistive neuroprosthesis for persons with incomplete SCI who lack strength to support independent ambulation (Field-Fote 2001; Ladouceur and Barbeau 2000; Stein et al. 1993). Implantable neuroprostheses for those without spared motor function have been used experimentally (Graupe and Kohn 1997; Triolo et al. 1996) and brought to market using surface electrical stimulation of the quadriceps and gluteus muscles (figure 13.3) (Brissot et al. 2000; Klose et al. 1997). Muscle activation for the latter system is sequenced by a microprocessor worn on the belt, with activation of step initiated by a finger-sensitive control switch located on a rolling walker used by ambulating subjects. When pressed, the electrical stimulator sends current to the stance limb that initiates contraction of the quadriceps and gluteus muscles. Contralateral hip flexion is then achieved through exploitation of an ipsilateral flexor withdrawal reflex obtained as a nociceptive electrical stimulus is introduced over the common peroneal nerve at the fibular head. This allows the hip, knee, and ankle to move into flexion followed by extension of the knee joint accompanying electrical stimulation to the quadriceps. As muscle fatigue occurs, increasing levels of stimulation can be provided by a switch mounted on the handle of the rolling walker.

Use of an ambulation neuroprosthesis is made less-efficient by postinjury muscle weakness and poor endurance, much like the challenges experienced in early electrically stimulated cycling. These limitations need to be overcome before ambulation training is undertaken. Electrically activated resistive knee extension exercise and conditioning of the gluteal muscles with electrically produced hip bridging (in supine position) will enhance performance once ambulation is initiated. It is inadvisable to undertake electrically stimulated ambulation training until the ability to stand with electrical stimulation for at least 3 to 5 min has been demonstrated.

Once electrically stimulated ambulation is successfully achieved, the ambulation rates are relatively slow and distances of ambulation relatively limited (Phillips et al. 1995). Community use of these devices remains limited to a small percentage of training subjects. Despite the limitations of ambulation velocity and distance, ambulation distances of up to 1 mile have been reported after training in some subjects (Phillips et al. 1995), and upper extremity fitness is enhanced following

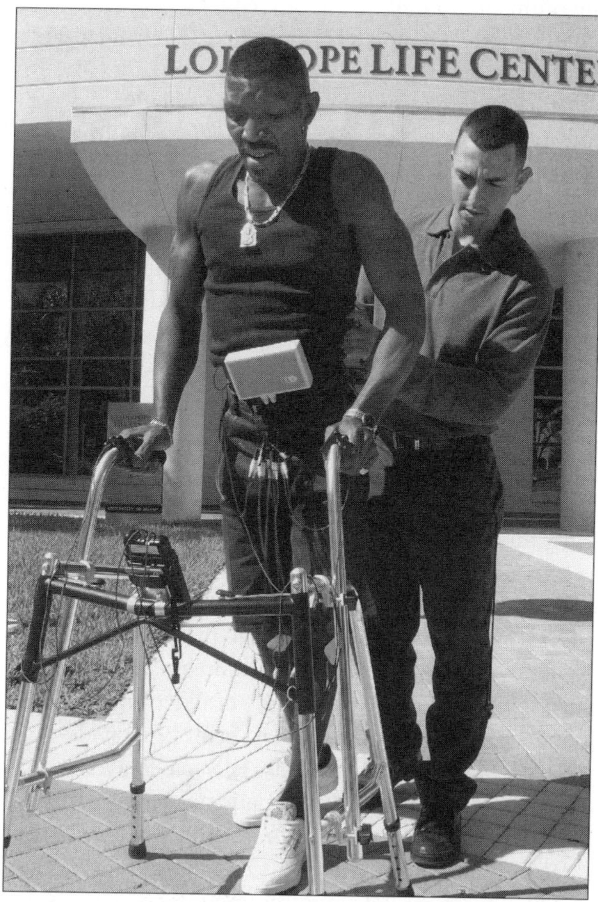

Figure 13.3 Walking with an ambulation neuroprosthesis and a walker by an individual with complete paraplegia. Patient controls to initiate stepping and adjust stimulation parameters are located on the handles of the walker.

Courtesy of Robert Camarena, the Miami Project to Cure Paralysis.

ambulation training (Graupe and Kohn 1998; Jacobs et al. 1997). Other beneficial adaptations to training include enhanced lower extremity muscle mass (Jaeger 1992), improved resting blood flow (Nash et al. 1997), and an augmented hyperemic response to an experimental ischemic stimulus (Nash et al. 1997). Ambulation training has failed to increase lower extremity bone mineralization (Needham-Shropshire et al. 1997), although most subjects began training beyond the time in their injury when substantial bone loss had already occurred.

Restoration of Function Following Long-Standing Paralysis

While persuasive evidence supports a role for exercise in health maintenance after SCI, much less is known of the role played by exercise in recovery of lost motor function. A thorough review of this topic is beyond the scope of this chapter, although several comprehensive monographs have summarized the current understanding of this important investigative theme (Barbeau et al. 1998; Bregman et al. 1997; Field-Fote 2004; Field-Fote and Tepavac 2002).

Most scientists and clinicians acknowledge the possibility for spontaneous recovery of sensorimotor function until 12 to 18 months following injury (Ditunno et al. 1992; Marino et al. 1999). This recovery may be due in part to resolution of "spinal shock" following injury (Ditunno et al. 2004). Also, because the spinal cord is rarely transected by injury, many individuals with SCI will have some sparing of white matter at the injury site even when the lesion appears neurologically complete by clinical criteria. This minimal tissue sparing is thought to influence segmental spinal cord function and recovery of motor ability (Basso 2000). Enhanced function may be facilitated by the presence of a central pattern generator that mimics locomotory patterns executed by persons with an intact neuraxis (Calancie et al. 1994; Pinter and Dimitrijevic 1999).

Despite long-standing dogma to the contrary, recent evidence in individuals with incomplete SCI suggests the potential for delayed recovery of function accompanying ambulation exercise (Dietz et al. 1998; Field-Fote 2001; Field-Fote and Tepavac 2002). Such delayed motor recovery has been observed in patients recovering from brain infarct and traumatic brain injury who aggressively recondition their paralyzed muscles. Whether this benefit is gained from training effects on muscle, reorganization of spinal reflexes, or reorganization of motor cortex is incompletely understood. However, spinal circuitry depends on the interplay of neuronal networks and reflexes that regulate motor output via their influence on spinal motor neurons. It is thought that the unique interplay of these two systems, as well as performance of activities that generate nervous activity from muscle afferents, is essential for developing, maintaining, or regaining motor function (Dietz et al. 1995, 2002; Wernig et al. 1999).

The best evidence for recovery of function following long-standing SCI involves individuals with incomplete spinal cord lesions who undergo locomotory training. Methods to achieve this training generally focus on unloading of the body with an overhead harness, with gaiting performed overground or on a treadmill (Dobkin et al. 1995; Field-Fote and Tepavac 2002; Gardner et al. 1998; Protas et al. 2001). Alternatively, gaiting can be performed using a driven gait orthosis as described in this chapter (Colombo et al. 2001). Evidence suggests that a single bout of treadmill training produces immediate increases in walking velocity and changes in reflex modulation during gaiting (Trimble et al. 1998). Chronic repetition of the reciprocal gait pattern enhances performance and provides cues to the spinal cord necessary to generate coordinated facilitated stepping. Given the importance of afferent feedback in generating purposeful movement, it has been hypothesized, and in some cases demonstrated, that coordinated reciprocated movements can enhance bipedal ambulation long after injury (Wirz et al. 2001).

Exercise Risks for Persons With Spinal Cord Injury

Special consideration is required when exercise is performed by persons with SCI. While typical risks of exercise injury and overuse apply, the consequences of risks may be far more serious and potentially irreversible, and will likely compromise daily activities to a far greater extent than similar injuries arising in persons without SCI. Risks of exercise participation are summarized in table 13.3.

- **Autonomic dysreflexia.** Individuals having cord injuries either at, or above, the T6 spinal level are prone to potentially life-threatening episodes of autonomic hyperreflexia (Erickson 1980). The neurological basis for these episodes involves loss of supralesional sympathetic inhibition after injury, which suppresses the unrestricted autonomic reflex in persons having an intact neuraxis. Absent central inhibition, the adrenals release high concentrations of epinephrine under reflex control, and their infralesional adrenergic targets express excessive noradrenergic stimulation (Comarr and Eltorai 1997). The most common stimuli evoking autonomic dysreflexia are bladder and bowel distension before their emptying. Other stimuli include venous thromboembo-

Table 13.3 Summary Risks Imposed by Exercise in Persons With Spinal Cord Injury: Causes and Prevention

Risk	Cause	Prevention
Fracture	More than 50% of sublesional bone is lost within the first six months after injury. Sublesional bone remains permanently rarefied and susceptible to fracture with even trivial injury.	No systematic evaluation for fracture susceptibility has been developed. Care should be exercised in wheelchair seating and those with severe chronic muscle spasm.
Musculoskeletal overuse/injury	Musculoskeletal overuse is occult in areas where sensation of pain is diminished. For the upper extremities, use of the arms to propel the wheelchair may cause injury or irreversible disability.	The lower extremities should be monitored for cardinal signs of injury. Heightened spasticity may cue injury even if swelling, pain, warmth, or erythema are not observed. Adequate range of motion of the upper extremities, strength, and balance must be achieved and maintained. Individuals using the upper extremities for sports must be skilled in the mechanics of ballistic wheelchair locomotion. Use a wheelchair that will minimize injury.
Thermal dysregulation	Loss of vasomotor and sudomotor responses below the level of injury. Altered blood flow redistribution during exercise. Absence of sweating reflex below level of injury.	Exercise in intemperate environment should be avoided. Attention should be placed on hydration, clothing, and signs and symptoms of heat stress.
Autonomic dysreflexia	Loss of central autonomic control results in reflex adrenergic responses to noxious stimuli.	Bowel routine and bladder emptying should be performed on schedule. External catheters should be inspected for outflow obstruction. Exercise should be avoided when autonomic episodes are increasing. Boosting of exercise responses using intentional urinary outflow obstruction must be discouraged.
Skin burn	Use of poorly hydrated or gelled conducting electrodes. Use of galvanic current for long duration or use of intense stimulation increases risks of burn.	Replace electrodes regularly and inspect for bubbles or drying at the edges.
Pressor decompensation during and after exercise	Loss of sympathetic reflex responses to exercise or postexercise pooling of blood in the lower extremities.	Careful prevention of orthostatic decompensation through conservative exercise progression. Active cool-down after exercise to support venous return. Anticipation of the need to recline subjects to prevent syncope.

lism, bone fracture, sudden temperature change, febrile episodes, and exercise. The disposition to autonomic dysreflexia during exercise is especially heightened when electrical current is used to generate muscle movement, or when people exercise while febrile or during bladder emptying. Episodes of autonomic dysreflexia are characterized by hypertension and bradycardia, supralesional erythema, piloerection, and headache (Comarr and Eltorai 1997). In some cases hypertension can rise to the point where crisis headache results, and cerebral hemorrhage and death ensue. Recognition of these episodes, withdrawal of the offending stimulus, and the possible administration of a fast-acting peripheral vasodilator may be critical in preventing serious medical complications. Prophylaxis with a slow calcium channel antagonist or $alpha_1$-selective adrenergic antagonist may be needed prior to exercise (Chancellor et al. 1994; Vaidyanathan et al. 1998). It is known that wheelchair racers have intentionally induced dysreflexia as an ergogenic aid by restricting urine outflow through a Foley catheter (Webborn 1999), which represents a dangerous and possibly life-threatening practice.

- **Musculoskeletal injury.** Persons with SCI risk fracture and joint dislocation of the lower extremities and serious injury to the upper extremities. The former might be caused by asynergistic movement of spastic limbs against cocontractive forces imposed by electrical stimulation of paralyzed muscles, or by inertia developed by devices used for exercise (Hartkopp et al. 1998). This explains why these activities are contraindicated for individuals having severe spasticity when at rest or uncontrolled spastic responses when electrical current is introduced. Precautions to prevent overuse injuries of the arms and shoulders are essential for those participating in upper extremity exercise (Burnham et al. 1993; Curtis et al. 1999; Olenik et al. 1995). As the shoulder joints are mechanically ill suited to perform locomotor activities but must do so in individuals using a manual wheelchair for transportation, these injuries may ultimately compromise performance of essential daily activities including wheelchair propulsion, weight relief, and depression transfers (Ballinger et al. 2000; Bayley et al. 1987).

- **Exercise hypotension.** Risks of postexercise hypotension (King et al. 1992, 1994) are associated with lost vasomotor responses to orthostatic repositioning (Lopes et al. 1984), although these episodes usually abate after upper limb training.

- **Thermal dysregulation.** Loss of sublesional vasomotor and sudomotor control after SCI poses a special challenge to exercise thermoregulation for those with SCI, and often results in hyperthermia (Gass et al. 1988; Ishii et al. 1995; Sawka et al. 1989). Hyperthermia is more pronounced in persons with higher-level injuries (Muraki et al. 1995, 1996) and during exercise in a hot, humid environment (Ishii et al. 1995; Price and Campbell 1999). Thus, attention should be paid to clothing, hydration, and limiting the duration and intensity of activities performed in intemperate environments.

- **Pain.** Persons with paraplegia must depend on their upper extremities for transportation, body transfers, and other activities. Thus, the consequences of and necessary treatments for shoulder pain and injury ultimately influence their independence. While some report that surgical repair of the shoulder results in full recovery of musculoskeletal function and remedy of pain (Robinson et al. 1993), others report not (Goldstein et al. 1997). Notwithstanding, those who advocate surgical invention as a management strategy for shoulder dysfunction fail to address how these individuals will manage during their convalescence with an immobilized limb, or how functions required during normal daily activities (e.g., manual wheelchair locomotion, weight shift and depression transfers, toileting, and driving) will be accomplished by persons with paraplegia while using one arm. These factors make pain prevention an essential part in planning for exercise by those with SCI.

Medications That May Influence Exercise Performance After Spinal Cord Injury

Many medication families are known to alter exercise responses of persons without SCI. The most commonly cited of these families are beta-adrenergic receptor antagonists, which are typically prescribed to treat hypertension, congestive heart failure, myocardial infarction, and angina. While beta-adrenergic blockers suppress maximal heart rate and lower exercise capacity, they are seldom prescribed for persons with SCI, although ironically they have effects that mimic the attenuated chronotropic responses to acute exercise experienced by persons with cervical SCI (Nash et al. 1995). While no studies have examined effects of drugs on exercise responses and capacities after SCI, the pharmacopoeia for persons with SCI typically contains specific medications used to treat spasm (Priebe et al. 1996), central pain (Ahn et al. 2003), anxiety (Lundqvist et al. 1997), and depression (Krause et al. 2000). In many cases the known adverse responses to treatment in persons without disability form sufficient basis for special caution in use by persons with SCI undergoing acute exercise and exercise training.

Various drugs are used as maintenance therapies to control elevated muscle tone and spasm accompanying SCI. These are usually classified as either central or direct-acting agents. The most commonly prescribed drug for this indication is Lioresal (Baclofen) (Kirshblum 1999; Taricco et al. 2000), a gamma-aminobutyric-acid (GABA) receptor agonist that enhances neuronal membrane chloride influx and promotes hyperpolarization of spinal tracts mediating muscle tone. Similar spasm reduction is achieved by the alpha-2 adrenergic agonist tizanidine (Zanaflex) (Taricco et al. 2000), which controls spasticity by enhancing presynaptic inhibition of motor neurons in the brainstem. Adverse responses to treatment with central antispasmodics typically include sedation, muscle weakness, and hypotension, all of which may adversely influence exercise performance of persons with SCI. Greater muscle weakness but less sedation is associated with use of the direct antispasmodic agent dantrolene (Dantrium) (Taricco et al. 2000), which inhibits myofibril excitation coupling by altering calcium ion flux in skeletal fibers. Benzodiazepines such as Diazepam (Valium) have also been used to treat muscle spasm after SCI (Priebe et al. 1996), although Lioresal and tizanidine afford better spasm relief with less sedation, tolerance, and addiction.

Depression is a common complication experienced early after SCI that sometimes persists into the chronic phase of recovery. Tricyclic antidepressants such as Elavil (amitriptyline) are often prescribed for treatment, although they are highly sedating, have a carryover effect in the morning after treatment, and exert anticholinergic effects that include bradycardia and orthostatic hypotension. Elavil has also been used as a first-line therapy for dysesthetic pain accompanying SCI (Cardenas et al. 2002), although second-generation voltage regulators such as gabapentin (Neurontin) appear safer and more effective (Ahn et al. 2003). Notwithstanding, persons taking gabapentin may still experience somnolescence, dizziness, ataxia, and fatigue. Gabapentin may also cause dysarthria, which might impair functional abilities in persons with SCI having marginal strength. Both Baclofen and tizanidine are also used to treat central pain (Ahn et al. 2003), and their adverse responses to treatment and exercise caveats are noted.

Although adverse effects of various medication families might depress exercise responses or make exercise participation more hazardous, several agents might actually benefit those exercising with SCI. While beta$_2$-selective adrenergic agonists are thought to exert performance-enhancing effects for those without disability (van Baak et al. 2000), the bronchodilator drug metaproteronol (Alupent) enhances upper limb strength and muscle mass for those with incomplete tetraplegia (Signorile et al. 1995) and also enhanced responses to electrically stimulated exercise (Murphy et al. 1999). Further, recent pilot data suggest that use of the alpha$_1$-selective adrenergic agonist midodrine (ProAmatine) (Mukand et al. 2001) enhances arm exercise performance of persons with SCI, most likely by a peripheral vasoconstrictor effect that elevates blood pressure during exercise. This drug-induced effect mirrors previous reports of enhanced exercise performance by persons with SCI when they undergo mechanical compression of the lower limbs (Houtman et al. 1999).

SUMMARY

Dysfunction of most body organs and regulatory systems is common after SCI. Persons recovering from injury are left with varying degrees and patterns of cardiocirculatory dysregulation, autonomic dysfunction, skeletal decline, and muscle weakness. These factors challenge performance efficiency and safety of exercise, and need to be carefully considered when one is planning exercise for persons with SCI.

Despite special exercise needs, equipment, and warnings, many persons with SCI currently benefit from a lifestyle that incorporates habitual physical activity. Efforts should be intensified by health care professionals to encourage therapeutic or recreational exercise after SCI as a health-enhancing strategy for those who have adopted a sedentary lifestyle. Individuals with higher levels of cord injury may require electrical stimulation to perform exercise, which poses special restrictions on use as well as unique risks from participation. Individuals with spared motor control of the upper extremities can perform arm or wheelchair exercises and participate in recreational sport so long as pain and incipient disability are anticipated and avoided.

Strengthening of the upper extremity to preserve shoulder and arm functions is critical and should be considered in the exercise plan insofar as spared function allows. Risks of injury or illnesses associated with imprudent exercise must be managed to ensure that physical activity and daily activities can be sustained without interruption by injury. If carefully prescribed, exercise has the demonstrated ability to enhance the activity, life satisfaction, and health of those with disability from SCI.

CHAPTER 14

STROKE

Joel Stein, MD

CASE STUDY

A 73-year-old man came to the hospital after sudden onset of right-sided weakness and dysarthria. Charles had a history of hypertension and admitted to noncompliance with his medication. Finding a left internal capsule lacunar infarct, his neurologist started him on aspirin for prevention of recurrent stroke and transferred him to a rehabilitation facility. There he enrolled in a multidisciplinary program of rehabilitation, with extensive physical, occupational, and speech therapy. His dysarthria resolved, but he continued to experience a persistent hemiparesis. Because of his inadequate ankle dorsiflexion, we fitted Charles with a plastic ankle–foot orthosis (AFO). His exercise program was primarily functionally oriented, and he made steady gains in both his activities of daily living (ADLs) and his mobility. Two weeks after his initial stroke, we discharged him to his home. He could walk independently with a straight cane and his AFO, but still needed assistance with bathing and cooking. He initially received home care services, but is now able to perform his ADLs independently. He received outpatient physical and occupational therapy, which have been completed. Guided by his rehabilitation team, he has been participating in a regular exercise program at a local gym and working to improve his endurance and lower limb strength. He reports that he is able to walk longer distances as a result of this program, and feels steadier on his feet, though he continues to require an AFO and cane and can only use his upper right upper limb as a gross assist. Despite his persistent deficits, Charles reports satisfaction with his recovery and has resumed an active lifestyle, including working as a volunteer in a hospital.

Charles's case illustrates both the successes and challenges of stroke rehabilitation. Many individuals achieve considerable functional improvement after stroke, yet both the mechanisms of this improvement and the most effective treatment programs remain poorly understood. Improvement after stroke frequently falls substantially short of premorbid function, leaving considerable impairments. This chapter reviews current knowledge of the mechanisms of stroke recovery, and the role that exercise can play in facilitating this recovery.

SCOPE OF THE PROBLEM

Stroke remains a major cause of morbidity and mortality in the United States, with approximately 700,000 new strokes occurring in the United States each year and 4,700,000 survivors alive today (American Heart Association 2002). Exercise in asymptomatic individuals at risk for cerebrovascular disease is an important public health issue, as exercise favorably affects risk factors for stroke such as hypertension, plasma lipids, obesity, and reduced insulin sensitivity (Bronner et al. 1995). Studies by Gillum and colleagues (1996), Kiely and colleagues (1994) and Shinton (1997) have found an association between physical inactivity and the risk of stroke. Meta-analysis has confirmed that moderate and high levels of exercise are associated with a reduced risk of both ischemic and hemorrhagic stroke (Lee et al. 2003). The magnitude of risk reduction associated with exercise and other lifestyle modifications is substantial, with estimates that 79% of strokes could be averted through regular exercise and avoidance of both smoking and obesity (Shinton 1997).

For individuals who sustain a stroke, exercise forms a large part of the rehabilitation program, despite limited data on its efficacy and uncertainty about how best to design exercise programs for the stroke survivor. In this chapter, I summarize current knowledge regarding the efficacy of various forms of exercise and related therapies for recovering function poststroke, and make recommendations for designing such exercise programs.

How Much Exercise?

With the emphasis on containing health care costs, the issue of what constitutes the optimal amount of exercise and overall rehabilitation poststroke has become a much discussed, if not well-studied, issue. Much of the research in this area has examined the amount of rehabilitation provided, and the setting in which it is provided. Due to the physical and cardiovascular limitations present in many stroke survivors, it is difficult to examine the effects of varying the intensity (training load) of exercise programs. In contrast, the length of each exercise session, their frequency, and the overall duration of the exercise training program can be more easily manipulated, and there is substantial variation in clinical practice in these areas. The intensity (therapy hours/week) of the overall rehabilitation program affects outcome (Kwakkel et al. 1997; Seitz et al. 1987; Sivenius et al. 1985), with intensive, hospital-based rehabilitation programs showing better functional outcomes than less intensive nursing home programs (Keith et al. 1995; Kramer et al. 1997). Despite these data, many individuals receive their rehabilitation in less intensive, nursing home-based rehabilitation programs (Retchin et al. 1997). There are also multiple reports (Indredavik et al. 1997; Kalra and Eade 1995; Kaste et al. 1995; Stevens et al. 1984; Strand et al. 1985), as well as a meta-analysis based largely on European studies (Stroke Unit Trialists 1997), indicating that structured stroke units have better outcomes than general medical units (see figures 14.1 and 14.2). Although some research suggests that the benefits of structured stroke units apply to individuals with both intermediate and severe disability (Kalra et al. 1993; Kalra and Eade 1995), these European studies have limited applicability to the United States because they generally do not distinguish between acute and rehabilitative phases of treatment. Comparing rehabilitation care to conventional medical care, another meta-analysis confirmed improved rates of discharge home but not other long-term benefits (Evans et al. 1995). While these studies help to validate the benefits of rehabilitation, they do not attempt to determine the

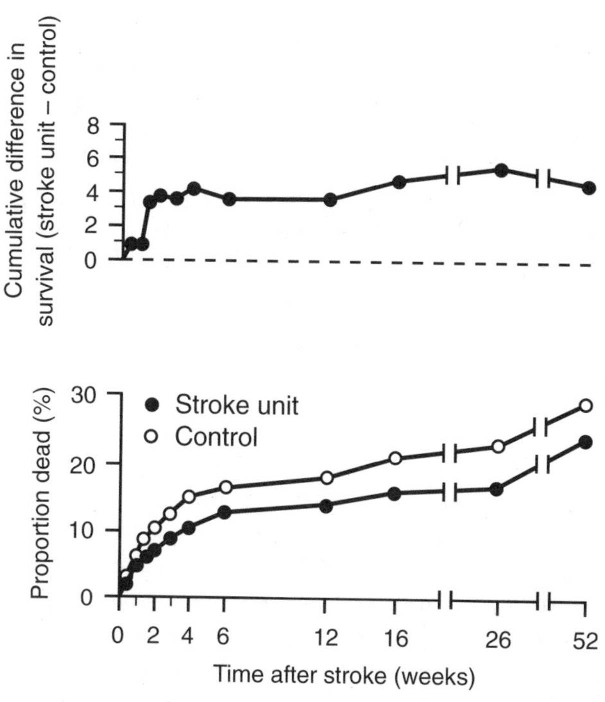

Figure 14.1 Proportion of patients known to have died after a stroke with the cumulative difference between those treated on stroke units and on control (general medical) units.

This figure was first published in the BMJ Stroke Unit Trialists' Collaboration, 1997, "Collaborative systematic review of the randomized trials of organized inpatient (stroke unit) care after stroke," *BMJ* 314:1151-1159, and is reproduced by permission of the *BMJ*.

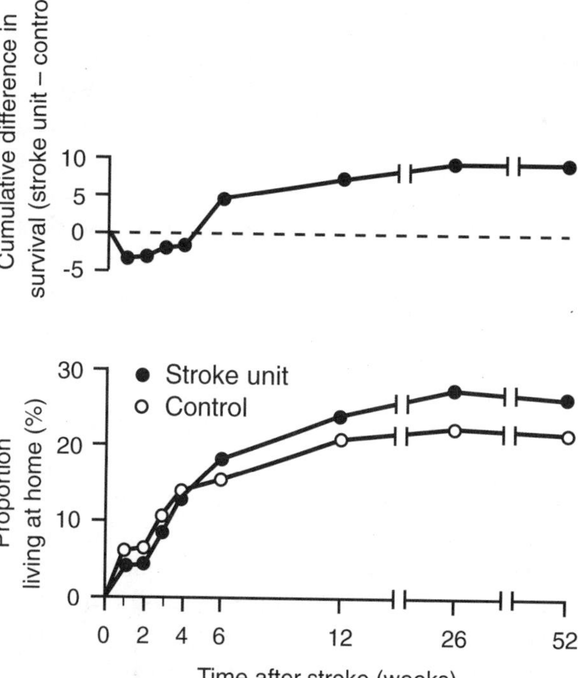

Figure 14.2 Proportion of patients living at home after a stroke, with the cumulative difference between those treated on stroke units and on control (general medical) units.

This figure was first published in the BMJ Stroke Unit Trialists' Collaboration, 1997, "Collaborative systematic review of the randomized trials of organized inpatient (stroke unit) care after stroke," *BMJ* 314:1151-1159, and is reproduced by permission of the *BMJ*.

optimum quantity and duration of exercise for individuals poststroke.

Interventions directed at increasing the amount (increased therapy time) of gait training early after stroke (Richards et al. 1993) have shown only transient benefits. Others have found a dose-response effect in therapy for ambulation, with greater amounts of weight-bearing exercise correlated with better ambulation status (Nugent et al. 1994). Sunderland and colleagues (1994) found that an "enhanced" physical therapy program (consisting of increased therapy time and efforts to increase functional use of the upper extremity) in the acute phase poststroke improved function at six months poststroke; after one year, however, there was no significant difference between the conventional and enhanced therapy groups.

Kwakkel et al. (1999) performed a well-controlled trial of therapy intensity in individuals with recent middle cerebral artery strokes and found that higher-intensity exercises for the legs led to improved mobility-related ADL ability. Only small improvements in dexterity were seen for individuals receiving higher-intensity upper limb exercise, however. The beneficial effects of intensive exercise were attenuated over time, and distinctions between the groups were no longer statistically significant by six months after the stroke (Kwakkel et al. 2002). A systematic review of exercise therapy for arm function after stroke concluded that insufficient data are available to allow any definitive statement regarding the effectiveness of this exercise or the optimal intensity or duration (van der Lee et al. 2001). In spite of continued uncertainty regarding the optimal intensity or duration of exercise after stroke, it appears that a dose–response relationship exists. Until more definitive data are available, physicians must base stroke rehabilitation exercise programs on clinical judgment, tempered by the limitations imposed by insurance coverage.

Recovery Versus Compensation

Individuals who sustain a stroke are, as a rule, more interested in recovery of neurologic function than in learning compensatory strategies. Rehabilitation exercise programs, however, tend to combine these two goals to varying degrees, in part because recovery of neurologic function is often unsatisfactory. It remains unclear to what extent exercise or other rehabilitation interventions can influence ultimate recovery. In competing for scarce rehabilitation resources, clinicians designing poststroke exercise programs must balance the goals of recovery versus compensation. For example, they can train an individual who has partially lost ankle dorsiflexion to try to recruit the tibialis anterior through cueing or biofeedback; or they can train the person to compensate by using a brace. The compensatory strategy of bracing may achieve more rapidly the functional goal of independent ambulation; but the cost may be less effort devoted to correcting the underlying motor deficit. Despite the centrality of this issue in the design of rehabilitation exercise programs, financial pressures, rather than scientific data, are determining the balance between these two approaches. The strong impetus to achieve independent functioning as quickly as possible has led to increased emphasis on compensatory approaches, rather than on attempts to facilitate recovery. While it may be argued that society should choose the least expensive approach (compensatory training) in the absence of evidence supporting a more expensive approach (facilitating recovery), the importance of continuing to examine this issue is paramount.

Physicians prescribe exercise for a variety of impairments that result from stroke. This chapter focuses on the use of exercise to improve motor control, strength, gait, balance, ataxia, sensation, and endurance. The use of exercise to learn compensatory strategies, per se, will not be discussed, though in practice this is intermingled with all of the above exercise programs.

Effects of Stroke on Neuromuscular Function

The effects of hemiparesis secondary to stroke on neuromuscular function are intertwined with the effects of deconditioning of the affected limb. Another confounding factor is the effects of stroke on motor strength on the limbs ipsilateral to the stroke (the "nonparetic" limbs) (Colebatch and Gandevia 1989; McCrea et al. 2003), as many studies use the nonparetic muscles as the basis of comparison. Landin et al. (1977) found paretic leg muscles to have a reduction in blood flow, increased lactate production, and higher glycogen consumption than nonparetic leg muscles. Some of these effects may be due to changes in the proportion of fiber types (Potempa et al. 1996), though cause and effect are not clear even if the correlations are valid.

Motor neuron firing patterns are a major determinant of muscle fiber myosin isoform composition (Lomo 1989; Pette and Vrbova 1992; Salmons and Sreter 1976). Motor neuron firing rates and recruitment are reduced in hemiparetic individuals (Gemperline et al. 1995), perhaps explaining the observed changes in muscle fiber type composition.

Studies of fiber type proportions have yielded apparently conflicting results. Most have observed selective atrophy of type II muscle fibers (Brooke and Engel 1969; Dattola et al. 1993; Dietz et al. 1986; Scelsi et al. 1984; Slager et al. 1985). A few studies, however, revealed an increased prevalence of type IIa fibers in paretic muscles (Frontera et al. 1997; Jakobsson et al. 1991), and one study showed no difference in fiber composition between affected and unaffected limbs (Sunnerhagen et al. 1999). While biopsy studies have mostly revealed atrophy, at least one researcher has reported some focal hypertrophy (Slager et al. 1985). Some of the observed variability in muscle histochemistry and morphometry may result from factors that experimenters did not control—specifically the severity of the weakness, the presence or absence of spasticity, patterns of compensation, and which specific muscle was studied. There is little information on the fiber composition of muscles of the nonparetic side poststroke, though one report found an increased proportion of type I fibers (Frontera et al. 1997). We do not know the effects of exercise on the fiber type proportions in muscle poststroke, and a trial of resistive and/or endurance exercises would be interesting.

MECHANISMS OF MOTOR RECOVERY POSTSTROKE

The natural history of stroke usually includes a significant degree of recovery, including recovery of motor function. Animal models (Johansson et al. 1996; Ohlsson and Johansson 1995) suggest that environment plays a significant role in the recovery of motor function, though we do not fully understand the mechanism(s) and optimal timing of such environmental stimulation. A major, largely unrealized, goal of stroke treatment is to use a combination of medical, surgical, and exercise treatments to enhance this natural recovery of function poststroke.

LEARNING VERSUS RECOVERY

Assessing the effectiveness of exercise therapy for recovery is complicated by the simultaneous motor learning that undoubtedly occurs. There are no data to contradict the supposition that individuals poststroke can "learn" new motor skills in their involved limbs in a fashion similar to the way healthy individuals do (though attenuated). The ability to learn new motor skills appears to represent a continuum based on the severity of neurologic deficits—it is likely better preserved in those with less severe neurologic deficits and may be absent in the densely plegic. Multiple studies have shown that individuals with chronic, stable motor deficits due to stroke can improve their motor functioning after specialized intensive training (Fasoli et al. 2003; Kunkel et al. 1999; Lehmann et al. 1975; Miltner et al. 1999; Tangeman et al. 1990; Taub and Wolf 1993; van der Lee et al. 1999; Werner and Kessler 1996; Wolf et al. 1989). The degree of recovery correlates with the amount of rehabilitation therapy provided (Langhorne et al. 1996; Nugent et al. 1994; Smith et al. 1981). Does this represent late recovery, or is it learning? Can the two phenomena truly be distinguished?

Cortical mapping has shown that, in both the intact (Nudo, Milliken et al. 1996; Pascual-Leone et al. 1994) and the injured (Levy et al. 2001; Liepert et al. 2000; Nudo, Wise et al. 1996) brain, learning motor tasks leads to changes in the organization of the cerebral cortex. Advances in functional imaging techniques may eventually enable us to separate the phenomena of learning and recovery. It is possible that the conceptual distinction between motor recovery and motor learning reflects an artificial dichotomy, with both phenomena occurring through similar patterns of reorganization of the cerebral cortex.

MECHANISMS OF MOTOR RECOVERY

The mechanisms of stroke recovery are incompletely understood. One mechanism involves assumption of lost function by adjacent areas of undamaged brain tissue. Detailed topographic maps of the primary motor cortex have provided considerable information about the elements forming the well-known motor homunculus. The reorganization of cortical maps after cortical injury occurs in the motor system (Asanuma 1991; Jacobs and Donoghue 1991; Nudo, Wise et al. 1996) as well as in the sensory (Pons et al. 1988), visual (Kaas et al. 1990), and auditory systems (King and Moore 1991). This remapping of adjacent cortical tissue is influenced by retraining (i.e., rehabilitation) of the animal through practice of previously acquired motor tasks (see figure 14.3), and may not appear without this activity (Nudo, Wise et al. 1996). Indeed, there is evidence that the undamaged adjacent cerebral cortex may experience a shrinkage of the cortical map for the affected limb

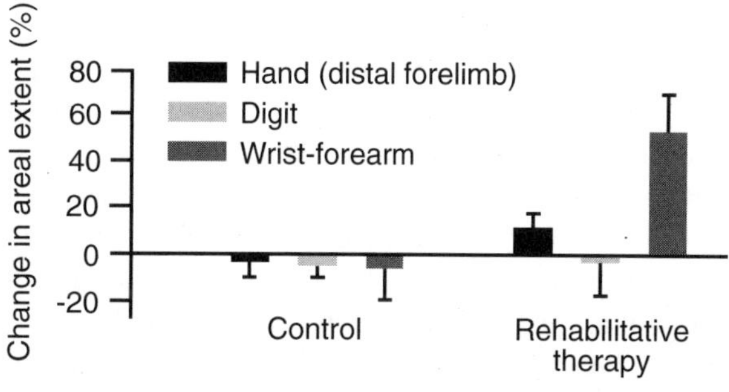

Figure 14.3 Changes in the cortical area size for the upper extremities in squirrel monkeys recovering from experimental cortical lesions. Comparison of rehabilitative therapy with control animals.

Reprint Neural substrates for the effects of rehabilitation training on motor recovery after ischemic infarct with permission from R.J. Nudo, B.M. Wise, F. SiFuentes, and G.W. Milliken, *Science* 272:1791-1794. Copyright 1996 AAAS.

in the absence of any rehabilitative efforts (Nudo and Milliken 1996).

In another mechanism of functional recovery, homologous regions of the unaffected contralateral cerebral hemisphere substitute for the infarcted brain tissue (Fisher 1992; Glees 1980; Sabatini et al. 1994). The unaffected ipsilateral hemisphere may control motor function through uncrossed pyramidal fibers, which may constitute as many as 25% of the pyramidal tracts (Nyberg-Hansen and Rinvik 1963). Functional MRI studies have found increased cortical activity in homologous areas contralateral to the stroke, as well as in undamaged regions adjacent to those affected by the stroke, suggesting that both mechanisms may play a role in recovery of motor function poststroke (Cramer et al. 1997). The functional MRI changes associated with recovery and rehabilitation have been recently reviewed (Schaechter 2004).

Exercise appears to have a broad, general effect on neurogenesis, by increasing levels of brain-derived neurotrophic factor (BDNF) and other growth factors (Cotman and Berchtold 2002). In principle, exercise should be capable of enhancing the brain's ability to respond to insults such as stroke by stimulating neurogenesis and overall plasticity, though this has not yet been demonstrated empirically in stroke survivors.

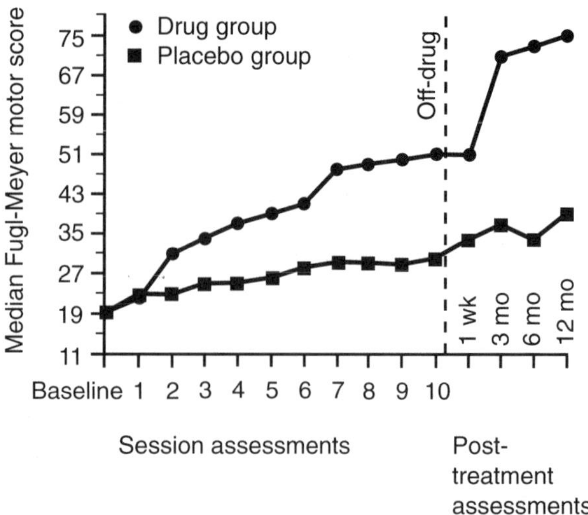

Figure 14.4 Median Fugl-Meyr motor scale scores over the course of combined amphetamine and exercise therapy sessions, with follow-up at one week after drug cessation and at 3, 6, and 12 months after stroke onset.

Reprinted, by permission, from D. Walker-Batson, P. Smith, S. Curtis, H. Unwin, and R. Greenlee, 1995, "Amphetamine paired with physical therapy accelerates motor recovery after stroke. Further evidence," *Stroke* 26:2254-2259.

Medical Interventions to Enhance Recovery

A variety of medical interventions have been studied in attempts to limit damage or enhance recovery during the acute stroke period. With the exception of thrombolytic therapy (NINDS Stroke Study Group 1995), these therapies have not been found useful in well-controlled clinical trials (Clark et al. 1997; Fisher and Schaebitz 2000).

Medications have also been studied in attempts to enhance motor recovery in the postacute phase. Amphetamines and related drugs are among the most promising of these agents, with both animal (Feeney et al. 1982; Hovda and Feeney 1984) and limited human data (Crisostomo et al. 1988; Grade et al. 1998; Walker-Batson et al. 1995) suggesting that they may enhance recovery. Interestingly, the human studies have combined exercise therapy with the administration of amphetamine, following the lead of animal studies that showed the effectiveness of combination therapies in stimulating motor recovery (Feeney et al. 1982; Hovda and Feeney 1984) (see figure 14.4). Other researchers (Martinsson and Wahlgren 2003; Sonde et al. 2001) have failed to confirm benefit from amphetamines, however, and definitive studies are needed. Other medications continue to be studied for this purpose. Levodopa was combined with physical therapy and found to enhance recovery in one study (Scheidtmann et al. 2001).

The use of biological modulators or stimulants of recovery is a promising and growing area of research. Growth factors also enhance recovery in animal models of acute stroke (Bethel et al. 1997; Kawamata et al. 1997) and appear effective even when administered several days after the stroke. Stem cell grafts have been found to be efficacious in correcting stroke-induced deficits in animal models (Veizovic et al. 2001).

Animal data (Feeney et al. 1982) and limited human data (Goldstein 1995) suggest that some commonly used medications—including clonidine, prazosin, phenobarbital, phenytoin, dopamine receptor antagonists, and benzodiazepines—may hinder recovery from stroke.

Environmental and Behavioral Interventions to Enhance Motor Recovery

Environmental and behavioral interventions, with particular emphasis on exercise, are the primary rehabilitative techniques for enhancing recovery poststroke. Several factors have limited direct study of the impact of rehabilitation interventions for enhancing motor recovery. These include

- the normal tendency for spontaneous recovery for several months poststroke,
- the heterogeneity of motor impairments and extent of brain tissue damage after stroke,

- the confounding effects of cognitive and perceptual impairments, and of medical complications after stroke,
- the difficulty in distinguishing clinically between recovery and motor learning,
- limitations in noninvasive assessment of subtle neurologic changes in living humans poststroke,
- difficulty in standardizing treatment, and
- difficulty conducting well-controlled studies during the early phase of recovery, where using an untreated control group (i.e., no rehabilitation) is considered unethical.

Hemispatial neglect, aphasia, confusion, and dementia can all impact attempts to enhance motor function after stroke and complicate efforts to perform well-designed clinical trials in this population. Concurrent medical illnesses, such as pneumonia or deep venous thrombosis, can also interfere with rehabilitation efforts. For these reasons, animal studies have been very helpful in understanding the influence of activity and exercise on recovery.

Animals provided with an enriched environment poststroke have better recovery of motor function (Johansson 1996; Ohlsson and Johansson 1995). Increased use of a paretic limb after experimental cortical injury can lead to a more normal pattern of dendritic arborization of pyramidal neurons (Jones and Schallert 1994).

Some limited animal data suggest, however, that excessive use of a paretic limb after experimental cortical injury can actually impede recovery, possibly due to the toxic effect of neurotransmitter release in the peri-infarct area. The researchers in this experiment created "excessive use" by immobilizing the nonparetic forelimb of a rat immediately after the cortical injury, and maintaining the forced use of the paretic limb for a 15-day period (Kozlowski et al. 1996). While extrapolating these data to humans is difficult, they suggest that extreme efforts to increase use of paretic limbs in the early poststroke period may be hazardous (Schallert et al. 1997). Intensive (CIMT) upper limb training during inpatient poststroke rehabilitation has been found beneficial (Dromerick et al. 2000), suggesting that current exercise programs do not exceed a safe threshold.

Some researchers have studied sensory stimulation as a possible mediator of recovery in poststroke patients. Several studies showed acupuncture to be helpful (Johansson et al. 1993; Magnusson et al. 1994; Naeser et al. 1992), though others have not demonstrated benefit (Sze et al. 2002b); and a recent meta-analysis failed to find any benefit for motor recovery (Sze et al. 2002a). Functional electrical stimulation (discussed later) may also exert its effects through increased sensory stimulation. The mechanisms by which acupuncture or other sensory stimulation modalities might influence stroke recovery remain speculative.

Exercise for Motor Control

The history of poststroke exercise for motor control is notable for the widespread clinical application of unproven treatment approaches. Multiple attempts to demonstrate the benefits of a particular therapeutic approach over a "standard" functionally oriented approach have failed to demonstrate any benefit. Dickstein et al. (1986) compared a functionally oriented program, proprioceptive neuromuscular facilitation (PNF) techniques, and the Bobath (neurodevelopmental or NDT) approach in 131 stroke patients. They found no differences among the three groups in functional ability, ambulation status, muscle tone, or isolated motor control. Hesse, Jahnke et al. (1994) found little benefit from an intensive four-week program of NDT-based exercise; and Butefisch and colleagues (1995) observed the NDT approach to be less effective in restoring motor control than a program of resisted flexion and extension exercises. Several trials have similarly failed to demonstrate any benefit of PNF techniques over conventional functionally oriented therapy (Logigian et al. 1983; Lord and Hall 1986; Stern et al. 1970). One comparison of NDT versus PNF showed no significant benefits of one treatment approach over the other (Wagenaar et al. 1990). Variations of these techniques, such as sensorimotor integrative treatment, apparently are no more effective than functionally oriented therapy programs (Jongbloed et al. 1989). Researchers continue to examine other techniques, such as ballistic movements, resisted agonist, and resisted antagonist movements (Trombly et al. 1986), but so far have found them to have no advantage over generally accepted techniques.

The Standard Approach

Despite its widespread application, there is no universally accepted definition of the "standard" functional approach: essentially, it involves providing physical assistance and encouragement for the stroke patient during functional or pre-functional tasks, and then gradually withdrawing this support as the individual's ability to perform desired activities improves. The therapeutic program typically incorporates instruction in compensatory techniques to improve functional abilities. Problems in defining this approach include the highly individualized nature of the treatment program, with variable emphasis on the "quality" of movement, and variable ratios of retraining paretic muscle groups versus encouraging compensation by unaffected muscle groups. Clinicians often fail to document the amount of time spent performing actual exercises, thus complicating efforts to determine a "dose–response" relationship between the amount of exercise and recovery.

Taub et al. (1993) have theorized that a portion of the decreased function after stroke may be due to a mechanism he terms "learned disuse," in which initial weakness of the paretic limb leads to failure to complete functional tasks with that limb. This failure leads in turn to a cessation of attempts to use the paretic limb, even as some neurologic improvement occurs. Thus this theory maintains that the continued failure to use the paretic limb is in part a learned behavior. Taub et al. (1993) and Wolf et al. (1989) examined restraint of uninvolved upper extremities in individuals with chronic stable hemiparesis (constraint induced movement therapy or CIMT). They coupled use of upper-extremity restraints with intense training programs consisting of six hours per day of various functional activities using the affected upper extremity (eating, writing, card games, etc.). The paretic limbs significantly improved in motor function after intensive two-week training periods and maintained the gains throughout a two-year follow-up (see figure 14.5). Several small replication studies have been performed (Kunkel et al. 1999; Miltner et al. 1999; van der Lee et al. 1999) in patients with chronic stable hemiparesis after stroke, and one study in patients early after stroke (Dromerick et al. 2000). One animal study has suggested that combining CIMT with rehabilitation exercises not only improves motor function, but may actually reduce the brain volume lost after stroke (DeBow et al. 2003). Modifications of this approach have been proposed (Page et al. 2002a, 2000b), but not yet extensively studied.

Other studies (Sterr and Freivogel 2003; Taub 1997) suggest that similar results may obtain through intensive physical training of the paretic limb without use of constraints in the normal upper extremity. These results are particularly intriguing given that the historical outcomes of therapeutic exercise for upper-extremity function have been quite disappointing. Only 5% of individuals who receive intensive therapy for upper-extremity weakness poststroke regain functional use of the upper extremity during rehabilitation (Gowland 1982). A larger multicenter study is currently under way to examine the value of this constraint-induced movement therapy more definitively (Winstein et al. 2003). If this study confirms the preliminary results suggesting benefit from this technique, important questions remain. Foremost among these is whether this technique is unique in its effects, or simply reflects the benefits that may be achieved through many hours of practice of a well-defined high-repetition ("massed practice") therapeutic exercise program (van der Lee 2001).

Other studies have demonstrated that intensive therapeutic exercise programs can improve functional ability in patients with chronic stable deficits poststroke (Duncan et al. 2003; Fasoli et al. 2003; Luft et al. 2004; Rodriquez et al. 1996; Tangeman et al. 1990), although some have shown that, not unlike what occurs in healthy subjects, the benefits of exercise are temporary and are not maintained after cessation of treatment (Wade et al. 1992). While it is possible that these improvements are due to motor learning rather than neurologic recovery, there are no data to reveal the mechanism of this improvement in function. Regression to prior functioning after cessation of the formal exercise program in some studies may indicate that the intervention was not effective in individuals with chronic deficits poststroke; or it may simply point to the need for some form of maintenance therapy.

Meaningful exercise appears more effective than meaningless exercise. The therapeutic advantages of functionally oriented training compared with nonmeaningful motor task training have been demonstrated in the upper limb for both normal individuals (Ferguson and Trombly 1997; Wu et al. 2000) and individuals after stroke (Ma and Trombly 2002; Nelson et al. 1996; Trombly and Wu 1999; Wu et al. 2000). Moreover, performance is improved when training occurs with actual rather than simulated functional tasks. In a supination

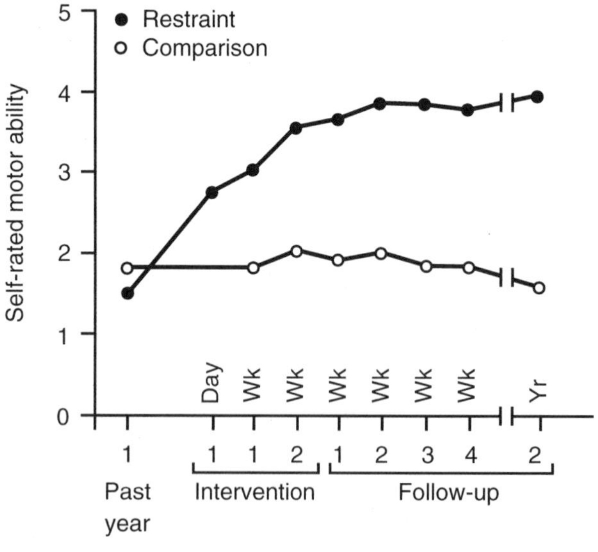

Figure 14.5 Self-rated motor ability based on activity logs for chronic stable poststroke subjects after paretic upper-extremity training. Comparison of subjects who had training with restraint of the unaffected arm versus control group.

task, Nelson et al. (1996) found that use of a simple dice game provided significantly more rotation than a rote, meaningless task. Training in complete functional tasks, such as bringing a pen to paper and writing, has been found to be more effective than training in the component parts of these tasks individually (Ma and Trombly 2001).

There are a number of possible mechanisms by which functional task training may provide advantages over nonfunctional training. These include increases in motivation and attention, enhanced tactile sensory feedback, and specificity of training. This motivational impact has been demonstrated by adding a functional task to a dynamic standing and reaching task, with the result that subjects engaging in the functional task spontaneously perform an increased number of repetitions (Hsieh et al. 1996). Based on these observations, therapeutic exercise programs should be designed to incorporate functional type tasks instead of routine "mat" exercises whenever possible. Training should focus on the functional tasks that are of the most personal relevance to the stroke survivor, since carryover to unrelated functional tasks is likely to be limited.

Biofeedback and Functional Electrical Stimulation

Multiple approaches have been used to ehnhance the efficacy of therapeutic exercise poststroke. Providing enhanced feedback via monitoring of EMG or other activity has had particular appeal. Many researchers have examined the utility of biofeedback (BFB) to facilitate improved neuromuscular control (see table 14.1), and there have been three meta-analyses of data on this subject. Schleenbaker and Mainous (1993) reviewed eight controlled trials of biofeedback for hemiplegia, totaling 192 subjects, and found a significant benefit to EMG-BFB compared with conventional treatment or no treatment ($p < .00001$). Another meta-analysis on the same subject failed to demonstrate significant benefit of biofeedback (Moreland and Thomson 1993). A third and more recent meta-analysis (Glanz et al. 1995) also failed to demonstrate benefit using the outcome measure of improved range of motion. The limitations in study design and comparability and variations in biofeedback training techniques of the studies included in these meta-analyses raise the possibility of a type II error (inadequate sample size) (Glanz et al. 1995). The correlation between results of meta-analyses and those from large randomized clinical trials is only fair (LeLorier et al. 1997), and the conflicting results of these meta-analyses suggest the need for a large randomized clinical trial for biofeedback poststroke.

Most trials of biofeedback have focused on "standard" EMG biofeedback, in which a surface electrode is placed over the agonist muscle (and in some cases the antagonist muscle), and the patient receives visual and/or auditory feedback when EMG activity is produced in the agonist muscle. Other forms of biofeedback have been examined as well, though not as extensively. Biofeedback of joint position obtained via an electrogoniometer has been used in several studies involving the upper extremity (Greenberg 1980) and the lower extremity (Colborne et al. 1993; Mandel et al. 1990; Morris et al. 1992). These studies have consistently reported some improved control of movement as reflected by joint position when compared to control groups. The limited data comparing positional biofeedback to EMG biofeedback suggest that the former is superior (Mandel et al. 1990). Neither Morris and colleagues (1992) nor Colborne and colleagues (1993), however, have demonstrated improved gait velocity from biofeedback when comparing it with conventional physical therapy. With advancing technology, increasingly sophisticated positional biofeedback systems have been developed that measure movement trajectory rather than simply joint position (Maulucci and Eckhouse 2001). Force feedback using static dynamometers was helpful in improving gait velocity in one study (Bourbonnais et al. 2002).

Another form of biofeedback has utilized force feedback via force plates in an effort to more equally distribute weight over the paretic leg (Cheng et al. 2001; Engardt 1994; Engardt et al. 1993; Geiger et al. 2001). While this approach does allow for better force distribution and better performance on a sit-to-stand task, only one study has shown an overall impact on functional status (Cheng et al. 2001).

Functional electrical stimulation (FES) has also been studied using a variety of techniques, including low-level stimulation below the motor threshold and higher degrees of stimulation intended to induce a muscular contraction. Intramuscular electrodes for delivering FES are also under study, and represent an intriguing alternative to surface FES (Chae 2003). Table 14.2 lists many of the published FES trials. A meta-analysis (Glanz et al. 1996) and systematic review (de Kroon et al. 2002) both found evidence that FES appears to promote recovery of muscle strength poststroke.

An interesting combination of FES and biofeedback is EMG-triggered FES. In this technique, the target muscle surface EMG signal is monitored, and when it exceeds a preset threshold, an electrical volley is generated that causes completion of the desired movement. This technique shares features of both FES and biofeedback and appeared to produce some benefit in an uncontrolled case series (Fields 1987) and in one small controlled study (Kraft et al. 1992). No research has demonstrated any benefit of this approach over standard FES techniques. A small pilot trial demonstrated

Table 14.1 Biofeedback Trials

Author	Trial design	Treatment focus	Intervention	Duration of treatment	Length of follow-up	Results
Basmajian 1975*	RCT n = 20 >3 months post-stroke	Ankle dorsiflexion	EMG-BFB + conventional PT vs. conventional PT	3 ×/week × 5 weeks	Variable	No benefit.
Mroczek 1978	Nonrandomized crossover design n = 9 >1 year poststroke	Wrist extension, elbow flexion	EMG-BFB vs. conventional PT	3 ×/week × 4 weeks	None	Both beneficial in restoring AROM, no difference between treatments.
Shiavi 1979	RCT n = 22 <1 month poststroke	Lower extremity	EMG-BFB + conventional PT vs. conventional PT	Varied	Variable	Improved muscle control; no functional assessment performed.
Hurd 1980#	RCT n = 24 Mean 76 days post-stroke	Deltoid or tibialis anterior (each 1/2 of subjects)	EMG-BFB vs. sham BFB vs. untreated control muscles. All continued usual therapy program.	5 ×/week × 2 weeks	None	EMG-BFB and sham BFB equivalent, though both superior to control.
Prevo 1982	Nonrandomized n = 18 >1 year poststroke	Upper extremity	EMG-BFB vs. conventional PT	28 sessions over 10 weeks	None	No benefit on agonist function, though decreased abnormal cocontraction.
Basmajian 1982*	RCT n = 37 2-5 months post-stroke	Upper extremity	EMG-BFB vs. conventional therapy	3 ×/week × 5 weeks	None	No benefit.
Burnside 1982*	RCT n = 22 0.5-12 years post-stroke	Ankle dorsiflexion	EMG-BFB vs. conventional PT	2 ×/week × 6 weeks	6 weeks	Increased strength in BFB group, no change in gait or range.
Wolf 1983a*	Controlled, nonrandomized n = 31 >1 year poststroke	Upper extremity	EMG-BFB of UE vs. no treatment	2-3 ×/week × 26 weeks	None	No functional benefit.
Wolf 1983b*	Controlled, nonrandomized n = 36 >1 year poststroke	Lower extremity	EMG-BFB of LE vs. no treatment vs. EMG-BFB to UE only vs. relaxation training	5 ×/week × 12 weeks	None	Improved AROM, decreased ambulatory aids. No change in walking speed.

Inglis 1984*	RCT w/crossover of control group n = 30 >6 months post-stroke	Upper extremity	EMG-BFB vs. conventional PT	3 ×/week × 7 weeks	None	Improved AROM and muscle strength.
John 1986#	Crossover n = 12 12-280 (mean 75.5) days poststroke	Lower extremity	EMG-BFB + conventional PT vs. conventional PT	Daily × 3 weeks for 20 minutes	None	No benefit.
Mulder 1986#	RCT n = 12 Duration poststroke not given	Ankle dorsiflexion	EMG-BFB vs. neurodevelopmental treatment	3 ×/week × 5 weeks	None	No benefit.
Basmajian 1987	RCT n = 29 1-12 months post-stroke	Upper extremity	EMG-BFB + behaviorally oriented PT vs. conventional PT	3 ×/week × 5 weeks	9 months	No benefit.
Cozean 1988*#	RCT n = 36 Mixed duration post-stroke	Gait	EMG-BFB vs. FES vs. EMG-BFB+FES vs. conventional treatment	3 ×/week × 6 weeks	None	Improved gait velocity in EMG-BFB+FES group compared with control.
Crow 1989*	RCT n = 40 2-8 weeks poststroke	Upper extremity	EMG-BFB for UE vs. conventional therapy	6 weeks	6 weeks	No benefit.
Mandel 1990#	RCT n = 37 >6 months post-stroke	Gait	EMG-BFB vs. positional BFB vs. no treatment control	2 ×/week × 6 weeks	3 months	Positional BFB improved walking speed compared with EMG-BFB, nontreated control.
Colborne 1993	Crossover n = 8 >7 months post-stroke	Gait	EMG-BFB vs. positional BFB vs. conventional PT	2 ×/week × 4 weeks	1 month	Some improvement in certain parameters of gait, but walking speed improved equally with all treatments.
Intiso 1994	RCT n = 16 Mean 9.8 months poststroke	Gait	EMG-BFB + conventional PT vs. conventional PT	15 sessions	None	Improved gait parameters, but no change in velocity.
Bradley et al. 1998	RCT n = 21 Acute poststroke	Gait	EMG-BFB + conventional PT vs. sham EMG-BFB + conventional PT	18 sessions	None	No difference between groups.

* Included in meta-analysis by Schleenbaker et al. 1993.
# Included in meta-analysis by Glanz et al. 1995.
BFB = biofeedback; EMG = electromyography; PT = physical therapy; RCT = randomized clinical trial.

Table 14.2 Functional Electrical Stimulation Trials

Author	Design	Treatment focus	Intervention	Duration of treatment	Length of follow-up	Results
Merletti 1978*	RCT n = 49 0.5-15 months post-stroke	Ankle dorsiflexion	FES + conventional PT vs. conventional PT	1 month	3 months	Improved strength in FES group, no functional outcomes documented.
Bowman 1979*	RCT n = 30 3-16 weeks post-stroke	Wrist extension	Electrogoniometer-triggered FES + conventional PT vs. conventional PT	2 × daily × 4 weeks	None	Increased wrist extensor torque and active ROM.
Winchester 1983*	RCT n = 40 <6 months poststroke	Knee extension	Electrogoniometer-triggered FES + conventional PT vs. conventional PT	4 weeks	None	Increased knee extensor torque, but no change in isolated knee extension control.
Kraft 1992	Nonrandomized controlled trial n = 18 >6 months poststroke	Upper extremity	EMG-triggered FES vs. low-intensity continuous FES, vs. proprioceptive neuromuscular facilitation vs. no treatment	3 months	9 months	3 treatment groups all improved motor function compared with control. No difference among treatment modalities.
Levin 1992*	RCT, with crossover of some "placebo" subjects n = 13 >8 months poststroke	LE spasticity and ankle dorsiflexion	TENS to common peroneal nerve vs. low-intensity TENS	5 ×/week × 3 weeks	None	Decreased spasticity and increased dorsiflexion strength in treatment group.
Faghri 1994	RCT n = 26 11-21 days poststroke	Shoulder subluxation, pain, and function	FES + conventional PT vs. conventional PT	7 days/week × 6 weeks	6 weeks	Reduced pain, subluxation, and improved motor function.
Bogataj 1995	Crossover n = 20 1-9 months post-stroke	Gait	FES + conventional PT vs. conventional PT	3 weeks	None	Improved gait parameters, but poor correlation with Fugl-Meyr.
Hummelsheim 1997	Prospective case series n = 12 3-4 months post-stroke	Wrist flexion and extension	FES to ECR and FCR + therapy	2 × daily × 2 weeks	None	No benefit to FES, but therapy improved function.
Chae et al. 1998	RCT n = 28 Acute stroke rehabilitation	Wrist and finger extension	FES + conventional therapy vs. sham FES + conventional therapy	1 hour daily × 15 sessions	3 months	Improved motor function, but no change in functional status.

* Included in meta-analysis by Glanz et al. 1996.

ECR = extensor carpi radialis; EMG = electromyography; FCR = flexor carpi radialis; FES = functional electrical stimulation; PT = physical therapy; RCT = randomized clinical trial; TENS = transcutaneous electrical stimulation.

efficacy of this technique over control treatment in acute stroke patients (Francisco et al. 1998). A similar technique of triggered FES has been used with positional rather than EMG feedback (Bowman et al. 1979; Winchester et al. 1983).

Although scientists have studied biofeedback for 20 years, its overall utility and most appropriate application remain unclear. Combining the technologies of EMG, FES, kinesiologic information, and force generation information may ultimately provide the best results with these techniques. At present, the available data on these techniques are inconclusive.

Balance Training

Although standing balance appears to correlate strongly with several measures of gait (Bohannon 1995), there is no conclusive evidence that exercise to improve balance leads to improved functional ambulation. Platform training for balance impairments in hemiplegic stroke patients can help increase the magnitude of postural deviations tolerated on a perturbed platform (Hocherman et al. 1984), and can reduce lateral sway (Shumway-Cook et al. 1988) and standing symmetry (Winstein et al. 1989). The improvement in static standing balance does not appear to lead to improved gait symmetry or speed, however (Winstein et al. 1989). One study has suggested that training with a standing biofeedback trainer can reduce the risk of falls poststroke (Cheng et al. 2001).

Sitting balance is important both functionally and prognostically (Feigin et al. 1996). One study found that devices providing feedback regarding sitting angle can be useful (Dursun et al. 1996). Training programs involving seated reaching tasks appear to help improve sitting balance, but without any carryover into ambulatory ability (Dean and Shepherd 1997). In general, balance training appears useful to the extent that it is task-specific for a functional activity (e.g., sitting balance training to improve sitting balance). There is no convincing evidence that balance training carries over from one activity to another, such as from standing balance to ambulation.

Treadmill Training

Partial body weight-supported gait training using a treadmill has been found to help restore ambulatory ability in nonambulatory hemiparetic patients in a number of studies (Barbeau and Visintin 2003; Dobkin et al. 1991; Hesse et al. 1994; Hesse et al. 1995; Visintin et al. 1998). Other studies, however, have failed to show significant benefit of this technique when compared with conventional gait training (Kosak and Reding 2000; Nilsson et al. 2001). Treadmill speed appears to influence the efficacy of this technique, with higher walking velocities appearing more effective (Pohl et al. 2002; Sullivan et al. 2002). While a recent Cochrane review failed to find an overall benefit to this technique (Moseley et al. 2003), there appears to be sufficient evidence to justify continued research. A major limitation of this technique is the requirement for multiple therapists to assist with training. The use of mechanical aids to assist with this form of training has been explored (Hesse et al. 1999; Werner et al. 2002), and may ultimately dovetail with lower-extremity robot-aided rehabilitation techniques.

Robot-Aided and Virtual Reality Based Exercise

The use of robots as an exercise aid to facilitate motor recovery is a promising area of research. Robot-assisted arm exercises provide force, visual, and in some cases auditory feedback to enhance accuracy of movement (see figure 14.6). Robots can be programmed to gradually withdraw support of the movement as patient performance improves, and even provide resistance when motor control and strength allow (Stein et al. 2004). Studies have shown improved motor control

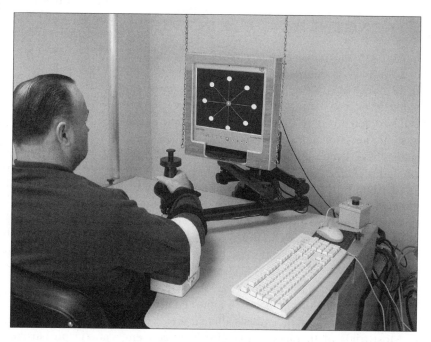

Figure 14.6 Robot-aided rehabilitation using the InMotion2 robot (Interactive Motion Technologies, Cambridge), based on the MIT-Manus robot.

with robot-aided training for individuals with recent stroke (Aisen et al. 1997; Volpe et al. 2000) and those with chronic, stable deficits after stroke (Fasoli et al. 2003; Ferarro et al. 2003; Lum et al. 2002). These improvements appear durable in some studies (Fasoli et al. 2004; Ferraro et al. 2003; Volpe et al. 1999), but not in others (Lum et al. 2002). While most reports of robotic training aids for stroke patients have focused on upper limb retraining, electromechanical training devices have been developed for lower limb training (Hesse et al. 2001), and robots are under development for this purpose. Whether robotic training will be found to have advantages over conventional exercise training remains to be established. Many robotic training devices are capable of recording kinematic data on the quality of movement, and have provided evidence that the quality of movement improves with robot-aided upper limb rehabilitation, becoming "smoother" with training (Rohrer et al. 2002).

Virtual reality systems have been developed for facilitating exercise training after stroke (Jack et al. 2001). Pilot studies have shown the feasibility and possible benefits of this approach for stroke and brain injury patients (Holden et al. 2001; Merians et al. 2002). Studies of normal individuals have shown that tasks learned using virtual reality training show attenuation of training effects when carried over to physical (i.e., nonvirtual) environments (Kozak et al. 1993). Whether incorporating haptic (touch) feedback into virtual reality systems will overcome this reduced generalization of training remains to be determined.

Strengthening Exercises

Impairments of strength are a key issue in many individuals who have sustained a stroke, but are notoriously difficult to separate from impairments of motor control. As would be expected, the best predictor of motor strength at the completion of rehabilitation is the motor strength at admission (Bohannon and Smith 1987). While some studies have demonstrated a correlation between muscle strength and functional ability (Bohannon and Andrews 1990; Hamrin et al. 1982; Sunderland et al. 1989), strength per se does not appear to be an independent predictor of gait performance after stroke (Bohannon 1995). A stroke survivor's ability to generate isokinetic torque at high velocities correlates better with his/her ambulatory function than does his/her ability to generate isometric torque (Nakamura et al. 1985), possibly reflecting the relationship between motor control and speed of movement in individuals after stroke.

Most trials of therapeutic exercise have concentrated on restoration of motor control rather than motor strength, and few have incorporated resistive exercises. Historically, some physicians have argued that resistive exercises might interfere with developing improved motor control (Bobath 1990), though no published evidence exists to support this contention. Studies of resistive upper limb exercises are limited, but have not shown advantages to this approach in improving motor control (Stein et al. 2004; Trombly and Quintana 1983; Trombly et al. 1986). Several studies have confirmed that resistive training results in strengthening of the paretic limb(s) poststroke (Badics et al. 2002; Ouellette et al. 2004; Sharp and Brouwer 1997; Teixeira-Salmela et al. 1999; Weiss et al. 2000). Beneficial effects of lower-extremity strength training on walking speed and stair climbing have been found in some studies (Teixeira-Salmela et al. 2001), but not others (Ouellette et al. 2004; Sharp and Brouwer 1997); however, self-reported physical functioning has consistently improved in all of these studies. Limited data also suggest that resistive exercises may accelerate the rate of functional improvement when compared with a standard functionally oriented program early after stroke, though not the ultimate functional outcome (Inaba et al. 1973).

In studying the relative benefits of concentric versus eccentric strengthening, Engardt et al. (1995) found both types of muscle actions equally effective for increasing muscle strength in the hemiparetic limb. Conflicting results have been found for the value of isokinetic strength training of the lower extremity poststroke: one study (Glasser 1986) observed no additional functional benefit to combining isokinetic training with standard physical therapy; another (Sharp and Brouwer 1997) reported that isokinetic strengthening of knee flexors and extensors in chronic stable poststroke individuals can increase both muscle strength and gait velocity, without adverse effects. Some investigators have noted a modest correlation between spasticity and motor strength in the same muscle in hemiplegic stroke patients (Bohannon et al. 1987), but others have not seen the correlation (Nakamura et al. 1985). Spasticity does not correlate well with gait speed (Bohannon and Andrews 1990). Resistance training and strengthening of hemiparetic muscles do not affect spasticity in those muscles (Badics et al. 2002; Brown and Kautz 1998; Miller and Light 1997; Sharp and Brouwer 1997; Teixeira-Salmela et al. 1999), and the importance of spasticity in designing exercise programs poststroke appears limited.

Exercise for Ataxia

A small but significant number of individuals develop ataxia poststroke, most commonly after cerebellar injury. There is a paucity of scientific literature on the use of therapeutic exercise for rehabilitation of cerebel-

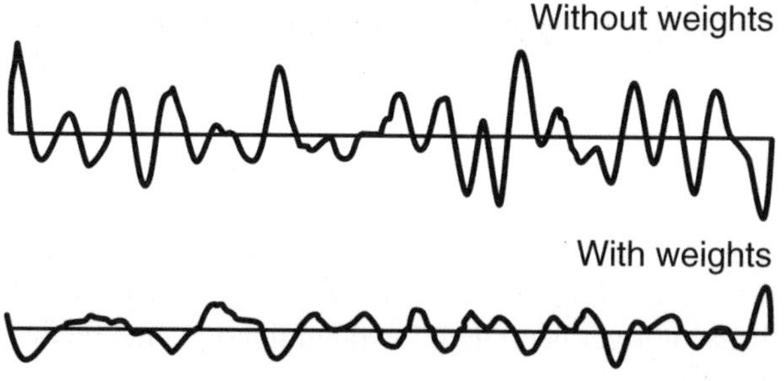

Figure 14.7 Accelerometer traces recording hand movement toward a target in an ataxic individual, with and without wrist weights.

Reprinted, by permission, from M.H. Morgan, 1975, "Ataxia and weights," *Physiotherapy* 61:332-334.

lar ataxia. While physicians have advocated Frenkel's exercises for many years to treat ataxia (Urbsheit and Oremland 1990), there are few objective data to support their use. Limb weights appear to provide some benefit both for upper-extremity functional tasks and for ambulation (Morgan 1975) (see figure 14.7). The optimal amount of weighting is patient-specific, with lighter or heavier weights reducing benefits. Case reports suggest that exercise training during both outpatient physical therapy (Gill-Body et al. 1997) and during comprehensive inpatient rehabilitation (Sliwa et al. 1994) provides some benefit for cerebellar ataxia. A small case series (Balliet et al. 1987) suggests that individuals with chronic stable ataxia may benefit from an exercise program that reduces the amount of weightbearing through the upper extremities. There are case reports of the utility of EMG biofeedback for ataxia (Davis and Lee 1980; Guercio et al. 1997) but no controlled trials.

EXERCISE FOR AEROBIC CONDITIONING

Deconditioning is highly prevalent poststroke, due in many cases to neurologic impairments that interfere with the ability to participate in aerobic conditioning exercise. Stroke patients are unable to achieve the same workload as age-matched control subjects during lower-extremity ergometry (Monga et al. 1988) or partial body weight-supported treadmill testing (MacKay-Lyons and Makrides 2002b). While standard physical and occupational therapy sessions may not provide adequate intensity to achieve cardiovascular training effects (MacKay-Lyons and Makrides 2002a), well-designed aerobic exercise programs for this population can reduce this deconditioning. Using an adapted bicycle ergometer, Potempa et al. (1995) found that a 10-week training period with gradually increasing workload resulted in significant improvements in maximal O_2 consumption, workload, and exercise duration in experimental subjects as compared with controls. Subjects also showed a significant reduction in systolic blood pressure at submaximal workloads. Other studies have confirmed the ability to successfully increase aerobic fitness in stroke survivors, with improved function resulting (Duncan et al. 2003; Katz-Leurer et al. 2003; Macko et al. 2001; Rimmer et al. 2000).

The safety of aerobic and other physiologically stressful exercise has been a concern in stroke patients. Coronary artery disease (CAD) shares many of the risk factors for stroke, and the two conditions frequently coexist. In one angiographic series, 35% of individuals with transient ischemic attack (TIA), stroke, or asymptomatic carotid bruit had evidence of severe CAD (>70% stenosis of one or more coronary arteries), with only 7% having normal coronary arteries (Hertzer et al. 1985). Roth (1993) estimated that approximately 75% of individuals who have sustained a stroke have heart disease. The fact that cardiac disease is the most common cause of death in long-term poststroke survivors (Matsumoto et al. 1973) argues for both the importance of aerobic exercise in this population, as well as some caution in implementing such a program.

Because of the high prevalence of cardiac disease in the stroke population, exercise stress testing may be necessary to assess the presence and severity of coronary artery disease in poststroke patients. Treadmill exercise testing appears reliable for hemiparetic stroke patients who are capable of undergoing this type of testing (Dobrovolny et al. 2003). For patients who are unable to undergo conventional treadmill or bicycle ergometry testing due to neurologic deficits, a variety of adapted exercise testing techniques offer suitable substitutes. These include arm, leg, or combined arm and leg ergometry, supine bicycle ergometry (Moldover et al. 1984), wheelchair ergometry, and low-velocity treadmill testing (Macko et al. 1997). Others (Roth 1993) have used cardiac monitoring during physical therapy to check for possible ischemia or arrhythmia. Finally, Dipyridamole thallium^{201} testing or Dobutamine echocardiography can identify ischemia without exercise. Despite the availability of these techniques, however, no large-scale studies have demonstrated improved outcomes as a result of routine cardiac testing in individuals poststroke.

OTHER BENEFITS OF EXERCISE

Stroke with resulting hemiplegia decreases bone mass on the hemiplegic side (Hamdy et al. 1993, 1995; Jorgensen and Jacobsen 2001), with resulting increased risk of osteoporotic fractures. Individuals who recover walking ability have a reduced rate of bone loss compared to nonambulatory stroke survivors (Jorgensen and Jacobsen 2001). Although no published reports have directly examined the effects of increased exercise on bone mineral density in the hemiplegic leg, it is reasonable to hypothesize that it may be of some benefit in this population. See chapter 15 for a more detailed discussion of the role of exercise in the rehabilitation of osteoporosis.

Home- and Community-Based Exercise

Among the major barriers to providing exercise therapy after stroke have been the logistic and financial challenges of providing this in an institutional setting. This is particularly problematic for the stroke survivor with residual motor deficits who might benefit from long-term exercise. Home-based exercise has been found to be practical and effective (Disler and Wade 2003; Duncan et al. 1998, 2003; Monger et al. 2002; Outcome Service Trialists 2003). Community-based group treatment has also been found to improve functional capacity (Eng et al. 2003). A greater reliance on home- and community-based exercise programs seems likely in the future.

Summary

More than 35 years ago, a review of stroke treatment in the *New England Journal of Medicine* concluded, "It has not yet been demonstrated that patients receiving formal physical therapy after strokes recover more quickly or more completely than those who receive no therapy" (Browne and Poskanzer 1969). While this statement is no longer considered true, there remains much in the use of therapeutic exercise poststroke that is not scientifically based. Given the high human costs of stroke and the financial pressures to reduce unproven or unnecessary care, the need for definitive studies of rehabilitation interventions in stroke has never been more acute. The community of rehabilitation professionals needs to establish recommendations—based on evidence—that provide the most effective and efficient programs of therapeutic exercise for stroke survivors. Documentation of functional outcomes will be essential to convince third-party payers to continue coverage of the current array of rehabilitation programs and new exercise treatments being developed.

CHAPTER 15

OSTEOPOROSIS

David M. Slovik, MD

CASE STUDY

A 73-year-old woman, R.D., came to us with acute back pain after lifting a heavy object. She was independent, in general good health with occasional back pain, and participated in many outside activities.

She had a normal menarche at age 13 and had two children. She had no history of eating disorders or chronic illnesses. She considered herself nonathletic and rarely had participated in sport activities. Her nutritional status was "average" when growing up, although she liked milk and dairy products.

She had a natural menopause at age 50 but refused hormone replacement therapy. She occasionally took calcium supplements and walked at the local mall one-half hour several times each week.

R.D.'s height was 61 inches (usual height 64 inches) and she weighed 105 pounds. She had a dorsal kyphosis and tenderness over several lumbar vertebrae and in the lumbar paravertebral area. Lumbosacral X rays showed end-plate compression of L1 and L3 vertebral bodies. Thoracic spine X rays also showed anterior wedge deformities of T10 and T12 vertebrae.

A femoral neck bone density by dual X-ray absorptiometry (DXA) showed a *t* score (compared to young female adult mean) of –3.2 standard deviations and a *z* score (compared to age-matched females) of –0.8 standard deviations. Additional workup revealed no secondary causes of osteoporosis.

We initially treated R.D. with analgesics and bed rest, progressing to activity as tolerated in subsequent weeks. We placed her on calcium supplementation, a multivitamin containing vitamin D, and antiresorptive therapy to slow bone loss. We also referred her to a physical therapist to begin a program of gentle abdominal and back-strengthening exercises and to learn how to care for her back and avoid future falls. After three months she had occasional low back discomfort late in the day, but was back to her independent state and able to participate in prior activities. A follow-up bone density measurement one year later was similar to the first reading, indicating no further bone loss.

Osteoporosis is a major public health problem because it leads to fractures with resultant morbidity, loss of independence, chronic suffering, and increased mortality. Osteoporosis affects more than 25 million people in the United States, and predisposes to more than 1.3 million fractures annually including over 500,000 vertebral, 250,000 hip, and 240,000 wrist fractures (Consensus Development Conference 1993; Riggs and Melton 1986). The lifetime risk of fracture is 40% for white women and 13% for white men from age 50; among those who live to be 90 years old, 33% of women and 17% of men suffer a hip fracture (Melton et al. 1992). Perhaps 90% of all hip and spine fractures among elderly white women are attributed to osteoporosis (Melton et al. 1997). The annual cost of caring for osteoporosis-related fractures in the United States in 1995 was \$13.8 billion (Ray et al. 1997). As the elderly population grows, the incidence of fractures will increase. Any means of increasing bone mass, slowing bone loss, and lessening the likelihood of falling will have major long-term health benefits.

Osteoporosis has been defined as a systemic skeletal disease characterized by low bone mass and microarchitectural deterioration of bone tissue, with consequent increase in bone fragility and susceptibility to fracture (Consensus Development Conference 1993). An updated version (NIH Consensus Development Panel 2001) defines osteoporosis as a skeletal disorder characterized by compromised bone strength predisposing a person to an increased risk of fracture. Bone strength primarily reflects the integration of bone density (determined by peak bone mass and amount of bone loss) and bone quality (determined by architecture, turnover, damage accumulation, and mineralization). The World Health Organization proposed that an individual with bone mineral density (BMD) or bone mineral content (BMC) more than 2.5 standard deviations below the young adult mean value has osteoporosis (Kanis et al. 1994).

Bone strength and health are related to many factors including genetics, nutrition, hormones, environmental influences, and physical activity. All of these factors are important to

- achieve the maximal amount of bone at the time of skeletal maturity (peak bone mass),
- maintain bone mass in adulthood, and
- slow the rate of bone loss in postmenopausal women.

Physical activity may be especially important, because it is something that most individuals can control. The prevention and treatment of osteoporosis involves nonpharmacologic and pharmacologic approaches. The former includes calcium and vitamin D supplementation, nutrition, lifestyle changes, and exercise. The latter includes hormone replacement, bisphosphonates, calcitonin, selective estrogen receptor modulators (SERMs), and parathyroid hormone. A beneficial program often combines both.

Bone adapts to physical and mechanical loads by altering its mass and strength. Although the physiological mechanisms are unknown, the bones appear to change either as a result of direct impact from the weight-bearing activity or of the action of the muscles attached to bone. High levels of physical activity and loading can increase bone mass, while low levels may lead to less bone. This chapter explores the effects that physical activity and exercise have on the skeleton at various stages of life and in various populations.

Mechanical Properties of Bone: Effects of Exercise

The primary function of the skeleton is to provide structural support; a secondary role, however, is to act as a source of minerals. In serving these functions, bone responds to many factors, including mechanical loading; sufficient force can lead to increased bone density.

In normal individuals, bone architecture (mass, shape, and internal arrangement) is primarily determined by the individual's genetic inheritance and the response to functional load bearing (Lanyon 1996). Lanyon also states that when a load is applied to a structure, it deforms until the intermolecular forces within the structure prevent further deformation. These intermolecular forces are the stresses, which approximately equal the applied load divided by the load-carrying area (stress = force per unit area). The deformation produced by the applied load can be resolved into strains, with each strain defined as the ratio of change in the relevant dimension to the original dimension. Very high repetitive strains can lead to damage and fractures.

Studies in animals have demonstrated that the osteogenic response to dynamic compressive forces is related to the magnitude of the load (Rubin and Lanyon 1985) and the rate of loading (O'Connor et al. 1982).

Although the mechanisms are unclear, it appears that mechanical loads stimulate bone cells (osteoblasts and osteocytes) in the loaded bones to change calcium fluxes to increase production of prostacyclin, prostaglandin E2, nitric oxide, and glucose-6-phosphate dehydrogenase (G6PD) and to increase RNA synthesis, with subsequent release of growth factors (American College of Sports Medicine 1995; Lanyon 1996).

Schwarz et al. (1996) reported that brief low- and high-intensity exercise by ten males (mean age 28 years) led to a significant increase in circulating insulin-like growth factors. The response was greater in the high-intensity group.

Disuse, Weightlessness, and Immobilization

The most dramatic example of the effect of physical activity on bone is the rapid, dramatic, and extensive loss of bone seen with any type of immobilization and disuse (Giangregorio and Blimkie 2002). Krolner and Toft (1983) reported that BMC of the spine decreased 0.9% per week in 34 patients aged 18 to 60 years who were hospitalized with low back pain due to protrusion of a lumbar intervertebral disk. Reambulation resulted in a gain in BMC, with restoration to nearly normal levels after four months. Goemaere et al. (1994) studied 53 patients with complete traumatic paraplegia of at least one year's duration. Compared to controls, the BMD of paraplegic patients was preserved in the lumbar spine but was markedly decreased in the proximal femur (–33%) and femoral shaft (–25%). In those performing passive weight-bearing standing with the aid of a standing device, BMD of the femur was significantly higher than in those not performing these activities. Del Puente and colleagues (1996) found significant bone loss in the femoral neck in the paralyzed limbs of 48 hemiplegic subjects; the degree of bone loss directly correlated with the length of immobilization. Of interest, in a study of 24 patients with a unilateral stroke, there was loss of BMD in the paretic extremities, but an increase in the nonaffected ultra-distal radius, perhaps due to increased compensatory activity in the arm (Ramnemark et al. 1999). Early studies with astronauts during spaceflight showed a significant increase in urinary calcium excretion and a decrease in BMC at the os calcis (Rambaut and Good 1985). In cosmonauts, Vico et al. (2000) found a decrease in BMD at the weight-bearing tibial site, with the loss evident as early as one month. Bone mineral density was preserved in the radius. The mechanism of bone loss and immobilization is not understood. Immobilization can lead to rapid increases in osteoclastic bone resorption, urinary calcium excretion, and bone loss. The alterations in bone metabolism occur rapidly, and bone resorption becomes elevated within the first few weeks of unloading. In fact, one study showed an increase in bone resorption within 24 hours of bed rest in healthy subjects (Baecker et al. 2003). In part, lack of muscle contraction against gravity may play a role. Bone mineral density that has been lost due to disuse or reduced weight bearing can be restored with resumption of normal activity. However, the recovery may be incomplete and may take much longer than the time required to have lost bone.

Physical Activity and Bone Mass

The effects of physical activity and exercise have been studied in many populations, at various ages, with different exercise regimens (some with confounding variables) and in cross-sectional and longitudinal studies. It is thus very difficult to answer the question, "Does exercise prevent bone loss, promote bone gain, or have any role in bone physiology?" without considering the specific population studied, the age and menopausal status of women included, and the type and intensity of the exercise program.

Athletes

Athletic training programs often include intense mechanical loading of specific bones or skeletal regions. The response to loading differs according to the magnitude of the load, the type of physical activity, and the level of exertion within the activity. Table 15.1 summarizes many studies of intense exercise training in different athletic groups.

BMD is higher in the dominant playing forearm compared to the nondominant forearm of lifetime tennis players. In 35 active male tennis players aged 70 to 84 years, Huddleston et al. (1980) found that the bone mass of the radius midshaft ranged from 4% to 33% greater in the playing arms compared with the nonplaying arms.

In a study of 51 professional tennis players, Jones and colleagues (1977) reported higher cortical bone density in the humerus of the playing arm. Haapasalo et al. (1996) found similar results in both young and older tennis players. A study by this same group (Haapasalo et al. 1998) showed that BMD was also greater in the playing arm of female junior tennis players, with the benefit of unilateral activity becoming evident at the time of the adolescent growth spurt.

Kannus et al. (1995) reported that, in a group of tennis and squash players, BMD was significantly greater in the playing versus the nonplaying arm compared to controls. The difference was two to four times greater in female players who started playing before or at menarche than in those who started more than 15 years after menarche. Kontulainen et al. (2003) published a similar report. Bass et al. (2002) also reported that in 47 competitive female tennis players ages 8 to 17 years, loading before puberty increased bone size by periosteal apposition and thus its resistance to bending, whereas after puberty, loading increased the acquisition of bone on the endosteal surface with little benefit in the bone's resistance to bending. Thus, high levels of activity before and during puberty have a larger impact on bone mass than activity started later and are region and surface specific.

Smith and Rutherford (1993) reported that male rowers have higher BMD of the lumbar spine and whole body compared with triathletes and sedentary controls. Each of the exercise groups devoted similar total hours to exercise each week, but the regimens differed: rowers used weights; the triathletes ran, swam, and cycled. Weightlifting appears to have a major influence on BMD.

Karlsson and coworkers (1993b) reported significantly higher BMD in hip, spine, and total body in weightlifters compared to controls. Similarly Conroy et al. (1993), using DXA to measure BMD in 25 elite junior Olympic weightlifters (mean age 17 years), found significantly greater BMD for the lumbar spine and proximal femur in the athletes compared with their age-matched controls, and also compared with an adult reference range (ages 20-39 years). BMD correlated with strength in this study, as it did in a report by Virvidakis et al. (1990), who observed higher BMC of the forearm in junior competitive male weightlifters than in age-matched controls. Hamdy and colleagues (1994) reported higher BMD in weightlifters' upper limbs but not in axial areas resulting, perhaps from a less intensive weightlifting program or from less axial loading compared to that of Olympic lifters.

Female weightlifters exhibit a similar response with significantly higher BMD (compared to controls) at the lumbar spine, distal radius, and several lower-extremity sites (Heinonen et al. 1993). BMC in young female body builders performing weightlifting resistance exercises

Table 15.1 Effects of Intense Training Programs on Bone Mineral Density in Athletes

Author	Type of exercise program	Sex	Age mean (years)	Number of subjects	Bone measurement	Results
Jones et al. 1977	Tennis (professional)	M F	27 24	48 30	X rays of humerus	Cortical thickness on playing arm was greater by 35% in men and 28% in women compared with control site.
Huddleston 1980	Tennis (lifetime)	M	70-84 (range)	35	BMC of forearm by SPA	Mean BMC 13% higher in playing than nonplaying arm.
Haapasalo et al. 1996	Tennis (competitive)	M F F	25 19 43	17 30 20	BMD of humerus by DXA	Young men and women: significantly greater values in BMD, BMC, and cortical wall thickness in playing vs. nonplaying arm in tennis players and compared to controls.
	Control	M F F	25 21 39	16 25 16		Older women: significant difference but smaller than for young.
Haapasalo et al. 1998	Tennis	F	9.4-15.5 (different Tanner Stage)	91	BMD of lumbar spine, humerus, and radius by DXA	1. In tennis players: BMD differences were significantly greater in the playing vs. nonplaying arm at all Tanner Stages (mean difference 1.6-15.7%). 2. In controls: mean difference –0.2 to 4.6% but significant at some humerus sites. 3. Players vs. control: difference (arms) significant at growth spurt (Tanner Stage III). Difference in lumbar spine significant at Tanner Stage IV. 4. Nonloaded, nondominant distal radius: no difference between players and controls at any Tanner Stage.
	Control	F	9.4-15.4 (different Tanner Stage)	58		
Kannus et al. 1995	Tennis and squash Controls	F F	28 27	105 50	BMC of radius, humerus, and calcaneus	Compared to controls, the players had significantly larger side-to-side differences at all measured sites.
Heinonen et al. 1993	Weightlifters Orienteers Cross-country skiers Cyclists Controls	F F F F F	25 23 21 24 23	18 30 28 29 25	BMD of lumbar spine, femur, patella, tibia, calcaneus, distal radius by DXA	Weightlifters had significantly higher BMD than controls at all sites except femoral neck and calcaneus. Orienteers had higher BMD than controls at distal femur and proximal tibia. Compared with other athlete groups, the weightlifters had higher BMD in lumbar spine, distal femur, patella, and distal radius.
Heinrich et al. 1990	Swimmers Collegiate runners Recreational runners Bodybuilders (weightlifting) Controls	F F F F F	22 20 30 26 25	13 5 11 11 18	BMC of lumbar spine and femur by DPA; forearm by SPA	BMC of bodybuilders significantly greater than in swimmers, collegiate and recreational runners, and controls.

Nilsson and Westlin 1971	Athletes: Weightlifters Throwers Runners Soccer players Swimmers Controls: Exercising Nonexercising	 M M M M M M M	 21 24 22 25 18 23 23	 11 4 25 15 9 24 15	BMD in distal end of femur by photon absorption method	Athletes had significantly denser femurs than nonathletes. BMD decreased with decreasing load. No difference between swimmers and controls. In controls, exercise group had significantly higher BMD than nonexercisers.
Gleeson et al. 1990	Weightlifting (modified Nautilus weightlifting program) Controls	F F	33 33	34 38	BMD of lumbar spine by DPA, and os calcis by SPA	BMD lumbar spine: weightlifters +0.8% ; controls –0.5%. No difference in os calcis.
Slemenda and Johnston 1993	Figure skaters Controls	F F	18 16	22 22	Total body bone mineral by DXA	Skaters had significantly higher BMD in legs and pelvis. BMD similar at upper body sites.
Karlsson et al. 1993a	Professional ballet dancers	M F	40 36	17 25	Total body and regional BMD by DXA, and BMD of forearm by SPA	Male dancers had higher BMD in femoral neck ($p < .05$). Female dancers had higher BMD in all hip measurements and in the legs ($p < .05$).
	Controls	M F	Age and sex matched to dancers	17 25		
Young et al. 1994	Ballet dancers Controls: Regular menses Amenorrhea/anorexia nervosa	F F F	17 17 18	44 23 18	Total body and regional BMD by DXA	Total body BMD and proximal femur sites in dancers similar to those in girls with regular menses and higher than in girls with anorexia nervosa ($p < .05$). Lumbar spine and non-weight bearing sites: BMD in dancers similar to that for anorexia nervosa. When corrected for weight, BMD at weight-bearing sites was higher in the dancers than in girls with normal menses ($p < .01$).
Conroy et al. 1993	Elite junior Olympic weightlifters Controls (no weightlifting)	M M	17 17	25 11	BMD of lumbar spine and proximal femur by DXA	BMD significantly higher in weightlifters at all sites compared to age-matched controls and adult reference range.
Virvidakis et al. 1990	Junior competitive weightlifters Controls (normal physical activity)	M M	15-20 (range) Age matched	59 91	BMC of forearm by SPA	BMC of distal and proximal forearm significantly greater in weightlifters.

(continued)

Table 15.1 *(continued)*

Author	Type of exercise program	Sex	Age mean (years)	Number of subjects	Bone measurement	Results
Hamdy et al. 1994	Weightlifting Running/jogging Cross-training (weightlifting and aerobic exercise) Recreational exercise	M M M M	27 29 31 28	11 12 8 9	BMC and BMD of lumbar spine and proximal femur by DPA	Upper limb BMD significantly greater in weightlifters compared to runners and recreational exercisers: similar to that in cross-trained athletes. No differences in spine or proximal femur.
Smith and Rutherford 1993	Rowing Triathletes Sedentary controls	M M M	21 29 22	12 8 13	BMD of lumbar spine and total body by DXA	Rowers: higher BMD of spine ($p < .01$) and total body ($p < .05$) compared to triathletes and controls. No difference in spine and total body BMD between triathletes and controls. Rowers: higher BMD of arms compared to controls ($p < .01$) but not triathletes.
Khan et al. 1996	Ballet dancers (retired) Controls	F F	51 52	101 101	BMD of lumbar spine, wrist, proximal femur, and total body by DXA	Dancers vs. controls: no difference in BMD at spine or hip. Lower BMD at ultradistal and mid-third radius in dancers ($p < .05$). No difference in the proportion of dancers and controls with osteopenia or osteoporosis (World Health Organization criteria).
Robinson et al. 1995	Gymnasts Runners Controls (exercise <3 hr/wk)	F F F	20 22 19	21 20 19	BMD of lumbar spine, femoral neck, total body by DXA	Oligo- and amenorrhea: gymnasts 47%; runners 30%; controls 0% BMD lumbar spine: lower ($p = .0001$) in runners compared to both gymnasts and controls BMD femoral neck: differed among all groups ($p = .0001$), gymnasts > controls > runners BMD total body: lower in runners compared to gymnasts and controls ($p < .01$)
Drinkwater et al. 1984	Athletes: runners and crew (amenorrheic) Athletes: runners and crew (eumenorrheic)	F F	25 26	14 14	BMD of lumbar spine by DPA, and radius by SPA	BMD of lumbar spine lower in amenorrheic athletes ($p < .01$). No difference in 2 radius sites.
Drinkwater et al. 1986	Athletes: runners and crew (amenorrheic who regained menses) Athletes: runners and crew (eumenorrheic) Athletes: runners and crew (amenorrheic)	F F F	28 28 ±28	7 7 2	BMD of lumbar spine by DPA, and radius by SPA	Regained menses group had an increase in BMD of spine of 6.2% ($p < .01$). Eumenorrheic group: no change. Amenorrheic group ($n = 2$) lost bone (–3.4%). No significant difference in radius.

Fisher et al. 1986	*Runners:* Amenorrheic Eumenorrheic	 F F	 25 30	 11 24	BMC of lumbar spine by DPA, and radius by SPA	BMD of spine: eumenorrheic > amenorrheic ($p = .02$). BMD of radius: no difference.
Marcus et al. 1985	*Elite distance runners:* Cyclic menses Amenorrhea Controls (nonathletes)	 F F F	 24 20 Similar to above	 6 11	BMD of lumbar spine by CT, and radius by SPA	BMD of spine: cyclic > amenorrhea ($p < .02$); controls > amenorrhea ($p < .05$). BMD of fore-arm: no difference.
Rencken et al. 1996	*Runners:* Amenorrheic Eumenorrheic	 F F	 26 26	 29 20	BMD of lumbar spine, proximal and shaft of femur, tibia, and fibula by DXA	BMD was lower in amenorrheic group at the lumbar spine, proximal femur sites, femoral shaft, and tibia ($p < .01$). No difference at fibula.
Myburgh et al. 1993	*Runners:* Amenorrheic Eumenorrheic	 F F	 29 28	 12 9	BMD of lumbar spine, proximal femur, total body by DXA, and radius by SPA	BMD was lower in the amenorrheic group at the lumbar spine, whole body, proximal femur sites, femoral shaft ($p < .05 – p < .005$). No difference at midradius and tibial shaft.
Fehling et al. 1995	*High impact:* Volleyball Gymnasts Active loading: Swimmers Controls (exercise <1 hr/wk)	 F F F F	 20 20 20 21	 8 13 7 17	BMD of lumbar spine, proximal femur, and total body by DXA	Impact group (volleyball and gymnasts) had greater BMD at lumbar spine, femoral neck, Ward's triangle, total body, legs, pelvis compared to active loading (swimming) and controls ($p < .05$). Gymnasts had greater BMD compared to all groups at right and left arm sites. No difference at any site between swimmers and controls.
Taaffe et al. 1997	*Cohort I (8 months):* Gymnasts Runners Controls (exercise <3 hr/wk) *Cohort II (12 months):* Gymnasts Swimmers Controls (exercise <3 hr/wk)	 F F F F F F	 20 21 20 19 20 19	 26 36 14 8 11 11	BMD of lumbar spine, femoral neck, and total body by DXA	Gymnasts from both cohorts had significant increases in BMD of the lumbar spine and femoral neck. Gymnasts from both cohorts had significantly greater increases in BMD than the other athletes or controls at the spine ($p < .01$) and compared to the other athletes at the femoral neck ($p < .05$). No difference among groups for change in whole body BMD.

(continued)

Table 15.1 *(continued)*

Author	Type of exercise program	Sex	Age mean (years)	Number of subjects	Bone measurement	Results
Heinonen et al. 1995	Aerobic dancers Squash players Speed skaters Controls (physically active) Controls (sedentary)	F F F F F	28 25 21 23 24	27 18 14 25 25	BMD lumbar spine, femur, patella, calcaneus, distal radius by DXA	Squash players had highest weight-adjusted BMD at all sites. Compared with sedentary controls: • Squash players had significantly higher BMD at lumbar spine (13.8%), femoral neck (16.8%), proximal tibia (12.6%), calcaneus (18.5%). • Aerobic dancers had significantly higher BMD at femoral neck (8.5%), proximal tibia (5.5%), calcaneus (13.6%), but significantly lower BMD in distal radius (–7.8%). • Speed skaters had significantly higher BMD at distal femur (7.2%). • No difference between physically active and sedentary controls in BMD at any site.
Hetland et al. 1993	Long-distance runners (>100 km/wk) Controls (≤5 km/wk) All subjects (0-160 km/wk)	M M M	32 31 32	22 12 120	BMC and BMD of lumbar spine, proximal femur, total body by DXA, and forearm by SPA	Long-distance runners had a significantly lower BMC in the lumbar spine, proximal femur, distal forearm, and total body than nonrunners. BMC of lumbar spine correlated negatively with weekly distance runners ($p < .0001$) and was 19% lower than in nonrunners. A similar relationship at other sites except femoral neck.
MacDougall et al. 1992	Runners: 5-10 mi/wk 15-20 mi/wk 25-30 mi/wk 40-55 mi/wk 60-75 mi/wk Controls (nonactive)	 M M M M M M	 28 29 28 30 36 33	 5 11 12 9 16 22	BMD of whole body and regions by DPA	BMD in lower legs was significantly higher ($p < .05$) in the 15-20 mi/wk group than in 5-10 mi/wk group or control. Cross-sectional area of tibia and fibula normalized to body weight tended to be larger with increasing mileage; 40-50 mi/wk significantly greater than control. No other differences in BMD.
Bilanin et al. 1989	Long-distance runners (>64 km/wk) Controls (nonrunners)	M M	29 27	13 11	BMD of lumbar spine and midtibia by DPA, and midradius by SPA	BMD of spine significantly lower in runners than nonrunners ($p < .05$). No difference between groups in tibia or radial BMD.
Aloia et al. 1978	Marathon runners Controls	M M	42 45	30 16	BMC of radius by SPA	No difference between groups.

Williams et al. 1984	Long-distance runners (9-month study): Consistent runners (mean 141 km/month) Inconsistent runners (mean 65 km/month) Controls (nonrunners)	 M M M	 48 50 47	 7 13 10	BMC of os calcis by SPA	"Consistent" runners but not "inconsistent" runners showed significant increase in BMC over controls.
Klesges et al. 1986	Basketball	M	20	11	BMC of total body and regions by DXA	From preseason to late summer, overall decrease of 6.1% in total BMC and 10.5% decrease in BMC of the legs.
Kontulainen et al. 2003	Tennis and squash: Young starters Old starters Controls	 F F F	 27 44 34	 36 28 27	BMD and bone strength by peripheral CT and DXA of humeral shafts and distal radius	Compared to controls, the players had significantly larger side-by-side differences, which were greatest in the young starters (before menarche).
Bass et al. 2002	Tennis: Prepuberty Peri-puberty Postpuberty	 F F F	 10 12 15	 17 11 19	BMC and humeral dimensions using DXA and MRI	BMC and resistance to torsion were 11-14% greater in the loaded arm than nonloaded arm in prepubertal players with no further increase in the other groups.
Flodgren et al. 1999	Kayaking Controls	M, F M, F	19 19	10 20	BMD total body, subregions, lumbar spine, proximal femur by DXA	Kayakers had significantly higher BMD in upper body sites.
Pettersson et al. 2000a	Cross-country skiers Controls	F F	16 16	16 16	BMD total body, subregions, lumbar spine, proximal femur by DXA	Compared with controls, the cross-country skiers had significantly higher BMD in the humerus, femoral neck, femur diaphysis.
Pettersson et al. 2000b	Competitive rope-skipping Soccer Controls	F F F	18 17 18	10 15 25	BMD total body, subregions, lumbar spine, proximal femur by DXA	Rope-skippers had 22% higher BMD at ultradistal site compared to control. Both high-activity groups had higher BMD at most loaded sites.
Sandstrom et al. 2000	Ice hockey Controls	F F	22 22	14 14	BMD total body, subregions including head, lumbar spine, proximal femur by DXA	Compared to controls, the ice hockey players had significantly higher BMD at all sites except the head.
Soderman et al. 2000	Soccer Controls	F F	16 16	51 41	BMD total body, subregions, lumbar spine, proximal femur by DXA	Compared with nonactive controls, the soccer players had significantly higher BMD of total body, lumbar spine, and multiple regions of hip.

BMC = bone mineral content; BMD = bone mineral density; CT = computerized tomography; DPA = dual photon absorptiometry; DXA = dual X-ray absorptiometry; MRI = magnetic resonance imaging; SPA = single photon absorptiometry.

was significantly higher than in nonexercising controls or in swimmers or runners who followed nonresistance exercise programs (Heinrich et al. 1990).

Resistance exercise comes in many forms. Slemenda and Johnston (1993) reported that 22 young female competitive skaters (ages 10-23), despite being thinner and having more oligomenorrhea or amenorrhea, had significantly greater skeletal densities compared to nonskaters in the lower part of the skeleton (pelvis and legs) and had similar densities at upper body sites. Karlsson et al. (1993a) measured BMD in 42 professional ballet dancers (17 men and 25 women), 28 of whom were still actively performing. After correcting for differences in body mass index, they found a significantly higher BMD in the lower extremities of female dancers and in the femoral neck of male dancers. In those dancers with a history of more than one year of amenorrhea, however, BMD of the spine was 7% lower than in the menstruating dancers.

Significant bone loss, along with menstrual irregularities and hypogonadism, often accompanies intense training programs or anorexia nervosa (AN) in young women. Young et al. (1994) studied the interrelationships of exercise, hypogonadism, and body weight in 44 female ballet dancers (mean age 17 years), 23 girls of comparable age with regular menstrual cycles (the controls), and 18 sedentary amenorrheic girls with AN. The total bone density in the dancers was similar to the controls and higher than that in girls with AN. At weight-bearing sites (proximal femoral), dancers had bone density higher than girls with AN ($p < .01$), and similar to controls, yet higher values compared to controls after adjustment for body weight. At non-weight-bearing sites (ribs, arms, and skull), on the other hand, dancers had BMD similar to the girls with AN and lower than the controls. After correction for age and weight, BMD did not differ from normal at non-weightbearing sites in the dancers, or in the girls with anorexia nervosa. The authors suggest that weight-bearing exercise may offset the effects of hypogonadism at predominantly cortical weight-bearing sites such as the proximal femur. While non-weightbearing sites and weight-bearing sites containing substantial trabecular bone may benefit little from weight-bearing exercise, they still benefit significantly by maintenance of body weight (figure 15.1).

BMD in 101 retired elite female ballet dancers (mean age 51 years, mean time since retirement 25.6 years) was lower than that of controls at non-weightbearing sites (ultra-distal and mid-third radius) but no different from that of controls at weight-bearing sites (hip and spine) in a study by Khan et al. (1996); the latter finding is particularly interesting, since in their youth the dancers had multiple risk factors for osteoporosis including greater prevalence of menstrual disturbances, greater lifetime alcohol intake, more smoking, and a lower calcium intake in adolescence. The retired dancers currently performed twice as much exercise as the controls. Note, however, that dancers who had experienced significant menstrual disturbance during their dancing years had 8% lower BMD of the lumbar spine, and 10%

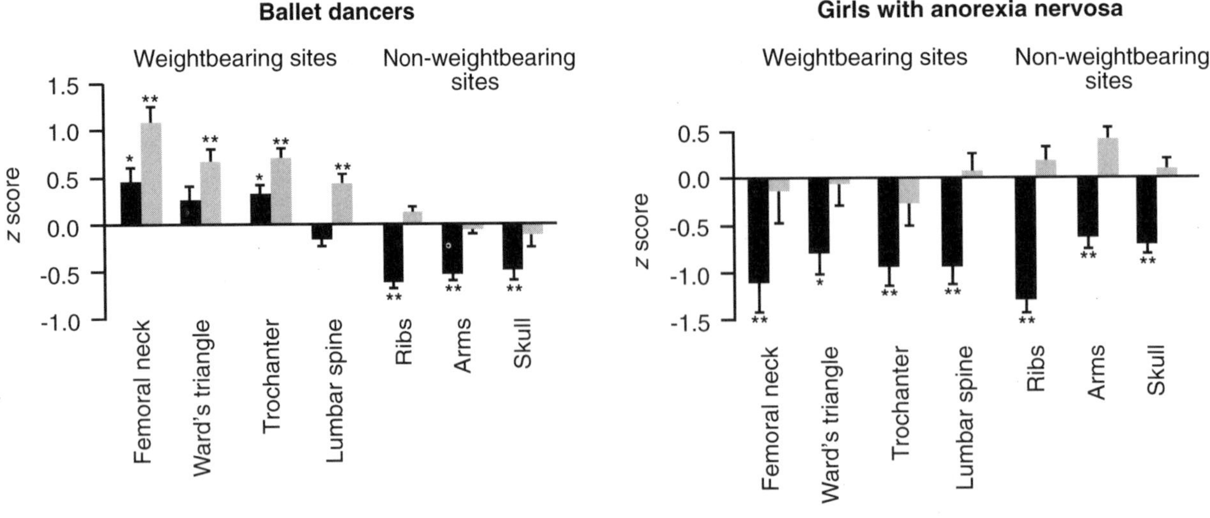

Figure 15.1 Bone density (mean ± SEM) expressed as a z score adjusted for age alone (■) and for both age and weight (■) in ballet dancers and girls with anorexia nervosa. In dancers, the z scores were normal or increased at weight-bearing sites and were reduced at non-weight-bearing sites before, but not after, adjustment for body weight. The z scores were negative at all sites in girls with anorexia nervosa before, but not after, adjustment for body weight. * $p < .05$, ** $p < .01$ (compared to zero).

lower BMD of the ultra-distal radius ($p < .05$), than their eumenorrheic-matched controls.

Gymnasts can achieve ground reaction forces as much as 18 times body weight (Taaffe et al. 1995). Robinson and colleagues (1995) studied bone mass and oligomenorrhea and amenorrhea in two groups of competitive female athletes with different skeletal loading patterns. They reported that, despite a similar prevalence of oligo- and amenorrhea, gymnasts had higher BMD than runners at the lumbar spine, proximal femur, and whole body, and higher BMD than controls at the femoral neck. Thus, high-impact exercises to the extent seen in female gymnasts may protect against bone loss associated with menstrual abnormalities.

Many young female athletes fit the female athlete triad characterized by disordered eating, menstrual dysfunction, and osteoporosis (West 1998). Drinkwater and coworkers (1984) observed that young amenorrheic athletes had decreased vertebral (but not radial) BMD compared to that of athletes with regular cycles. A follow-up study (Drinkwater et al. 1986) reported that six of the seven original amenorrheic athletes who resumed menses had a marked increase of vertebral BMD in 14.4 months. Fisher et al. (1986) reported that BMC of the lumbar spine was lower in amenorrheic runners, but positively correlated with estradiol levels in all women. Marcus et al. (1985) studied 11 elite women distance runners, mean age 20 years, with secondary amenorrhea. They found BMD of the lumbar spine in this group to be lower than that in similar runners with normal menstrual cycles and in age-matched nonathlete controls, but higher than in runners with secondary amenorrhea and less physical activity. Thus, although intense exercise may reduce the impact of amenorrhea on bone mass, these runners are still at high risk for exercise-related fractures. In a study of 49 female athletes (primarily runners), Rencken and colleagues (1996) compared bone loss at multiple skeletal sites in 49 women runners with either amenorrhea or normal menstrual cycles. Amenorrheic athletes had significantly lower BMD at the lumbar spine and at multiple areas of the proximal femur, the femoral shaft, and tibia including those sites that were subjected to impact loading during exercise. Myburgh et al. (1993) also reported significantly lower BMD in axial and appendicular sites in amenorrheic runners.

Several researchers have studied different loading exercises and training programs in collegiate female athletes. Fehling and colleagues (1995) compared BMD of collegiate female athletes who competed in impact-loading sports (volleyball and gymnastics) with that of athletes who participated in an active loading sport (swimmers), and also with nonathlete controls. The impact-loading group had significantly greater BMD at the lumbar spine, femoral neck, Ward's triangle, and total body compared to the active loading and control groups. Furthermore, oligomenorrhea and amenorrhea in the gymnastics group did not negatively affect BMD, supporting evidence that high magnitudes of mechanical loading may offset the detrimental effect of hormone deficiency. This is another example of the importance of site specificity in exercise programs. Taaffe et al. (1997) found comparable results. After either 8 or 12 months of training, the gymnasts (high-impact loading) in two separate studies had significant increases in BMD at the lumbar spine and femoral neck, compared to runners, swimmers, and controls. Again, these increases were independent of reproductive hormone status (figure 15.2).

Heinonen et al. (1995) examined 59 Finnish female athletes representing three sports with different skeletal

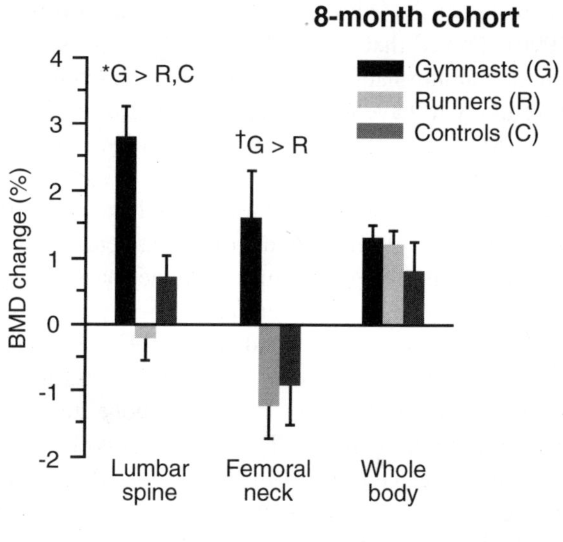

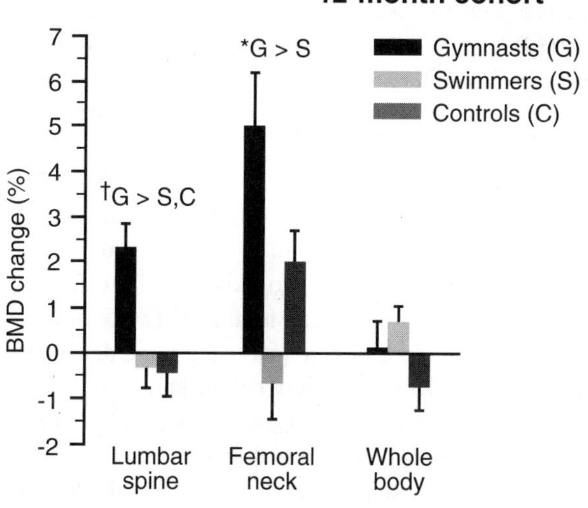

Figure 15.2 Percent change in lumbar spine, femoral neck, and whole-body BMD for 8-month and 12-month cohorts. * $p < .001$, † $p < .01$. Values are mean ± SEM.

From D. Taaffe et al., 1995, "High-impact exercise promotes bone gain in well-trained female athletes," *Journal of Bone Mineral Research* 12:255-260. Reprinted with permission of the American Society for Bone and Mineral Research.

loading (aerobic dancers, squash players, speed skaters). The highest BMD values were in sites receiving the highest impact, supporting the concept that high strain rates and high peak stresses are more effective in enhancing bone formation than low-force repetitions. Many other investigators have reported higher BMD in various sports at site-specific regions receiving very high skeletal loading. These include upper body sites in kayaking (Flodgren et al. 1999), arms and hip in cross-country skiing (Pettersson et al. 2000a), wrist and lower extremity in rope skipping (Pettersson et al. 2000b), most sites in ice hockey players (Sandstrom et al. 2000), and spine and hip in soccer players (Soderman et al. 2000).

Intensive training and exercise programs may also lead to skeletal problems. As noted previously, female athletes who have menstrual abnormalities may have low bone density. Moreover, Myburgh and coworkers (1990) showed that in athletes (mainly runners) with similar training habits, those with stress fractures are more likely to have lower bone density, lower dietary calcium intake, current menstrual irregularity, and lower contraceptive use.

The impact of intensive exercise and training programs has also been studied in male athletes. Investigating the impact of running on bone mass in 120 healthy physically active men (ages 19-56 years) who ran 0 to 160 km/week, Hetland et al. (1993) found that long distance runners had a lower bone mass at the spine, femur, and forearm, and higher bone turnover, than nonrunning controls. There was no evidence of gonadal failure in this group. In fact, lumbar BMC which was negatively correlated with the distance run weekly was 19% lower in the elite runners than in the healthy, active, but nonrunning controls. While Bilanin et al. (1989) observed a similar phenomenon, in this case that vertebral BMD was 9.7% lower in 13 male long distance runners than in controls, other data are contradictory: Aloia and colleagues (1978) found no difference in BMC of the radius in marathon runners; Williams et al. (1984) reported that BMC of the os calcis increased during a nine-month marathon training program; and MacDougall et al. (1992) found no BMD differences at multiple sites between male runners (5-75 miles/wk) and controls, although the lower leg bone density was higher in the 15 to 20 mile/week group.

A report by Klesges and coworkers (1996) illustrates how complicated this question is. These investigators measured BMC and calcium intake/losses in 11 members of a college Division I-A male basketball team. From preseason to late summer (approximately 11 months), total BMC decreased 6.1% and BMC of the legs decreased 10.5%, with dermal calcium losses of 422 mg per training session. Calcium supplementation was associated with increases in BMC. The authors concluded that bone loss is related to calcium intake, and that exercise is positively related to BMC but only if calcium intake is sufficient to offset dermal loss. Although this study was very small, its implications are significant, demonstrating the need for more extensive investigation into the changes occurring within intensive training programs.

Childhood and Adolescence

Although osteoporosis is considered a disease of the elderly, predisposition for it begins in childhood and adolescence. It is extremely important to attain the maximal amount of bone at skeletal maturity (peak bone mass), which typically occurs by the end of late adolescence (Bonjour et al. 1991; Matkovic et al. 1994) although slight increases in bone mass may occur after this. The major determinant of peak bone mass is genetic, contributing up to 70% to 80% of the variability. Environmental factors, including nutrition and exercise, are important for the remaining 20% to 30% (Recker et al. 1992; Slemenda et al. 1991).

In a prospective study of 59 pairs of white monozygotic twins (ages 5-14 years), Slemenda and coworkers (1991) investigated the influence of physical activity on BMD in children by using questionnaires filled out separately by the children and their mothers. Total time spent in weight-bearing activity was significantly related to BMD in the radius and hip, independently of age or gender. A weaker, yet still positive correlation was present for the lumbar spine. Increases in peak skeletal mass may carry through into adulthood and ultimately lessen the incidence of osteoporotic fractures. Zanker et al. (2003) measured BMD in 20 gymnasts and 20 untrained children (10 male and 10 female in each group) ages 7 to 8 years. Significant differences of 8% to 10% were observed between female gymnasts and untrained girls in the spine, arm, and total body with trends toward higher BMD within the pelvis and legs. Thus, gymnastics training before the age of 7 can enhance acquisition of bone mass, with the magnitude linked to cumulative volume of training. This would be very important if the increase can be maintained into adulthood.

In a three-year longitudinal study, Nurmi-Lawton (2004) followed 45 gymnasts (ages 8-17 years) and 52 normally active controls. They used quantitative ultrasound (QUS) and DXA and reported that the gymnasts had significantly higher QUS and axial and appendicular BMC and BMD across puberty. The gymnasts had up to 24% to 51% higher BMC and 13% to 28% higher BMD depending on skeletal site, thus showing that sustained impact loading exercise can continue throughout puberty.

In a cross-sectional study by Bass and colleagues (1998), BMD was measured in 45 active prepubertal female gymnasts (mean age 10 years), 36 retired female gymnasts (mean age 25 years), and controls for each group. Bone mineral density in the active prepubertal gymnasts was 0.7 to 1.9 SD higher at the weight-bearing sites than in controls and increased as the duration of training increased. During 12 months, the increases in BMD of the total body, spine, and legs in the active prepubertal gymnasts was 30% to 85% greater than in prepubertal controls. In the retired gymnasts, the BMD was 0.5 to 1.5 SD higher than in controls at weight-bearing sites (figure 15.3). There was no diminution of BMD during the 20 years after retirement (mean 8 years), despite lower frequency and intensity of exercise. Thus, increases in bone density in the prepubertal years may have long-term effects into adulthood.

In a nine-month controlled trial of high-impact exercises in 25 premenarcheal and 39 postmenarcheal girls, Heinonen et al. (2000) reported that bone gain above that attributed to growth itself could be obtained in exercising premenarcheal girls but not postmenarcheal girls, supporting the concept that the premenarcheal period is a critical time for additional bone mineral acquisition. In a 26-week randomized study of 32 postmenarcheal adolescent girls, resistance training produced increases in motor strength, as well as a trend toward a transient increase in spine BMD at 13 weeks but not at 26 weeks (Blimkie et al. 1996).

A seven- to nine-month jumping intervention program showed improvements in BMD, bone structure, and strength in prepubescent children (Fuchs et al. 2001), prepubertal boys (MacKelvie et al. 2002), pre- and early-pubertal girls (McKay et al. 2000; Petit et al. 2002; MacKelvie et al. 2001), and adolescent girls (Witzke and Snow 2000). In a single-blind prospective, randomized controlled 8.5-month study in 66 pre- and early-pubertal girls (mean age 8.8 years), a moderate-impact or low-impact (control) exercise program was assessed with or without calcium supplementation (Iuliano-Burns et al. 2003). Greater gains in bone mass at loaded sites were achieved when short bursts of moderate exercise were combined with increased dietary calcium. The former conferred region-specific effects and the latter produced generalized effects.

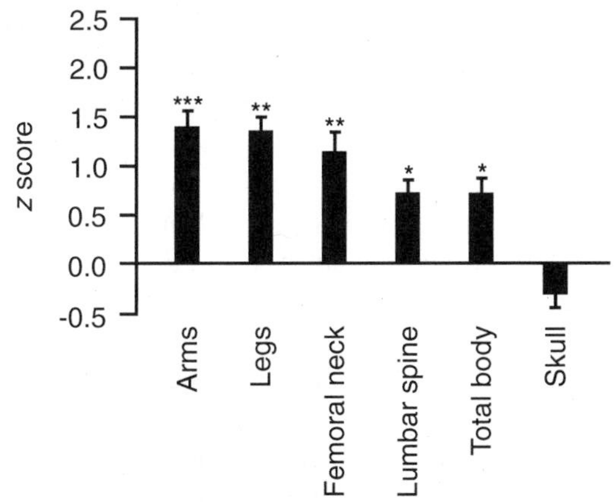

Figure 15.3 Cross-sectional data showing regional areal bone density expressed as a *z* score in retired female gymnasts. The *z* scores were higher than the predicted mean value in controls (represented by zero) at each site except the skull. * $p < .05$, ** $p < .01$, *** $p < .001$ compared to zero.

From S. Bass et al., "Exercise before puberty may confer residual benefits in bone density in adulthood: Studies in active prepubertal and retired female gymnasts," *Journal of Bone Mineral Research* 1998: 13:500-507l. Reprinted with permission from the American Society for Bone and Mineral Research.

In 101 women ages 20 to 35 years, McCulloch et al. (1990) reported that the mean bone density of the os calcis was significantly higher for those who participated in any kind of organized sport or fitness programs as children. Following 84 males and 98 females longitudinally from age 13 until age 28, however, Welten et al. (1994) found that only weight-bearing activity and body weight contributed significantly to lumbar BMD at age 27. Weight-bearing activity was the best predictor of BMD in males, and body weight was the best predictor in females. Greendale and coworkers (1995) investigated the association between BMD and lifetime physical activity in 1703 adults (mean age 73); she found that, although current and lifetime exercise (including during the teen years) was positively associated with BMD of the hip, it did not protect against fractures.

Cooper et al. (1995) reported that growth and physical activity in childhood were important determinants of peak bone mass in 21-year-old women (n = 153), suggesting that growth may primarily determine the size of the skeletal envelope, while activity modulates the mineral density within the skeletal envelope. Slemenda and colleagues (1994), following 90 children (ages 6-14 years) for three years, also described physical activity as a significant predictor of BMD at all skeletal sites in the prepubertal group. Prepubertal children in the highest activity quartile had 4% to 7% greater rates of mineralization than those in the lowest activity group. In contrast, Kroger et al. (1993) observed increases in BMD during adolescence but no significant relationship between physical activity and the increment rate of bone density. These studies generally underline the importance of physical activity in childhood and adolescence, in achieving the highest peak bone mass.

Young Adult and Premenopausal Women

Although most bone mass accumulates by age 17 to 18, additional small increases in bone mass may occur in young adults after linear bone growth has stopped. Rodin et al. (1990) reported a 5% increase in spinal bone density in premenopausal women between the age groups 18 to 22 and 33 to 37 ($p < .03$).

After following 156 healthy young adult women (ages 18-26 years) for up to five years, Recker et al. (1992) observed that the median gain in bone mass for the third decade of life was 4.8% for the forearm, 6.8% for lumbar BMD, and 12.5% for total body bone mineral. The rate of gain in spinal bone density was negatively correlated with age, but positively correlated with levels of physical activity as well as calcium intake. The authors suggest that lifestyle changes among college-aged women involving relatively modest increases in physical activity and calcium intake could effect a significant long-term reduction in the later risk of osteoporosis.

There are at present too many confounding factors in published research heterogeneity of populations, varying levels of exercise (both in intensity and loading stresses to specific bones), variability in methods for measuring bone density, and variability in the designs of research projects to permit an unambiguous claim that physical activity and exercise increase bone mass in young adult women. Despite the difficulties in interpreting these studies, however, several general principles are emerging. In particular: (1) there appears to be a positive correlation between activity level and BMD; and (2) activities that deliver high loads to specific bones appear most beneficial.

The effect of physical activity and exercise may vary with the groups studied. The previous sections addressed the effects of activity and exercise on the growing skeleton in childhood and adolescence. Another group to look at is young adult and premenopausal women. (Review articles of randomized and nonrandomized trials include Vuori 2001; Wolff et al. 1999; Kelley et al. 2001; and Wallace and Cumming 2000.)

Cross-Sectional Studies

Perhaps the best way to look at the data is to divide the studies into cross-sectional and interventional studies (Bouxsein and Marcus 1994; Ernst 1998; Gutin and Kasper 1992; Kelly et al. 2001; Marcus et al. 1992; Snow et al. 1996; Vuori 2001; Wallace and Cumming 2000; Wolff et al. 1999).

As discussed on pages 223-232, unilateral exercise programs have shown that tennis and racquetball players have higher bone mass in their dominant compared with nondominant arms. In addition, elite athletes and long-term exercisers have greater bone mass than nonexercisers, particularly at sites undergoing the greatest mechanical loading. In gymnasts, in fact, high-impact loads at the hip from tumbling and dismounting may override the potential deleterious effects on bone of low gonadal function (Robinson et al. 1995).

Less clear, however, is the effect of less intense recreational sports activities and regular physical activity on bone mass. Aloia et al. (1988) measured physical activity in 24 healthy premenopausal women (mean age 39) using a motion sensor worn at the waist. Total physical activity levels were significantly correlated with BMD of the spine and with total body calcium, but not with BMD of the radius. In 161 healthy Asian women (ages 19-25 years), Hirota and colleagues (1992) found that those with the longest prior history of physical activity had the highest radial BMD. Lifetime physical activity correlated with BMD at the radius for 181 premenopausal women (ages 20-50 years) surveyed by Halioua and Anderson (1989). Davee et al. (1990) studied 27 premenopausal women (ages 20-30 years) with different long-term exercise programs. Those who supplemented aerobic exercise with muscle-building activities for more than one hour per week had higher spine densities than those who were sedentary or who participated in aerobic exercises only. In addition, IGF-1 (insulin-like growth factor) levels were greatest in that group and correlated with hours of muscle building per week. In 38 premenopausal women (ages 24-28 years), Metz and colleagues (1993) found that 90 minutes of moderate physical activity weekly correlated positively with radial BMD.

Others have not found similar results. Kirk and colleagues (1989) studied 10 premenopausal female recreational runners who ran more than 20 miles/week for at least two years. The generally higher vertebral bone density in younger runners vs. sedentary controls was not statistically significant, although there was a significant positive correlation between vertebral bone density and physical fitness as assessed by $\dot{V}O_2$max. Jacobson and colleagues (1984) reported that a group of athletic women aged 20 to 40 years had higher BMD than controls at the radius and lumbar spine. Picard et al. (1988) found no differences in BMC between a low-exercise and high-exercise group of women, aged 40 to 50 years, who followed their usual exercise pattern. For two years, Mazess and Barden (1991) followed 300 premenopausal women (ages 20-39 years), assessing activity with pedometer and accelerometer measurements over 48-hour periods. They found no relationship between current physical activity and bone density at several sites. In a study using peripheral quantitative computerized tomography, physical activity did not preserve bone density in the non-weight-bearing radius in premenopausal women but was beneficial at the weight-bearing tibia. The effects became more apparent in the postmenopausal group (Uusi-Rasi et al. 2002).

In summary: based on cross-sectional studies, there appears to be no clear-cut relationship between current activity status and bone status in moderately active people.

Intervention Studies

Prospective and (especially) randomized studies provide the clearest way to determine the effects of any intervention.

NONRANDOMIZED STUDIES

The intensity and specificity of exercises may be most important. In a nonrandomized controlled 12-month study, Gleeson and coworkers (1990) compared 34 premenopausal women (mean age 33) who followed a modified Nautilus weightlifting program lasting 30 minutes three times per week with 34 matched controls. The weightlifting group had a nonsignificant increase in mean lumbar BMD; but when matched to the controls, which showed a small decrease, the difference between the groups was significant ($p < .05$). There was no difference in BMD of the os calcis. A more dramatic effect of weightlifting may not have occurred because (1) in contrast to the young elite weightlifters, these subjects' skeletons had stopped growing; or perhaps (2) the resistance exercises were not sufficiently strenuous. Smith et al. (1989) conducted a four-year nonrandomized aerobic and upper-body strength program in 142 (62 control and 80 exercise) pre- and postmenopausal women (mean age 50 years). Regardless of menopausal status, the exercise group who participated in 45 minutes of physical activity 3 days/week lost significantly less bone than controls in the radius, ulna, and humerus. In a 10-year longitudinal study from Amsterdam, 225 males and 241 females (ages 27-36 years) had lumbar bone density and two aspects of physical activity (mechanical and metabolic) measured (Bakker et al. 2003). Over a 10-year period, a positive correlation was found between physical activity expressed in terms of biomechanical ground reaction forces and lumbar BMD in males but not females, although in females a significant relationship was found for the first six years. A nonlinear relationship between the metabolic component of physical activity and lumbar BMD was found for both males and females, suggesting a metabolic threshold at which extra physical activity may be ineffective.

Winters and Snow (2000) studied 29 premenopausal women (ages 30-45 years) on a 12-month progressive impact (jump) plus lower body resistance training program. When compared to controls, the exercise group had a significant increase in BMD at the greater trochanter and showed a borderline increase at the femoral neck, but also had a 13% to 15% increase in strength and power. However, the positive benefits of impact plus resistance training were lost over a six-month period when training was withdrawn. Thus, continued training, even at a lower intensity, may be necessary to maintain the benefit of exercise.

In contrast to the previous positive studies, Rockwell et al. (1990) compared 10 premenopausal women (mean age 36 years) in a weightlifting program with seven sedentary women (mean age 40 years). After nine months of weight training aimed at loading the axial skeleton and strengthening large muscle groups, the exercise group had a 4% decrease in lumbar BMD while the control group did not lose bone. No significant change in femoral density occurred in either group.

RANDOMIZED STUDIES

Several researchers have conducted randomized intervention exercise studies in young women.

In an eight-month intervention trial, Snow-Harter and colleagues (1992) randomly assigned 52 healthy college-aged women (mean age 19.9 years) to a control group, to a group that jogged three times weekly, or to a weightlifting group. Lumbar spine BMD showed small but significant increases of 1.2% in the weight training and 1.3% in the jogging groups. Proximal femur BMD did not change in any group. More prolonged loading of the hip may be needed for increases in BMD to occur.

Bassey and Ramsdale (1994) reported that after six months, 14 young women in a high-impact exercise program (mean age 32) had a significant increase of 3.4% in trochanteric BMD compared with 13 women in a low-impact control group (mean age 30). In the second six months, the control group crossed over to the high-impact exercise and subsequently showed a significant increase of 4.1% in trochanteric BMD. Spinal BMD did not change. Heinonen et al. (1996) studied 98 premenopausal women (mean age 39) in a randomized 18-month trial of a high-impact exercise program. BMD at the femoral neck increased significantly more in the training group compared to controls ($p = .006$). Lohman et al. (1995) found similar results, wherein lumbar spine and femur trochanter BMD increased significantly for a group of premenopausal women (mean age 34) in a resistance exercise program. In a two-year randomized trial of 63 premenopausal women, Friedlander and coworkers (1995) found that an exercise program combining aerobics and weight training produced significant positive differences in BMD between the exercise and control groups at the spine, proximal femur, and calcaneus. A study by Bassey et al. (1998) was aimed at assessing a practical exercise regimen of 50 vertical jumps 6 days/week of mean height 8.5 cm that produced mean ground reactions of three times body weight in premenopausal women (mean age 38 years) and four times body weight in postmenopausal women (mean age 55 years). In the premenopausal women there was a significant increase of 2.8% in femoral BMD after five months, yet in the postmenopausal women there was no increase or difference when compared to controls after 12 and 18 months. Thus, even a brief high-impact exercise in premenopausal women may be helpful.

Contrary to the above studies, one randomized three-year study in 67 premenopausal women (mean age 36) reported that back extension and shoulder girdle weightlifting had no significant effect on BMD at the spine, hip, or radius (Sinaki et al. 1996).

These studies generally support a positive effect of physical activity on bone in premenopausal women, with high-impact programs having the most benefit. However, making any definitive statement is premature because of the wide differences among exercise programs, skeletal sites tested (e.g., spine, hip, forearm), and populations studied.

POSTMENOPAUSAL WOMEN

With advancing age after menopause, the most significant clinical consequence of bone loss is the occurrence of fractures. Low bone mass and falling are the two major risk factors for osteoporotic fractures later in life. A primary goal of exercise in postmenopausal women is to slow down and reverse bone loss, if possible, and to improve balance and motor strength in order to lessen the likelihood of falling and sustaining a fracture.

Determining the effects of exercise in postmenopausal women has not been simple. Results are often contradictory and difficult to compare because of many confounding variables including the ages of the subjects, their health and co-morbid conditions, and their nutritional status as well as differences in exercise regimens and methods, and sites of bone mass measurements. Table 15.2 summarizes many randomized studies on BMD in postmenopausal women. (Review articles of randomized and nonrandomized trials include Ernst 1998; Kelley et al. 2001; Wallace and Cumming 2000; Wolff et al. 1999; and Vuori 2001.)

CROSS-SECTIONAL STUDIES

The data from these studies in postmenopausal women are quite variable. Nelson et al. (1988) studied 18 sedentary and 15 endurance-trained postmenopausal women (mean age 62 years) who had run an average of 22.6 miles/week since menopause. The active women had significantly lower body weight, body fat, and estrone levels than the sedentary group; yet BMD of the spine, proximal femur, and radius did not differ between the two groups. When normalized for body weight, moreover, BMDs of the spine and radius were higher in the endurance-trained group.

Other studies of long-distance runners have also reported higher lumbar spine density. In 41 long-distance runners aged 50 to 72, Lane et al. (1986) observed that BMD of the lumbar spine was 40% higher than for matched controls. Michel and coworkers (1989) in a cross-sectional study found a strong correlation between lumbar BMD and moderate weight-bearing exercise (up to 300 min/wk) in 23 postmenopausal women (mean age 57). Five women who exercised even more than the five hours/week, however, had lower BMD than the other exercisers. In a two-year longitudinal study of 40 female and male subjects over age 50, Michel and colleagues (1991) again found a high positive correlation between changes in exercise and changes in bone density in a moderate exercise group. In a subset of "overexercisers" (>300 min/wk in females and >200 min/wk in males) a negative correlation between exercise levels and BMD was found. On the other hand, Kirk et al. (1989) reported no differences in vertebral bone density between controls and nine postmenopausal long-distance runners.

Greendale et al. (1995) evaluated the relationship between use of leisure time, BMD, and osteoporotic fracture in community-dwelling adults (1014 women and 689 men) with a mean age of 73. The researchers found positive associations between current exercise and BMD at the total hip, greater trochanter, intertrochanter, and femoral neck. Lifetime exercise was similarly associated, demonstrating as well a barely significant association with spinal BMD. These data suggested a protective effect of current and lifelong exercise on hip BMD, but not on osteoporotic fracture, in older men and women. In a study of 100 postmenopausal women (ages 50-68 years) by Ballard et al. (1990), those in a high-physical activity group had significantly greater BMD of the radial shaft, but not distal radius, than women in the low-activity group. Uusi-Rasi et al. (1998) reported on the effect of physical activity and calcium intake in 422 women in three age groups (25-30, 40-45, and 60-65 years). High physical activity and high calcium intake were associated with higher total body BMC compared to the low-activity and low calcium intake group. In addition, BMD of the weight-bearing femoral neck was 5% higher in the high physical activity group than the low physical activity group, but there was no difference in radius BMD. However, high physical activity was related to larger and mechanically more competent

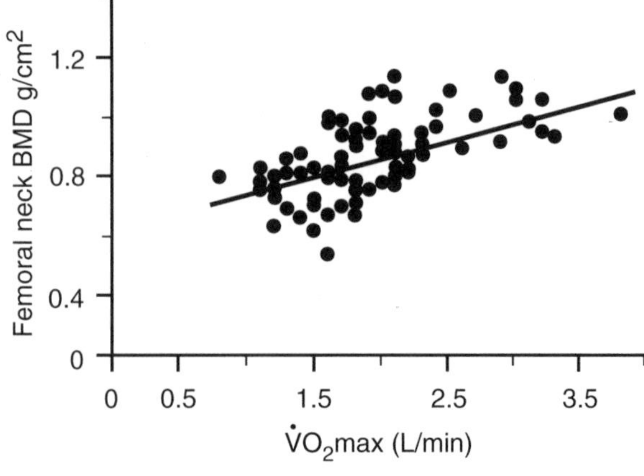

Figure 15.4 Plot of femoral neck BMD against physical fitness ($\dot{V}O_2$max) in 84 normal women. Equation for regression: femoral neck BMD = 0.61 + 0.13 ($\dot{V}O_2$max).

Reproduced from the *Journal of Clinical Investigation*, 1986, 78:618-621 by copyright permission of The American Society for Clinical Investigation.

Table 15.2 Effects of Exercise on Bone Mineral Density in Postmenopausal Women in Randomized Studies

Author	Type of exercise program	Duration of study (months)	Age (years)	Number of subjects	Bone measurement	Results
Bassey and Ramsdale 1995	High-impact exercise: 50 heel drops daily	12	54	20	BMD of lumbar spine, proximal femur, and radius by DXA	No significant increases in BMD at any site in either group. BMD at ultradistal radius site decreased in exercise group ($p < .001$).
	Control: flexibility and low-impact exercise		55	24		
Chow et al. 1987	Aerobic exercise: 30 min of walking, jogging, dance 3 d/wk	12	57	17	Calcium bone index by neutron activation analysis	Bone mass significantly higher in both exercise groups compared to controls. No difference between the exercise groups.
	Aerobics/strength training. Additional 10-15 min low-intensity strength training (free weights attached to wrists and ankles: 10 reps for each muscle group at 10 reps max 3 d/wk)		56	16		
	Control (maintain current activity level)		56	15		
Grove and Londeree 1992	High-impact group: supervised exercise ≥2 times their body weight, 20 min, 3 d/wk	12	57	5	BMD of lumbar spine by DPA	Control: –6.08% ($p = .002$). Both exercise groups: no change over time but both significantly different from control ($p < .05$). No difference between low- and high-impact group.
	Low-impact group: supervised exercise ≤1.5 times their body weight, 20 min, 3 d/wk		54	5		
	Control (nonexercise)		56	5		

(continued)

Table 15.2 (continued)

Author	Type of exercise program	Duration of study (months)	Age (years)	Number of subjects	Bone measurement	Results
Hatori et al. 1993	High intensity: work intensity above anaerobic threshold (110% heart rate) walking 3 d/wk	7	56	12	BMD of lumbar spine by DXA	Control: decrease of 1.7%; high intensity: increase of 1.1%; moderate intensity: decrease of 1.0% High intensity versus control: significant difference ($p < .05$); moderate intensity versus control: no significant difference.
	Moderate intensity: work intensity below anaerobic threshold (90% heart rate) walking 3 d/wk		58	9		
	Control		58	12		
Heinonen et al. 1998	Calisthenics: 3 sets of 16 reps of 8 different exercises to load muscles of lower extremities; additional wrist and ankle weight bands (1-2 kg) 4 d/wk	18	53	35	BMD of lumbar spine, femoral neck, calcaneus, and radius by DXA	Linear trend of maintaining BMD of femoral neck in endurance group compared to control ($p < .05$); calisthenics group: nonsignificant. BMD other sites: no training effect in either group, except distal radius BMD of endurance group showed significant negative trend ($p < .006$).
	Endurance: walking, jogging, ergometry, cycling, stair climbing, treadmill at 55-75% $\dot{V}O_2max$ 4 d/wk		53	32		
	Controls: stretching once per week		53	34		
Lau et al. 1992	Stepping up and down a block (9 in. in height) 100 times and then exercise (moving upper trunk while standing) 4 d/wk	10			BMD of lumbar spine and hip by DXA	Exercise did not have any significant effect on rate of bone loss at any site. Two-way analysis of variance showed significant interaction of calcium supplements and exercise at femoral neck ($p < .01$), but not at other sites.
	Placebo		75	12		
	Calcium (800 mg/d)		75	12		
	Exercise plus placebo		79	11		
	Exercise plus calcium (800 mg/d)		76	15		

Martin and Notelovitz 1993	Treadmill exercise to 70-85% of maximal heart rate 3 sessions/wk	12			BMD of lumbar spine by DXA and forearm by SPA	No increase in BMD; but training attenuated loss of lumbar BMD in women who were ≤6 years after the onset of menopause.
	1. 30-min session		60	20		
	2. 45-min session		58	16		
	3. Control (maintain normal daily activities)		57	19		
Nelson et al. 1994	High-intensity strength training (dynamic exercise including concentric and eccentric contractions): hip extension, knee extension, lateral pull-down, back extension, abdominal flexions (using pneumatic resistance machines); 3 sets of 8 reps at 80% of 1RM during 45-min session 2 d/wk	12	61	20	BMD of lumbar spine, femoral neck, and total body by DXA	Femoral neck: (p = 0.2) Exercise: +0.9% Control: 2.5% Lumbar spine: (p = 0.4) Exercise: +1.0% Control: –1.8% Total body bone mineral: (p = NS) Exercise: +0.0% Control: –1.2%
	Control (maintain current physical activity level)		57	19		
Notelovitz et al. 1991	Resistance circuit weight-training program using Nautilus equipment; 8 reps maximum for each exercise; 15-20 min sessions 3 d/wk	12			BMD of lumbar spine, total body by DPA, and midshaft radius by SPA	Spine: exercise plus estrogen +8.3% p = .002; estrogen +1.5% p = NS Total body: exercise plus estrogen +2.1% p = .003; estrogen +0.6% p = NS Midshaft radius: exercise plus estrogen +4.1% p = .01; estrogen –0.3% p = NS
	Estrogen		46	11		
	Exercise plus estrogen		43	9		

(continued)

Table 15.2 (continued)

Author	Type of exercise program	Duration of study (months)	Age (years)	Number of subjects	Bone measurement	Results
Prince et al. 1991	Supervised low-impact aerobic exercise for 1 hr/wk Two brisk 30-min walks/wk	24			BMD of three forearm sites by densiometer	Exercise: distal; –2.6%; median –2.4%; proximal –2.0% Exercise + calcium: distal –0.5%; median –1.3%; proximal –1.5% Exercise + estrogen: distal +2.7%; median +0.8%; proximal +0.7% Controls: distal –2.7%; median –1.9%; proximal –1.5% Bone loss similar in controls and exercise group. Bone loss significantly lower in exercise-calcium group at distal and median site. Increase in BMD in exercise-estrogen group at all sites and significant from changes in all other groups.
	Exercise		57	41		
	Exercise plus calcium		57	39		
	Exercise plus estrogen		55	40		
	Controls (normal bone density)		56	42		
Prince et al. 1995	Exercise 4 hr/wk: 2 hr supervised weight-bearing class; 2 hr walking; subjects asked to exercise at a rate to increase their heart rate to 60% of peak for age	24			BMD of lumbar spine, hip, and ultra-distal ankle by DXA	Femoral neck: exercise plus calcium: +0.28% ($p < .05$); calcium (both groups): –0.18% No significant bone loss at the spine in any group. Significant reduction in rate of bone loss at ultradistal site of tibia for all groups compared to placebo, but no difference between exercise plus calcium group and calcium group.
	Placebo		63	42		
	Exercise plus 1 g calcium (tablets)		63	42		
	Calcium 1 g (powder)		63	42		
	Calcium 1 g (tablets)		62	42		

Pruitt et al. 1995	High-intensity resistance training: 1 set of 14 repetitions at 40% 1RM as warm-up followed by 2 sets of 7 repetitions at 80% 1RM 3 d/wk	12	67	8	BMD of lumbar spine and hip by DXA	Spine: high intensity +0.7%; low intensity +0.5%; controls –0.1% Total hip: high intensity +0.8%; low intensity +1.0%; controls –0.9% Femoral neck: high intensity –0.2%; low intensity +1.8%; controls –0.9% No significant change in BMD of spine or proximal femur (despite effective muscle-strengthening program).
	Low-intensity resistance training: 3 sets of 14 repetitions at 40% 1RM; Nautilus and universal gym equipment used (10 exercises) 3 d/wk		68	7		
	Control (maintain current activity)		70	11		
Revel et al. 1993	Psoas training: in sitting position, with 5-kg sandbag on knee, 60 flexions of each hip daily	12	57	30	BMD of lumbar spine by CT	No significant change in either group. In subgroup of "assiduous" exercisers, BMD loss significantly greater in the control group.
	Deltoid training (control): in sitting position, 1-kg sandbag on each hand, 60 abductions of both arms daily		56	39		
Sandler et al. 1987	Walking: goal to achieve minimum walking of 7 mi/week (at least 3 mi/session) 2 d/wk	36			Bone density of midshaft radius using CT	No difference in change in bone tissue density. Walking group had a significantly greater increase in cross-sectional area of the radius than the control group, but only for those in a high-grip strength group ($p < .05$).
	Exercise		58	114		
	Control		57	115		

(continued)

Table 15.2 *(continued)*

Author	Type of exercise program	Duration of study (months)	Age (years)	Number of subjects	Bone measurement	Results
Sinaki et al. 1989	Back-strengthening exercises: backpack with weights equivalent to 30% of maximal isometric back muscle strength; in prone position, subject lifted backpack 10 times 5 d/wk	12			BMD of lumbar spine by DPA	Exercise: –1.4% $p < .001$ Control: –1.2% $p = .006$ NS difference between groups (back extensor strength increased more in exercise group than control ($p = .002$).
	Exercise		56	34		
	Control (no back exercises)		57	31		
Smidt et al. 1992	Progressive resistive program for the trunk muscles: at 70% maximal strength, 3 sets of 10 repetitions of 3 exercises (sit-up, double leg raise, prone trunk extension) 3-4 d/wk	12			BMD of lumbar spine and hip by DPA	No significant differences between the exercise and control groups.
	Exercise		57	22		
	Control (maintain current lifestyle)		55	27		
Humphries et al. 2000	Weight training 2 times/wk Progressive increase to 90% 1RM (2-4 repetitions): No HRT HRT Walking 2 sessions of 50 min: No HRT HRT	 6 6 6 6	 50 58 54 55	 21 14 20 9	BMD of lumbar spine by DXA	No significant group differences in lumbar BMD. However, in the walking group significant 1.3% decrease.

Kerr et al. 2001	Strength training, additional weight training	24	60	42	BMD of hip, lumbar spine, forearm, and whole body by DXA	No difference between group in BMD at forearm, lumbar spine, or whole body sites. Increase in BMD at total and intertrochanteric hip sites in the strength training group.
	Fitness training, stationary bicycle	24	59	42		
	Controls	24	62	42		
Maddalozzo and Snow 2000	3 × wk all muscle groups High-intensity free weight final stage 3 sets, 2-4 reps, 90+% 1RM	6	54	9	BMD of hip, lumbar spine, and whole body by DXA	No significant difference in BMD between groups at any bone site. Training programs resulted in improvements in total body strength, but no change in circulating IGF-1.
	Moderate-intensity machine weight 3 sets, 10-13 reps, 40-60% 1RM	6	55	9		
Bravo et al. 1996	3 ×/wk, 1 hr weight-bearing exercises (walking, stepping up and down from benches, aerobic dancing, flexibility exercises) to reach 60-70% of heart rate reserve	12	60	61	BMD of lumbar spine and hip by DXA	No significant change in spine or femoral neck BMD in exercising group, but significant decrease in spine in controls.
	Controls	12	60	63		

BMC = bone mineral content; BMD = bone mineral density; CT = computerized tomography; DPA = dual photon absorptiometry; DXA = dual energy X-ray absorptiometry; RM = repetition maximum; SPA = single photon absorptiometry.

bones in the femoral and radial shafts, an effect that was stronger with increasing age.

Clinicians and researchers usually have assessed aerobic fitness by measuring maximal oxygen consumption ($\dot{V}O_2max$). Evaluating 84 normal women, Pocock and coworkers (1986) found that aerobic fitness was the only significant predictor of femoral neck BMD in the 46 who were postmenopausal. Weight and fitness predicted lumbar BMD (figure 15.4).

Chow and colleagues (1986) studied 31 postmenopausal women (ages 50-59 years) and found a significant correlation between physical fitness and bone mass of the trunk and proximal femur; using neutron activation analysis (NAA), they expressed their data as a calcium bone index. Bevier et al. (1989) reported that, in 55 women aged 61 to 84 years, there was no relationship between aerobic capacity ($\dot{V}O_2max$) and BMD of the spine or forearm. However, in 36 men aged 63 to 80 years there was a significant correlation between $\dot{V}O_2max$ and BMD of the lumbar spine. In a cross-sectional study of 55 postmenopausal women (mean age 73.5 years), Vico and colleagues (1995) reported that $\dot{V}O_2max$ was the strongest predictor of proximal femur BMD, accounting for 10.8% to 18.3% of the BMD variability. In addition, at the vertebral level, psoas surfaces constituted the best predictor of lumbar BMD. The anatomic connections between psoas muscles and vertebrae can explain such a relationship. Jacobson et al. (1984) reported significantly higher BMD in the radius in a group of women aged 55 to 70 years who regularly exercised, as compared to age-matched controls.

In addition to physical fitness, body composition and muscular strength appear positively correlated with BMD. Reid, Plank, and Evans (1992) found that, in premenopausal women, and Reid et al. (1992) found that, in postmenopausal women, total body fat mass was positively correlated to BMD throughout the skeleton. Bevier and colleagues (1989) found a significant correlation between fat mass and lean mass with each other and to spine BMD but not radius BMD in postmenopausal women aged 61 to 84 years. Grip strength correlated significantly with forearm density and spine density, yet the researchers found no correlation between back strength and lumbar BMD. This contrasts with the report by Sinaki et al. (1986), who found a significant correlation between lumbar spine BMD and back extensor strength in a younger postmenopausal group, aged 49 to 65 years. In this group, they also reported a positive correlation between lumbar spine BMD and the level of physical activity (Sinaki and Offord 1988). Sinaki et al. (1974) also found a significant correlation between midradius BMC and grip strength.

Snow-Harter and colleagues (1990) found muscle strength to be an independent predictor of BMD in 59 women aged 18 to 31 years; they theorized that muscle groups with attachments distant from the spine and hip may strongly affect BMD at these sites. In a group of 181 men and women aged 45 to 77 years, Hughes et al. (1995) observed significant associations between elbow extensor strength and radial BMD in both men and women and between knee flexor muscle strength and lumbar BMD in women. Madsen et al. (1993) reported highly significant correlations between quadriceps strength and BMD of the proximal tibia in 66 healthy women, aged 21 to 78 years, including 24 women aged 60 to 78 years.

Interventional Studies

The best way to avoid the biases in cross-sectional studies is to use a prospective randomized intervention trial. This avoids the possibility that people predisposed to a type of exercise will self-select for participation in that exercise.

Nonrandomized Studies

In a group of nine postmenopausal women (mean age 53) who followed an exercise program using the guidelines of the President's Council on Physical Fitness three times a week for one year, Aloia et al. (1978) found an increase in total body calcium compared to a decrease in the control group. Cavanaugh and Cann (1988) reported that a moderately brisk walking program of one year's duration by 17 postmenopausal women (ages 49-64 years) did not prevent the loss of spinal bone density. Nelson and colleagues (1991) studied the effect of a one-year supervised walking program and increased calcium intake in 36 postmenopausal women (mean age 60 years). Subjects wore leaded belts (3.1 kg) around their waists and walked for 50 minutes four times a week. Trabecular BMD of the lumbar spine, as measured by computed tomography, increased 0.5% in the exercising women and decreased 7.0% in sedentary women. There was no significant change in femoral neck or radius BMD. The lack of response at some sites in these studies may be due to inadequate mechanical forces being applied.

In a study by Krolner and colleagues (1983), 16 postmenopausal women (mean age 61) participated for eight months (one hour twice weekly) in a moderate program of walking, running, and sitting/standing exercises. Lumbar spine BMC increased 3.5% in the training group and declined 2.7% in the controls ($p < .005$ between groups). There was no difference between the groups in forearm BMC. Dalsky et al. (1988) studied 35 postmenopausal women, aged 55 to 70 years, 17 of whom were in a weight-bearing exercise training program consisting primarily of walking, jogging, and stair climbing. BMC of the lumbar spine significantly increased 5.2% in the exercise group after 9 months and 6.1% after 22 months. In those who stopped exercising, lumbar BMC fell to baseline, suggesting that exercise must be maintained to retain its benefit. Pruitt et al. (1992) studied 17 postmenopausal women (mean age 54) in a weight training program using Universal Gym equipment, free weights, and ankle weights, 3 days/week for nine months. Lumbar BMD increased 1.6% and was significantly different from that of the control group, who lost 3.6%. There were no differences at the femoral neck or distal wrist.

A nine-month strength training program prevented the loss of calcaneal bone in older women (mean age 72) in a study by Rundgren and colleagues (1984). Ayalon et al. (1987) studied 14 osteoporotic women (mean age 63) in a five-month program that specifically loaded the distal forearm. During the year prior to the study, BMD of the distal forearm significantly decreased in both the exercise and control group; but during the exercise period, it increased in the exercise group (+3.8%) while significantly decreasing in the control group (–1.9%). In 54 women (ages 36-67 years), Peterson and coworkers (1991) compared the effects of an endurance dance program, a program that combined endurance dance and resistance weight training, and a control sedentary program. Although muscle strength increased with weight training, there were no significant changes in BMD of the lumbar spine, hip region, or appendicular skeleton with either training program.

Kohrt and colleagues (1997) assigned 39 older, sedentary women (ages 60-74 years) to one of three groups:

- Exercises providing stress to the skeleton through ground-reaction forces (GRF) (i.e., walking, jogging, stair climbing)
- Exercises through joint-reaction forces (JRF) (i.e., weight lifting, rowing)
- Sedentary control group

Both the GRF and JRF exercise programs resulted in significant and similar increases in BMD of the whole body, lumbar spine, and Ward's triangle region of the proximal femur. The GRF program also produced a 3.5% increase in BMD of the femoral neck ($p < .01$). Although the JRF program did not increase BMD of the femoral neck, it increased lean body mass ($p < .01$) and strength ($p < .01$) and thus may still be important in reducing the risk for falls.

Iwamoto et al. (1998) found that in 35 postmenopausal women (ages 53-77 years), a daily exercise program of outdoor walking and gymnastics training produced a 4.48% increase in lumbar spine BMD at 12 months.

Randomized Studies

Chow and coworkers (1987) used NAA to measure bone mass in 48 postmenopausal women (ages 50-62 years), randomly assigning subjects to an aerobic exercise program, to a program of aerobic exercise plus strength training, or to a control group. At the end of one year the exercise groups did not differ significantly from each other, but both had greater bone mass than controls ($p < .05$).

Grove and Londeree (1992) randomly assigned 15 early postmenopausal women (ages 49-65 years) to a control group, a low-impact exercise group, or a high-impact group. Each exercise group had 20 minutes of supervised exercise three times a week. After one year, the control group had a significant decrease in lumbar BMD (–6.08%). Both exercise groups maintained BMD, and this was significantly different from the controls. Hatori and colleagues (1993) reported a significantly higher lumbar spine BMD in a high-intensity exercise group relative to control subjects after a seven-month program, while those in a moderate-intensity group did not differ significantly from controls. The high-intensity group walked three times per week for seven months with heart rates at about 110% of anaerobic threshold. Martin and Notelovitz (1993) reported that in 18 postmenopausal women within six years after the onset of menopause, those assigned to treadmill walking for one year had reduced spinal BMD loss compared with nonexercising similar women ($p < .05$).

In a study of 39 postmenopausal women (ages 50-70 years), Nelson and coworkers (1994) randomly assigned 20 women to a high-intensity strength training program of workouts 2 days/week for one year, using five different exercises. The other 19 women were sedentary controls. Muscle mass, muscle strength, and dynamic balance significantly increased in the strength-trained women and decreased in the controls. Femoral neck BMD and lumbar spine BMD increased by 0.9% and 1.0%, respectively, in the strength-trained women, and decreased by 2.5% and 1.8%, respectively, in the controls ($p = .02$ and .04). Not only did the exercise program strengthen bone, but by improving muscle function and balance it probably lessened the likelihood of falling and sustaining a fracture as well (figure 15.5).

Notelovitz and colleagues (1991) randomly assigned 20 surgically menopausal women to receive either estrogen (mean age 46 years) or estrogen plus a variable-resistance weight training program involving Nautilus muscle strengthening/endurance equipment (mean age 43 years). After one year, lumbar spine BMD increased 8.3% in the exercise group, total body BMD increased 2.1%, and midshaft radial BMD increased 4.1%, compared to nonsignificant changes in the nonexercising group. Thus, variable-resistance training in estrogen-replete women added bone to both the axial and appendicular skeleton. Perhaps the difference between the beneficial results from resistance training in this study compared to other studies is that the patients in the Notelovitz study were younger and able to train at an intensity needed to maximally stress the muscle.

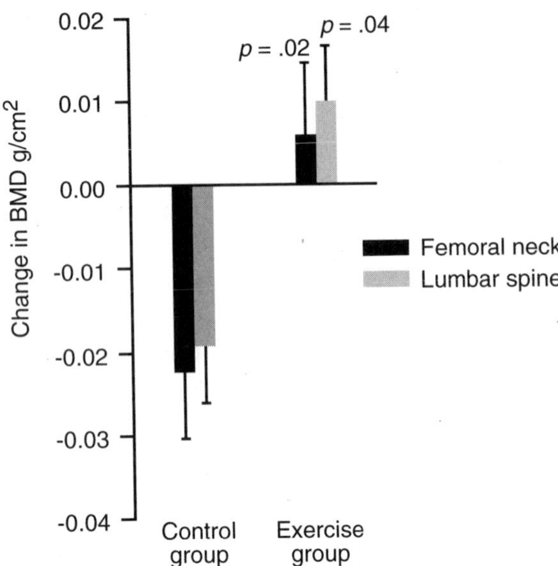

Figure 15.5 Changes in bone after the interventions (either no exercise or high-intensity strength training). The values are means ± SE for individual changes in bone adjusted for age, smoking, and baseline bone mineral density, using analysis of covariance. BMD = bone mineral density.

Reprinted, by permission, from M.E. Nelson et al., 1994, "Effects of high-intensity strength training on multiple risk factors for osteoporotic fractures: A randomized controlled trial," *JAMA* 272:1909-1914. Copyrighted 1994, American Medical Association.

In a study of 120 postmenopausal women (mean age 56) who had low forearm bone density, Prince and colleagues (1991) randomly assigned them to an exercise program, to exercise plus calcium (1 gram daily), or exercise plus estrogen. Exercise alone did not prevent bone loss at the forearm. When combined with calcium, exercise slowed bone loss; but when combined with estrogen, exercise significantly increased BMD (figure 15.6).

Pruitt et al. (1995) compared the effects of 12-month high-intensity and low-intensity resistance training programs in 26 older postmenopausal women aged 65 to 79 years. Despite an effective muscle-strengthening program, resistance training did not produce significant changes in spine or proximal femur BMD in either the high- or low-intensity groups. The women in this study possessed good BMD on entrance, and the majority had taken hormone replacement therapy for at least one year prior to participation. The authors suggest that the resistance training in this study may not have differed sufficiently from activities (particularly of the lower limb) normally carried out by older, active women, thus being insufficient to produce increases in bone density. Yet such training may still confer benefits by improving strength and possibly balance, lessening the likelihood of falling or sustaining fractures.

Revel and coworkers (1993) evaluated 78 postmenopausal women half in a psoas muscle training program,

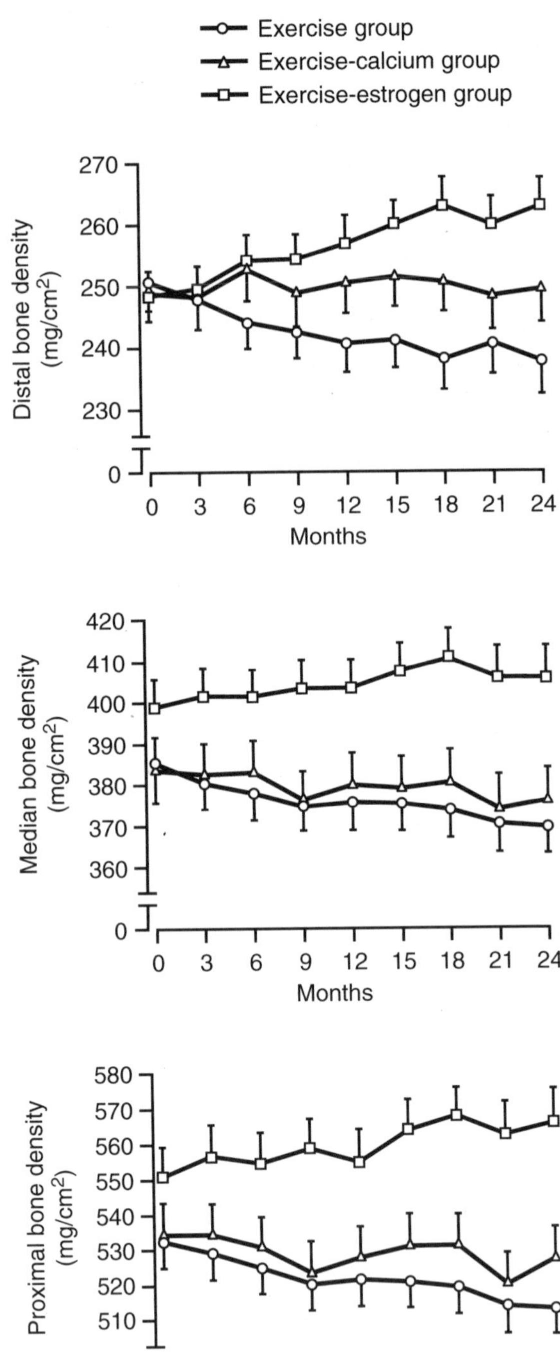

Figure 15.6 Effects of three interventions on bone density at distal, median, and proximal forearm sites during a two-year study period. Values are means ± SE for all women remaining in each group at the time indicated. After two years there were 35 women remaining in the exercise group, 36 in the exercise-calcium group, and 32 in the exercise-estrogen group.

Reprinted, by permission, from R.L. Prince et al., 1991, "Prevention of postmenopausal osteoporosis: A comparative study of exercise, calcium, supplementation, and hormone replacement therapy," *N Engl J Med* 325:1189-1195. Copyright 1991 Massachusetts Medical Society. All rights reserved.

half in a deltoid training program (the control group). The psoas muscle attaches to the lumbar vertebrae. Losses in lumbar spine BMD were comparable in both groups after one year. However, in the subgroup of women who performed the psoas exercises assiduously for one year, there was a significantly smaller loss than in the controls. Sandler and colleagues (1987) studied 229 postmenopausal women: half were sedentary controls, and half walked more than seven miles a week for three years. Bone loss in the radius was similar in both groups, but changes in the cross-sectional area of the radius were significantly greater in the walkers with high grip strength than in controls with comparable high grip strength. The significance of this finding is not clear, but may indicate that some local muscular loading was involved. Sinaki et al. (1989) studied the effect of back-strengthening exercises on spinal BMD in 34 postmenopausal women, mean age 56. Despite an increase in back extensor muscle strength in the exercise group, there was no difference in the rate of bone loss between the exercise and control group. Perhaps the load generated on the back extensors was insufficient to adequately load the skeleton. Smidt et al. (1992) also investigated the effect of a progressive resistance training program for trunk muscles in 22 early postmenopausal women (mean age 57). They found no significant differences in BMD between the exercise and control groups at the lumbar spine and proximal femur at the end of one year.

Humphries et al. (2000) found in 64 women age 45 to 65 that there was no significant difference in lumbar spine BMD at 24 weeks in those subjects performing high-intensity strength training or low-intensity walking, whether or not they were receiving hormone replacement therapy. However, in the walking subgroup there was a 1.3% decrease from baseline when a within-group analysis was performed.

Kerr et al. (2001) examined the effect of a two-year exercise intervention and calcium supplementation on BMD in 126 postmenopausal women (mean age 60 years). In the strength training group, there was a progressive increase in loading; and in the fitness group, additional stationary bicycle riding occurred with no change in loading. Although no difference was seen between groups in BMD at the forearm, lumbar spine, or whole-body sites, there was a significant increase in BMD at the total and intertrochanteric hip sites in the strength training group.

In summary, these prospective studies offer modest but variable evidence that increased activity either through dynamic exercises or high-intensity weight training may improve bone mass, muscle strength, and/or balance, possibly translating into fewer falls and fractures. The data are often contradictory, and we need to learn much more about specific exercises (both in type and intensity) in specific populations. Kelley (1998) used meta-analysis to examine the effects of exercise on regional BMD in postmenopausal women, analyzing 11 randomized trials yielding 40 outcome measures in a total of 719 subjects (370 exercise, 349 nonexercise). Kelley concluded that exercise may slow the rate of bone loss in postmenopausal women, but that it is premature to form strong conclusions regarding the effects of exercise on regional BMD. We need additional, well-designed studies.

Physical Activity, Fall Prevention, and Fractures

In 1990, there were an estimated 1.7 million hip fractures worldwide, most resulting from falls (Melton 1993). In a community of 336 elderly persons at least 75 years of age in New Haven, Connecticut, 32% fell during one year, 24% had serious injuries, and 6% had fractures (Tinetti et al. 1988). One out of every six white women in the United States will have a hip fracture during her lifetime (Cummings et al. 1989); among Americans aged 65 years or older, falls are the leading cause of death from injury (Sattin 1992). The incidence of hip fracture increases exponentially after age 65, and the rate of hip fracture among white women is twice that of white men (Sattin 1992). Those who survive often suffer long-term disability.

Low bone density is a major risk factor for hip fracture during a fall (Chandler et al. 2000). Important risk factors for falling include lower- and upper-extremity weakness, low physical activity, gait abnormalities, poor balance, poor transfer skills, visual impairment, sedatives and other prescription medications, cognitive impairment, neurologic disorders, anxiety, and depression (Cummings et al. 1995; Dhesi et al. 2002; Greenspan et al. 1994; Grisso et al. 1991; Johnell et al. 1995; Rubenstein et al. 1994; Sudarsky 1990; Tinetti et al. 1988).

Changes in any of these risk factors may have important long-term clinical implications. The most significant benefit of exercise may be to modify some of these factors, improve neuromuscular function, and reduce the likelihood of falling. Johnell et al. (1995) felt that 50% of hip fractures result from potentially reversible risk factors. For older individuals, Greenspan et al. (1994, 1998) emphasized that the characteristics of falls, including the direction, are at least as important as BMD in determining hip fracture risk. They suggest that reducing the odds of falling directly on a hip, or enhancing the hip's ability to withstand such an impact, could decrease the severity of falls and the risks of fractures. Interventions for these purposes include exercises to improve quadriceps strength, neuromuscular function, and gait.

Province and coworkers (1995) did a meta-analysis of the seven FICSIT studies (Frailty and Injuries:

Cooperative Studies of Intervention Techniques). These are independent, randomized, controlled clinical trials assessing intervention efficacy in reducing falls and frailty in elderly patients. All included an exercise component for 10 to 36 weeks, with follow-ups for falls and injuries continuing for the two to four years of the study. A total of 2328 subjects participated, including residents of two nursing homes and five community-dwelling sites. Although the minimum ages differed at the study sites, the youngest was 60 years. Female participation in the seven centers ranged from 42% to 81%. While the exercise component varied across the studies, all subjects trained in one or more areas of endurance, flexibility, balance platform, tai chi (dynamic balance), and resistance. Those subjects assigned to the interventions that included exercise or balance training had significantly fewer falls. Thus, exercise by elderly adults can reduce the risk of falls.

Fiatarone et al. (1994) conducted a randomized placebo-controlled trial comparing progressive resistance exercise training, multinutrient supplementation, both interventions, and neither in 100 frail nursing home residents (mean age 87.1 years) over a 10-month period. In the subjects who underwent exercise training, muscle strength increased by 113%, gait velocity by 11.8%, stair-climbing power by 28.4%, and thigh muscle areas by 2.7%. Levels of spontaneous activity also increased. Nutritional supplement had no effect on any primary outcome measure. Thus, even in a frail elderly population, high-intensity exercise training is a feasible and effective way to counter muscle weakness and physical frailty.

Using a multiple risk factor intervention that included an exercise program in 301 subjects over age 70, Tinetti et al. (1994) found a significant reduction in the risk of falling. In a one-year randomized controlled trial, Lord and coworkers (1996) studied 179 postmenopausal women (ages 60-85 years) who engaged in twice-weekly structured general aerobic exercise. The exercise group showed significant improvements in quadriceps strength and postural sway, but not BMD, when compared with the control group. Indices of fracture risk also decreased significantly in the exercise group, despite lack of improvement in BMD, implying that it is possible to lower fracture risk without improving bone density. Gerdhem et al. (2003) reported on 1004 women age 75 years from the Malmo Osteoporosis Prospective Risk Assessment study. Physical activity and muscle strength accounted for a very small part of bone mass variability. In the elderly, the authors felt that the major fracture-preventive effect of physical activity was unlikely to be mediated through increased bone mass but rather due to improvements in balance, coordination, and mobility.

Elderly subjects, even the frail elderly, appear to tolerate exercise well (even mild high-impact programs) when the activity is appropriate—particularly when health professionals take into consideration the participants' other medical conditions and properly supervise the programs. Thus, lifestyle changes, exercise (even higher levels of leisure-time physical activity), and rehabilitation programs should significantly reduce falls and fractures (American College of Sports Medicine 1998; DiPietro 2001; Gardner et al. 2000; Gregg et al. 2000; Karlsson 2002; Sinaki 2003; Tinetti 2003).

Summary

The studies described in this chapter show that an exercise program can be established for nearly anyone, and that such programs may be helpful in building and maintaining bone mass, strengthening muscle, improving balance, and preventing falls and fractures. It is not yet clear precisely how to individually tailor exercise programs according to specific individuals' needs, or how long such programs should last. Yet it is important to individualize exercise programs that should begin (when appropriate) only after medical clearance and under the supervision of a physician and a physical therapist.

Although there is much that we need to learn about the effect of exercise on bone health and osteoporosis, at this time we can make several general statements:

1. Many studies support the beneficial effects of exercise.
2. Bone adapts to alterations in mechanical loading.
3. The skeleton responds in a site-specific manner to mechanical loading.
4. If the load is high enough, bone will respond.
5. To see an increase in BMD in specific areas, it is important to load the specific bones.
6. Physical activity may increase peak bone mass in childhood and adolescence, maintain bone mass in young adulthood, and slow bone loss in older subjects.
7. Young bones respond more favorably to mechanical loading than older bones.
8. Exercise may improve balance, strength, mobility, and gait, and lessen the likelihood of falling and sustaining a fracture.
9. Older postmenopausal women and even the frail elderly can tolerate appropriately designed strength training and resistance exercise programs, potentially improving both muscle strength and BMD.

Acknowledgments

I wish to thank Christine Carr and Donna MacDonald for their typing of this manuscript.

CHAPTER 16

HUMAN IMMUNODEFICIENCY VIRUS

Susan D. Driscoll, MPH, MSN, ANP; and Steven Grinspoon, MD

CASE STUDY

A college-educated, 50-year-old, human immunodeficiency virus (HIV)-positive Caucasian male with severe HIV lipodystrophy, insulin resistance, hypertriglyceridemia, low high-density lipoprotein (HDL) cholesterol, and a history of renal cell carcinoma, status postnephrectomy 1 1/2 years prior, and on a stable highly active antiretroviral therapy (HAART) for 10 months and on no other medications, completed an aerobic and progressive resistance training (PRT) regimen. Exercise consisted of 30 min of aerobic exercise at 75% of maximal heart rate on a stationary bike followed by three sets of 10 repetitions at 80% of 1-repetition maximum (1RM) three times a week for various muscle groups. The 1RM was adjusted every two weeks. The patient also began treatment with metformin at a dose of 850 mg twice a day for the 12-week intervention.

At baseline, the patient was overweight with a body mass index (BMI) of 27.7 kg/m^2, a waist-to-hip ratio (WHR) of 1.04, and waist circumference of 99.7 cm. His serum lactic acid level and kidney and liver function were normal. His CD4 count was 557 cells/mm^3, and HIV viral load was undetectable (<50 copies). The patient was 100% compliant with the exercise regimen and metformin. As expected with metformin treatment, abnormal insulin and glucose response was completely corrected. However, in addition to improved insulin and glucose metabolism, there were major improvements in body composition, aerobic endurance, strength, and cardiovascular indices seen with the addition of exercise in this patient. Body mass index decreased from 27.7 kg/m^2 at baseline to 22.8 kg/m^2, with a corresponding decrease in WHR, a 4.9-cm decrease in waist circumference, a 1.7-cm decrease in neck circumference, and an increase of 2.5 cm for midthigh circumference. Measures of body composition by dual X-ray absorptiometry (DEXA) also improved significantly, with a decrease in fat and increase in lean body mass in the arms and legs and a decrease in trunk fat. The patient demonstrated significant decreases in both visceral and subcutaneous abdominal fat as measured by computerized tomography (CT) scan.

There were improvements in strength as measured by all six upper and lower body resistance exercises and an increase in aerobic capacity measured by an increase in exercise time and increase in percentage submaximal heart rate attained with maximal exertion. In terms of cardiovascular indices there was a decrease from a triglyceride level of 243 to 223 mg/dL, a decrease in total cholesterol by 13 mg/dL, a decrease in low-density lipoprotein (LDL) cholesterol of 9 mg/dL, no change in HDL cholesterol, a decrease in C-reactive protein, and a decrease in both systolic and diastolic blood pressures at rest. In terms of safety, the regimen was well tolerated, with CD4 counts, HIV viral loads, and lactate levels remaining stable. There was also a reported improvement in Beck Depression Inventory score, suggesting improved quality of life with participation in an aerobic and PRT regimen.

THE HIV PANDEMIC

Since the first case of acquired immunodeficiency syndrome (AIDS) was identified in 1981 in San Francisco, HIV/AIDS has grown into a full pandemic. According to a United States Agency for International Development (USAIDS) report, there were an estimated 42 million people in the world living with HIV/AIDS in 2002, and less than 1% of these persons received HAART. In the United States, the number of newly diagnosed AIDS cases increased to a high of approximately 80,000 per year in 1993 (Centers for Disease Control [CDC] 2002). Since the advent of HAART, the numbers of AIDS cases and AIDS-related deaths have decreased to approximately 40,000 per year and 15,000 per year, respectively (CDC 2002). Despite decreases in the number of AIDS cases and AIDS-related deaths, the number of persons living with HIV/AIDS continues to rise, demonstrating that HIV/AIDS has progressed from a once fatal to a more chronic disease in Western Europe and North America. The changing nature of HIV/AIDS treatment, newly associated comorbidities, and increased disease chronicity have led to new challenges in the treatment of persons with HIV/AIDS.

Clinicians must now consider the optimal treatment strategies for the long-term complications of HIV and HAART. These complications include the metabolic and body composition changes of HIV lipodystrophy, an inability to gain lean body mass in AIDS wasting syndrome (AWS), and the accompanying psychosocial and quality of life issues, such as decreased physical functioning and body image disturbances. Preliminary research has shown that exercise may be an important primary treatment strategy or adjunctive treatment strategy (or both) for the long-term complications of HIV and HAART. This chapter summarizes data on the role of exercise in the treatment of HIV- and AIDS-related complications.

EXERCISE TO IMPROVE PHYSICAL FUNCTION IN HIV-INFECTED PATIENTS

Chronic disease is often associated with fatigue. In a cross-sectional study of 15 adolescents with HIV and 15 age-, gender-, and activity level-matched controls, peak oxygen consumption ($p < .003$), peak treadmill stage ($p < .003$), exercise duration ($p < .004$), and oxygen pulse ($p < .009$) were lower in those infected with HIV compared to controls (Cade et al. 2002). These data illustrate that similar to other chronic disease states, chronic HIV infection affects endurance in HIV patients.

AEROBIC TRAINING AND EXERCISE FUNCTION IN HIV

A number of studies have investigated whether aerobic training can improve exercise function in HIV-infected individuals (table 16.1).

In an early study by MacArthur et al. (1993), 32 primarily male HIV-infected patients were randomly assigned to low-intensity aerobic exercise (four 10-min intervals at 50-60% of $\dot{V}O_2max$) or high-intensity exercise (six 4-min intervals at 75-85% of $\dot{V}O_2max$) on a treadmill, stationary bike, rowing machine, or stair stepper three days a week for 24 weeks. In the six compliant subjects, $\dot{V}O_2max$ increased from 33.2 to 41.2 $ml \cdot kg^{-1} \cdot min^{-1}$, a 24% improvement from baseline. However, the small size of the study and poor compliance rate limited the conclusions that could be drawn. Smith et al. (2001) studied 60 healthy HIV-infected men and women on stable antiretroviral therapy in a randomized, wait-listed, controlled study. Subjects were randomized to an aerobic exercise training program, three times a week for 12 weeks, consisting of a 20-min warm-up and 30 min of aerobic exercise on a stationary bike, stair stepper, or cross-country machine at 60% to 80% of subject's $\dot{V}O_2max$.

Experimental subjects participated in a minimum of 28 (78%) of the 36 possible exercise sessions and demonstrated significant increases in aerobic capacity, as measured by increased time on a treadmill in minutes, in comparison to the control group. There were also significant decreases in BMI (kg/m^2); triceps, central, and peripheral skinfold measurements; umbilical waist circumference; and WHR measurements in the aerobic exercise group in comparison to the control group. In addition, there was a trend toward improved $\dot{V}O_2max$ in the exercise group in comparison to the control group. These data suggest that aerobic exercise improves aerobic capacity and body composition measures in HIV-infected patients, but the optimal exercise regimen and intensity level remain unknown in this population.

Stringer et al. (1998) investigated aerobic exercise regimens of varied intensity in 26 HIV-infected patients. Subjects performed a moderate-intensity exercise program three times a week for six weeks, consisting of 1 hr of aerobics at an intensity equivalent to 80% of the lactic acidosis threshold (LAT) or high-intensity aerobic training at 50% of the difference between the LAT and $\dot{V}O_2max$, in comparison to a control group receiving no exercise intervention. The high-intensity group performed a proportionally shorter amount of exercise while maintaining the total work per session identical to that of the moderate-intensity group. There was a 91% compliance rate for all subjects completing the study. The LAT increased significantly in both exercising groups ($p < .01$), but the $\dot{V}O_2max$ and maximal power

Table 16.1 Summary of Aerobic Exercise Studies in HIV-Infected Subjects

Author	Subjects	Design	Intervention	Major Findings
MacArthur et al. 1993	32 HIV+ ♂ (30) and ♀ (2)	Randomized pilot study	Randomized to: Low intensity aerobic exercise: four 10 min intervals at 50-60% of $\dot{V}O_2max$ High intensity aerobic exercise: six 4 min intervals at 75-85% of $\dot{V}O_2max$ 3 d/wk × 24 wks on a treadmill, stationary bike, rowing machine, or stair stepper, adjusted q2wks with HR and perceived exertion.	6 subjects compliant (>80% of sessions attended). $\dot{V}O_2max$ increased 24% in compliant subjects (33.2 to 41.2 $ml \cdot kg^{-1} \cdot min^{-1}$). Minute ventilation increased 13% in compliant subjects (91 to 103 L/min). Oxygen pulse increased 24% in compliant subjects (13.4 to 16.6 ml/beat). No significant changes in CD4 count with treatment. Comments: Unable to statistically compare treatment groups, as only 6 subjects (3 in each group) were included in analysis.
Smith et al. 2001	60 HIV+ ♂ and ♀ on stable HAART with no AIDS defining illnesses or wasting (<85% of IBW)	Randomized, wait-listed, controlled study	20 min of walking/jogging for warm-up followed by aerobic exercise on a stationary bike, stair stepper, or cross-country machine for 30 min at 60-80% of $\dot{V}O_2max$ 3 d/wk × 12 wks. Duration and intensity adjusted at intervals to maintain prescribed HR.	30 control and 19 treatment subjects completed initial 12 wks of study with a minimum of 78% compliance (28/36 possible sessions) in first 12 wks. Significant increase in time on treadmill (1 vs. 0.2 min) and significant decreases in BMI (–0.5 vs. 1.2 kg/m^2), triceps skinfold (–2.2 vs. 1.2), central skinfolds (–6.2 vs. 0), peripheral skinfolds (–9.9 vs. –2.1), umbilical waist (–0.01 vs. 0.01), and weight (–1.5 vs. 0.5 kg) in the exercise group vs. the control group. 15 control subjects completed the exercise protocol from wk 12-24 with significant decreases in weight (–2.4 ± 3.6), BMI (–0.8 ± 1.1 kg/m^2), and triceps skinfold (–4.9 ± 7.4). No significant changes in CD4 count.

(continued)

Table 16.1 (continued)

Author	Subjects	Design	Intervention	Major Findings
Stringer et al. 1998	34 HIV+ ♂ and ♀ (11%) with CD4 count between 100-500 cells/mm^3)	RCT	Randomized to: Control – asked to maintain current activity. Moderate intensity: 1 hr 3 d/wk × 6 wks at 80% of LAT work rate. Heavy intensity: 3 d/wk × 6 wks at 50% of LAT-$\dot{V}O_2$max, leading to proportionally shorter exercise time (30-40 min avg.) with total work/session = moderate intensity group. All sessions done on cycle ergometer.	26 subjects completed with exercise compliance of 91%. Significant increase in LAT in both exercise groups. $\dot{V}O_2$max and WRmax increased significantly in heavy intensity group only. No significant changes in CD4 count. Significant improvements in QOL questionnaire in both exercise groups in comparison to control group. Comment: Training intensity not adjusted over time and HR not monitored during training.
Terry et al. 1999	31 inactive HIV+ subjects (17 ♂ and 14 ♀)	Randomized trial	15 min warm-up followed by 30 min of aerobic exercise intervals (walk/run interval training 5/1 min), then a 15 min stretching routine 3 d/wk × 12 wks, with randomization to: Moderate intensity at 55-60% of maximal HR. High intensity at 75-85% of maximal HR.	21 subjects completed protocol. Eleven in high intensity and 10 in moderate intensity group. Significant increases in exercise time seen in both groups (70 s in moderate and 190 s in high intensity group). Maximal systolic BP increased significantly in the high intensity group (29 mmHg). No significant changes in CD4 count. Comment: High drop out rate (68%), but 100% compliance in those completing regimen.

Note: ♂ = men; ♀ = women; BMI = body mass index; BP = blood pressure; d = days; HR = heart rate; HAART = highly active antiretroviral therapy; hr = hour; IBW = ideal body weight; LAT = lactic acid threshold; min = minutes; q2wks = every two weeks; QOL = quality of life; RCT = randomized controlled trial; s = second; $\dot{V}O_2$max = maximal oxygen uptake; wk(s) = week(s); WRmax = maximal work rate.

output increased significantly only in the high-intensity group ($p < .01$), suggesting that the intensity and not the amount of exercise is important to improve aerobic capacity in this population (Stringer et al. 1998).

In another study of aerobic exercise intensity in Brazil, healthy HIV-infected men and women completed a 12-week exercise program consisting of 36 sessions (1 hr each) three times a week, at either a moderate intensity (60% of maximal heart rate) or a high intensity (84% of maximal heart rate) (Terry et al. 1999). Aerobic capacity increased significantly in both moderate-intensity and high-intensity groups, but the high-intensity group achieved a significantly larger incremental gain in aerobic capacity ($p < .01$).

Taken together, these data suggest that aerobic exercise training improves aerobic capacity and endurance in HIV-infected patients. As anticipated, increased intensity of training results in more significant improvements in aerobic capacity in the HIV population.

EXERCISE IN AIDS WASTING SYNDROME

Exercise training programs with a focus on resistance training have been investigated to see if they can reverse muscle atrophy and weakness (sarcopenia) and increase lean muscle mass in the AIDS Wasting Syndrome.

EFFECTS OF THE AIDS WASTING SYNDROME

The AIDS Wasting Syndrome is defined by the CDC as a net weight loss of at least 10% (CDC 1987). However, Wheeler et al. (1998) found that weight loss of as little as 5% is associated with increased morbidity and mortality in HIV patients. AIDS wasting is a common and serious complaint in persons with HIV, despite treatment of HIV/AIDS in the era of HAART. In a cohort of HIV-infected subjects followed longitudinally, 18% of patients demonstrated a sustained weight loss of >10% of body weight for at least a year, 21% demonstrated >5% loss of body weight, and 8% had a BMI of <20 kg/m^2 (Wanke et al. 2000). Among patients followed at the Johns Hopkins AIDS Service from 1994 to 1998, the incidence of AIDS wasting did not decrease after the introduction of HAART (Moore and Chaisson 1999). These data suggest that AIDS wasting remains a serious clinical concern in HIV/AIDS, even among those treated with potent antiretroviral therapy.

Clinical manifestations of AIDS wasting, particularly the loss of metabolically active lean tissue, have been associated with impaired strength and functional status, accelerated disease progression, and increased mortality, illustrating the necessity for physical rehabilitation in this population (Grinspoon et al. 1999; Guenter et al. 1993; Palenicek et al. 1995; Schwenk et al. 2000; Suttmann et al. 1995; Thiebaut et al. 2000; Wheeler et al. 1998). Using weight as a predictor of survival, Wheeler et al. (1998) showed that the risk of death nearly doubled in patients with a weight loss of 5% to 10% in comparison with a weight loss of 0% to 5% over four months. Similarly, Guenter et al. (1993) demonstrated an 8.3-fold increase in risk of death in HIV-infected patients at <90% of their ideal body weight (IBW). Palenicek et al. (1995) demonstrated a significantly reduced survival in men who had lost >4.5 kg three to nine months before the development of AIDS (1.05 vs. 1.48 years, $p = .0001$).

More recently, a study showed adjusted survival hazard ratios (HR) of 1.9 (95% CI, 1.4-2.6), 3.3 (95% CI, 2.4-4.4), and 6.7 (95% CI, 5.2-8.6) for weight loss of <5%, 5% to 10%, and >10% from baseline, respectively, over a mean follow-up period of 19.9 months (Thiebaut et al. 2000). In addition, a BMI between 16.0 and 18.4 kg/m^2 was associated with a 2.2-fold (95% CI, 1.6-3.0) increased risk of death, and a BMI of <16 kg/m^2 was associated with a 4.4-fold (95% CI, 3.1-6.3) increased risk of death in HIV-infected adults. Other measures of body composition, such as phase angle and body cell mass (BCM) by bioelectric impedance analysis (BIA), have also been shown to predict mortality in HIV patients (Schwenk et al. 2000; Suttmann et al. 1995). Rehabilitative and therapeutic strategies to increase weight and lean body mass are important in HIV-infected patients with the wasting syndrome.

RESISTANCE EXERCISE AND AIDS WASTING

Exercise has been investigated as a potential treatment strategy to increase weight and lean body mass (LBM) and improve functional status in patients with AIDS wasting (table 16.2). In particular, resistance exercise has been shown to increase lean tissue in HIV-infected patients (Bhasin et al. 2000; Roubenoff et al. 1999a, 2001; Yarasheski et al. 2001). In a small study of 10 patients with AIDS wasting, whole-body protein synthesis rates increased after acute exercise on a stair stepper, indicating that the ability to respond to exercise with increased protein synthesis is maintained in AIDS wasting (Roubenoff et al. 2001). In an early controlled study of PRT three times a week for six weeks for HIV-infected men recovering from pneumocystis pneumonia, Spence et al. (1990) demonstrated significant increases in weight (1.7 kg) in exercising patients versus a loss of weight (1.9 kg) in nonexercising patients.

In a study of six subjects who met the criteria for AIDS wasting and participated in an eight-week PRT program three times a week at 80% of their 1RM, there was an even greater increase in LBM of 2.8 kg in exercisers versus 1.4 kg in nonexercisers ($p < .08$) (Roubenoff et al. 1999a). Roubenoff et al. (1999a) demonstrated a significantly greater weight gain in the AIDS wasting group compared to those in the PRT program without AIDS wasting. In addition, dietary energy and protein intake was increased in the AIDS wasting group, suggesting appetite stimulation with PRT in the wasting group (Roubenoff et al. 1999a).

Although studies of exercise in AWS patients have focused largely on men, a recent study of PRT was performed in 12 women with BCM ≤90% by BIA. Progressive resistance training, consisting of three sets of 10 repetitions at 75% of 1RM over 14 weeks, increased fat-free mass by 1.6 kg, decreased fat mass by DEXA scan and magnetic resonance imaging (MRI), and increased muscle strength (Agin et al. 2001). These studies indicate that exercise regimens may work to improve LBM, strength, appetite, and metabolic indices in patients with AIDS wasting.

Exercise, Testosterone Analogs, and AIDS Wasting

A number of studies have investigated exercise in combination with testosterone analogs in the treatment of AIDS wasting (table 16.3). In a four-arm study of eugonadal men with AIDS wasting, subjects were randomized to receive placebo (N = 12), placebo and exercise (N = 10), testosterone (N = 10), or testosterone and exercise (N = 11) for 12 weeks (Grinspoon et al. 2000). Exercise was thrice weekly and consisted of 20 min of aerobic training at 60% to 70% of age-predicted maximum heart rate followed by a PRT program. The PRT program had patients increase resistance for six upper and lower body exercises as follows: weeks 1 and 2, two sets of eight repetitions at 60% of 1RM; weeks 3 through 6, two sets of eight repetitions at 70% of 1RM; weeks 7 through 12, three sets of eight repetitions at 80% of 1RM. Grinspoon et al. found that the exercise program alone significantly increased LBM (+2.3 kg), arm and leg muscle cross-sectional area determined by CT, and HDL cholesterol compared to baseline ($p < .01$). Patients receiving combined testosterone enanthate (200 mg intramuscularly [IM] once a week) and exercise demonstrated significant improvements in weight, LBM, fat mass, muscle area, and strength, but no improvement in HDL cholesterol compared to baseline.

Similarly, Bhasin et al. (2000) performed a 16-week study of 49 HIV-infected men with low testosterone and weight loss of ≥5% over six months, randomized to placebo and no exercise (N = 14); testosterone enanthate (100 mg per week IM) and no exercise (N = 17); placebo and exercise (N = 15); or testosterone and exercise (N = 15). Those treated with exercise alone or with both testosterone and exercise showed significant increases in muscle strength. Lean body mass increased by 2.6 kg ($p < .001$) in the testosterone and exercise group. Body weight increased significantly by 2.2 kg ($p = .02$) in men in the exercise-only group, but did not change in men receiving placebo (–0.5 kg, $p = .55$) or testosterone and exercise (0.7 kg, $p = .08$).

Strawford et al. (1999) conducted a double-blind, randomized, placebo-controlled, eight-week trial in 22 HIV-infected men with weight loss undergoing PRT, consisting of three sets of 10 repetitions set at 80% of 1RM for six upper and three lower body exercises, and receiving replacement doses of testosterone enanthate (100 mg IM every week). Groups were randomized to treatment with oxandrolone at a dose of 20 mg per day orally (N = 11) or placebo (N = 11). Weight, LBM, and strength increased, whereas fat mass decreased, in both treatment groups. In contrast, Sattler et al. (1999) studied a group of asymptomatic HIV-infected men randomized to receive PRT in combination with supraphysiologic doses of nandrolone (600 mg IM every week) (N = 15) or nandrolone alone. Exercise was three times a week for 12 weeks with free weights, followed by a warm-up of one set of five to eight repetitions at 50% of 1RM and three sets of 10 repetitions at 80% of 1RM, adjusted every two weeks. Subjects randomized to nandrolone and PRT demonstrated significantly greater increases in strength in comparison to the nandrolone-only treatment group. Body weight increased significantly in both groups (nandrolone group increased 3.2 ± 2.7 kg, and combined treatment group increased 4.0 ± 2.0 kg); however, there was a greater net increase in LBM of 5.2 kg in the combined treatment group compared to 2.9 kg in the nandrolone-only group. Total thigh muscle area, quadriceps muscle area, and hamstring muscle area increased significantly in both treatment groups. Body cell mass increased significantly in both groups. Fat mass did not change in the nandrolone-only group, but there was a significant reduction in the combined treatment group by 1.2 kg.

In addition to improved body composition with combined testosterone and exercise treatment, Sattler et al. (2002) found an effect of treatment on metabolic measures, including cholesterol and glucose. Metabolic measurements of 14 subjects in the nandrolone-only group and 14 in the combined treatment group were made at 12 and 24 weeks, after the study intervention. LipoA was significantly reduced in all subjects at week 12, but not at week 24. High-density lipoprotein significantly decreased at week 12 for all subjects and remained decreased at week 24 for all subjects in the combined treatment group. Fasting insulin and homeostasis model assessment (HOMA-IR) were significantly lower in the combined treatment group at week 12. Progressive resistance training may significantly increase LBM to a greater degree in combination with anabolic therapies, such as testosterone. Combined anabolic/PRT regimens may be useful for subjects with AIDS wasting;

Table 16.2 Summary of Exercise Studies in AIDS Wasting Syndrome

Author	Subjects	Design	Intervention	Major Findings
Roubenoff et al. 2001	31 HIV+ subjects with or without AWS	Non-controlled, non-randomized, treatment study	15 min on 60 cm step at 1 step/s.	22 subjects completed (10 with AWS, 12 without AWS). No differences at baseline between groups in leucine flux, oxidation, or NOLD. NOLD, 6 d post exercise, was significantly higher in AWS group compared to non-wasting group. Comment: Main conclusion was that AWS patients retain the anabolic response to exercise seen in non-wasting HIV+ subjects.
Roubenoff et al. 1999	20 HIV+ ♂ and 5 ♀	Non-randomized, non-controlled treatment study	PRT 3 d/wk × 8 wks at 75-80% of 1 RM adjusted q2wks for leg press, leg extension, chest press, and seated row exercises in 3 sets of 8 reps.	24 subjects completed with >90% compliance. Significant increase in all 4 measures of strength and increases remained significant at 16 wks. Significant increases seen in LBM (1.75 ± 1.94 kg) and decreases in fat (–0.92 ± 2.22 kg) by DEXA. 6 subjects with AWS. Fat mass significantly increased in the AWS group in comparison to the non-wasting group (0.95 vs. –1.5 kg), which persisted at 16 wks. Weight significantly increased in AWS group in comparison to non-wasting group (3.8 vs. –0.2 kg), which persisted at 16 wks. Trend toward increased dietary energy and protein intake in AWS group in comparison to non-wasting group.
Spence et al. 1990	24 HIV+ men recovering from PCP Pneumonia	RCT	Randomization to: PRT 3 d/wk × 6 wks, consisting of 1 set of 15 reps to 3 sets of 10 reps for knee, chest-arm, and shoulder-arm exercises. Non-exercise.	Significant increase in weight (1.7 kg) in exercise subjects vs. weight loss (–1.9 kg) in non-exercising subjects. Increased muscle strength for all subjects.

(continued)

Table 16.2 *(continued)*

Author	Subjects	Design	Intervention	Major Findings
Grinspoon et al. 2000	54 eugonadal men with AWS	RCT with 2 × 2 factorial design	Randomization to: Testosterone enanthate 200 mg/wk or placebo IM PRT and aerobics consisting of 20 min aerobics on a stationary bike at 60-70% of age predicted maximal HR with 15 min cool down followed by 2 sets of 8 reps at 60% of 1 RM wks 1-2, 2 sets of 8 reps at 70% of 1 RM wks 3-6, 3 sets of 8 reps at 80% of 1 RM wks 7-12 for leg extension, leg curl, leg press, lateral pull down, arm curl, and triceps extension 3 d/wk × 12 wks or no exercise training.	78% compliance in 21 patients completing exercise regimen. Significant increases in LBM (2.3 ± 2.2 kg), arm muscle area (346 ± 147 mm^2), and leg muscle area (797 ± 654 mm^2) from baseline in the placebo and training group (N = 10). Significant increase in HDL (0.08 ± 0.16 mg/dl) from baseline in the placebo and training group (N = 10). Patients receiving combined exercise and testosterone enanthate had significant improvements in weight, LBM, fat mass, muscle area, and strength.
Agin et al. 2001	37 HIV+ ♀ with BCM ≤ 90%	RCT with subjects being their own control group thru assessment wks 0-6	Randomization to: Whey protein 1 g/kg per day (PRO) PRT 3 d/wk × 14 wks consisting of 3 sets of 10 reps at 50% of 1 RM for wk 1, then 75% of 1 RM with weight increases of 2.5 lbs., if patients finished 10 reps without undue fatigue (PRE). PRO/PRE	30 ♀ completed the protocol with > 94% compliance in those completing PRT. PRE group had significant changes from baseline for BCM (0.74 kg), muscle by MRI (1.2 kg), fat mass by MRI (–1.71 kg), and fat mass by DEXA (–1.8 kg). Fat free mass by DEXA increased by 1.6 kg (p = .06). PRO/PRE group had significant changes from baseline in BCM (0.61 kg) and fat free mass by DEXA (1.4 kg). Significant changes in fat mass by MRI in the PRE vs. PRO/PRE group (–1.7 vs. 0.7 kg). Significant changes in fat mass by DEXA in the PRO vs. PRE group (2.1 vs. –1.8 kg).

Note: ♂ = men; ♀ = women; AWS = AIDS wasting syndrome; BCM = body cell mass by body impedance analysis; d = days; DEXA = dual energy X-ray absorptiometry; HDL = high density lipoprotein; HR = heart rate; IM = intramuscular; LBM = lean body mass; min = minutes; MRI = magnetic resonance imaging; NOLD = non-oxidative leucine disposal; PCP = pneumocystis carinii; PRT = progressive resistance training; q2wks = every two weeks; RCT = randomized controlled trial; reps = repetitions; RM = repetition maximum; s = second; wk(s) = week(s).

Table 16.3 Summary of Trials of Combined Steroid and Exercise Treatment in Aids Wasting

Author	Subjects	Design	Intervention	Major Findings
Bhasin et al. 2000	61 HIV+ ♂ with serum testosterone < 349 ng/dl and weight loss of 5% or > in previous 6 mo	Randomized, double blind, placebo controlled trial	Randomized to Placebo and no exercise Testosterone enanthate 100 mg/wk IM and no exercise Placebo and exercise Testosterone enanthate 100 mg/wk IM and exercise Exercise consisted of 3 sets of 12-15 reps at 60% of initial 1 RM wks 1-4, then periodized exercise, 4 sets of 4-6 reps at 90% on heavy, 80% on medium, and 70% of 1 RM on light days wks 5-10, then 5 sets of 4-6 reps at loads increased by 7% for upper body and 12% for lower body wks 11-16, 3 d/wk × 16 wks.	49 patients completed (12 in group 1, 15 in group 2, and 11 in groups 3 and 4) with > 16 patients having > 90%, 5 with 75-89%, and 1 with 70% compliance with exercise sessions. 29-36% increase in muscle strength in 5 exercises in the exercise group and 10-32% in the testosterone and exercise group. No advantage to combination testosterone and exercise over treatment with exercise alone. Significant increase in thigh muscle volume in exercise group (62 cm^3) and in testosterone and exercise group (44 cm^3) and this change was significantly greater in the exercise group in comparison to the placebo group. Significant increase in LBM with testosterone and exercise (2.6 kg). Significant increase in BW (2.2 kg) in ♂ who exercised and this change was significantly > placebo group.
Sattler et al. 2002	Same as above	Same as above	Same as above	30 subjects completed study with 98.5% compliance with PRT in exercisers. Significant decrease in Lipoprotein a (–7.2, –6.9, and –7.1 mg/dl) and decrease in HDL (–8.7, –10.7, and –8.7 mg/dl) in the nandrolone only, nandrolone and PRT group, and overall, respectively. Significant decreases in fasting glucose (–15.1 mg/dl), fasting insulin (–12 μU/ml), and HOMA-IR (–3.3) and a significant increase in QUICKI (0.027) from baseline in the nandrolone and PRT group.
Grinspoon et al. 2000	Refer to table 16.2			

(continued)

Table 16.3 *(continued)*

Sattler et al. 1999	33 HIV+ ♂ with CD4 counts between 50-400 mm^3 and BMI of 20-27.5 kg/m^2	Randomized, open label trial	All subjects received nandrolone deconoate 200 mg IM wk 1, 400 mg IM wk 2, and 600 mg IM wk 3-12 and were randomized to: 1. PRT 2. No PRT. PRT was 3 d/wk × 12 wks with 5-8 reps at 50% of 1 RM for warm-up, followed by 3 sets of 8 reps at 80% of 1 RM with adjustments to 1 RM q2wks for bench press, pull downs, military press, biceps curls, triceps extensions, leg press, calf raises, leg curls, and leg extension exercises.	30 subjects completed the study with 98.5% PRT compliance in those completing exercise. Significant increases from baseline in the nandrolone only and nandrolone and PRT group for body weight, LBM, BCM, total thigh muscle, quadriceps muscle, and hamstring muscle area. The magnitude of change for LBM was significantly greater in the nandrolone and PRT group in comparison to the nandrolone only group (5.2 vs. 3.9 kg). Fat mass decreased significantly from baseline in the nandrolone and PRT group (–1.2 kg). Significant increases in all measures of strength in both treatment groups. There were significantly greater gains in strength in the nandrolone and PRT group in comparison to the nandrolone only group.
Strawford et al. 1999	24 eugonadal men with at least a 5% weight loss in the previous 2 years	Double-blind, randomized, placebo-controlled trial	All subjects received testosterone enanthate 100 mg/wk IM and PRT 3D/wk × 8 wks, consisting of 3 sets of 10 reps for 6 upper and 3 lower body exercises at 80% of 1 RM that was adjusted at wk 4. Randomization was to: 1. Oxandrolone 20 mg qd 2. Placebo	22 completed the trial. Significant increases from baseline for cumulative nitrogen retention in both groups, but greatest in oxandrolone group (5.6 vs. 3.8 g/d). Significant increase from baseline for weight (6.7 vs. 4.2 kg) and LBM (6.9 vs. 3.8 kg) in both groups, but greater increases in the oxandrolone group. Fat mass decreased significantly in both the oxandrolone (1.7 kg) and placebo group (1.6 kg) and bone density increased in both the oxandrolone (105 g) and placebo group (80 g). Significant improvements in all 6 measures of strength from baseline in both groups with significantly higher increases for chest press, biceps pull, triceps push, and leg press in the oxandrolone group in comparison to the placebo group. Significant improvements in flexion, extension, and total work measured by dynamometer testing of both the shoulder and knee muscle in both groups with changes in shoulder strength being significantly greater in the oxandrolone group in comparison to the placebo group for both flexion and extension. Note: Exercise compliance not reported.

Note: ♂ = men; BCM = body cell mass by body impedance analysis; BMI = body mass index; BW = body weight; d = days; wk(s) = weeks; HDL = high density lipoprotein; HOMA-IR = homeostasis model assessment; IM = intramuscular; LBM = lean body mass; mo = month; PRT = progressive resistance training; q2wks = every two weeks; qd = once daily; QUICKI = quantitative insulin sensitivity and in this context, exercise may counteract the potential negative effects of anabolic treatment on HDL, insulin, and glucose.

Exercise in HIV Lipodystrophy

HIV lipodystrophy is another long-term complication of HIV and HAART. Lipodystrophy syndrome is characterized by fat redistribution and metabolic abnormalities, including dyslipidemia and impaired glucose tolerance, and has a reported prevalence ranging from 35% to 62% in HIV patients exposed to HAART and approximately 12% in HAART-naive patients (Carr et al. 1999; Friedl et al. 2001; Lichtenstein et al. 2001). The fat redistribution in HIV lipodystrophy is characterized by a loss of fat in the face and extremities and fat accumulation in the abdomen, breasts, and neck, including a "buffalo hump" on the back of the neck in some patients (Lo et al. 1998). The body composition and metabolic abnormalities of HIV lipodystrophy are similar to the changes seen in syndrome X or metabolic syndrome (a cluster of clinical characteristics including increased waist circumference, hypertriglyceridemia, decreased HDL cholesterol, hypertension, or hyperglycemia [National Cholesterol Education Program 2001]) and may be associated with increased risk for cardiovascular disease and diabetes in the HIV population.

Numerous studies have documented metabolic abnormalities in association with potent antiretroviral therapy in HIV-infected patients. For example, Behrens et al. (1999) reported that 57% of 98 protease inhibitor recipients experienced hyperlipidemia, with 19% demonstrating increased LDL, 44% demonstrating hypertriglyceridemia, and 37% demonstrating combined lipid abnormalities. Intra-abdominal fat accumulation is known to be highly predictive of cardiovascular disease and diabetes in HIV-negative subjects (Fujioka et al. 1987; Bjorntorp 1988; Matsuzawa et al. 1995). In HIV-negative obese subjects with central adiposity, both weight reduction and intensive aerobic exercise reduce serum triglycerides, raise HDL, lower blood pressure, and decrease the risk of diabetes (Franz et al. 1994). Therefore exercise may be beneficial to improve metabolic and body composition abnormalities in HIV lipodystrophy patients (table 16.4).

In a case report, a 44-year-old HIV-infected white male with self-reported fat loss in the arms and legs, increased abdominal girth, and increased breast size underwent four months of exercise training, including PRT and 20 min of aerobic exercise three times a week (Roubenoff et al. 2002). A diet of 1.3 times resting energy expenditure was provided, with 30% of calories from fat, ≤10% from saturated fat, >25 g of fiber per day, and low glycemic index foods. The patient's BMI decreased by 2.87 kg/m^2, WHR by 0.1, percentage body fat by 8.6%, and percentage trunk fat by 5.7%. Total abdominal fat, subcutaneous abdominal fat, visceral abdominal fat, and waist circumference were reduced. Low-density lipoprotein decreased by 30 mg/dL; HDL decreased by 23 mg/dL; and total cholesterol decreased by 52 mg/dL, in association with improved HOMA IR.

In a small study of 10 men with increased abdominal girth who participated in 20 min of aerobic exercise on a stationary bike or treadmill and a PRT program at 80% of 1RM thrice weekly over 16 weeks, Roubenoff et al. (1999c) observed significant increases in strength for three of four exercises and a significant decline in total body fat by 1.5 kg, with predominant fat loss in the trunk (–1.1 kg). In another small prospective study of six HIV lipodystrophy patients participating in a combined aerobic and resistance training program three times a week for 10 weeks, Jones et al. (2001) found significant improvements ($p < .05$) in body mass, percentage body fat, WHR, arm and leg circumferences, aerobic endurance, and composite strength. In addition, there was an 18% decrease in total cholesterol ($p = .001$) and a 25% decrease in triglycerides ($p = .05$) at 10 weeks compared to baseline. Similar improvements in body composition and lipids were seen in a four-month study of an aerobic exercise program consisting of three 45-min sessions on a cycle ergometer, at a heart rate corresponding to ventilatory threshold (VO_{2VTh}), in 17 lipodystrophic and two dyslipidemic HIV-infected adults (Thoni et al. 2002). Thoni et al. (2002) observed a 13% reduction in total abdominal fat ($p < .001$), a 12% reduction in visceral abdominal fat ($p < .01$), a 23% reduction in total cholesterol ($p < .01$), a 43% reduction in triglycerides ($p < .01$), and a 6% increase in HDL ($p < .01$). Calculation of the estimated relative risk of cardiovascular disease in subjects studied by Thoni et al. (2002) demonstrated a 13% reduction in risk ($p < .01$) from baseline to the end of the four-month intervention.

Recently we conducted a prospective study designed to determine the additional benefit of a 12-week combined aerobic and PRT program in 25 HIV-infected patients with fat redistribution and insulin resistance who were receiving the diabetic drug metformin at a dose of 850 mg twice a day. Significant improvements in body composition, strength, and aerobic capacity with exercise in the combined treatment group compared to the metformin-only group were noted (Driscoll et al. 2004a). In addition, there were significant improvements in both systolic and diastolic blood pressure and larger decreases in insulin levels in the combined treatment group. These data suggest that exercise may work to improve glucose and insulin metabolism, in addition to improving cardiovascular disease indices and body composition in patients with HIV lipodystrophy.

Table 16.4 Summary of Exercise Studies in Patients With HIV Lipodystrophy

Author	Subjects	Design	Intervention	Major Findings
Roubenoff et al. 2002	44-year-old ♂ with self report of fat redistribution	Case study	Aerobic and resistance training 3 d/wk × 16 wks consisting of 20 min of aerobic exercise on an elliptical machine at 80-85% of maximal HR followed by 3 sets of 8 reps for leg press, chest press, leg extension, seated row, and knee flexion exercises. 1/3 of sessions were supervised. Dietary intake was set at 1.3 × REE, with 15% of total caloric intake from protein, 30% from fat, ≤ 10% from saturated fat, ≥ 25g of fiber per day, and low glycemic index foods. He participated in weekly nutrition counseling sessions.	He completed the protocol with 90% compliance. Maximal dynamic strength (average for all 5 exercises) increased by 54% and $\dot{V}O_2max$ increased by 16.8%. BMI and WHR decreased by 10%, body fat decreased by 33%, trunk fat decreased by 39%, TAT decreased by 43%, SAT decreased by 38%, and VAT decreased by 52%. LDL decreased by 16%, HDL decreased by 33%, total cholesterol decreased by 18%, fasting insulin decreased by 45%, and HOMA IR decreased by 52%.
Roubenoff et al. 1999	14 HIV+ ♂ with self-report of increased abdominal girth	Open label, pilot study	Aerobic and resistance training 3 d/wk × 16 wks consisting of 20 min of aerobic exercise on a treadmill or stationary bike followed by approximately 1 hour of resistance training for 4 upper and lower body exercises at 80% of 1 RM.	10 completed the protocol with an average compliance of 77% (range 53-98%). Significant decreases in total body fat (–1.5 kg) and trunk fat (–1.1 kg). Significant increases in 3 out of 4 measures of strength [leg press (13%), leg extension (19%), and chest press (18%)]. No significant improvement in seated row exercise (7%).
Jones et al. 2001	5 ♂ and 1 ♀ with HIV and lipodystrophy (self report and MD confirmation of fat redistribution)	Prospective study	90 min of aerobic exercise and PRT 3 d/wk × 10 wks. Aerobics was 20 min of cycling at 70% of peak HR followed by 60 min of resistance training consisting of 3 sets of 10 reps for 3 lower and 3 upper body exercises. Muscle strength and aerobic function were assessed weekly and the exercise regimen was adjusted accordingly.	6 subjects completed with 80-100% compliance. Total cholesterol and triglyceride concentrations decreased by 17.6 and 25.3% respectively. Significant improvements were seen in % body mass (5.5%), body fat (–13.93%), WHR (–4.67%), arm (9.32%), and leg (7.93%) circumferences. % Aerobic endurance (21.8%) and composite strength (94%) increased significantly.

Driscoll et al. 2004a	37 HIV+ ♂ and ♀ on stable antiretroviral therapy for > 3 mo with hyperinsulinemia (fasting insulin ≥ 104 pmol/L or 120 min insulin ≥ 521 pmol/L) and evidence of fat redistribution (WHR > 0.9 in ♂ and > 0.85 in ♀ and lipodystrophy score > 2)	Prospective, randomized study	All subjects given metformin 850 mg PO BID and randomized to: No PRT Combined aerobic and PRT 3 d/wk × 12 wks, consisting of a 5 min warm-up on a stationary bike and flexibility routine, then 20 min of aerobic exercise at 60% of maximal HR × 2 wks, then 30 min at 75% of maximal HR thereafter. This was followed by a PRT program consisting of 3 sets of 10 reps at 60% of 1 RM × 2 wks, then 70% of 1 RM × 2 wks, then 80% of 1 RM thereafter with adjustment to 1 RM q2wks for 3 lower & upper body exercises.	25 subjects completed the study with an average compliance with sessions of 93 ± 2%. Significant increases in 5 out of 6 measures of strength in the metformin and exercise group in comparison to metformin only. Significant improvements in WHR (–0.02 vs. –0.01), thigh muscle area by CT (3 vs. 7 cm^2), and SAT by CT (–13 vs. –1 cm^2) in the metformin and exercise group vs. the metformin only group. Significant decreases in both systolic (–12 vs. 0 mmHg) and diastolic (–10 vs. 0 mmHg) blood pressures, fasting insulin (–42 vs. 0 pmol/L) and insulin AUC (–298808 vs. –8917 pmol/L) in the metformin and exercise group in comparison to the metformin only group.
Thoni et al. 2002	19 HIV+ ♂ and ♀ with self-report and MD confirmation of fat redistribution or dyslipidemia	Open label study	Aerobic exercise on a cycle ergometer for 45 min at HR corresponding to VO_{2VTh}, 2 d/wk × 4 mo.	19 subjects finished with > 85% compliance. 2 patients without fat redistribution were taken out of the analysis leading to results similar to those below. Significant improvements in $\dot{V}O_2$max (193 ml/min), WRmax (9.3 watts), VO_{2VTh} (144.4 ml/min), and RE O_2max (–6.7). Significant decrease in TAT (–30.7 cm^2) and VAT (–11.9 cm^2).

Note: ♂ = men; ♀ = women; AUC = area under the curve; BID = twice a day; BMI = body mass index; CT = computed tomography; d = day; HDL = high density lipoprotein; HOMA-IR = homeostasis model assessment; HR = heart rate; LDL = low density lipoprotein; min = minutes; mo = months; PO = orally; PRT = progressive resistance training; q2wks = every two weeks; REE = resting energy expenditure; RE O_2max = respiratory equivalent; reps = repetitions; RM = repetition maximum; SAT = subcutaneous abdominal fat by CT; TAT = total abdominal fat by CT; VAT = visceral abdominal fat by CT; $\dot{V}O_2$max = maximal oxygen uptake; VO_{2VTh} = ventilatory threshold; WHR = waist-to-hip ratio; wk(s) = weeks; WRmax = maximal work rate.

In the metformin and exercise study previously described (Driscoll et al. 2004a), there was a significant improvement in intramuscular adiposity ($p = .04$) as measured by CT scan in the metformin and exercise group in comparison to the metformin-only group (Driscoll et al. 2004b). The change in muscle adiposity correlated with measures of insulin and remained a significant predictor of insulin in a model comprising other measures of body composition, including WHR, trunk fat as measured by DEXA scan, subcutaneous leg fat, and visceral abdominal fat (Driscoll et al. 2004b). To investigate the relationship between exercise history and metabolic abnormalities in HIV-infected patients, Gavrila et al. (2003) conducted a cross-sectional study of 120 HIV-infected men and women with greater than six months of HAART exposure, 29 of whom demonstrated fat redistribution. Subjects were asked to complete multiple choice questionnaires on intensity, frequency, and duration of current exercise.

Gavrila et al. (2003) found that the total exercise index (equal to exercise intensity × duration of exercise × number of exercise sessions per week) was inversely correlated with triglycerides ($p < .008$) and HOMA IR ($p < .008$) in a model adjusting for age, sex, tobacco and alcohol use, fat percentage, WHR, CD4 count, duration of HAART exposure, presence of fat redistribution, blood pressure, HDL, and LDL cholesterol. These data suggest that exercise correlates with measures of cholesterol and insulin in patients with HIV lipodystrophy and that this relationship may be driven by the changes in fat distribution seen with exercise. Further studies are necessary to elucidate the specific physiologic mechanism relating fat distribution and exercise performance to insulin resistance in the HIV population. Nonetheless, current data suggest that exercise has clear beneficial effects on body composition and metabolic measurements in patients with HIV lipodystrophy.

Exercise to Improve Psychosocial and Quality of Life Issues in HIV

The chronic complications and symptoms of HIV disease can significantly affect quality of life (QOL), and the effects of exercise to improve QOL have been studied in the HIV population. Fourteen HIV lipodystrophy patients from a clinic in London were interviewed about their perceptions of life with HIV (Power et al. 2003). Subjects commented on the physical effects of the condition and the pains associated with particular movements, but were largely concerned with body image. Patients complained of being self-conscious of their appearance and reported reduced self-esteem and reduced confidence leading to depression and isolation. In a cross-sectional study of 175 HIV-infected patients, 83 with lipodystrophy, lipodystrophic patients had significantly lower scores in physical functioning, role function, and physical health summary scores by Medical Outcomes Study (MOS)-HIV questionnaire (Orlando et al. 2002).

Several investigators have looked at the impact of exercise on measures of QOL in HIV-infected patients. Fifty-four men completed a 12-week open trial of testosterone (400 mg IM biweekly) and were asked about current exercise habits (Wagner et al. 1998). Twenty-nine men reported exercise during the trial with a mean frequency of three to four days per week for an average of 87 min; 10 subjects reported resistance training only; 2 subjects reported only cardiovascular workouts; and 17 subjects reported both aerobic and resistance training. The Endicott Quality of Life Enjoyment and Satisfaction Questionnaire, a 16-item self-report measure of perceived satisfaction in various life domains, showed significant improvement in satisfaction in 12 of the 16 domains assessed, including physical health, mood, household activities, social relationships, leisure activities, sexual interest and activity, overall well-being, and overall life satisfaction, in exercisers compared to the testosterone-only group. In addition, a recent study of women participating in a 14-week PRT program showed significant improvements in MOS-HIV physical activity scores and increases in general health perceptions and vitality (Agin et al. 2001). Exercise may contribute to overall well-being and QOL in HIV-infected populations.

Fatigue is another common complaint in patients with HIV. In an analysis of responses to 422 voluntary online or mailed questionnaires collected at multiple sites in Europe and North America, fatigue—which was distinguished from other related concepts like weakness—was the HIV symptom listed sixth most often by HIV-infected patients; and exercise was listed as a successful treatment in this regard (Corless et al. 2002). In a meta-analysis of several studies of HIV-infected patients, the incidence of fatigue ranged from 55% to 98%, and several causes of HIV-related fatigue were noted, including anemia, impaired liver or thyroid function, malnutrition, wasting, AIDS dementia, HIV myopathy, immunosuppression, hormonal deficiencies, depression, lack of exercise, pain, infection or fever, nutritional deficiencies, excessive inactivity or rest, and growth hormone dysregulation (Corless et al. 2002).

In addition to problems with physical functioning and QOL, HIV-infected patients may suffer from clinical depression. The prevalence of major depression has been reported at approximately 22% to 32% in persons with HIV, twice that observed in the general population (Neidig et al. 2003). Several studies have shown more rapid immune decline, increased mortality, and nonadherence to HAART in HIV-infected patients with signs and symptoms of depression (Neidig et al. 2003). In HIV-negative populations, regular exercise has proven an effective therapy for mild to moderate depression and helpful as an adjunct to medical therapy in severe depression (Neidig et al. 2003). In a study of 60 HIV-positive patients on stable treatment receiving three 1-hr aerobic sessions per week with 30 min of aerobic activity at 60% to 80% of $\dot{V}O_2$max or no exercise, there were significant improvements in two validated measures of depression (the Center for Epidemiological Studies Depression Scale and the Profile of Mood States) and a trend toward decreased Beck Depression Inventory scores ($p = .064$) in the exercise group in comparison to the nonexercise group (Neidig et al. 2003). These data suggest that exercise may benefit HIV patients with clinical depression, but further studies are needed.

EXERCISE EFFECTS ON IMMUNE STATUS AND LACTIC ACID

An important question for HIV patients is the effects of exercise on immune function. An acute bout of exhaustive exercise in healthy adults has been shown to activate the immune system, leading to leukocytosis, neutrophilia, and lymphopenia, with variable effects on rate of infection with respiratory viruses (Cannon 1993; Cohen et al. 1991; Nieman et al. 1990; Nieman 1997). Acute exercise has also been found to increase the production of inflammatory cytokines, including interleukin-1B and tumor necrosis factor alpha, which can increase HIV replication (Angel et al. 1995; Cannon and Kluger 1983; Fielding et al. 1993; Granowitz et al. 1995, 1996). An important question is whether acute or chronic exercise (or both) could affect immune function in patients infected with HIV.

One hundred fifty-six HIV-positive homosexual men in a New York City cohort, followed from 1985 to 1991, were asked to fill out questionnaires in an effort to investigate the relationship of disease progression to exercise history (Mustafa et al. 1999). Based on participant answers to the questionnaires, subjects were classified as self-reported exercisers (exercising at least three times per week) (70%) or nonexercisers (30%). Self-reported exercisers had a slower progression to AIDS at one year (HR = 0.68, 90% CI) and a slower progression to death from AIDS at one year (HR = 0.37, 90% CI). Exercisers also showed increased CD4 counts after one year. The protective effect of exercise in this cohort of men was lost after the first year, and exercise habits were not reassessed longitudinally.

In vitro studies of the effects of exercise on immune response have also been performed (Rohde et al. 1995). An in vitro study of lymphocytes from eight HIV-positive and seven HIV-negative subjects was performed while patients were at rest, during exercise, and 2 hr after exercise (Rohde et al. 1995). Exercise consisted of 1 hr at 75% of $\dot{V}O_2$max on a stationary bike. The investigators found that proliferation of lymphocytes was lower in all conditions in HIV-infected versus HIV-negative patients and that the percentage of CD4 cells did not significantly change in relation to exercise in either group. In 1992, Rigsby et al. showed that an aerobic and strength training regimen for 12 weeks in 13 HIV-infected subjects resulted in no significant differences or changes from baseline in CD4 cell counts.

Similar results were noted in vivo by Ullum et al. (1994). Eight HIV-positive and eight HIV-negative age- and sex-matched controls exercised on a bicycle ergometer at 75% of $\dot{V}O_2$max for 1 hr. Neutrophil counts increased more in the control group. Lymphocytes increased significantly in both groups with exercise and then recovered to baseline levels at 2 and 4 hr postexercise. As with leukocytes and neutrophils, the percentage and total numbers of CD4 cells were significantly lower in the HIV group in comparison to controls at baseline, but the percentage of CD4 cells did not change in response to exercise. In 1999, Perna et al. demonstrated a 13% increase in CD4 cells in 11 HIV-infected compliant exercisers compared to an 18% decline seen in 7 noncompliant exercisers in response to aerobic interval training at 70% to 80% of maximal heart rate three times a week.

In another in vivo study of acute exercise, Roubenoff et al. (1999b) investigated 25 HIV-infected subjects performing a one-time 15-min bout of exercise on a stair stepper at a cadence of one step per second while on a meat-free diet for one week. The study showed increased neutrophil counts 2 hr after acute exercise ($p < .06$) that then decreased to pre-exercise levels. In contrast, mean HIV RNA (ribonucleic acid) did not increase during the week after exercise ($p = .12$). In a randomized study of exercise in 60 healthy HIV-infected men and women, CD4 cell counts, CD4 percentage, and HIV-1 RNA copy numbers did not change significantly during the study for the experimental or control groups (Smith et al. 2001). In a six-week study of aerobic exercise in 26 healthy HIV-infected patients, there were no significant changes in CD4 count or HIV RNA in any of the treatment groups (Stringer et al. 1998). Taken together, the evidence from a number of studies suggests that acute or chronic exercise does not alter immune status or enhance HIV replication in HIV-infected patients.

Lactic acid levels are increased in HIV-infected patients, perhaps as a result of mitochondrial toxicity due to nucleoside reverse transcriptase inhibitor (NRTI) therapy. An important question is whether exercise will increase lactate levels to a greater degree in HIV-infected subjects. Roge et al. (2002) investigated eight HIV patients treated with HAART, demonstrating either fat redistribution or elevated p-lactate. Subjects were exposed to increasing exercise intensity until exhaustion. HIV-infected patients demonstrated elevated levels of lactate at rest; but maximal serum lactate values did not increase relative to the control group with exercise, and the decline in blood lactate in the recovery period was similar between groups. In our study of HIV-infected patients with lipodystrophy receiving combined metformin and PRT, significant lactic acidosis did not occur (Driscoll et al. 2004a). Preliminary data from several exercise studies in HIV-infected adults suggest that exercise is safe for HIV-infected adults in terms of immune function and lactic acidosis.

SUMMARY

Since the development of HAART, HIV has evolved from a deadly infectious disease to a chronic condition. Chronic infection with HIV/AIDS is associated with long-term complications, including fatigue, AIDS wasting, lipodystrophy, and an overall lower QOL in such patients. Although further research into the role of exercise in HIV-infected patients is needed, current research demonstrates the efficacy of both aerobic training and PRT for treatment and rehabilitation of the chronic complications of HIV and HAART in this population. Aerobic exercise improves aerobic capacity and body composition in HIV-infected patients. Progressive resistance training alone or in combination with aerobic exercise in patients with AIDS wasting increases LBM, weight, and strength and decreases fatigability, and may help to increase HDL cholesterol and appetite in such patients. The addition of PRT in patients with AIDS wasting treated with testosterone may increase LBM and strength beyond increases with testosterone alone and may counteract the negative effects of anabolic treatments on cholesterol, insulin, and glucose metabolism. Improvements in weight and lean mass should in turn reduce the morbidity and mortality seen in AIDS wasting.

Combined aerobic training and PRT regimens in patients with HIV lipodystrophy improve body composition, WHR, waist circumference, visceral and subcutaneous abdominal fat, strength, aerobic capacity, cholesterol profiles, and insulin and glucose metabolism. There is also significant evidence to suggest that aerobic or resistance training, or the combination, can improve QOL and symptoms of depression in HIV-infected populations. Exercise has also been well documented to be a safe and well-tolerated treatment in HIV patients and does not seem to alter immune status or precipitate lactic acidosis. Further studies of the benefits of exercise in HIV patients are still needed, particularly in regard to optimal frequency, intensity, and duration of aerobic and resistance training, alone or in combination, for the treatment of various chronic disease states observed in HIV-infected populations. However, data to this point suggest that exercise in any form will benefit the health and well-being of HIV-infected patients.

CHAPTER 17

OBESITY

Ronenn Roubenoff, MD, MHS

CASE STUDY

Charles L., a 48-year-old white insurance agent, weighs 258 pounds (122 kg), and is 5′9″ (175 cm) tall. When he played football in high school, he weighed 205 pounds (93 kg), then reduced to 190 pounds (86 kg) by age 24. At age 30 he again weighed 205 pounds (93 kg), and by age 40 he was 230 pounds (105 kg). He says he "watches what he eats," and is surprised to hear his current weight. Mr. L. becomes short of breath walking down the hall from the waiting room to the examining room. He says that he gets up to urinate once or twice per night. He denies smoking, but drinks "a couple of beers" each night. Blood pressure is 150/96 mmHg (with a large cuff), and his heart rate is 88 bpm. A repeat blood pressure after sitting quietly is 148/96 mmHg. General examination is unremarkable. Waist circumference is 46 inches, and hip circumference is 42 inches. Initial laboratory evaluation shows that his CBC and electrolytes are normal, his random glucose is 167 mg/dL, and urinalysis is unremarkable. He returns for further tests, including a fasting glucose of 128 mg/dL, and glucose two hours after an oral glucose load is 192 mg/dL.

Twenty-five mg daily of hydrochlorothiazide is prescribed for hypertension, and Mr. L. is sent to the dietitian for diet therapy of his metabolic disorders and obesity. The dietitian determines that Mr. L's usual dietary intake is 2500 calories/day. His diet contains 42% of calories from fat. He is instructed in a diet that reduces his energy intake to 2000 kcal, with 30% of calories from fat, and 2 grams of sodium.

At one-month follow-up, blood pressure has improved to 132/84, and weight to 254 pounds (115 kg). Mr. L's rate of weight loss (1 pound/week) is good, but exercise is added to ensure continued loss and ability to stabilize at a satisfactory level. He is counseled to begin a walking program, taught how to take his pulse, and asked to walk 1 mile/day 3 times a week for four weeks, increasing to 2 miles/day 3 to 5 times per week. The pace should be brisk enough to reach a target heart rate of about 140 beats per minute ([220 – age] × 0.85). He is encouraged to do this outdoors or indoors, and to consider joining a health club where he can use treadmills, bicycles, and other machines, swim, or do aerobics.

One year later, his weight is 217 pounds, his fasting glucose is 108 mg/dL, and his blood pressure is 130/80. He states he feels much better and did not realize before that he had been suffering from low energy and fatigue until these symptoms had resolved.

The prevalence of obesity is increasing rapidly in the United States and other developed countries, as well as in some developing countries. In June 1998, the National Institutes of Health (NIH) and National Heart, Lung, and Blood Institute (NHLBI) adopted a new scheme, which now aligns the United States with the World Health Organization for classifying overweight and obesity (NHLBI 1998). Overweight is defined as a body mass index (BMI) of 25.0-29.9 kg/m^2, and obesity is defined as a BMI ≥30.0 kg/m^2. According to the most recent National Health and Nutrition Examination Survey (NHANES III), 39.4% of adult American men and 24.7% of adult American women are overweight, while 19.9% of men and 24.9% of women are obese (see "Definitions of Overweight," page 266).

Since these surveys were begun in 1960, the prevalence of overweight (utilizing the new criteria) has remained relatively stable, while the prevalence of

Table 17.1 Trends in the Prevalence of Overweight and Obesity in the United States 1960-1994

	BMI (kg/m²)			
Survey	25-29	30-34	35-39	40+
NHES I (1960-62)	30.5%	9.6%	2.4%	0.8%
NHANES I (1971-74)	32.0%	10.1%	2.8%	1.3%
NHANES II (1976-80)	31.5%	10.1%	3.1%	1.3%
NHANES III (1988-94)	32.0%	14.4%	5.2%	2.9%

Data shown are the proportion of the U.S. population in each BMI category.

obesity has increased substantially (table 17.1). These increases in the prevalence of obesity have occurred during a time when dietary intake of fat as a percent of energy intake in the United States has been stable or falling slightly, and dietary intake of fruits and vegetables has increased; however, the total intake of energy (and thus total fat intake) may have increased despite the compositional changes of the diet. Moreover, there has been a progressive decline in physical activity in the United States, which coincides with the increase in obesity, suggesting that inadequate physical activity may play an important role in developing and maintaining obesity. If correct, this hypothesis provides an important rationale for aggressively prescribing exercise to prevent and treat obesity.

Health Implications of Obesity

Obesity is a major public health problem in the developed world, and there is evidence that it is rapidly becoming a problem in the developing world. Obesity is a risk factor for diabetes, coronary artery disease, hypertension, gallstones, gout, and osteoarthritis, as well as cancer of the breast, colon, and prostate (Colditz et al. 1995; Hubert et al. 1983). These comorbidities increase the risk of premature mortality; they also increase risks of longer hospital stays and of more difficult recovery from various acute medical problems and from surgery. Even reductions as small as 5% in weight can reduce the risks of developing these comorbidities, or at least reduce their severity. It is not necessary to reduce weight to the level of ideal body weight in order to see clinically significant improvements in blood pressure or glycemic control. Moreover, it is unlikely that most obese individuals can achieve and maintain a loss of more than 10% to 15% of starting weight with nonsurgical treatment. Thus, it is neither necessary nor realistic for most obese adults to slim down to published or perceived definitions of "ideal weight." People also are more likely to maintain a gradual weight loss, avoiding the wide swings in weight that occur with more restrictive diets, known popularly as "yo-yo" dieting. Increased physical activity is important to maintain reduced weight after an initial reduction phase.

Definitions of Overweight

	BMI (kg/m²)
Overweight	25-29.9
Obese	30-39.9
Extreme obesity	40+

Body Composition Through the Life Cycle

Of a healthy newborn child's total weight, 10% to 15% is fat and approximately 25% is muscle. In contrast, a healthy young adult has 15% to 25% fat and 40% muscle. With age, the ratio of fat to muscle increases even in healthy adults who maintain their weight throughout their lives. By the eighth decade, it is not unusual to see adults with 40% body fat even though their weights are within 20% of ideal. Most adults in the developed world gain weight between their twenties and their sixties, after which there is a slow decline in weight. During this time period, a gain of only one pound per year would lead to a 40-pound weight gain, of which 30 pounds are expected to be fat. After the 7th decade, weight tends to stabilize and then decline as sarcopenia sets in.

Comparing Weights: The Body Mass Index

The simplest way to assess obesity is to weigh a person. Because weight alone can be misleading, however—150 pounds is low for a 6-foot tall man, but excessive for a

5'2" woman—researchers developed ways to compare weight for height, usually using one of several **body mass indices (BMIs).** The most common such measure is the Quetelet index (weight in kg divided by the square of the height in meters), to which the simple term **BMI** typically refers. Because the BMI is designed to compare weights of people of different heights, it has a greater correlation with body weight than with height (Micossi and Harris 1990). Although useful, the BMI exhibits important age and gender biases: a BMI of 25 kg/m^2 does not represent the same body composition in men as in women, or in young persons as in old persons. Clinicians have often used BMI to indicate body fatness: weight gain in adults is mostly fat, and BMI correlates reasonably well ($r \sim .5$-$.7$) with fat mass (Micossi and Harris 1990; Roubenoff et al. 1995). However, it correlates equally well with lean mass. Calculation of BMI allows clinicians to assign initial classification of weight for height, but only after they consider mitigating factors. For example, there are obviously great differences between a 200-pound linebacker, who may be heavy but has a low percentage body fat and is very physically fit, and a 200-pound sedentary man with a protuberant abdomen and poor physical conditioning. Yet each may have the same BMI. Fortunately, such dramatic differences in body composition are usually apparent even to untrained observers.

BMI has been useful as an indicator of increased mortality risk. Risk of death increases with age; and when this risk is plotted against BMI, it is clear that a BMI greater than about 27 kg/m^2 is associated with an increased risk of death (Metropolitan Life Insurance Company 1980; Roberts 1989). This increased risk is attributed to the excess body fat of people with high BMIs, and their attendant reduced physical activity. Thus the **ideal body weight** is the range of weights (or BMIs) associated with the lowest risk of mortality in the population. Although some believe there is also increased risk of death at low BMIs (below 20 kg/m^2) due to insufficient lean mass, such a discussion is beyond the scope of this chapter (see Forbes 1987). In reality, BMI is only a fair measure of body fatness: to use it as a surrogate for fatness may be necessary in a busy clinical practice and in large-scale epidemiological studies, but it should not be encouraged or accepted uncritically. The best use of BMI lies in assessing individuals' weights, not their fatness.

ETIOLOGY OF OBESITY

Development of obesity is a multifactorial process involving genetic, metabolic, and environmental factors. Genetic factors confer the potential for obesity, but it is the interaction between genetic and environmental factors, such as diet and level of physical activity, that result in weight gain. Gains in body weight by definition represent an imbalance between energy intake and energy expenditure; to maintain body weight, an individual must match intake and expenditure. To illustrate just how precise this regulation is, consider a small energy imbalance of +2% (or +50 kcal/day for an individual with total maintenance needs of 2500 kcal/day), an imbalance that can easily occur. That small imbalance, if persisting over one year, would result in a gain in body weight of approximately five pounds. In epidemiological studies, the average weight gain in adults is between 0.5 and 2.0 pounds/year (Jeffrey and French 1997; Williamson 1993; Williamson et al. 1993), suggesting that most persons chronically maintain energy balance to greater than 99% tolerance. Discussion of the role of energy intake in obesity is well beyond the scope of this chapter; Schoeller (1998) reviewed the contribution of energy intake and dietary factors to energy balance.

Total energy expenditure (TEE) comprises resting energy expenditure, the thermic effect of food, and energy expended on physical activity. **Resting energy expenditure (REE)** accounts for approximately 60% to 75% of TEE, and represents the energy cost of essential biological functions such as respiration, cardiac function, and maintaining membrane potentials and ion gradients. The viscera and the brain contribute disproportionately to REE. While skeletal muscle at rest expends less energy per unit mass than many other tissues, the large total mass of muscle translates to a significant contribution to REE. The thermic effect of food (TEF) usually provides about 10% of TEE, reflecting the energy required to digest and assimilate ingested food. Energy expenditure for activity (EEA) is the most variable part of TEE, and can range from approximately 15% of TEE in sedentary persons to over 50% in active persons or athletes. The ratio of TEE:REE can be considered an index of physical activity (termed **physical activity level,** or **PAL**). Since both TEE and REE can be elevated in obesity (see below), using absolute values of these measures may be confusing; it is therefore important to normalize levels of activity to REE.

In addition to being the most variable component of energy expenditure, energy spent on physical activity is the most difficult to measure accurately. Techniques employed include questionnaires and inventories, heart-rate monitoring, accelerometers worn on the belt or at other body sites, indirect calorimetry performed in a metabolic chamber over 24 hours, and the doubly labeled water method (DLW). Because subjects are restricted to a metabolic chamber environment during calorimetry testing, and therefore may not follow habitual levels of activity, this approach may underestimate TEE. DLW measures CO_2 production in free-living persons by administering stable isotopes of hydrogen and oxygen and following the disappearance of these isotopes in urine, blood, or sputum (Roberts 1989). While DLW is the most accurate way to determine TEE, it is also by far the most expensive and technically challenging, requiring expertise in administration and laboratory analysis of isotopes. As will be discussed later, measuring TEE by DLW while measuring REE by indirect calorimetry permits calculation of nonresting energy expenditure (or TEE minus REE), which includes energy expenditure associated with daily activities as well as with exercise.

Regulation of Energy Intake

There has been an explosion of knowledge about the neuroendocrine regulation of food intake in the past decade. It is now clear that obesity is not merely a failure of willpower, but a hormonally driven disorder in brain control of energy balance. Many different genetic mutations have been found to explain up to 5% of cases of childhood obesity, but in general no simple genetic explanation has emerged for obesity. The key pathways regulating dietary intake and physical activity are shown in figure 17.1. For a more detailed discussion, please see the review by Korner and Aronne (2003). The emerging biology of obesity indicates that leptin, a hormone made by fat cells in the periphery, acts along with insulin in lean persons to reduce dietary intake by suppressing the orexigenic neuropeptide Y (NPY) and stimulating the anorexic neuropeptide melanocortin at the same time. These two peptides, with overlapping support from MCH, orexins, CART, and others, regulate food intake and energy expenditure to achieve energy balance. When fat mass expands, leptin levels rise, but a relative resistance to both leptin and insulin in the brain develops that slowly limits the ability of leptin to brake positive energy balance. At the same time, insulin resistance is thought to be at least partially responsible for many of the deleterious health effects of obesity, such as diabetes, hypertension, and cardiovascular disease.

Schwartz et al. (2003) have suggested that the balance of these hormones favors weight gain and failure of energy-restricted diets (see figure 17.2). They propose that in the basal state, the weight-losing (catabolic) pathways (primarily via melanocortin) are activated by leptin and insulin, while the weight-gaining (anabolic) pathways (primarily NPY) are suppressed to maintain weight. With weight loss, the reverse happens, and activation of the anabolic pathways and inhibition of the catabolic ones occur. This response is inherently stronger than the response to weight gain, which leads to the attempted further stimulation of the already basally stimulated catabolic pathways and further inhibition of the already suppressed anabolic pathways. Thus, over time, in developed societies where energy expenditure is relatively low and energy availability is high, most people tend to gain weight. Almost 50 years ago, Jean Mayer hypothesized that the mechanisms controlling energy balance are accurate at high levels of physical activity, but that there is a threshold below which these mechanisms become imprecise and this leads to obesity; recent data suggest that this hypothesis is valid. Thus, an important role of exercise in treating obesity may be to increase daily caloric needs to a level where the body's regulatory mechanisms are better able to function.

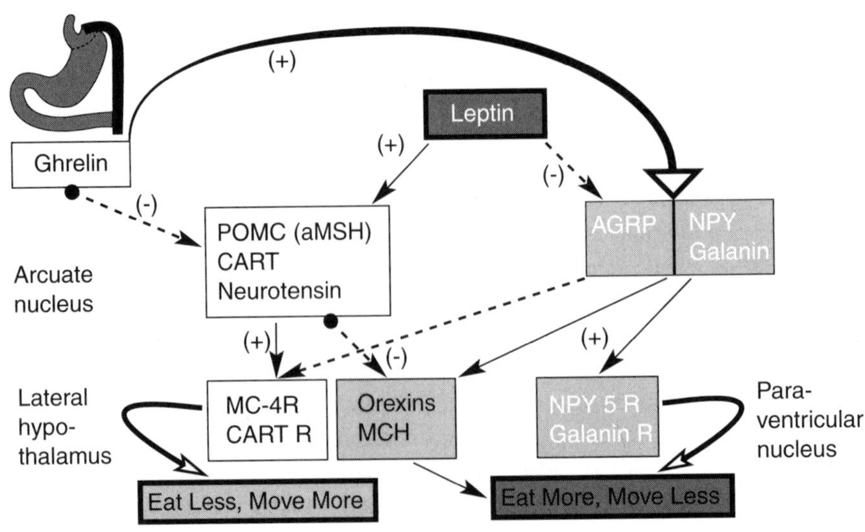

Figure 17.1 Major pathways regulating energy balance in humans. AGRP = Agouti-related protein; CART = cocaine- and amphetamine-related transcript; MC = melanocortin; MCH = melanin concentrating hormone; MSH = melanocyte stimulating hormone; NPY = neuropeptide-Y; POMC = proopiomelanocortin; R = receptor.

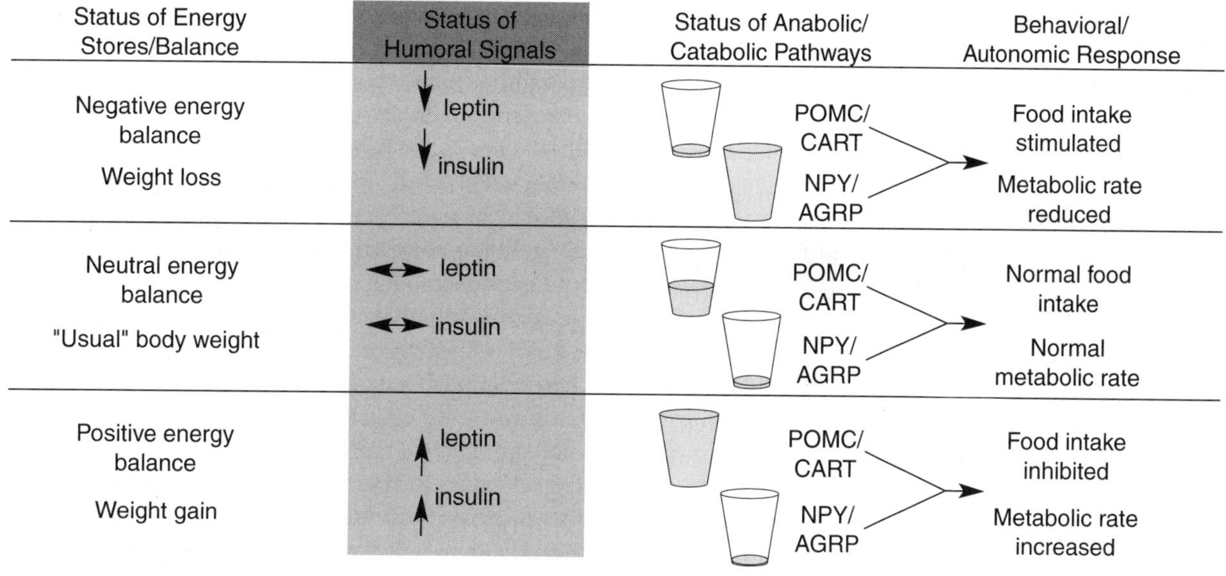

Status of Energy Stores/Balance
Status of Humoral Signals
Status of Anabolic/ Catabolic Pathways
Behavioral/ Autonomic Response
Negative energy balance
Weight loss
leptin
insulin
POMC/ CART
NPY/ AGRP
Food intake stimulated
Metabolic rate reduced
Neutral energy balance
"Usual" body weight
leptin
insulin
POMC/ CART
NPY/ AGRP
Normal food intake
Normal metabolic rate
Positive energy balance
Weight gain
leptin
insulin
POMC/ CART
NPY/ AGRP
Food intake inhibited
Metabolic rate increased

Figure 17.2 Model for the relationship between levels of leptin and insulin and activity of brain neuropeptide regulators of energy balance. At baseline, usual levels of leptin and insulin stimulate a higher steady state production of catabolic pathways (POMC/CART) than anabolic ones (NPY/AGRP). During starvation, low leptin and insulin promote positive energy balance vigorously, because there is a great deal of unused capacity to increase NPY and AGRP and moderate leeway to suppress POMC and CART. However, during positive energy balance, elevation in leptin and insulin has relatively less capability to either suppress NPY and AGRP (which are already relatively suppressed at baseline) or to increase POMC and CART, which are already at relatively higher levels than NPY and AGRP during neutral energy balance.

Reprinted, by permission, from M.W. Schwartz et al., 2003, "Is the energy homeostasis system inherently biased toward weight gain?" Copyright © 2002 American Diabetes Association from *Diabetes*, Vol 52, 2002: 232-238. Reprinted with permission from The American Diabetes Association.

ENERGY EXPENDITURE: RELATIONSHIP TO OBESITY

Two questions logically arise when one considers the relationship between obesity and energy expenditure: (1) Do obese persons expend less energy than their lean counterparts, thus allowing maintenance of the obese state? (2) Does a deficit in energy expenditure or any of its components promote obesity?

Cross-sectional studies reveal that, in absolute value, both total and resting energy expenditure are increased in the obese in comparison to lean counterparts. As measured by DLW, TEE is positively correlated with body weight (Rising et al. 1994; Schulz and Schoeller 1994). REE increases with weight gain, although in some regression models other factors (such as fat mass and genetics) account for additional variability of REE. While REE rises absolutely in the obese, its value per unit of lean mass is not appreciably different from that of leaner people.

Despite the absolute increase in TEE observed in obesity, the amount of energy expended on physical activity when normalized to the REE is actually lower in obese persons than in lean persons. Using DLW in combination with REE measured by indirect calorimetry, Roberts et al. (1995) observed an inverse relationship between percent of weight as body fat (%BF) and TEE/REE. Other investigators using DLW have also found inverse relationships between fatness and energy spent on physical activity normalized for REE (Rising et al. 1994; Schulz and Schoeller 1994). Cross-sectional comparison of PAL from different studies does not consistently show a lower PAL for the obese; but within individual studies, the inverse relationship between obesity and PAL appears more consistently. This apparent discrepancy is possibly due to methodological differences between labs in using DLW to measure TEE. Using questionnaires to measure energy spent on leisure time activities, Gardner and Poehlman (1994) found that energy spent on leisure time activity (again normalized to REE) decreases as body fat increases. TEF is also measured as part of TEE; and although TEF appears to be lower in the obese, the actual significance of this deficit in relation to body weight remains unclear. It is likely that the overall small contribution of TEF to TEE, and the small magnitude of the differences observed with obesity, make TEF a relatively minor factor in energy balance in comparison to REE and EEA.

Thus, although absolute levels of TEE and REE are increased in obese persons, nonresting energy expenditure is likely to be depressed relative to REE. Theoretically, the increased expenditure needed to support movement of excess weight (especially in weight-bearing exercise) will partially offset this deficit. The cause of this low nonresting energy expenditure in obesity remains speculative; but in extreme obesity, deconditioning, dyspnea, and joint pain are likely contributors. In terms of overall energy balance, low nonresting energy expenditure is likely to contribute to maintenance of the obese state (Schoeller 1998).

Energy Expenditure: Development of Obesity

The mere association between obesity and decreased PAL or EEA (relative to REE) provides no information about cause and effect. To evaluate if obesity results from low energy expenditure, some researchers have conducted prospective studies or studies in individuals who are no longer obese. Large epidemiological studies attempting to prospectively link levels of physical activity to weight gain have rendered mixed results. In the NHANES I Epidemiological Follow-Up Study, Williamson and coworkers (1993) evaluated recreational physical activity and body weight at baseline as well as changes in these parameters after 10 years. As expected, baseline activity was inversely related to baseline weight, but baseline activity did not predict changes in weight at follow-up. Levels of activity at follow-up were inversely related to weight gain over 10 years, and a decrease in activity or maintenance of a low level of activity over 10 years was also associated with risk of weight gain. Similarly, in the Healthy Women Study, Owens et al. (1992) observed an inverse relationship between baseline physical activity and weight gain over three years. In the Health Professionals Follow-Up Study (Coakley et al. 1998), the men most likely to gain weight over four years were those who maintained a low level of activity or decreased activity, or who increased time spent watching television. As reviewed by Williamson (1996), a number of methodological and other issues (including the difficulty of accurately measuring physical activity) may hamper the ability of these observational studies to reach a consensus regarding predictive factors for weight gain.

Prospective trials utilizing 24-hour calorimetry or DLW may better estimate TEE (and hence activity, if REE is also measured), but such trials have been rare to date. Ravussin and colleagues (1988) examined 24-hour energy expenditure using a room calorimeter (respiratory chamber) in 95 Southwestern American Indians, and then followed the subjects' weight gain for up to two years. There was a significant inverse correlation between TEE at baseline and subsequent weight gain ($r = -.33, p < .001$). Fifteen of the 95 subjects gained at least 7.5 kg during the follow-up period. Subjects who expended 200 kcal/day less than the group mean at the initial examination had a fourfold higher probability ($p < .02$) of gaining at least 7.5 kg over the next two years. To emphasize the previous discussion about the small difference between positive and negative energy balances, note that the mean difference in 24-hour energy expenditure between subjects who gained at least 7.5 kg and those who did not was only 87 kcal/day (2262 ± 194 kcal/day, vs. 2349 ± 133; $p = .12$).

Using the DLW method, Roberts and coworkers (1988) measured TEE in infants at three months of age and then assessed weight gain over the next nine months. At 12 months of age, infants who exceeded the 90th percentile of weight for height were considered overweight. At three months, the weight of infants who subsequently became overweight did not differ significantly from that of infants who did not become overweight (5.97 kg vs. 5.56 kg); but infants who eventually became overweight had a lower TEE than the other infants (61 kcal/kg vs. 80 kcal/kg, $p < .05$). These studies, along with the few others that measured TEE (Davies et al. 1991; Griffiths and Payne 1976; Griffiths et al. 1990) suggest that deficits in TEE may contribute to subsequent gains in weight.

Regular exercise seems to attenuate the increase in fat mass with age. Van Pelt et al. (1998) found that postmenopausal female runners (mean age 56 years; average 28 miles/week) averaged 23.4% body fat, compared to 15% body fat in premenopausal female runners (mean age 30 years; average 38 miles/week). Although this observation suggests that fat mass increases substantially with age even among highly active runners, note how these results compare with those of sedentary women studied at the same time: the postmenopausal sedentary women (mean age 61 years) had 40% body fat while the premenopausal sedentary women (mean age 29 years) had 27% body fat. Thus, the athletes had an age-related difference in their body fatness of 8.4%, while the sedentary women had a difference of 13.0%. These data suggest that habitual exercise reduced the age-related increase in body fatness by about 35% (13.0 – 8.4 divided by 13.0). In addition, the habitual exercisers were also significantly more fit than the sedentary women at any age ($\dot{V}O_2max$ 55 ± 0.9 vs. 42 ± 1.5 ml · kg^{-1} · min^{-1}). Although some caution is appropriate in interpreting cross-sectional rather than longitudinal data, these observations suggest that high levels of physical activity can prevent obesity.

While a large portion of TEE is determined by REE (and hence by lean mass), energy spent on physical activity remains an effective way to increase total expenditure. Since (as is often pointed out) a couple of cookies can overcome the caloric expenditure of an hour of exercise, it is relatively difficult to create a negative energy balance by physical activity alone. It is true that exercising an extra 100 or 200 calories/day amounts to only about 10% of the day's energy intake. Nevertheless, as discussed previously, the difference between

Table 17.2 Energy Costs of Moderate Physical Activity

	METs	Cost (kcal) of 1 hour of activity for a 70-kg woman	100-kg man
Walking @ 3 mph	3.5	245	350
Running @ 6 mph	10	700	1000
Raking lawn	4	280	400
Pushing power mower	4.5	315	450
Slow freestyle swim	8	560	800
Doubles tennis	6	420	600
Volleyball	3	210	300
Golf/pulling clubs	5	350	500

A MET is equal to a multiple of resting energy expenditure (REE). Assigned MET value × body weight (kg) × (duration of activity/60 minutes) = kcal.

positive and negative energy balance in most individuals is relatively small, so that even a small increase in physical activity can influence whether that day's balance is positive or negative. As table 17.2 shows, even moderate physical activity can lead to important caloric expenditures, especially in more obese people who require more energy to perform work on their body mass (i.e., to move).

Effect of Exercise on Dietary Intake

In contrast to evidence that a sedentary lifestyle predisposes humans to gain weight, physical activity level does not seem to affect food intake appreciably, either in terms of quantity or quality. In general, exercise does not appear to consistently influence the amount or the macronutrient composition (energy, protein, and fat) of ad libitum diets (King et al. 1997). It has been hypothesized, but not proven, that a more physically active lifestyle could entrain other healthy lifestyle choices (e.g., smoking cessation, reduced intake of dietary fat, and increased intake of fruits and vegetables). Because they expend more energy than sedentary people, athletes also tend to consume more energy and protein. In a study of nonobese women, increased energy intake compensated for increasing energy expenditure from exercise (Pi-Sunyer and Wood 1985). In several trials with obese persons, exercise without dietary restriction resulted in small losses of weight, but the energy imbalance was attributable to the additional energy expended on physical activity and not due to decreases in energy intake (Pi-Sunyer and Wood 1985). However, responses differed in other trials. Nieman and Onasch (1990) examined the effect of moderate exercise training (45 min, or about 5 km, of brisk walking five days a week for 15 weeks) on dietary quality in 36 sedentary, mildly obese women who were randomly assigned to attend supervised exercise sessions or remain sedentary. All the women were encouraged to eat ad libitum. The women in the exercise group did not change their weights, while the control subjects gained about 1.1 kg ($p < .002$). The women in the exercise group tended to reduce their total energy intake, largely due to lower carbohydrate intake, while there was a mild increase in the control subjects' energy intake ($p < .09$).

It has been postulated that exercise and energy intake in the obese (but not in normal-weight adults) may be dissociated because the large fat mass, with its corresponding large energy store and leptin production, acts as a buffer to prevent exercise from triggering hyperphagia. Another mechanism by which exercise may contribute to diminished energy intake is by increasing compliance with a hypocaloric diet. Racette et al. (1995) evaluated the effect of inclusion of aerobic exercise on weight loss over 12 weeks in subjects instructed to consume energy at a level of 75% of basal metabolic rate. Exercising subjects were instructed to consume additional energy to compensate for the cost of exercise. Subjects who exercised lost 10 ± 3.2 kg, while the nonexercising group lost 8.1 ± 2.3 kg ($p < .05$). Exercising subjects consumed energy (determined by DLW) at a level closer to the prescribed amount. Dietary compliance was inversely correlated with anxiety and depression ($r = -.5$, $p = .05$), both of which frequently accompany dieting. This study suggests that inclusion of exercise may facilitate compliance with, and psychological tolerance of, a hypocaloric diet.

Effect of Exercise on Energy Expenditure

Resting energy expenditure increases with body size, and the increased absolute REE in obese people reflects that 25% of their excess weight is lean mass (Forbes 1987). When REE is expressed per kilogram of lean mass (or normalized to lean mass by other statistical means), there is no consistently observed difference between obese and leaner persons (suggesting that total quantity of cell mass, rather than the proportions or metabolic state of different types of cells, is the major determinant of REE in the obese (Ravussin et al. 1988)). However, there are probably other small but important effects on REE, such as from genetic factors and fat mass. Ravussin et al. (1988) observed that people with low REE were more prone to develop obesity than people with higher REE; this difference withstood adjustment for lean body mass. People in the lowest tertile of REE gained an average of 2.75 kg/year, while those in the middle and upper tertiles had no significant gain per year ($p < .01$). The difference in total 24-hour energy expenditure between the low REE group and the other groups was only about 90 kcal/day.

Despite the benefits of exercise, most other studies failed to demonstrate increases in REE in response to aerobic training (Broader et al. 1992; Wilmore et al. 1998). Meredith and coworkers (1989) found no change in REE after 12 weeks of endurance training in either young (mean age 24; mean body fat 21%) or older (mean age 65; mean body fat 37%) healthy adults. Broader et al. (1992) also found no change in REE in 15 healthy nonobese men (ages 18-35; mean body fat 18%) who trained aerobically for 12 weeks. More recently, a large and methodologically rigorous study of a 20-week aerobic cycling training program (60%-75% of $\dot{V}O_2max$ for 30-50 min/day, three times per week) caused no change in REE in mildly overfat men (24% body fat) and women (35% body fat) despite a large improvement (18%) in aerobic fitness measured by $\dot{V}O_2max$ (Wilmore et al. 1998).

Even if aerobic training can indeed increase REE in normal-weight individuals, there is reason to doubt that overweight adults can achieve similar increases. First, it is more difficult to achieve high absolute work loads in sedentary, obese adults, because they often have comorbid conditions (heart disease, lung disease, arthritis) that limit exercise capacity, and because they often must overcome a personal history of not exercising, perhaps even of disliking exercise. Second, there is evidence that obese adults have an impaired catecholamine response to exercise, with lower epinephrine (but not norepinephrine) production and greater postexercise insulin resistance compared to lean subjects (Yale 1989). Specific approaches to exercise prescription in the elderly have recently been reviewed by Jakicic and Gallagher (2003).

Effects of Weight Loss on Energy Expenditure

Loss of body weight, regardless of how it is lost, leads to decreases in TEE, REE, and EEA. TEE decreases because its individual components decline. Although loss of metabolically active lean mass leads to a reduction in REE, the decrease is greater than predicted by simple loss of lean mass. As would be expected, the thermic effect of feeding decreases in proportion to the hypocaloric energy intake usually recommended for weight loss. Energy expended on physical activity also declines, in part due to the decreased energy cost of moving a smaller body mass, and in part due to other factors.

Negative energy balance achieved through a hypocaloric diet decreases REE substantially (often by 10%-15%). This drop is greater than would be expected from the loss of lean mass (Saltzman and Roberts 1995); and it is proportional to the actual caloric deficit (energy needed to maintain weight minus actual intake). Some researchers have observed that measured REE remains below that predicted by lean mass during weight stabilization following loss (Saltzman and Roberts 1995). Teleologically, we can view the below-predicted REE associated with weight loss as the body's attempt to defend its existing weight. While only a few studies have addressed the issue of whether exercise can overcome these decreases in REE, limited data suggest it is unlikely that aerobic exercise can completely overcome the metabolic down-regulation that underfeeding engenders.

An alternative approach, which has been studied to a lesser extent, is whether resistance training can increase REE. Unlike aerobic training, which is thought to increase REE (at least transiently) by increasing sympathetic nervous system outflow, resistance training may increase REE by increasing body cell mass, especially muscle mass. Ballor and colleagues (1996) compared 12 weeks of thrice-weekly aerobic or weight training in 18 men and women (aged 56-70 years) who had recently lost an average of 9 kg by dieting. At the end of the 12 weeks, REE of the aerobic training group had declined 12 ± 41 kcal/day, versus an increase of 79 ± 37 kcal for the resistance training group ($p < .07$). The aerobic training group lost more weight than the resistance training group (2.4 kg loss vs. 0.3 kg gain, $p < .05$)—but this is because the resistance training group gained 1.5 kg of lean mass and lost 1.2 kg of fat mass, while the aerobic group lost 0.6 kg of lean mass and 1.8 kg of fat mass (all $p < .05$). In addition, Van Etten et al. (1997) observed that resistance training increased not only REE but also energy expenditure of physical activity outside the training sessions, a phenomenon we have seen several times in our laboratory (Campbell et al. 1994; Rall et al. 1996).

These studies indicate the profound differences between aerobic and resistance training in their effects (outlined in more detail later) both on metabolism and on body composition. Nelson (1998) has written a valuable book for the lay public, outlining how to reduce fat mass through strength training.

Negative energy balance also reduces EEA, which decreases to a greater extent than REE during weight loss (Leibel et al.1995; Saltzman and Roberts 1996; Weigle et al. 1988). To determine the role of lost body mass on EEA, Weigle and colleagues (1988) estimated EEA for walking before and after weight loss of 22% in obese men. After the weight loss, the men wore lead-filled vests to replace lost weight, permitting the authors to calculate the energy cost of carrying that weight. Weigle estimated that approximately 56% of the decline in TEE resulted from reduced energy cost associated with lower body mass. Other suggested reasons for lower EEA after weight loss include decreases in spontaneous activity and increases in the efficiency of movement. Given the reductions in energy expenditure during and following weight loss, exercise may compensate by contributing its own costs directly to EEA, by increasing REE (in the case of resistance training), and by helping to preserve lean mass. We further discuss these concepts below.

Exercise for Treatment of Obesity

In the absence of a hypocaloric diet, light to moderate exercise is unlikely to result in loss of substantial body weight or fat mass. The energy cost of such activity (see table 17.2) is unlikely to induce an adequate and uncompensated energy deficit over the long term; individuals create deficits sufficient to induce weight loss much more readily by reducing energy intake. However, exercise itself may induce small losses of weight. In comparing worksite-based exercise and diet programs, for example, Pritchard et al. (1997) found that the exercise program resulted in a decrease of 2.6 ± 3.0 kg of body weight.

Effect of Exercise on Weight Loss and Preservation of Lean Body Mass During Hypocaloric Feeding

In a meta-analysis evaluating the effects of exercise during dieting, Miller et al. found that the mean one-year weight loss in 493 studies was 10.7 ± 0.4 kg with dietary restriction, 2.9 ± 0.4 kg with exercise alone, and 11.0 ± 0.6 kg with combined diet and exercise (Miller, Koceja et al. 1997). Although some researchers have observed improved weight loss when exercise accompanies dieting, the above meta-analysis increases the difficulty of interpreting these data. However, there does seem to be a dose response of exercise effect on both weight loss and regain: patients who exercised at least 200 min/week lost 12 kg at 6 months versus 6.5 kg in subjects who exercised less than 150 min/week, and were better able to maintain their weight loss at 18 months (Jakicic et al. 1999). In trials in which exercise increased lost weight beyond dieting alone, it is not clear whether the loss was due to the effects of exercise on energy output, the effects of exercise on REE, the effects of exercise on energy intake, or some combination of these factors.

While exercise does not appear to dramatically increase the amount of weight lost, it does appear that exercise while dieting helps to preserve lean mass. Just as accretion of lean mass accompanies gains of fat mass, loss of weight is characterized by loss of both fat and lean. In underfeeding studies that measured body composition changes during weight loss, approximately 25% of lost weight was lean mass (Saltzman and Roberts 1995). A meta-analysis by Ballor and Poehlman (1994) showed significant preservation of lean mass when exercise accompanied weight loss, in terms of absolute amount of lean mass and of lean loss as a percentage of weight loss. Sweeney et al. (1993) found that aerobic and resistance exercise were equally beneficial during weight loss (compared to no exercise) in preserving lean mass. While we need further effort to clarify the optimal nature and intensity of exercise to accompany hypocaloric diets, strong evidence suggests that exercise will allow preservation of lean mass with weight loss. This phenomenon may be especially important to those with sarcopenic obesity (i.e., reduced lean mass in the setting of increased fat mass) which often characterizes the obese state in older persons.

Effect of Exercise and Physical Activity on Weight Regain After Weight Reduction

Following loss of weight, maintenance of reduced weight is consistently associated with participation in regular supervised (Pace and Rathburn 1945; Pavlou et al. 1989; Sahakian et al. 1983; Saris et al. 1992; Vallejo 1957) or self-initiated (Schoeller et al. 1997) exercise. Klem and colleagues (1997) described factors associated with successful maintenance of lost weight in the National Weight Control Registry, a study of individuals who had lost at least 30 pounds and had maintained that loss for at least one year. These subjects reported, on average, energy spent on physical activity equal to walking 45 miles/week. Using DLW along with measurement of REE, Schoeller et al. (1997) observed the relationship in women between energy expenditure and weight regain

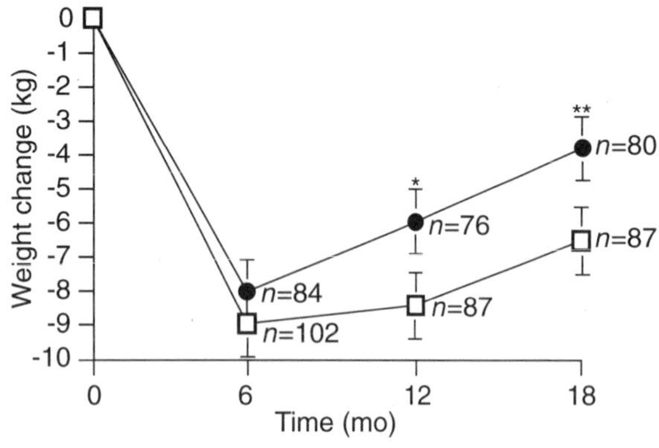

Figure 17.3 Mean weight change over time by treatment group (●, 1000 kcal/wk exercise; □, 2500 kcal/wk exercise). * $p < .07$; ** $p < .04$.

Reprinted, by permission, from R.W. Jeffrey, R.R. Wing, N.E. Sherwood, and D.F. Tate, 2003, "Physical activity and weight loss: Does prescribing higher physical activity improve outcomes?" *American Journal of Clinical Nutrition* 78:684-689.

after an average loss of 23 kg. PAL was inversely related to weight gain. The relationship between energy spent on activity and weight regain was not linear, but showed a threshold effect. Recently, Jeffery et al. (2003) compared the effects of a moderate exercise program (1000 kcal/week expenditure) and a high physical activity program (2500 kcal/week), in addition to a behavioral weight loss dietary program. Dietary intake was the same in both groups, falling from about 2100 kcal/day at baseline to 1500 to 1600 kcal/day over an 18-month period. As shown in figure 17.3, both groups achieved the same degree of weight loss over the first 6 months (8.1 vs. 9.0 kg), but the high physical activity group kept significantly more weight off at 12 and 18 months. Thus, exercise appears to have an important role in the maintenance of weight loss, but the amount of activity needed may exceed what has been previously recommended.

Effect of Exercise on Serum Lipoproteins and Glucose Metabolism

Weight loss per se is only one goal of weight reduction: amelioration of weight-related risk factors for diseases such as coronary artery disease and diabetes are also important effects of weight loss. Lowering serum LDL-cholesterol and triglycerides is an important benefit of weight loss, and even small changes in weight can markedly reduce the risk of heart disease. Several authors have examined whether exercise offers additional benefits beyond those conferred by weight loss through dieting. Schwartz (1987) showed that exercise could improve HDL-cholesterol and apolipoprotein A-1 levels in obese men, despite relatively little weight loss. Wood et al. (1988) studied the effects of weight-reduction diet (mean of 336 kcal/day lower intake after one year than at baseline, $p < .01$; n = 42) versus a supervised aerobic exercise program (walking and jogging a mean of 18.9 km/week; n = 47) versus a usual diet and activity control group (n = 42) over one year. All participants were men with 120% to 160% of ideal body weight. There was no significant change in total or LDL-cholesterol in any study group, but triglyceride levels fell significantly in both groups (exercise: –0.16 mmol/L; diet: –0.27 mmol/L; control +0.08 mmol/L; $p < .05$ for both interventions vs. control). In addition, HDL-cholesterol increased significantly in both exercise and diet groups (see figure 17.4), and there was no difference between the two interventions in their ability to raise HDL-cholesterol.

In a follow-up study, Wood and colleagues (1991) examined the effect of adding aerobic exercise to a hypocaloric National Cholesterol Education Program (NCEP) Step 1 diet (figure 17.5). This is a more realistic question to study, since most overweight persons are counseled to both reduce their food intake and exercise more. In the follow-up study, the authors randomly assigned 132 overweight men (BMI 28-34 kg/m^2) and 132 overweight premenopausal women (BMI 24-30 kg/m^2) to an NCEP weight-reduction diet alone, to the diet with aerobic exercise, or to a control group for one year. All subjects were between ages 24 and 49. The exercise intervention was brisk walking or jogging three times a week at 60% to 80% of maximal heart rate for 25 min per session initially,

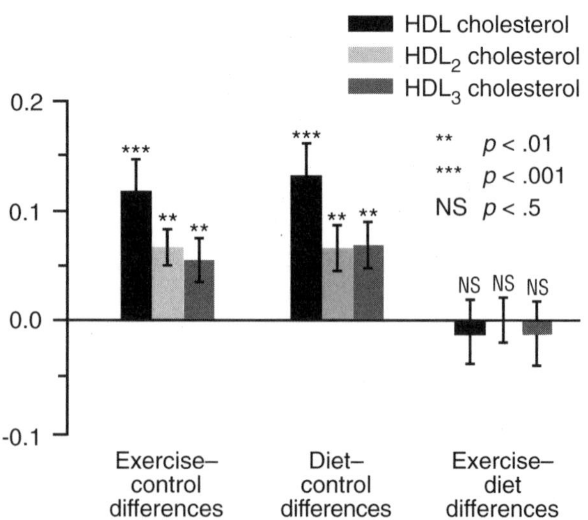

Figure 17.4 One-year changes in plasma concentrations of HDL-cholesterol, HDL_2-cholesterol, and HDL_3-cholesterol: differences in response between aerobic exercise, dietary restriction, or neither. Error bars indicate standard errors.

Reprinted, with permission, from P.D. Wood et al., 1988, "Changes in plasma lipids and pioproteins in overweight men during weight loss through dieting as compared with exercise," *New England Journal of Medicine* 319:1173-1179.

increasing to 45 min per session by the fourth month of the study. After one year, both intervention groups had a similar mean decline in their total energy intake of about 470 kcal/day in the women and about 590 kcal/day in the men. There was a significant reduction in body fat in both intervention groups (–4.3 ± 5.2 kg [mean ± SD] in the diet group; –7.8 ± 4.6 kg in the diet + exercise group; +1.2 ± 3.8 kg in the control group). As in the authors' previous study, HDL-cholesterol increased, but in the current study the increase was significantly higher in the diet plus exercise group compared to the diet alone group only among the men (see figure 17.4). Serum triglycerides fell in both intervention groups among the men, but not among the women. LDL-cholesterol fell with both diet and exercise in both men and women. This study confirms that both diet and exercise reduce lipoprotein risk factors for heart disease in men, but that the effects in premenopausal women are much smaller. In fact, the men in this study had significantly higher total cholesterol (5.41 ± 0.87 mmol/L in the men vs. 4.98 ± 0.73 mmol/L in the women) and LDL-cholesterol at baseline than did the women, whose premenopausal status further put them at lower risk of heart disease. Thus, the women with normal blood cholesterol at baseline showed less responsiveness to the intervention, but they were at lower risk of coronary artery disease in any case. The effect of diet or diet plus exercise in the men was to lower their cholesterol to the women's baseline mean level, while the women's response to the intervention lowered their cholesterol by an additional 10% or so.

As in the report by Wood et al. (1991) on premenopausal women, Fox and coworkers (1996) also observed limited effects of exercise and diet on serum lipids of postmenopausal women with relatively low risk for coronary disease. In this study, 41 healthy postmenopausal women (mean age 66 years; mean weight 120% to 140% of ideal) were assigned to diet (500 kcal/day deficit) plus supervised exercise (aerobic exercise at 60%-70% of $\dot{V}O_2$max one day per week, plus resistance training using 12 major muscle groups at 80% of 1 RM two days per week); 500 kcal/day deficit diet alone; or 700 kcal/day deficit diet alone. The last group had an energy deficit equal to that of the diet plus exercise group. Assignment was evidently not random, as the availability of time to exercise was a factor in choice of study groups. The study lasted 24 weeks. All groups lost weight to a comparable extent (6.5 kg). None of the study groups exhibited changes from baseline in total cholesterol, LDL-cholesterol, HDL-cholesterol, or triglycerides. However, all three treatment groups significantly improved their insulin responses to oral glucose tolerance tests, suggesting that the weight loss decreased insulin resistance both with and without exercise. Again, these data suggest that in overweight adults who do not have significant hyperlipidemia, there is little effect of diet or exercise on serum lipids.

In contrast, persons who have elevated cholesterol levels appear to benefit from weight reduction, and have an additional benefit from exercise (Wood et al. 1991). The effect seen by Fox's group on glucose metabolism is larger in persons who have more severe insulin resistance at baseline, and can occur with exercise alone in the absence of weight change. Katzel et al. (1995) randomly assigned 170 men to weight-reducing diet,

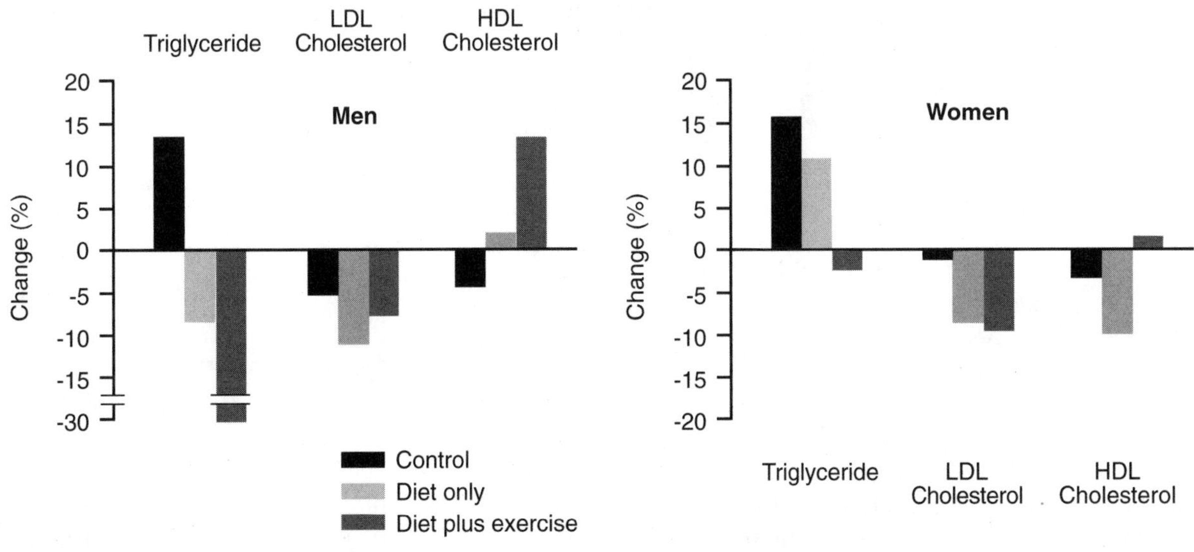

Figure 17.5 Percent change in plasma triglyceride and lipoprotein cholesterol concentrations in response to dietary restriction, diet plus aerobic exercise, or neither in men and women.

Reprinted, with permission, from P.D. Wood et al., 1991, "The effects on plasma lipoproteins of a prudent weight-reducing diet, with or without exercise in overweight men and women," *New England Journal of Medicine* 325:461-466.

aerobic exercise (treadmill or stationary bicycle training three times per week for 45 min per session), or a weight-maintaining control group (figure 17.6). Only 111 men (65%) completed the study. For those in the exercise group, $\dot{V}O_2max$ increased by 17%, and weight did not change; weight declined by 10% among the dietary restriction group, but $\dot{V}O_2max$ did not change; neither measurement changed in the control group. Weight loss led to a significant 13% increase in HDL-cholesterol, decreased blood pressure, and improved glucose and insulin levels both in the fasting state and in response to an oral glucose tolerance test (OGTT). In contrast, the aerobic exercise group had a smaller improvement in OGTT insulin response, but without changes in fasting glucose or insulin resistance, HDL-cholesterol, or blood pressure. The authors concluded that weight loss was more effective than exercise in reducing coronary artery disease risk factors in obese men. However, the increase in aerobic fitness shown with the exercise intervention indicates that exercise causes unique changes in physiologic status that are independent of the effects of weight loss. In this sense, it is clear that weight loss and exercise prescriptions are synergistic and should be considered part of a complete package of lifestyle alterations to improve quality of life and prevent degenerative diseases in obese adults.

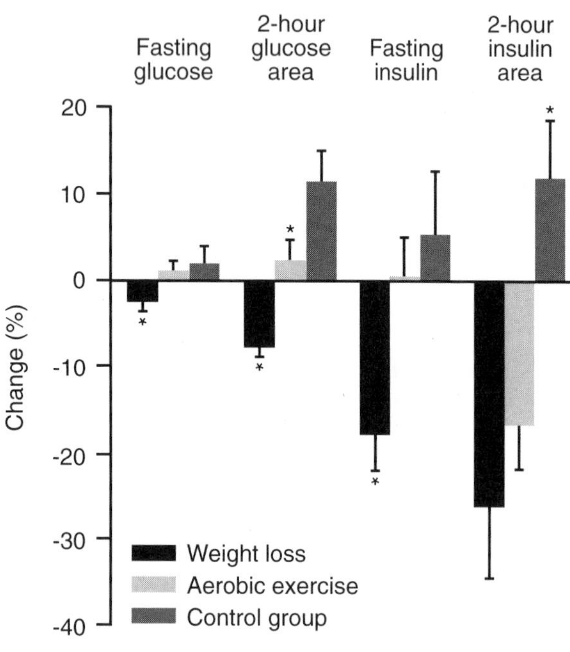

Figure 17.6 Percent change in fasting plasma glucose and insulin concentrations and 2-hour plasma and insulin concentrations during an oral glucose tolerance test, in men undergoing a weight reduction diet, aerobic exercise, or neither. Error bars indicate standard errors of the mean.

Reprinted, by permission, from L.I. Katzel et al. "Effects of weight loss vs. aerobic exercise training on risk factors for coronary disease in healthy, obese, middle-aged and older men," *Journal of the American Medical Association* 274: 1915-1921.

SUMMARY

Over half of American men and women are either overweight or obese. Obesity is a risk factor for many serious disabilities and diseases, some of them fatal. It is natural and probably unavoidable that the ratio of fat to muscle will increase as adults age, and the neuroendocrine basis for this epidemic is now becoming clearer. Exercise, however, can significantly slow the rate of increase.

There appears to be an inverse correlation between total energy expenditure and subsequent weight gain, whether for infants or for adults. Preventing weight gain by increasing exercise levels appears easier than losing gained weight once it exists. High levels of physical activity, higher than most researchers have heretofore thought, apparently can largely prevent obesity.

Obese people have higher absolute values of total and resting energy expenditure than leaner people. It is difficult to create a negative energy balance (taking in less energy than that expended) through exercise alone. There is evidence, however, that increasing lean mass through resistance exercise can increase resting energy expenditure. And although neither aerobic nor resistance exercise appears to strongly abet weight loss, which primarily occurs through dietary restrictions, resistance exercise appears to help maintain weight loss by increasing lean mass and thereby increasing both resting energy expenditure and the general energy expenditure of physical activity.

Apart from weight loss, aerobic exercise has important effects on a number of cardiac risk factors, especially those related to blood lipids. Even in the absence of significant weight loss, in obese individuals with hyperlipidemia (but not so much in the nonobese or in obese individuals with normal blood lipids) aerobic exercise may increase levels of HDL and lower triglyceride levels.

Obese individuals are best served by well-designed hypocaloric diets and by exercise programs that include vigorous aerobic and resistance components.

ACKNOWLEDGMENTS AND DISCLOSURE

This material is based upon work supported by the U.S. Department of Agriculture, under Agreement No. 58-1950-9-001. Any opinions, findings, conclusion, or recommendations expressed in this publication are those of the authors and do not necessarily reflect the view of the U.S. Dept. of Agriculture. Also supported in part by NIH Grants DK45734 and AG15797, and General Clinical Research Center Grant M01-RR-00054. Dr. Roubenoff is an employee of Millennium Pharmaceuticals, Inc.

CHAPTER 18

CANCER

Kerry S. Courneya, PhD; Lee W. Jones, PhD; and John R. Mackey, MD

CASE STUDY

A 45-year-old female office worker was diagnosed in 1993 with breast cancer involving the axillary lymph nodes. She underwent a modified radical mastectomy followed by adjuvant chemotherapy and locoregional radiotherapy. Her cancer recurred with symptomatic bone metastases in 2003, at which time she began palliative chemotherapy. After two cycles of chemotherapy, she became mildly anemic (hemoglobin = 105 g/L), making her eligible for a clinical trial examining the effects of adding exercise training to an erythropoiesis-stimulating protein for the treatment of mild to moderate anemia in cancer survivors. Upon study entry, her hemoglobin was 107 g/L and her peak oxygen consumption was 16.2 $ml \cdot kg^{-1} \cdot min^{-1}$ (4.6 METs). Nevertheless, her overall quality of life was still quite good (174/188 on a self-report scale). The exercise program consisted of 12 weeks of cycle ergometry, three times a week, for 15 to 45 min at 60% to 85% of peak aerobic capacity. She attended 35 of the 36 scheduled exercise sessions (97% adherence rate). At 12 weeks, the woman's hemoglobin level had increased 20% to 128 g/L, and her peak oxygen consumption had increased 78% to 28.9 $ml \cdot kg^{-1} \cdot min^{-1}$ (8.3 METs). Moreover, despite her excellent quality of life at baseline, the woman experienced a further 7-point increase in quality of life after the exercise program (181/188).

WHAT IS CANCER?

Unlike normal cells, cancer cells have undergone genetic changes that allow them to grow and divide indefinitely (Gribbon and Loescher 2000). As cancer cells accumulate, they often cling together and develop into a mass called a tumor or neoplasm. Although benign tumors grow and enlarge only at the site where they began, cancerous tumors destroy the normal tissue that surrounds them. Additionally, many cancers are able to spread (i.e., metastasize) throughout the body via the bloodstream or lymph system and form "colony" tumors at new sites. As the cancer continues to spread, it typically invades and destroys vital organs (e.g., brain, lung, liver), which ultimately causes death.

The term *cancer* represents over 100 diseases that can occur in virtually any tissue or organ in the body. Most cancers, however, fall into one of four major classifications based on the type of cell from which they arise. Carcinomas are cancers that develop from epithelial cells that line the surfaces of the body, glands, and internal organs. They compose 80% to 90% of all cancers and include the most common types of cancer such as prostate, colon, lung, cervical, and breast cancer. Cancers can also arise from the cells of the blood (i.e., leukemias), the immune system (i.e., lymphomas), and connective tissues such as bones, tendons, cartilage, fat, and muscle (i.e., sarcomas).

EPIDEMIOLOGY OF CANCER

Cancer is a major public health burden worldwide (Parkin et al. 2001), with about 11 million new cases of cancer diagnosed each year (Ferlay et al. 2004). In the United States alone, over 1.35 million new cases of cancer were expected to be diagnosed in 2004, and the lifetime probability of developing the disease is about 41% (American Cancer Society 2004). Globally, cancer causes over 6 million deaths annually (Ferlay et al. 2004). Cancer is the second leading cause of death in the United States, with over 560,000 deaths from cancer expected in 2004. The four most common cancers—

Table 18.1 Estimated New Cancer Cases and Deaths for the Major Cancer Sites by Sex, United States, 2004

	Estimated new cases			Estimated new deaths		
Site	Total	Male	Female	Total	Male	Female
All sites	1,368,030	699,560	668,470	563,700	290,890	272,810
Breast	217,440	1,450	215,990	40,580	470	40,110
Prostate	230,110	230,110	–	29,900	29,900	–
Lung	173,770	93,110	80,660	160,440	91,930	68,510
Colorectal	146,940	73,620	73,320	56,730	28,320	28,410

Note: Excludes basal and squamous cell skin cancers and in situ carcinomas except urinary bladder.

Adapted from the American Cancer Society, 2004, *Cancer facts & figures 2004*. Atlanta, GA: American Cancer Society.

Table 18.2 Five-Year Relative Survival Rates for the Most Common Cancers by Stage at Diagnosis, United States, 1992-1999

Site	All stages (%)	Local (%)	Regional (%)	Distant (%)
Prostate	97.5	100	100	34.0
Breast	86.6	97.0	78.7	23.3
Colorectal	62.3	90.1	65.5	9.2
Lung	14.9	48.7	16.0	2.1

Note: Rates are adjusted for normal life expectancy and are based on cases diagnosed from 1992 to 1999 followed through 2000.

Adapted from the American Cancer Society, 2004, *Cancer facts & figures 2004*. Atlanta, GA: American Cancer Society.

prostate, breast, colorectal, and lung—account for over 50% of all new cancer cases and deaths each year in the United States (table 18.1). In terms of demographics, men are slightly more likely to develop and die from cancer than women, but it is age that really drives cancer incidence and mortality. About 76% of all cancers are diagnosed in persons aged 55 and older.

The chances of surviving cancer have improved substantially over the past few decades due to earlier detection and more effective therapies. The five-year relative survival rate across all cancers and disease stages is 63% (American Cancer Society 2004); this figure climbs to over 90% for certain cancers if detected early (table 18.2). The high incidence rates and improved survival rates have resulted in almost 10 million cancer survivors currently alive in the United States. Incidentally, a cancer survivor is defined by the National Coalition for Cancer Survivorship as any individual diagnosed with cancer, from the time of discovery and for the balance of life.

Medical Treatments for Cancer

The most common treatment modalities for cancer are surgery, radiation therapy, and systemic (i.e., drug) therapy. These medical interventions produce advantages in disease-free and overall survival; however, they are commonly associated with significant toxicities that can impact quality of life (QOL). Surgery is the oldest and most common cancer therapy (Frogge and Cunning 2000). More individuals are cured by surgery than by any other cancer therapy. Unfortunately, surgery is successful only if the cancer is localized to a small area. There can be significant morbidity associated with surgery depending on the location and extent of the operation, including wound complications, infections, loss of function, decreased range of motion, diarrhea, dyspnea, pain, numbness, lymphedema, fatigue, and anxiety.

Radiation therapy has been used to treat cancer since the early 1900s (Hilderley 2000). Approximately 60% of cancer survivors will receive radiation therapy at some point as part of their treatments (Maher 2000). Radiation therapy can cure some cancers if they are localized and can also provide palliative relief if the cancer is incurable. External beam radiation therapy is the most common method of delivering radiation. Radiation given for curative purposes is typically delivered in repeated small doses (i.e., fractions) over a five- to eight-week period in order to maximize the killing of cancer cells and minimize the damage to normal cells. Nevertheless, toxicity to healthy tissues does occur and is dependent on the dose and the site that is irradiated (Maher 2000). Radiation therapy can cause side effects such as pain, blistering, reduced elasticity, decreased range of motion, nausea, fatigue, dry mouth, diarrhea, lung fibrosis, and cardiomyopathy (Maher 2000).

Unfortunately, up to 60% of cancer survivors have micrometastatic disease at the time of diagnosis (Frogge and Cunning 2000). Micrometastatic disease means that the disease has already spread from the original site but is undetectable by standard diagnostic methods. Consequently, many cancer survivors are offered systemic therapy (i.e., drugs). The three major types of systemic therapy are chemotherapy, endocrine or hormone therapy, and biologic therapy. Chemotherapy is usually administered intravenously or orally and is given in repeated courses or cycles two to four weeks apart over a three- to six-month period. Chemotherapy may cause significant side effects including fatigue, anorexia, nausea, anemia, mucositis, neutropenia, thrombocytopenia, peripheral neuropathies, ataxia, alopecia, and cardiotoxicity (Camp-Sorrell 2000). The incidence and severity of these side effects depend on the type of drugs, mechanisms of drug action, drug dosage, administration schedule, presence of other comorbidities, and the application of supportive care interventions (Camp-Sorrell 2000). As with all treatments, the side effects from chemotherapy can be acute (i.e., appear almost immediately) or late-appearing (i.e., appear within a few weeks, months, or even years after treatments). Moreover, the side effects can dissipate quite quickly after treatment cessation or can become chronic.

Hormone therapy is usually administered orally (continuously or intermittently) for many months or years and can have significant side effects such as weight gain, muscle loss, proximal muscle weakness, fat accumulation in the trunk and face, osteoporosis, fatigue, hot flashes, and increased susceptibility to infection. Lastly, biologic therapies, the newest treatments, are designed to take aim at the molecular targets underlying a cancer cell's ability to grow, spread, and evade the body's defenses. For example, immunologic therapy uses the body's own defense mechanisms to act against cancer cells and to potentiate the effects of other drugs (Battiato and Wheeler 2000). Antiangiogenic therapies attempt to stop cancer cells from triggering new blood vessel formation. Inhibiting the formation of new blood vessels can prevent a microscopic tumor from growing into a dangerously large tumor and can potentially improve cancer survival. Such biologic treatments tend to be better tolerated than chemotherapy but can still produce significant side effects such as cardiotoxicity, loss of lean body mass, fatigue, and high blood pressure.

Increasingly, combinations of cancer therapies (i.e., surgery, radiotherapy, and systemic therapy) are used to treat cancer. The timing and sequence of the treatments vary depending on the cancer. It is possible for some cancer survivors to be treated on multiple occasions with multiple modalities, either concurrently or sequentially, for many months or even years. Moreover, in addition to these therapeutic medical interventions, many cancer survivors receive supportive care therapies that are also associated with side effects (e.g., anti-emetics, analgesics, colony-stimulating factors, erythropoietic therapy, antidepressants). In totality, a cancer diagnosis and its associated prolonged and intensive therapies can have a significant impact on the functional and emotional well-being of cancer survivors.

Exercise in Cancer Survivors

Research on the role of exercise in cancer rehabilitation is relatively recent compared to research on cancer prevention (Courneya 2003) or research on the rehabilitation of other chronic diseases (e.g., heart disease, chronic obstructive pulmonary disease). Nevertheless, there have been many recent reviews on this topic, and the reader is referred to these reviews for details concerning the approximately 50 studies published prior to 2002 (Courneya 2003; Courneya et al. 2002b). In this chapter, we provide a summary overview of 16 studies published in 2002 and 2003 (table 18.3) and a detailed review of five controlled clinical trials in the field.

Summary of Studies Published in 2002 and 2003

Sixteen studies were published in 2002 and 2003 on the effects of exercise in cancer survivors (table 18.3). The cancer survivor groups studied were breast, prostate, colorectal, and mixed (i.e., more than one cancer). The ages of participants ranged from the early 20s to the 80s, but most participants were between 40 and 69 years old. Most of the studies included cancer survivors at multiple stages of the cancer experience (e.g., during treatments, soon after treatments, long-term survivors). Study designs consisted of nine randomized controlled trials with usual-care controls, two nonrandomized controlled trials with usual-care controls, and four pre-post designs with no controls. The sample sizes ranged from 9 to 135. In 13 studies the exercise program was supervised, whereas in 3 it was home based.

Nine studies tested an aerobic exercise training program; six tested a combined aerobic and resistance training program; and one tested resistance training alone. The majority of studies followed traditional exercise prescription guidelines in terms of frequency,

Table 18.3 Studies of Exercise in Cancer Survivors, January 2002 Through December 2003

Authors, year	Sample	Design	Exercise program	Outcome variables	Results
		OBSERVATIONAL STUDIES			
Pinto et al. 2002	69 breast cancer survivors, % on treatment not reported	Prospective cohort	Self-reported over 12 months	Mood states, symptoms, social support, QOL, coping, exercise participation	Exercising at or below recommended levels vs. no exercise associated with higher levels of physical functioning.
		INTERVENTION STUDIES			
Burnham and Wilcox 2002	18 posttreatment breast/colon patients	Randomized controlled trial	Supervised low-intensity (25-35% HRR) or moderate-intensity (40-50% HRR) aerobic exercise program, 3 times/wk for 10 weeks	Aerobic capacity, body fat, flexibility, QOL, symptoms	Exercise groups ↑ aerobic capacity, flexibility, ↓ body fat, ↑ QOL compared with control. No differences between exercise groups.
Kolden et al. 2002	40 postsurgical breast cancer survivors; 65% were receiving chemotherapy	Pre-post test	Supervised group exercise training including aerobic and resistance training, 3 times/wk for 16 wk	Aerobic capacity, QOL, body fat, anxiety, depression, strength, flexibility	Exercise training ↑ flexibility, aerobic capacity, strength, and multiple QOL subscales.
Coleman et al. 2003	16 multiple myeloma cancer survivors receiving HDC and BMT	Randomized controlled trial	Combined aerobic and strength training program, 3 times/wk for 30-60 min for 6 months	Mood states, sleep, body composition, aerobic capacity, and strength	Exercise training ↑ lean body composition vs. control. Trends toward a difference for multiple QOL outcomes.
Courneya et al. 2003a	93 postsurgical colorectal cancer survivors; 66% were receiving adjuvant therapy	Randomized controlled trial	Home-based exercise program, 3-5 times/wk, moderate intensity for 20-30 min	QOL, SWL, depression, anxiety, aerobic fitness, fatigue, body composition, flexibility	Primary analysis revealed no significant differences. Ancillary analyses (↑ vs. ↓ fitness), differences on overall QOL and multiple subdomains.
Courneya et al. 2003b	96 mixed cancer survivors attending group therapy; 44% were receiving radiation or chemotherapy	Randomized controlled trial	Home-based aerobic exercise program, 3-5 times/wk, moderate intensity for 20-30 min	QOL, SWL, depression, anxiety, aerobic fitness, fatigue, body composition, flexibility	Exercise group showed ↑ in FWB, ↓ fatigue, body composition compared with control.

Authors, year	Sample	Design	Exercise program	Outcome variables	Results
Courneya et al. 2003c	52 postmenopausal breast cancer survivors, 46% on hormone therapy	Randomized controlled trial	Supervised moderate-intensity (70-75%) aerobic exercise program, 3 times/wk for 15 wk	Aerobic capacity, QOL, body composition	Exercise group showed ↑ in VO_2peak, QOL, and multiple QOL subdomains vs. control.
Dimeo et al. 2003	66 mixed cancer survivors receiving conventional or HDC	Pre-post test	Daily supervised moderate-intensity aerobic exercise program during hospitalization (30 ± 10 days)	Physical performance (walking speed, RPE), hemoglobin concentration	Physical performance remained unchanged during hospitalization, hbg ↓ during this time.
Fairey et al. 2003	52 postmenopausal breast cancer survivors, 46% on hormone therapy	Randomized controlled trial	Supervised moderate-intensity (70-75%) aerobic exercise program, 3 times/wk for 15 wk	Fasting insulin; glucose; IGF-1, 2; IGFBP-1, 3; and molar ratio	Exercise group showed ↓ IGF-1, ↑ IGFBP-3 and molar ratio vs. control.
Hayes et al. 2003a	12 mixed cancer patients receiving HDC	Nonrandomized controlled trial	Combined supervised moderate aerobic and resistance training program, 3 times/wk for 12 wk. Controls performed stretching.	Energy expenditure—singly and doubly labeled water technique and body composition	Exercise led to ↑ in TEE, FFM vs. control.
Hayes et al. 2003b	12 mixed cancer patients receiving HDC	Nonrandomized controlled trial	Combined supervised moderate aerobic and resistance training program, 3 times/wk for 12 wk. Controls performed stretching.	White blood cell count, lymphocyte function, CD3+, CD4+, CD8+	No significant effects of exercise on any immunologic outcome vs. control.
McKenzie and Kalda 2003	14 posttreatment breast cancer survivors with unilateral upper extremity lymphedema	Randomized controlled trial	Supervised progressive 8-week upper body resistance and aerobic exercise training program	Lymphedema and QOL	Exercise resulted in no changes in arm circumference or arm volume. Exercise ↑ in 4 SF-36 subdomains vs. control.
Oldervoll et al. 2003	9 posttreatment fatigued Hodgkins cancer survivors	Pre-post test	Home-based aerobic exercise training program 3 times/wk, 40-60 min for 20 wk	Aerobic capacity, lung function, fatigue, QOL	Exercise led to ↑ in aerobic capacity and physical functioning and ↓ in fatigue.

(continued)

Table 18.3 *(continued)*

Authors, year	Sample	Design	Exercise program	Outcome variables	Results
Pinto et al. 2003	21 posttreatment breast cancer survivors, % receiving treatment not reported	Randomized controlled trial	Supervised moderate-intensity aerobic exercise program, 3 times/wk for 12 wk	Aerobic capacity, mood states, affect, body esteem	Exercise led to ↑ in body image and trends for fitness and distress vs. control at posttreatment.
Segal et al. 2003	155 prostate cancer survivors on androgen deprivation therapy	Randomized controlled trial	Supervised progressive, moderate-intensity resistance training program, 3 times/wk for 12 wk	Fatigue, QOL, strength, body composition	Resistance training led to ↓ fatigue, ↑ QOL and upper and lower body strength vs. control.
Young-McCaughan et al. 2003	46 mixed cancer survivors; 24% were undergoing treatment	Pre-post test	Combined aerobic and strength training program, 2 times/wk for 12 wk	Aerobic capacity, sleep patterns, and QOL	Exercise led to ↑ in aerobic capacity, sleep patterns, and QOL.

CD = cluster designation; FFM = fat free mass; FWB = functional well-being; HDC = high dose chemotherapy; HRR = heart rate reserve; IGF = insulin-like growth factor; IGFBP = IGF binding protein; RPE = rating of perceived exertion; SWL = satisfaction with life; TEE = total energy expenditure.

intensity, and duration. The length of the exercise interventions ranged from 3 to 24 weeks. The studies examined a wide range of biopsychosocial outcomes including functional outcomes (e.g., aerobic capacity, body composition, flexibility, strength, energy expenditure), QOL, mood states (e.g., anxiety, depression), sleep patterns, and biologic outcomes (e.g., hemoglobin, immune function). In terms of results, almost all studies showed some statistically significant improvements after completion of the exercise program, including improvements in exercise capacity, body composition, overall QOL, QOL subdomains, mood states, metabolic hormones, and fatigue.

Generally speaking, the recent studies on the effects of exercise in cancer survivors were of good quality, consisting of mostly randomized controlled trial (RCT) designs with appropriate controls, supervised exercise sessions, an appropriate exercise stimulus, objective fitness assessments, and validated psychometric scales. The primary methodological limitations of these studies include (a) small convenience samples, (b) poorly described RCT methodology (e.g., randomization, blinding), (c) significant loss to follow-up, (d) less than optimal exercise adherence rates, (e) failure to use intention to treat analyses, (f) relatively short exercise interventions, and (g) heterogeneous participants that spanned the survivor continuum from the time during adjuvant treatment to several months or many years posttreatment.

Selected Controlled Clinical Trials of Supervised Exercise

Winningham and colleagues (1989) conducted one of the early seminal studies in the field. These researchers examined the effects of supervised aerobic interval training on functional capacity in early-stage breast cancer survivors receiving chemotherapy. They randomly assigned 62 participants to an exercise, placebo, or control group (the number assigned to each group was not provided). Participants assigned to the exercise group performed aerobic interval training on a cycle ergometer that oscillated between 60% and 85% of heart rate reserve, three times a week, for 10 weeks. Exercise duration was not specified. Participants assigned to the placebo group performed stretching and flexibility exercises for 10 weeks, but the frequency and duration were not reported. The control group were instructed to maintain their normal activities. The primary endpoint was functional capacity, assessed by a graded exercise test using gas exchange analysis.

The authors reported a 27% (17/62) loss to follow-up and a final sample in each arm of 18 (exercise group), 11 (placebo group), and 16 (control group). Adherence rates in the exercise and placebo groups were not reported. Results showed that the exercise group had significantly higher scores at posttest (covaried for baseline scores) for peak oxygen consumption, maximum test time, and maximum workload compared to the placebo and control groups. More specifically, the exercise group experienced a mean improvement in the functional capacity measures of 40% whereas there were small declines in both the placebo and control groups.

Another early important contribution to the field was a study by Dimeo and associates (1997) that examined the effects of exercise in cancer survivors with solid tumors who were receiving high-dose chemotherapy and an autologous peripheral blood stem cell transplant. Seventy participants were allocated to an exercise training group (n = 33) or usual-care control group (n = 37) on their first day of hospitalization. Participants assigned to the exercise group performed daily aerobic interval exercise training on a supine cycle ergometer for 30 min a day (alternating 1-min bouts of exercise and rest) at an intensity of at least 50% of their heart rate reserve for the length of their hospitalization (M = 14.4 days; SD = 2.9 days). The primary endpoint was physical functioning, assessed by maximal speed on a treadmill stress test. Secondary endpoints were the incidence and severity of complications, assessed according to standard World Health Organization criteria. The authors reported a 9% (6/70) loss to follow-up for the physical performance posttest assessment and an 82% adherence rate in the exercise arm. Results showed that the exercise group had a significantly higher maximal physical performance at posttest compared to the control group (13% difference). In terms of change scores, the exercise group declined in maximal physical performance by 13% whereas the control group declined by 19%. Posttest differences were also observed for duration of neutropenia and thrombopenia, platelet transfusion rate, duration of hospitalization, and severity of pain and diarrhea.

In the first large-scale RCT, Segal et al. (2001) compared the effects of supervised and self-directed exercise to usual-care in early-stage breast cancer survivors receiving adjuvant therapy (radiation, chemotherapy, hormone therapy). Participants (N = 123) were stratified by type of adjuvant therapy (chemotherapy vs. no chemotherapy) and randomly assigned to self-directed exercise (n = 40), supervised exercise (n = 42), or a usual-care control group (n = 41). Participants assigned to the self-directed and supervised exercise groups were asked to perform a progressive walking program at 50% to 60% of their predicted maximal oxygen uptake, five times per week, for 26 weeks. Exercise duration was not reported. The supervised exercise group were asked to perform three supervised and two home-based exercise sessions per week whereas the self-directed exercise group were asked to perform all five exercise sessions at home. The usual-care group were advised to exercise if they felt well enough but did not receive a specific prescription. The primary endpoint was physical functioning as assessed by the Medical Outcomes Survey Short-Form-36 (SF-36). Secondary endpoints were physical fitness, body weight, and other dimensions of health-related QOL as assessed by the Functional Assessment of Cancer Therapy-Breast (FACT-B) scales.

The authors reported a 20% (24/123) loss to follow-up and a 72% adherence rate in both exercise arms among the 99 participants who completed the trial. Intention to treat analyses were conducted on all randomized participants using last-observation-carried-forward for missing data. Results revealed significant differences among the groups for the primary endpoint of physical functioning. More specifically, physical functioning decreased by 4.1 points in the control group whereas it increased 5.7 points and 2.2 points in the self-directed and supervised exercise groups, respectively. Post hoc tests revealed that only the self-directed exercise group was statistically superior to the control group in terms of change in physical functioning. No significant differences were reported for other QOL indices. Secondary stratified analysis showed improvements in aerobic fitness and body weight in the subset of women in the supervised exercise group who did not receive chemotherapy.

In the largest RCT to date, Segal et al. (2003) examined the effects of supervised resistance exercise training on muscular fitness and QOL in prostate cancer survivors being treated with androgen deprivation therapy (a common hormone treatment for prostate cancer survivors that depletes testosterone to castrate levels). Participants (n = 155) were randomly assigned to an exercise (n = 82) or control (n = 73) group. The exercise group performed nine resistance exercises three times per week at 60% to 70% of 1-repetition maximum for a 12-week period. The primary endpoints were fatigue and QOL (assessed by self-report scales), and the secondary endpoints were upper body and lower body muscular strength (assessed by standard load tests for the chest press and leg press). The authors reported a 13% loss to follow-up (20/155) and a 79% adherence rate among all participants randomized to the exercise arm (including dropouts). Intention to treat analyses using last-observation-carried-forward for missing data showed statistically significant differences in change scores favoring the exercise group for fatigue, QOL, and upper body and lower body muscular fitness. The fatigue change was 3.0 points, and the QOL change was 5.3 points—changes that the authors argued were clinically meaningful based on guidelines for the scale. In terms of muscular strength, the exercise group increased upper body strength by 41% and lower body strength by 32% compared to the control group's decline in these measures by 8% and 4%, respectively. Moreover, subgroup analyses showed that these favorable effects were present for men who were being treated with palliative versus curative intent and for men who had been treated with the therapy for shorter versus longer than one year. No data were presented on the effects of the intervention on disease progression.

Finally, Courneya et al. (2003c) examined the effects of supervised aerobic exercise training on cardiopulmonary and QOL endpoints in postmenopausal breast cancer survivors who had recently completed all treatments except hormone therapy. Participants (N = 53) were randomly assigned to an exercise (n = 25) or control (n = 28) group. The exercise group trained on cycle ergometers three times per week at a moderate intensity (70%-75% peak capacity) and progressed from 15 to 35 min over a 15-week period. The primary endpoints were peak oxygen consumption (assessed by a graded exercise test using gas exchange analysis) and QOL (assessed by self-report scales). Only one participant failed to complete the trial, and there was a 98% adherence rate in the exercise group. Results for the cardiopulmonary and QOL endpoints showed statistically significant differences in change scores favoring the exercise group for peak oxygen consumption, peak power output, QOL, happiness, fatigue, and self-esteem (Courneya et al. 2003c). More specifically, peak oxygen consumption increased by 17.4% in the exercise group compared to a 3.4% decline in the control group. The QOL and fatigue change score differences were 8.8 points and 7.3 points, respectively, both of which may be considered clinically meaningful changes for the self-report scales that were used. Moreover, multiple regression analyses demonstrated that some of the changes in QOL were mediated by changes in peak exercise capacity.

From the same trial, Fairey et al. (2003) reported on the peptide hormone endpoints of insulin, insulin-like growth factors (IGFs), and insulin-like growth factor binding proteins (IGF-BPs). The results showed that exercise training had no significant physiologic effects on fasting insulin, glucose, insulin resistance, IGF-2, or IGFBP-1 in postmenopausal breast cancer survivors. Significant effects in favor of the exercise group were found, however, for IGF-1, IGFBP-3, and the IGF-1: IGFBP-3 molar ratio, suggesting that the intervention may have implications for disease recurrence and long-term survival.

Overall, the literature to date has demonstrated that exercise is safe, feasible, and beneficial to QOL for many cancer survivors both during and after treatments. Moreover, the recent research on this topic has improved in both quantity and quality. There is still no direct evidence, however, that exercise can reduce the risk of recurrence or improve survival after a cancer diagnosis. We now turn our attention to guidelines for exercise testing and prescription in this population.

Exercise Testing and Prescription Guidelines for Cancer Survivors

It is important to take into account the unique aspects of cancer and its treatments when developing exercise testing and prescriptions guidelines for cancers survivors. These guidelines should address many factors, including the goals of the exercise testing, possible screening requirements, modifications to the exercise tests, the planned mode of exercise, the necessary volume of exercise, the optimal physical and social context for benefits and adherence, any exercise precautions, and effective motivation and behavior change strategies. Taking all these factors into account will increase the likelihood of the cancer survivor's obtaining optimal benefits from exercise with minimal risk, while at the same time maximizing long term motivation and adherence.

Testing Guidelines

Exercise testing in cancer survivors may serve several important functions including

- quantifying the physical condition of a person prior to a given treatment,
- quantifying the short- and long-term functional effects of the disease and its treatments,
- identifying any comorbid conditions that may cause exercise limitations (e.g., cardiovascular disease),
- developing/modifying an exercise prescription, and
- determining the benefits of the prescribed exercise program.

Given that cancer and its treatments may affect all aspects of health-related fitness in cancer survivors (i.e., cardiorespiratory endurance, muscular strength and endurance, flexibility, anthropometry and body composition, gait and balance), a comprehensive fitness assessment is warranted. If possible, exercise testing should be performed before treatment, during treatment lasting longer than three months, immediately after treatment, and three to six months posttreatment. Exercise testing in cancer survivors requires special precautions and considerations in addition to those recommended for middle-aged and older adults in general. These special precautions arise from the significant morbidity experienced by cancer survivors during and immediately following the cessation of therapy (table 18.4).

Screening

Prior to exercise testing, it is important to screen cancer survivors for any major health conditions that

Table 18.4 Exercise Testing Precautions for Cancer Survivors

Complication	Precaution
Complete blood counts	
Hemoglobin level <8.0 g/dl	Avoid tests that require significant oxygen transport (i.e., maximal aerobic tests).
Absolute neutrophil count ≤0.5 × 10 * 9/l	Ensure proper sterilization of equipment and avoid maximal tests.
Platelet count <50 × 10 * 9/l	Avoid tests that increase risk of bleeding (e.g., high-impact exercises).
Fever >38° C	May indicate systemic infection and should be investigated. Avoid exercise testing.
Ataxia/dizziness/peripheral sensory neuropathy	Avoid tests that require significant balance and coordination (e.g., treadmill, free weights).
Cachexia (loss of >10% of premorbid weight)	Loss of muscle mass usually limits exercise to mild intensity depending on degree of cachexia. Avoid exercise testing altogether.
Mouth sores/ulcerations/xerostonia	Avoid mouthpieces for aerobic tests. Use face mask and keep hydrated.
Dyspnea	Avoid maximal tests.
Bone pain	Avoid tests that increase risk of fracture (e.g., high-impact/stress tests such as treadmill and 1RM).
Severe nausea/vomiting	Avoid maximal tests.
Extreme fatigue/weakness	Begin tests at lower power output, use smaller incremental increases, and avoid maximal tests.
Surgical wounds/tenderness	Select a test that avoids pressure/trauma to the surgical site.
Radiation burns	Wear loose clothing. Avoid equipment with straps (e.g., heart rate monitors).
Poor functional status	Avoid exercise testing altogether if Karnofsky Performance Status (KPS) score ≤60%.
Self-consciousness	Avoid testing procedures and facilities that may heighten self-consciousness (e.g., limited clothing, observation by others, challenging tests).

Adapted from Courneya, Mackey, and Jones 2000.

may affect exercise safety and performance (e.g., heart disease, diabetes, musculoskeletal conditions). These conditions are often more prevalent in cancer survivors because of their disease and treatments, their older age at diagnosis, and the fact that many of the risk factors for developing cancer are similar to those for other chronic diseases and health conditions (e.g., smoking, obesity, inactivity). In addition, it is important to have cancer survivors complete a cancer history questionnaire (figure 18.1). The cancer history questionnaire should assess information on important disease and treatment variables such as cancer site, disease stage, treatment protocol, supportive care medications, and any known or suspected side effects of treatments (e.g., ataxia, cardiomyopathy, pulmonary complications, orthopedic conditions). The survivor's oncology team may need to be consulted to provide complete and accurate information.

Testing Modifications

In principle, the exercise tests should stress the person to at least the level that will be experienced during the exercise program so that any symptoms might be identified under a more controlled environment. Moreover, it is desirable to stress the person as close to maximum capacity as is safely possible to provide better diagnostic information about cardiorespiratory function and a more accurate and reliable basis for exercise prescription. Notwithstanding the special precautions and considerations highlighted in table 18.4, most otherwise healthy cancer survivors can safely perform symptom-limited maximal testing.

The decision concerning what types of exercise tests to use will depend on the specific limitations imposed by each disease and treatment combination. As one example, cancer survivors who have recently undergone rectal or prostate surgery may prefer a treadmill

1. Date of cancer diagnosis (day/month/year): ______________________
2. Type of cancer (e.g., breast, colon): ______________________
3. Stage of cancer at diagnosis (i.e., I, II, III, IV): ______________________
4. Did/will treatment include surgery? (please circle) Yes No

   If yes:

   (a) Type of surgery: ______________________

   (b) Date of surgery (day/month/year): ______________________

   (c) Limitations imposed by surgery: ______________________
5. Did/will treatment include radiation therapy? (please circle) Yes No

   If yes,

   (a) Beginning and end dates (day/month/year): ______________________

   (b) Treatment schedule: ______________________

   (c) Sites of the body irradiated: ______________________

   (d) Acute/chronic side effects: ______________________
6. Did/will treatment include drugs/medications? (please circle) Yes No

   If yes,

   (a) Beginning and end dates (day/month/year): ______________________

   (b) Treatment schedule: ______________________

   (c) Class/type of drugs: ______________________

   (d) Acute/chronic side effects: ______________________

Anything else about your cancer diagnosis or treatment that we missed? Please add it here.

____

____

____

____

____

Figure 18.1 Sample cancer history questionnaire.

Modified from K.S. Courneya, J.R. Mackey, and H.A. Quinney, 2002, Neoplasms. In *ACSM's resources for clinical exercise physiology: Musculoskeletal, neuromuscular, neoplastic, immunologic, and hematologic conditions*, eds. J.N. Myers, W.G. Herbert, and R. Humphrey. (Baltimore, MD: Lippincott Williams & Wilkins), 187.

test to assess functional capacity as opposed to a cycle ergometer test for obvious reasons. Similarly, cancer survivors presenting with specific limitations in range of movement in the upper extremities following surgery or radiation therapy (e.g., breast, head, and neck) will likely be unable to perform tests involving upper body movements (e.g., arm ergometer tests, bench press). Moreover, cancer survivors who have neurological complications from chemotherapy that affect sensation, coordination, or balance (e.g., ataxia, peripheral neuropathies) will require stable tests (e.g., recumbent cycle ergometer, guided weight machines) as opposed to less stable tests (e.g., treadmill test, step test, free weights). Finally, some cancer survivors will experience severe nausea and fatigue at certain times during treatments and will not likely tolerate maximal testing. In these situations, submaximal tests should be considered with lower initial power outputs and smaller incremental increases.

Body composition tests may also have to be modified. More specifically, skinfold tests may need to be modified based on the surgical or radiation sites as well as any side effects (e.g., blistering, lymphedema). Existing prediction equations have not been validated in cancer survivors and may not be accurate in this population. Moreover, hydrostatic weighing is contraindicated for cancer survivors who are neutropenic or myelosuppressed because of increased risk of infection. The

Table 18.5 General Aerobic Exercise Recommendations for Otherwise Healthy Cancer Survivors

Parameter	Guideline/comment
Mode	Most exercises involving large muscle groups are appropriate, but walking is especially preferred. Key is to modify exercise mode based on acute/chronic disease and treatment effects and participant preferences. Also consider activities that are enjoyable, build confidence, facilitate perceptions of control, and develop new skills.
Frequency	At least 3 to 5 times per week, but daily exercise may be optimal for deconditioned cancer survivors performing lighter-intensity/shorter-duration exercises. Key is to exercise regularly while allowing for missed days due to treatment toxicities.
Intensity	Moderate intensity depending on current fitness level and severity of side effects from treatments. Guidelines include 50-75% $\dot{V}O_2max$ or HRreserve, 60-80% HRmax, or 11-14 RPE. HRreserve is best guideline if HRmax is estimated rather than measured. It may be necessary to consider RPE because of tachycardia.
Duration	At least 20-30 continuous minutes, but this goal may have to be achieved through multiple intermittent shorter bouts (e.g., 5-10 min) with rest intervals in deconditioned participants or those experiencing severe side effects of treatment.
Progression	Initial progression should be in frequency and duration, and only when these goals are met should intensity be increased. Progression should be slower and more gradual for deconditioned participants or those experiencing severe side effects of treatment. Progression may not always be linear. It may be cyclical with periods of regression.
Context	One that incorporates social interaction and involves an environment that engages the mind and spirit. Be aware of issues of privacy and self-consciousness when providing a context (e.g., public change rooms, showers, and washrooms; younger, athletic clientele).

Adapted from Courneya, Mackey, and Jones 2000.

bottom line for fitness professionals is that creativity will be needed to select (and perhaps modify) a testing protocol that is comprehensive yet personalized for a given cancer survivor.

Exercise Prescription Guidelines

On the basis of current evidence, the American Cancer Society has made a general recommendation that cancer survivors should be encouraged to exercise regularly (Brown et al. 2003). Specific exercise prescription guidelines, however, are challenging for this population because cancer comprises over 100 different diseases with an ever-growing arsenal of treatment protocols that produce a wide constellation of side effects varying with each individual. Consequently, the appropriate exercise prescription will vary depending on the cancer site (e.g., prostate, colon, lung), the treatment protocol (e.g., surgical procedure, specific drugs), individual responses to treatment (e.g., level of fatigue, nausea, pain, cachexia, ataxia), comorbid conditions (e.g., heart disease, musculoskeletal conditions), baseline fitness, and participant preferences. To date, only breast cancer survivors have received any sustained research attention; but even for this population, the optimal type, frequency, duration, intensity, progression, and context of exercise are not known. Nevertheless, some general guidelines can be provided based on the literature as well as our own clinical experience (table 18.5).

Goals

Exercise goals for cancer survivors will vary depending on the phase of the cancer experience (Courneya and Friedenreich 2001). If feasible, it may be useful to begin an exercise program prior to treatment to enhance physical conditioning as much as possible. During treatment, exercise goals should emphasize exercising regularly, preventing functional decline, and managing specific symptoms and side effects. Immediately after treatment, the goals may shift to rehabilitation of specific impairments incurred during treatment. After recovery from the acute effects of cancer treatments, goals may become more long-term, including the optimization of general health and reduction of the risk of disease recurrence and other diseases for which cancer survivors are at higher risk (e.g., osteoporosis, second cancers, cardiovascular disease). For those in palliative care, the goals may include pain relief and the maintenance of independent living for as long as possible.

Mode

With respect to exercise mode, the majority of studies on cancer survivors have tested walking or cycle ergometer interventions. Walking has been prescribed for the home-based programs and is preferred by over 80% of cancer survivors (Jones and Courneya 2002). Most studies prescribing cycle ergometry have been laboratory based, and the most likely reason for prescribing this modality is the availability of the equipment. The advantages of cycle ergometry include a sitting position with leg exercises that minimize the effects of ataxia (i.e., coordination and balance problems) and limitations in upper extremity movement (e.g., shoulder problems, arm lymphedema). In the study noted earlier, however, only 4% of cancer survivors preferred this mode of exercise (Jones and Courneya 2002).

The key point when prescribing activity mode in cancer survivors is to take into account any acute or chronic physical impairments that may have resulted from medical treatment. At present, there is no evidence that one type of aerobic exercise is superior to another for the general rehabilitation of cancer survivors. As with all older, chronic disease populations, safety is the primary concern. Swimming should be avoided by those survivors with nephrostomy tubes, non-indwelling central venous access catheters, and urinary bladder catheters. High-impact exercises or contact sports should be avoided in cancer survivors or palliative care patients with primary or metastatic bone cancer or rheumatism. From a clinical perspective, walking is probably the most appropriate modality to prescribe. Although evidence for the efficacy of weight training is only beginning to emerge (Segal et al. 2003), the optimal rehabilitation program for older persons with chronic diseases, including cancer, will likely combine aerobic and weight training.

Volume

The volume of exercise (i.e., frequency, intensity, and duration) prescribed for cancer survivors has closely followed the American College of Sports Medicine's (1998) more traditional guidelines for "vigorous" exercise. Most studies have prescribed moderate- to vigorous-intensity exercise (e.g., 60-80% of maximal capacity) performed three to five days per week for 20 to 30 min per session. The more recent guideline of accumulating 30 min of moderate-intensity exercise on at least five days of the week has not been tested in cancer survivors, but this prescription also appears appropriate. Either prescription may need to be modified based on fitness level and morbidity resulting from medical treatments. Many cancer survivors will not be able or willing to exercise at certain times during treatment because of severe side effects such as fatigue, nausea, pain, diarrhea, and general malaise. Given that the type and severity of side effects vary from survivor to survivor, it is essential to build flexibility into the exercise prescription. This flexibility allows cancer survivors to modify the frequency, intensity, or duration of their exercise depending on how well they are tolerating treatments.

High-intensity exercise should probably be avoided during cancer treatment because of the potential immunosuppressive effects. This concern may be moot because the vast majority of cancer survivors prefer low- to moderate-intensity exercise (Jones and Courneya 2002). The more likely challenge, therefore, is reassuring cancer survivors that moderate- to vigorous-intensity exercise is safe, feasible, and beneficial for them. Moreover, the challenge of prescribing intensity is exacerbated by the fact that many cancer survivors receiving treatments (especially chemotherapy) experience tachycardia, which makes heart rate alone an unreliable indicator of exercise intensity. We recommend that intensity also be monitored by a rating of perceived exertion scale using the range of "somewhat hard" to "hard."

From a duration perspective, it is likely that many cancer survivors will not be able to tolerate 30 min of continuous exercise at the start of their treatments, especially if they were previously sedentary. Some researchers have used intermittent or interval training (i.e., alternating short sessions of exercise and rest) as a way of accumulating the 30 min. This approach is recommended for older deconditioned persons with chronic diseases and may also be optimal for cancer survivors who have been sedentary, are deconditioned, are experiencing significant side effects, or are receiving palliative care.

Physical and Social Context

A recent survey has provided valuable information on the preferences of cancer survivors regarding the physical and social aspects of exercise (Jones and Courneya 2002). For example, the study indicated that 44% of cancer survivors prefer to exercise alone, 27% prefer to exercise with other cancer survivors, and 11% prefer to exercise with noncancer survivors (19% had no preference). Clearly, there is a market for offering exercise classes specifically for cancer survivors, especially for women. Moreover, 40% of cancer survivors prefer to exercise at home, 19% at a cancer center, 16% outdoors, and 13% at a community center (12% had no preference). This finding suggests that home-based exercise programs will also be popular among cancer survivors. As a final example, 48% of cancer survivors prefer to exercise in the morning compared to 23% in the afternoon and only 5% in the evening (24% had no preference). This finding may reflect the fact that fatigue tends to accumulate over the course of the day in cancer survivors and that they are most energetic in the mornings.

It is also important to recognize that cancer and its treatments can make many cancer survivors self-conscious about their ability to exercise (e.g., limited strength, poor endurance, lack of coordination), their appearance (e.g., surgical scars, removal of a breast, lymphedema, prostheses, loss of all body hair), and the possibility of unpleasant behaviors at any time (e.g., diarrhea, vomiting, fainting). To address these concerns, it is imperative to have staff that understand and are empathetic to the cancer experience. It may also be helpful to have a facility where the other exercise clientele are also dealing with disease or physical challenges (e.g., older adults, other chronic diseases). Lastly, issues of privacy may be of greater concern for cancer survivors, and exercise programs should attempt to accommodate this concern (e.g., private change rooms, private shower stalls, single washrooms, limited mirrors).

Psychological Factors and Benefits

It is also important for the fitness professional to understand that cancer survivors exercise as much for psychological health as for physical health. Consequently, it is important to take psychological benefits into account when prescribing exercise for cancer survivors. As a general guideline, fitness professionals should prescribe exercise that is enjoyable, builds confidence, facilitates perceptions of control, develops new skills, incorporates social interaction, and takes place in a physical environment that engages the mind and spirit. We have previously discussed dragon boat racing as an example of an exercise that may optimize psychological health (Courneya et al. 2002a). Research has shown that cancer survivors can, in fact, experience significant psychological benefits with an appropriately designed exercise program, including improvements in anxiety, depression, self-esteem, and happiness (see table 18.3; Courneya 2003).

Additional Precautions

Finally, although exercise is generally a safe supportive therapy for cancer survivors, there are certain precautions in addition to those related to age and other comorbid conditions that should be heeded to avoid unnecessary risks. One of the most important precautions is the presence of metastatic bone disease, which occurs at some point in approximately 50% of all cancer survivors. Although bone metastases most commonly occur in the vertebra, pelvis, femur, and skull, the most common site of major fracture is the hip. Survivors at particular risk of hip fracture have hip pain that is worse on activity, lytic lesions in the peritrochanter area of the femur, and metastases that measure more than half the diameter of the bone on plain films. Such survivors should be referred to their oncologist and should avoid contact sports or high-impact exercise. Cancer survivors should also stay well hydrated, because the combination of exercise and cancer treatments may lead to significant dehydration. Other important precautions are listed and described in table 18.6.

Exercise Motivation in Cancer Survivors

The effectiveness of exercise as a supportive care intervention for cancer survivors will depend to a large extent on the motivation and adherence of participants in such a program. Exercise adherence is a major challenge in the general population and is likely even more difficult during and after cancer treatments. Studies have shown that there is a significant decline in the volume of physical exercise performed by cancer survivors during treatments that is not recovered even years after treatments are completed (Courneya and Friedenreich 1997a, 1997b). Nevertheless, 84% of cancer survivors are interested in receiving exercise counseling at some point during the cancer experience (Jones and Courneya 2002). Moreover, research has started to examine the major incentives and barriers to exercise in cancer survivors (Courneya and Friedenreich 1997c, 1999; Nelson 1991; Young-McCaughan and Sexton 1991). Although some general conclusions can be made, the specific incentives and barriers are likely to vary depending on the type of cancer, extent of disease, type of medical treatments, existence of other comorbid conditions, timing of the exercise, and other personal factors. The key point for fitness professionals is that cancer survivors will present with unique incentives and barriers to exercise that need to be understood and addressed. Creative exercise programming and adherence strategies will be required for this population.

Future Research Directions

The nascency and breadth of the exercise oncology field mean that significant research remains to be completed. Future research is needed using rigorous RCT methodology to definitively answer questions concerning the role of exercise in cancer survivors both during and after treatments. Research should be extended beyond breast cancer survivors to the many other cancer groups who may benefit from exercise. For breast cancer survivors, there is sufficient evidence to warrant second-generation studies focusing on more specific questions such as the optimal timing, type, frequency, intensity, duration, progression, and context for exercise. Research should also be extended beyond high-dose treatments with stem cell transplantation to the many other therapies that cancer survivors endure (e.g., radiation therapy,

Table 18.6 Exercise Prescription Precautions for Cancer Survivors

Complication	Precaution
Complete blood counts	
Hemoglobin level <8.0 g/dl	Avoid activities that require significant oxygen transport (i.e., prolonged or high intensity).
Absolute neutrophil count <0.5 × 10 * 9/l	Avoid activities that may increase risk of bacterial infection (e.g., swimming).
Platelet count <50 × 10 * 9/l	Avoid activities that increase risk of bleeding (e.g., contact sports or high-impact exercises).
Fever >38° C and >40° C	May indicate systemic infection and should be investigated. If neutropenic, avoid exercise altogether. If not, avoid high-intensity exercise if fever >38° C and all exercise if fever >40° C.
Ataxia/dizziness/peripheral sensory neuropathy	Avoid activities that require significant balance and coordination (e.g., treadmill, free weights).
Cachexia (loss of >10% of premorbid weight)	Loss of muscle mass usually limits exercise to mild intensity depending on degree of cachexia.
Dyspnea	Investigate etiology. Exercise to tolerance.
Bone metastases/pain	Avoid activities that increase risk of fracture at the location of the bone pain/metastases.
Severe nausea	Investigate etiology. Exercise to tolerance.
Extreme fatigue/muscle weakness	Exercise to tolerance.
Severe lymphedema	Avoid exercises with the affected limb.
Dehydration	Ensure adequate hydration.
Self-consciousness	Avoid activities and contexts that may heighten self-consciousness (e.g., limited clothing, observation by others, challenging tests).

Adapted from Courneya, Mackey, and Jones 2000.

hormone therapy, biologic therapy). Lastly, studies are needed to further elucidate the mechanisms of change in QOL and to compare and integrate exercise with other currently accepted supportive care interventions.

SUMMARY

Over 11 million new cancer cases are diagnosed worldwide annually and the number of deaths from cancer is increasing. Treatments for cancer are intensive and cause significant acute and chronic reductions in physical functioning and QOL. Evidence from approximately 70 studies suggests that exercise may be a beneficial supportive therapy for many cancer survivors. Exercise testing and prescription in this population must take into account the diverse morbidities caused by the disease and treatments. Guidelines for exercise prescription include moderate- to vigorous-intensity exercise performed three to five times per week for 30 to 60 min in an environment that optimizes psychosocial health. Finally, facilitating exercise adherence among cancer survivors will require a good understanding of the unique incentives and barriers in this population and their preferences for exercise counseling and programming.

ACKNOWLEDGMENT

Kerry S. Courneya, PhD, is supported by the Canada Research Chairs Program and a Research Team Grant from the National Cancer Institute of Canada with funds from the Canadian Cancer Society and the Sociobehavioral Cancer Research Network. We would like to acknowledge the many colleagues, graduate students, and research participants who have contributed to this research.

CHAPTER 19

End-Stage Renal Disease

Pelagia Koufaki, PhD; and Tom Mercer, PhD

Case Study

RB was a 61-year-old white male retired high school teacher. He was living alone and was being treated by continuous ambulatory peritoneal dialysis (CAPD). RB enrolled in an exercise program after discussions with his consultant nephrologists in which he reported loss of sensation in his upper and lower limbs ("limbs were feeling cold and numb all the time") that limited his confidence in performing activities beyond basic activities of daily living. He reported difficulty walking, ascending and descending stairs, bathing himself, and driving, due primarily to the very limited sensation in his feet. He reported that he frequently felt weak and lethargic and rarely left the house. RB reported that he had a physically active background involving activities such as walking, rock climbing, and swimming, which he stopped after having a minor heart attack. He occasionally experienced chest pains that did not last long, and he attributed them to indigestion. However, he also reported that occasionally he had these pains in sudden exposure to very cold air.

His consultant nephrologist confirmed that RB had had a myocardial infarction seven years ago, and cardiac angiography revealed a small infarcted area as well as arteries that were blocked to some degree. The case notes indicated elevated levels of blood glucose and blood lipids that were currently being addressed through dietary interventions. RB's peripheral neuropathy was also confirmed from case notes.

On the day RB arrived for his pretraining exercise assessments, his resting blood pressure (BP) was 140/74 mmHg and his heart rate (HR) was 80 bpm. He had 2 L of fluid in the abdominal cavity. He was overweight (105 kg) with a body mass index of 32.7 kg · m^{-2}. He had been on dialysis for 34 months and had never had a renal transplant. He was not on any medication other than the usual renal nutritional supplementation, vitamins, and erythropoeitin (EPO). He had normal hemoglobin (Hb) levels (14.2 g · dl^{-1}), was well nourished (Subjective Global Assessment [SGA] = 6), and had not suffered from any medical complications in the three months prior to entering the program.

RB performed a step incremental exercise protocol on a cycle ergometer (2-min stages with ~25-W increments). He managed to complete 9 min on the cycle ergometer, achieving a peak workload of 108 W, peak HR of 120 bpm, and peak BP of 179/95 mmHg. The reasons he gave for terminating the test were muscle fatigue, breathlessness, and fear of the increased effort. His VO_2peak was measured at 17.4 ml · kg^{-1} · min^{-1}, and his VO_2 at ventilatory threshold (VT) was 10.5 ml · kg^{-1} · min^{-1}. The VT occurred after 3.3 min of exercise at a workload of ~45 W. Functional status, functional capacity, and quality of life were also assessed using the Duke activities of daily living (ADL) questionnaire, walking–stair climbing/descending test, chair sit-to-stands (STS), and a self-evaluated quality of life questionnaire (Schedule for Evaluation of Individual Quality of Life [SEIQOL]). When compared to an age-, gender-, and physical activity-matched healthy control person, RB presented with 35% deficit in VO_2peak, 74% in Duke-ADL, 45% in quality of life (QOL), 86% in walk test, 150% in stair climbing/descending, and 25% in STS.

RB was entered into an exercise class for CAPD patients. This class met three times per week and included continuous aerobic cycling and "body weight-resisted" local muscular endurance conditioning exercises. RB progressed to the point that he could complete 2 × 20-min bouts of continuous cycling by the end of three months. At this time he was also able to complete two circuits of local muscular endurance conditioning exercises, including step-ups, lunges, sit-ups, and squats. By six months of exercise training, RB could complete 40 min of continuous aerobic cycling and two muscular endurance circuits. At the six-month assessment point he completed 13 min of exercise on the cycle ergometer and had increased his VO_2peak to 22.9 ml · kg^{-1} · min^{-1} (>1 MET), which now reflected only a 15% deficit compared to a matched healthy control participant. Duke-ADL was improved by 46%, stair ascent/descent time by 26%, walking time by 27%, STS performance by 82%, and QOL by 142%. Compared to his matched healthy control counterpart, RB achieved better scores in STS performance and QOL by 55% and 25%, respectively. Also by the end of the exercise program he had lost 8 kg and reported better sensation in his limbs, and he had not felt chest discomfort for the last few months of his training program. His consultant also informed us that in his last routine cardiac angiogram there was evidence of spontaneous revascularization. Aside from the physiological and functional benefits he achieved, RB himself felt that the real value of the exercise rehabilitation program had been that it helped him to regain his self-confidence to be physically active and generally improved his QOL.

What Is End-Stage Renal Disease?

Chronic renal failure (CRF) is characterized by a progressive and irreversible destruction of the nephron mass leading to the deterioration of renal function. There are diverse potential causes of CRF, including diabetes mellitus, hypertension, autoimmune diseases (e.g., lupus, glomerulonephritis), obstructive uropathies, infections (e.g., cystitis), and genetic (e.g., polycystic kidneys) and congenital diseases (Bommer 1992; U.K. Renal Registry 2002). Although disease progression may often be gradual, it will typically result in end-stage renal failure (also referred to as end-stage renal disease [ESRD]).

The deterioration of renal function may even be asymptomatic in the early stages of CRF and recognizable only via clinical investigation. The glomerular filtration rate (GFR) is a clinically important index of renal function that reflects the rate at which kidneys filter waste products and equates to the percentage of normal kidney function remaining. It is typically estimated by calculating creatinine clearance rate on the basis of information about the patient's age, body mass, and serum creatinine levels. Table 19.1 illustrates how decreasing GFR is operationally used to describe the degree of impaired renal function and aid in the accurate identification of patients at each stage of the disease trajectory (National Kidney Foundation 2002).

The transition into end-stage renal failure, with the concomitant derangement of normal biochemical, metabolic, and endocrine functions, is accompanied by the development of the clinical syndrome of uremia. Uremic symptoms such as anorexia, generalized lethargy and fatigue, sleep disorder, neurological dysfunction, nausea, and vomiting are frequently evident. The appearance of these symptoms is remarkably consistent and appears to be largely cause independent. Indeed, abnormal plasma levels of many substances, including urea, creatinine, phosphate, and parathyroid hormone, have been identified as potential uremic toxins. Accompanying clinical signs of ESRD include fluid retention (peripheral and pulmonary edema), raised BP, diminishing hemoglobin levels, and abnormal biochemistry (creatinine, serum urea, and potassium). The pathologic effects of renal failure are multisystemic, with virtually no major body system unaffected. Common consequences of end-stage renal failure are well documented and include anemia, metabolic acidosis, secondary hyperparathyroidism, muscle weakness, peripheral neuropathy, hypertension, left ventricular hypertrophy, autonomic dysfunction, elevated triglycerides, and reduced high-density lipoprotein cholesterol (Bommer 1992). At this point, with the kidneys no longer able to perform their regulatory and excretory functions, some form of renal replacement therapy (RRT) is needed to maintain life (Department of Health Renal Team 2004).

Renal Replacement Therapy

Three methods of RRT are currently available: hemodialysis (HD), peritoneal dialysis, and renal transplantation. The term renal replacement therapy is used to describe treatments for end-stage renal failure in which, in the absence of kidney function, the removal of waste products from the body is achieved by dialysis. However, since neither form of dialysis corrects the loss of the hormones secreted by the normal kidney, synthetic EPO and vitamin D supplementation is often necessary. The term also covers the complete replacement of all

Table 19.1 Chronic Kidney Disease: A Clinical Action Plan

Stage	Description	GFR (mL/min/1.73 m^2)	Action*
	At increased risk	≥90 (with CKD risk factors)	Screening, CKD risk reduction
1	Kidney damage with normal or ↑ GFR	≥90	Diagnosis and treatment, treatment of comorbid conditions, slowing progression, CVD risk reduction
2	Kidney damage with mild ↓ GFR	60-89	Estimating progression
3	Moderate ↓ GFR	30-59	Evaluating and treating complications
4	Severe ↓ GFR	15-29	Preparation for kidney replacement therapy
5	Kidney failure	<15 (or dialysis)	Replacement (if uremia present)

Shaded area identifies patients who have chronic kidney disease; unshaded area designates individuals who are at increased risk for developing chronic kidney disease. Chronic kidney disease is defined as either kidney damage or GFR <60 mL/min/1.73 m2 for ≥3 months. Kidney damage is defined as pathologic abnormalities or markers of damage, including abnormalities in blood or urine tests or imaging studies.

* Includes actions from preceding stages.

GFR = glomerular filtration rate; CKD = chronic kidney disease; CVD = cardiovascular disease.

Source: National Kidney Foundation. 2002. KDOQI clinical practice guidelines for chronic kidney disease: Evaluation, classification, and stratification. Kidney Disease Outcome Quality Initiative. *Am J Kidney Dis* 39(2 Suppl. 2):S1-S246.

kidney functions by transplantation. Although international variations exist, HD remains the most frequently employed form of RRT, with >60% of patients receiving this treatment in countries like Germany and the United States. In contrast, although only 33% of patients in the United Kingdom receive RRT via HD, almost 50% of prevalent U.K. ESRD patients are treated by renal transplant. Worldwide, typically fewer than 10% of ESRD patients are treated via peritoneal dialysis RRT, with the exception of the United Kingdom, where approximately 18% of patients receive this form of RRT (U.K. Renal Registry 2002).

Both "dialysis" methods actually involve the processes of dialysis and ultrafiltration. The former process ensures that waste substances are removed via the processes of diffusion and filtering of solutes across a semipermeable membrane, while the latter establishes and maintains fluid/water balance. Hemodialysis treatment requires patients to be attached to a dialysis machine via a permanent access to the circulation. This treatment usually takes place at a dialysis unit, where the patient's blood is passed through a dialyzer machine (a large filter) in small quantities. Warm, cleansing dialysate solution is pumped through the filter so that the waste products and excess water in the blood are drawn into the cleansing solution through the processes of diffusion and osmosis; thus over the course of the procedure, plasma composition is restored toward normal values. This form of dialysis usually requires patients to attend the renal unit three times a week, during which time they spend 4 to 5 hr dialyzing.

The second mode of dialysis is peritoneal dialysis (PD), with CAPD the predominant method. This technique requires the implant of a silastic catheter into the peritoneal cavity, with its end coming out from the side of the abdominal area. Dialysis occurs through the introduction of dialysate solution into the peritoneal cavity via the implanted catheter. The peritoneal membrane acts as a natural filter. After a period of around 5 hr, the waste-containing dialysate solution is drained from the abdomen and a new quantity of dialysate is introduced. Each exchange takes around 45 min and must be repeated four or five times daily.

RENAL TRANSPLANTATION

Renal transplantation replaces all the kidney's functions, so EPO and vitamin D supplementation is unnecessary. A single kidney is placed, usually in the pelvis close to the bladder, to which the ureter is connected. The kidney is attached to a nearby artery and vein. The immediate problem is the body's acute rejection of the foreign graft, which has largely been overcome during the first months using drugs such as steroids and cyclosporin. These drugs, and others that can be used for that purpose, have many undesirable side effects, including the acceleration of vascular disease, so myocardial infarcts and strokes are more common in transplant patients than in age-matched controls. Moreover, the effects of immunosuppressive medications, specifically glucocorticoids, cause wasting of proximal skeletal muscles and may contribute to the diminished exercise capacity of these patients (Horber et al. 1986). During subsequent years there is a steady loss of transplanted kidneys owing to a process of chronic rejection; treatment of this is quite unsatisfactory at the moment, so many patients require a second or even a third graft over several decades, with further periods of dialysis in between.

Scale and Nature of the Problem

Although in relative terms, ESRD does not account for a large proportion of total morbidity in the population, treatment with RRT (dialysis) consumes a disproportionately large amount of the health care budget in the developed world. In the United States ESRD patients represent about 0.12% of the total population of 270 million (approximately 380,000 people), but the cost of their care exceeds US$18 billion per year; around 6% of the total annual Medicare budget (U.S. Renal Data System 2001). A similar picture emerges from the United Kingdom, where the treatment of the 0.05% of the total population with renal failure is estimated to cost 1% to 2% of the total NHS budget (Department of Health Renal Team 2004, p. 13). Overall, it is estimated that worldwide there are approximately 1 million patients who require chronic dialysis (Sims et al. 2003).

The number of patients with ESRD is increasing at an alarming rate, with annual numbers of new patients starting RRT constituting between 17% (U.K.) and 24% (U.S.) of the total number of patients receiving treatment. Although reports suggest that the continuous increase in the incidence and prevalence of RRT (a proxy statistic for ESRD) is a worldwide phenomenon (Rayner et al. 2004; U.K. Renal Registry 2002; U.S. Renal Data System 2002), figure 19.1 illustrates the wide variation that exists in RRT treatment rates, with the rates in the United States much higher than in Europe.

In conjunction with this growth in RRT, the age demographic of the ESRD population has also shifted quite dramatically in the last 20 years. According to the U.K. Renal Registry (2002), only 1% of those accepted for RRT in the United Kingdom were over the age of 65 in 1978. This figure had risen dramatically to 23% by 1988 and more than doubled again to 47% by 1998, with the number of elderly patients receiving RRT expected to continue to rise in the future (Bevan 2000). Epidemiologic data now indicate that over 40% of all ESRD patients in the United States and 50% of all patients starting HD treatment in Europe are more than 60 years of age. These demographic trends may be partially explained by more relaxed and increased acceptance to therapy, as well as improved survival from other diseases or an increase in the true incidence of renal disease (or both). Improved dialysis techniques, such as ultrafiltration control and bicarbonate-based dialysate, have also made dialysis treatment more tolerable for the more vulnerable patient groups, including the elderly. As a result, once patients have started dialysis they have a longer life expectancy (Bhatnagar 1998). Indeed, with the introduction of RRT, some patients have enjoyed near-normal life span, surviving in reasonable health for more than 30 years, particularly if they have received a transplant (Department of Health Renal Team 2004, p. 6).

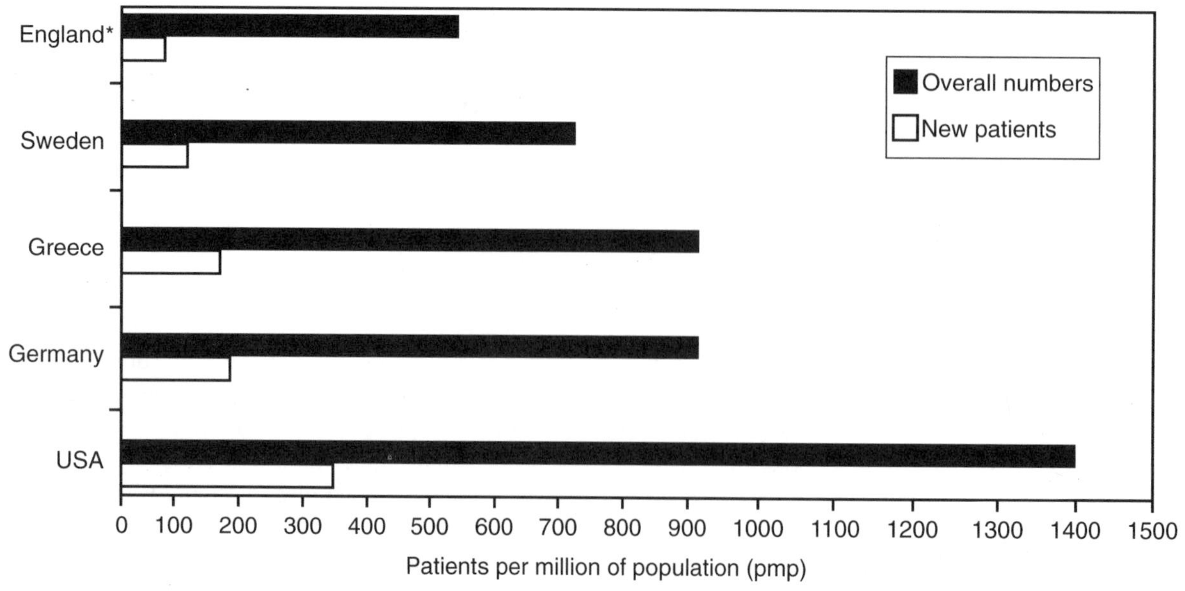

Figure 19.1 Selected international comparison of treatment rates for incident and prevalent patients receiving renal replacement therapy.

However, the increasing age of incident patients and the longer survival of patients receiving dialysis RRT also increase the prevalence of comorbid hypertension and diabetes. Historically, HD patients over the age of 70 present with, on average, twice the number of comorbid diseases compared with younger patients (Chester et al. 1979). Comorbidity in general, and cardiovascular comorbidity in particular, can greatly compromise the ability to cope with dialysis treatment, leading to a higher rate of mortality in these older patients (Kutner et al. 1997; Stack and Messana 2000). In addition, the added burden of comorbidity in older patients requires a disproportionate amount of medical and nursing care with a consequentially higher need for inpatient beds (Winearls 1999). Malnutrition and loss of muscle mass are prevalent in ESRD and are a devastating complication of chronic uremia (England et al. 1995). As muscle wasting also occurs with aging in the non-renal failure population (Porter et al. 1995), the muscles of elderly renal failure patients are likely to be subject to the combined deleterious effects of sarcopenia and uremia (Sakkas et al. 2003a), resulting in skeletal muscle wasting, derangement, and weakness (Kouidi et al. 1998; Sakkas et al. 2003b). These effects are also likely to be further compounded by lower and declining levels of habitual physical activity in this population (Johansen et al. 1999; Sugawara et al. 2002). The exposure to this "cocktail" of chronic uremia, sarcopenia, and disuse atrophy likely exacerbates the loss of functional independence of elderly patients with renal failure (Heiwe et al. 2001; Mercer et al. 2004).

PATHOPHYSIOLOGY AND PHYSICAL DYSFUNCTION IN END-STAGE RENAL DISEASE

Physical dysfunction in ESRD is an extremely complex problem. Renal patients have significantly reduced levels of exercise capacity. Typically, mean VO_2peak is around 18.8 ml · kg^{-1} · min^{-1} and ranges from 13 to 28 ml · kg^{-1} · min^{-1}, which corresponds to ~65% of that of age-, gender-, physically activity-matched healthy counterparts. Objectively measured functional capacity using reliable and validated tests reveals greater impairment in activities relating to daily living, with deficits ranging from 20% to 120%, especially in the older dialysis population (Koufaki 2001; Naish et al. 2000).

Several potential factors have been implicated in the reduced VO_2peak observed in patients with ESRD. In fact, ESRD could be either the result or the cause of medical conditions such as diabetes, for example, that lead to multisystemic dysfunction and which in turn provoke symptoms of various severity that finally limit exercise capacity. These factors include abnormalities in most of the major determinants of oxygen transport and utilization during rest and exercise conditions (see figure 19.2). Abnormalities of volume overload, that cause changes in cardiac function, in conjunction with metabolic abnormalities such as acidosis, electrolyte imbalance, and presence of uremic toxins in the blood, have been implicated in the impairment of oxygen transport and utilization and thus the reduced exercise tolerance of ESRD patients (Moore 2000). The mechanisms underlying the interactions and the effects of the aforementioned abnormalities on exercise capacity are not yet well understood, but it seems that fluid overload may reduce diffusional conductance of O_2 in all tissues. Fluid overload can also invoke mild congestive heart failure by increasing preload. Electrolyte imbalances (calcium, potassium) can alter myocardial contractility during exercise. It has been suggested that the presence of uremic toxins alters electrochemical potential across the sarcolemma and thus that excitation of the working muscles is less effective (Moore 2000).

Anemia-related left ventricular hypertrophy and congestive heart failure, mainly due to volume overload, arrhythmias, or both, can lead to myocardial dysfunction and in turn limit exercise capacity. Routine administration of EPO has partially reversed some of these mechanisms.

Defects in muscle structure and function have also been demonstrated, including muscle fiber atrophy, degenerative changes, capillary-to-fiber dissociation, mitochondrial myopathy (Diesel et al. 1993; Kouidi et al. 1998; Moore et al. 1993a, 1993c; Moore 2000; Sakkas et al. 2003a), all of which are implicated in impaired oxygen transport resulting in decreased exercise tolerance. Diesel et al. (1990) reported that VO_2peak was significantly correlated with isokinetic muscle strength and not with indices of blood oxygen-carrying capacity, suggesting that peripheral muscle function may be a more important determinant of VO_2peak in ESRD patients.

Over the years, attempts to identify the most important determinants of physical function (exercise capacity) only revealed additional new abnormalities and limitations. Predictors of physical function in ESRD include sedentary lifestyle, cardiovascular comorbidity, number of additional comorbidities, age, serum albumin, serum creatinine, dialysis dose, nutritional status, muscle atrophy, muscle strength, years of dialysis, functional capacity, and systemic inflammation (Diesel et al. 1990; Johansen et al. 2001, 2003; Moore et al. 1993c; Sietsema et al. 2002). While these observations confirm the multisystemic effects of renal disease, they also highlight the difficulties of establishing a single

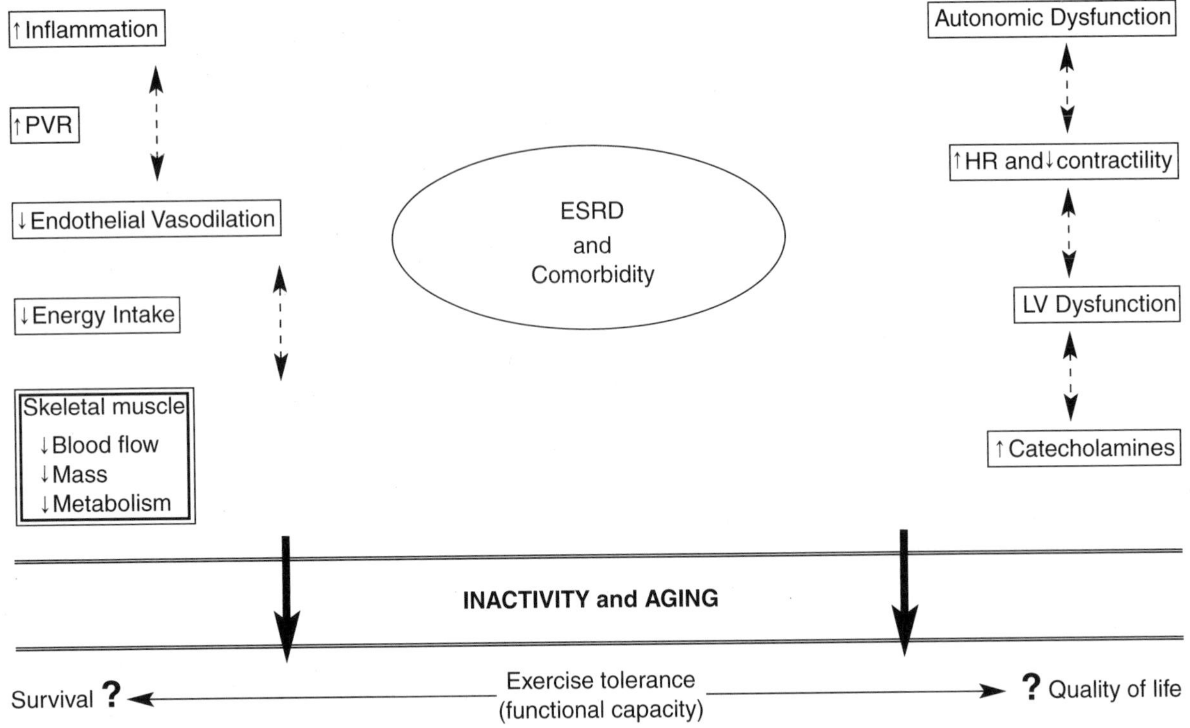

Figure 19.2 Factors affecting the exercise tolerance and rehabilitation outcome of patients with end-stage renal disease (ESRD). The pathophysiological abnormalities associated with ESRD, exacerbated by inactivity and process of aging, significantly affect functional capacity (functional independence), quality of life (QOL), and survival in ESRD, all three of which may serve as outcome variables for rehabilitation therapy. Several research investigations across different chronic medical conditions and in healthy populations have demonstrated that regular exercise significantly reduces manifestations of many of the pathophysiological mechanisms included in this schematic and also has a major positive effect on exercise/functional capacity. What remains to be established is whether exercise rehabilitation has a long-term positive effect on survival and QOL of patients with ESRD.

best approach to characterize physical dysfunction. A closer examination of the aforementioned relationships reveals that the parameters that explain the greater variability in exercise capacity are muscle function-related measures.

Exercise Rehabilitation Aims

Although there is an increasing interest in the role of exercise rehabilitation in patients receiving renal transplantation, data are available for only a small number of studies. As a result, this review focuses on the effects of exercise training on patients receiving dialysis RRT. Interested readers are directed to the review by Painter (1999), one of the very few available, for more information on the subject of exercise training post-transplantation. The focus of dialysis treatment itself, whatever the mode, is to sustain life. Although this has a major independent impact on survival outcome, it also adds a very heavy load of constraints and limitations on patients' everyday life. The physical, mental, and psychological shock associated with the initiation of dialysis is enormous, with patients struggling to cope with almost every aspect of it.

In addition, more often than not, ESRD is accompanied by other medical conditions. Reduced levels of O_2-carrying capacity due to renal anemia, metabolic/hormonal disturbances, impaired autonomic function, cardiac dysfunction, and in particular skeletal muscle abnormalities arising from underlying vascular and neuropathic defects only complicate renal replacement treatment and the overall clinical picture for the patient. Interactions among kidney failure and associated comorbid conditions compound and exacerbate the long-term deterioration of all bodily functions. Figure 19.3 illustrates how the presence of selected pathologies may possibly manifest as impairment, functional limitation, and ultimately disability for patients with ESRD (Tawney et al. 2003). The gradual loss of strength, endurance, and motivation, when combined with the process of aging and pronounced symptoms, adds to the burden of everyday life. Together, these factors trigger a spiral of fatigue, loss of confidence, fear, inactivity, functional disability, physical and mental dependency

Pathology	Impairment	Functional limitation	Disability
• Uremia	• Neuropathy	• Walking velocity	• Work or employment
• Anemia	• Low energy	• Gripping	• Leisure time activities
• Albumin	• Muscle atrophy	• Manual dexterity	• Health Assessment Questionnaire (26)
• Kt/V	• Sensory deficits	• Balance	• Arthritis Impact Measurement Scales (20)
• Acidosis	• Symptoms	• Corrdination	• Medical Outcomes Study Short Form (27)
• 1,25-OH_2)-vitamin D deficiency	• Range of motion	• Chair stands	
• Malnutrition	• Muscle weakness		
• Hyperparathyroidism	• Cardiorespiratory fitness		
• Amyloidosis			
• L-carnitine			

Figure 19.3 Examples of factors in the disablement process in end-stage renal disease.

Reprinted, by permission, from K.W. Tawney, P.J. Tawney, and J. Kovach, 2003, "Disablement and rehabilitation in end-stage renal disease," *Seminar in Dialysis* 16(6): 447-452. www.blackwell-syergy.com.

on others, and poor QOL. In the end, most patients with ESRD will die because of cardiovascular disease (~50% of all mortality) largely developed and worsened by the multisystemic derangement that accompanies their primary disease.

To date, there have been amazing therapeutic advances in the treatment of renal-cardiovascular syndrome, including early and improved management of anemia, better and more precise nutritional supplementation, and enhanced dialysis adequacy to more closely resemble kidney function. However, contemporary dialysis patients are still able to achieve, on average, only around 65% of the peak oxygen consumption (VO_2peak) of age-, gender-, and physical activity-matched asymptomatic controls (Koufaki et al. 2002a). VO_2peak is the single best indicator of integrated physiology from the single muscle cell to the mouth that represents coordinated function of all factors mentioned in figure 19.2; therefore it best demonstrates overall physiological, functional, and possibly motivational state. Moreover, contemporary ERSD patients, now more than ever, heavily rely on disability benefits to ensure acceptable living conditions. Therefore, it becomes clear that although the aim of ESRD treatment and care (survival) has been partially achieved, the optimization of treatment is not yet accomplished.

Exercise rehabilitation may offer the solution for achieving physically independent living and more symptom-free years of survival and thus maximizing potential for better QOL in patients with ESRD. Research evidence from the non-ESRD clinical exercise rehabilitation literature shows that physical training can positively affect the factors outlined in figure 19.2 (see chapters 2, 3, 8, 9, and 10). It has also been shown that regular physical training significantly diminishes and delays the effects of aging on physiological and functional capacity (chapter 20). In both healthy and diseased populations, active lifestyle and high VO_2peak constitute highly important factors leading to decreased morbidity and improved survival. It has also been shown that more active and fit people seem to enjoy life more. In the following sections, available research evidence is presented in an attempt to establish whether exercise rehabilitation in ESRD can positively modify the three most important aims of rehabilitation, which are capability for independent living, good QOL, and improved symptom-free survival.

Feasibility and Safety of Exercise Rehabilitation Options in End-Stage Renal Disease

The feasibility and safety of exercise training in patients with ESRD have been widely assessed. Most of the exercise-related information available comes from studies involving patients on HD. Although other RRT modes, such as CAPD, have been investigated, the few available comparison studies show that no significant differences exist between dialysis modes with regard to their effects on exercise tolerance and trainability characteristics (Painter et al. 1986a; Koufaki et al. 2001; Lo et al. 1998). Therefore, results from HD studies may reasonably be extrapolated to other dialysis modes.

Most of the early exercise trials involved the patient exercising on non-dialysis days and required attendance at rehabilitation centers where the exercise was performed under the supervision of an exercise specialist or physiologist. Soon it was realized that patients on HD had a logistical "advantage" over patients with other chronic disease conditions. They had to attend dialysis sessions on three occasions each week, during which they would have to spend 3 to 4 hr per day confined to a dialysis chair or bed. This feature of their treatment presented a theoretical opportunity to enhance exercise compliance. Recent reports (Konstantinidou et al. 2002; Kouidi et al. 2004) confirmed this notion in showing a lower dropout rate for exercisers on an on-dialysis program (~17%) compared to those participating in non-dialysis day outpatient programs (~23%).

These research-based observations showed that with modification of exercise equipment to accommodate the clinical environment and appropriately designed exercise prescription, it was possible to effectively rehabilitate dialysis patients without any adverse events. Moore and colleagues (1993b) addressed concerns about the potential threat posed by the interaction of exercise stress with the well-documented shift in body fluids seen toward the end of dialysis and its relation to episodes of hypotension, exercise intolerance, fatigability, tiredness, dizziness, and so on. Their investigations established that exercise responses recorded "off-dialysis" were not significantly different from those observed "on-dialysis" as long as exercise was performed within the first couple of hours of the dialysis session. This research endorsed both the safety and the physiological validity of off-dialysis exercise prescriptions as a basis for subsequent on-dialysis exercise (figure 19.4).

Other researchers had patients performing part of their exercise regime (weight training or cycling or device-assisted exercises) either just before or after the dialysis session (Akiba et al. 1995; DePaul et al. 2002; Ota et al. 1996). Although no adverse clinical effects were reported, the validity and effectiveness of such timing are questionable. These studies failed to demonstrate any substantial improvement in the research outcomes, and this may relate to the volume and intensity of exercise that patients were willing or able to accomplish immediately before or after dialysis. Hemodynamic status can be compromised at these time points given that HD patients typically come to dialyze with around 3.5 L of extra fluid and a disturbed acid-base relationship. These factors are reversed after dialysis, and this

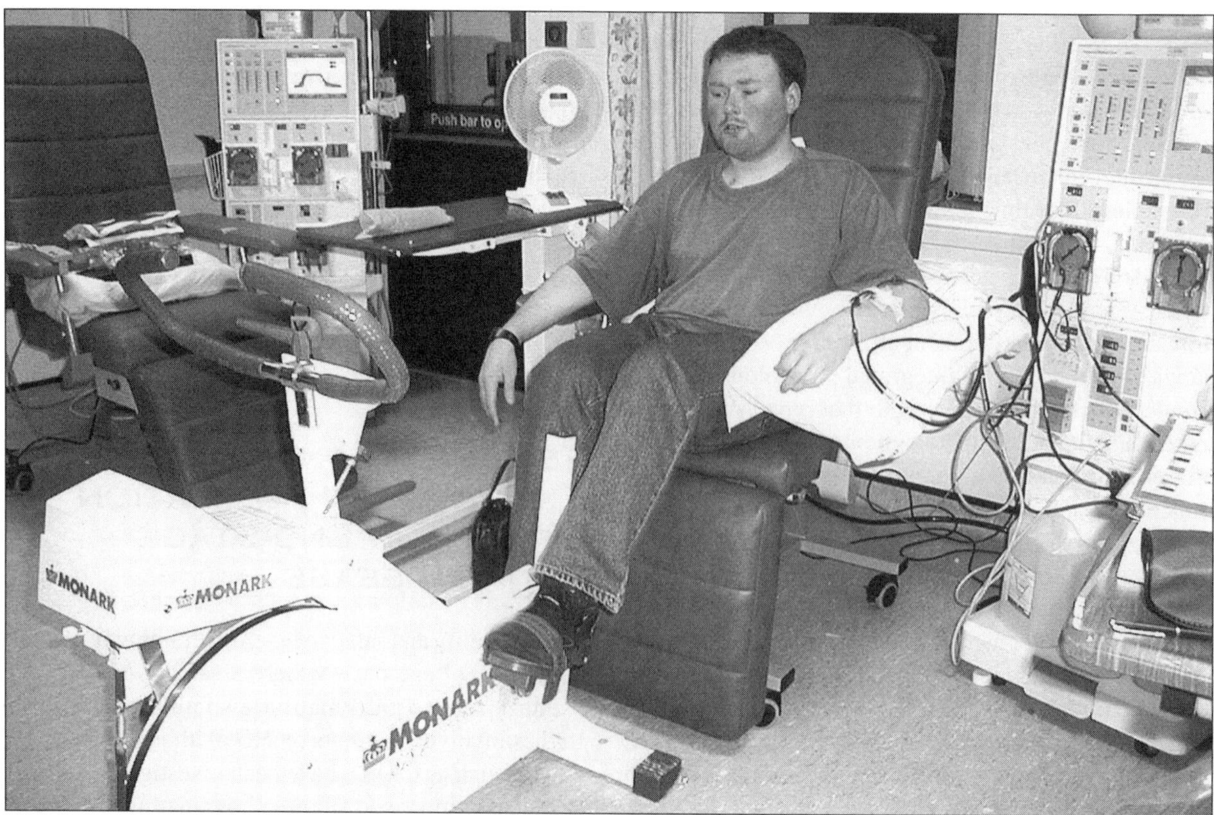

Figure 19.4 Cycle ergometer aerobic exercise during hemodialysis.

may cause transitional symptoms such as hypotension and dizziness that also may affect a patient's perception of exercise or willingness to exercise (or both).

What needs to be noted is that the state just before and after dialysis is a sensitive transitional phase for the restoration of body fluid homeostasis. The prescription of exercise during these transitional processes would appear to be both physiologically counterintuitive and probably counterproductive. Exercising on off-dialysis days does not appear to pose any dangers or limitations to patients' performance. Indeed, it may provide patients with more freedom and choice of activities. Conversely, some patients regard the idea of committing to exercise on their "free" (non-dialysis) days as too much of an intrusion.

Patients on PD usually dialyze at home three to four times a day or overnight. It may be suitable for these patients to engage in exercise training at rehabilitation centers or health clubs. Painter et al. (1986a) and Koufaki et al. (2001) have demonstrated that exercise test responses do not differ between patients on HD and PD modes. Moreover, the training responsiveness of PD patients is very similar to that of HD patients (Koufaki et al. 2002a; Lo et al. 1998; Mercer et al. 2002). Some reports suggest that patients using the CAPD mode may find it easier to exercise with their abdomen empty of the dialysate (Painter 1993). However, the presence of the fluid in the abdominal cavity does not appear to cause any major difficulties during conventional exercise modes such as walking or cycling. Greater consideration of the abdominal catheter exit area may be necessary during activities such as swimming. In general, with these patients, exertional tasks that may abnormally increase intrathoracic and intra-abdominal pressures, such as variations of abdominal sit-ups, back raises from prone position, and weightlifting exercises from supine positions, should be avoided. This is particularly important for exercise performed in nonsupervised environments.

The effectiveness of prescribed home-based exercise programs, and of "advice and encouragement" counseling programs designed to promote increased physical activity, has also been evaluated (Deligiannis et al. 1999b; Headley et al. 2002; Konstantinidou et al. 2002; Painter et al. 2000; Stephens et al. 1991; Tawney et al. 2000). No studies indicated complications or adverse effects for the home exercisers. However, the limited amount of information available seems to indicate that home exercisers may not be able to achieve similar magnitudes of benefit, reflected in smaller percentage improvements in VO_2peak, compared with patients exercising under direct supervision (Deligiannis et al. 1999b; Konstantinidou et al. 2002; Painter et al. 2000; Stephens et al. 1991). Functional capacity and health-related QOL were also not significantly improved following home rehabilitation (Painter et al. 2000; Tawney et al. 2000). The long-term benefits of home-based rehabilitation programs may be better evaluated after an initial period of in-center rehabilitation with professional instruction and guidance. In general, home rehabilitation options require the patients to be confident about monitoring and progressing their own exercise regime. Although home-based exercise is a very attractive option for the promotion of long-term health benefits, it may be practically useful, from a compliance perspective, only for highly motivated and relatively high-functioning patients who have some experience of physical activity.

Exercise Prescription in End-Stage Renal Disease

The vast majority of research trials have utilized conventional aerobic exercise training of moderate intensity using cycling or walking/jogging as preferred options. The average exercise program duration was about six months, with three exercise sessions performed per week in most cases. Target exercise intensities were usually derived from peak incremental exercise test data, with most studies using 50% to 85% of VO_2peak or HRmax ranges. Monitoring of intensity was typically achieved using HR and BP monitors and Borg's rating of perceived exertion (RPE) scales. In some cases in which ESRD is accompanied by heart failure or other cardiac disease with known rhythm abnormalities, electrocardiogram monitoring should always be used. Exercise prescription based on submaximal exercise responses (HR, VO_2, power output) associated with physiological anchor points, such as VT or lactate threshold (LT), might also be considered, as they reflect submaximal physiological changes and are less likely to be influenced by discomfort, tolerance, and motivation (Koufaki et al. 2002a). Exercise intensity corresponding to 80% to 90% of the predetermined VT/LT has been shown to be a safe and effective exercise prescription (Koufaki et al. 2002a). Periodic readjustments based on exercise training responses (HR, BP, patients' perceptions of exercise intensity [RPE scales, breathlessness scales] and repeat testing) should be made to assure stimulus maintenance. The effectiveness and validity of an exercise prescription based predominantly on RPE responses may be enhanced when the target RPE is anchored to a physiological index such as LT or VT (Mercer 2001).

More recent studies have utilized training modalities such as weight training, calisthenics, swimming, and sport games in fitter patients, with no adverse effects. The notion that inclusion of a variety of exercise activities may be needed to optimize physiological, functional, and psychosocial benefits in these patients is justifiable. Research evaluations have shown larger physiological benefits in groups of patients who performed multitask activities of varying intensities and for durations longer than three months (Deligiannis et al. 1999a; Konstantinidou et al. 2002; Kouidi et al. 1997). In contrast, other studies have shown enhanced benefits in functional tasks that are specific to the type of exercise training undertaken (Koufaki et al. 2002a). Thus, if the aim of the rehabilitation program is to improve walking ability of the patients, then some sort of walking activity should be incorporated.

Currently there is insufficient information to support any informed recommendation of weight training in the ESRD population. Although weight training or other forms of intermittent resistance exercise have been evaluated in other chronic medical conditions with no adverse effects and with significant improvements in rehabilitation outcomes (heart disease, pulmonary disease, etc.; for more information, refer to respective chapters in this book), further comprehensive studies are required for patients with ESRD. The possible advantage of weight training over conventional aerobic training is its potential to optimize benefits in bone mineral density, lean body mass, and muscle strength, all of which are important attributes for the patient with ESRD. However, the incorporation of weight training exercises in rehabilitation programs by some investigators (DePaul et al. 2002; Headley et al. 2002) did not yield conclusive results (see table 19.2). Observations made may also have been "contaminated" by interactive effects of other types of exercise. One major drawback for the application of conventional weight training for patients with ESRD concerns the practicalities of its implementation during dialysis. Thus, patients would have to perform weight training on off-dialysis days with the accompanying compliance and cost issues.

There have been some developments, however, in the clinical exercise rehabilitation techniques that may help to overcome the limitations to weight training during HD. Meyer et al. (1997) described a form of high-intensity interval cycling training that is performed at about 100% to 110% of peak workload for the work phases, lasting 30 sec, followed by longer active recovery phases. This type of exercise training was designed to develop muscle strength and cardiorespiratory fitness for patients with heart failure. Despite the high exercise workloads, the program was no more hemodynamically stressful (indeed, less so) than continuous aerobic exercise. This type of exercise intervention may provide a useful exercise prescription for patients on dialysis as it combines weight training characteristics (very short-duration exercise at high resistance) with aerobic exercise (high-intensity bouts intermittently matched with recovery phases at low resistance; overall prescription sustained for ~20 min or longer). Exercise trials are currently being undertaken to assess feasibility and effectiveness of this type of program for HD patients.

Effectiveness of Exercise Rehabilitation in End-Stage Renal Disease

The following section presents a summary overview of available research evidence in an attempt to establish the extent to which exercise rehabilitation interventions have been shown to impact positively on the key rehabilitation outcomes for people with end-stage renal disease. The evidence base reviewed is almost exclusively restricted to data generated by published controlled trials of exercise training in patients with end-stage renal disease. Although a detailed critique of the studies included is beyond the scope of this chapter, we have attempted to contextualize the importance of these observations whenever possible.

Peak Exercise Tolerance

Peak oxygen uptake (VO_2peak) is the most widely reported index of exercise capacity in exercise training studies of ESRD patients (see table 19.2). VO_2peak is generally considered an integrated measure of motivational drive and physiological responses to exercise stress and is modifiable by exercise training, indicating that physical conditioning may have a positive effect at multiple levels (see figure 19.2). Directly measured VO_2peak has long been considered a significant and independent marker of prognosis and outcome for patients with heart disease (AHA Science Advisory 2000). Recently, Sietsema and colleagues (2004) identified VO_2peak as one of the most important predictors of mortality in a sample of 175 ESRD patients. Patients were followed for 3.5 years. The average percentage improvements in VO_2peak (computed from studies included in table 19.2) observed in response to programs of structured, supervised exercise rehabilitation, performed either on (dialysis day) or off dialysis (non-dialysis day), were ~19% and ~ 26%, respectively. These improvements were noted following, on average, approximately six months of training.

Only one study has been located that has directly compared the effectiveness of on- and off-dialysis exercise programs for improving VO_2peak (Konstantinidou et al. 2002). These authors compared exercise training performed during HD sessions with (i) exercise training carried out in-center by outpatients on non-dialysis days and (ii) exercise at home by a third group, also on non-dialysis days. They observed that the outpatient program was the most effective, improving VO_2peak by 43% (see table 19.2). Nonetheless, the other intervention formats also significantly improved VO_2peak by 24% and 17%, respectively. These data translated into average improvements of >1 MET and <1 MET for exercise during HD and home-based exercise, respectively. Overall, it seems that outpatient programs were more effective in improving peak exercise tolerance by the clinically important threshold of 1 MET (3.5 ml $O_2 \cdot kg^{-1} \cdot min^{-1}$). The potential clinical significance of this threshold is underscored by the report of Myers and colleagues (2002), who observed a ~12% reduction in all-cause mortality for every 1-MET improvement in VO_2peak.

Kouidi and colleagues (2004) recently published their observations on the benefits of long-term exercise training. Two groups consisting of 16 and 18 patients exercising at outpatient programs and during dialysis, respectively, were exercise tested before and after four years of training. VO_2peak after that period had increased by an impressive 70% (3.5 METs) in the outpatient group and by 50% (2.4 METs) in the on-dialysis group. However, the group that exercised on off-dialysis days had a higher dropout rate (37%) compared to the on-dialysis group (21%).

In summary, it seems that outpatient rehabilitation programs are more effective in inducing a clinically meaningful improvement in short-term peak exercise capacity (VO_2peak). This is probably due to the variety of physical exercises and effort that patients can dedicate off dialysis and maybe also due to the fact that more mobile and more highly motivated patients are likely to take part in these programs. On the other hand, exercising off dialysis carries a greater risk for increased dropout. Promotion of exercise during dialysis should be targeted as a first line of approach, since evidence shows that it can also induce clinically important outcomes if maintained for long enough (Kouidi et al. 2004).

Submaximal Exercise Tolerance

The effects of exercise training on the responsiveness of submaximal indices of exercise tolerance are less well described in the literature. Measurements of submaximal exercise tolerance either during a transient phase (lactate threshold or its proxy ventilatory threshold, LT/VT) or during the rate of adjustment to steady state exercise (VO_2 kinetics) may better represent the ability to perform or tolerate ADL than peak exercise testing. Assessment of submaximal capacity may be particularly valuable in people with chronic disease, since these people very rarely approach their upper limits of exertion. A substantial improvement in these indices may translate into a significant delay of the onset of fatigue at higher absolute metabolic demand with the possible prevention of early cessation of a physical task (Basset et al. 2000). The average reported improvement in LT/VT following structured and supervised rehabilitation programs was ~19% (Konstantinidou et al. 2002; Koufaki et al. 2002b; Zabetakis et al. 1982). The rate of adjustment to steady state exercise did not improve significantly following three months of training (Koufaki et al. 2002a). An additional three months of training did, however, induce a significant improvement in VO_2 kinetics, which may indicate the need for sufficiently long duration of exercise training in clinical populations (Koufaki et al. 2002b). The findings of Kouidi and colleagues (2004), who reported impressive improvements in VT ranging from 42% to 52% after their four-year exercise program, would appear to support this observation.

Cardiovascular Function and Risk Markers

Only one randomized controlled study (Deligiannis et al. 1999b) has evaluated the effects of exercise training on cardiac function using resting and steady state exercise echocardiography. Although the limitations of exercise echocardiography are known, the investigators reported significant improvements in stroke volume index, cardiac output index, and ejection fraction during steady state exercise for groups of patients who completed programs of "during-dialysis" and "home-based" exercise training. In contrast, using a research design consisting of a "sham" exercise "control period," followed by 12 weeks of cycle ergometer exercise training, Moore et al. (1993c) observed no changes in stroke volume and cardiac output as measured invasively by the dye-dilution method during peak exercise testing. Deligiannis et al. (1999a) also demonstrated improved cardiovascular autonomic modulation, as assessed by 24-hr heart rate variability measures, for a group of patients who exercised during dialysis compared with a nonexercising control group. The latter report lends support to the potential beneficial effect of exercise training on restoring the disturbed cardiac autonomic function in ESRD by improving the dominance of vagal over sympathetic tone.

The effectiveness of exercise training in modifying other cardiovascular risk factors in patients with ESRD has not been decisively established. Goldberg et al. (1983) reported significant improvements for a group of exercisers in terms of triglyceride levels (33%), very-low-density lipoprotein cholesterol (16%), and high-density lipoprotein cholesterol (16%). Total cholesterol and low-density lipoprotein cholesterol did not change. In contrast, several other independent groups of researchers (Lo et al. 1998; Greene et al. 1979; Stephens et al. 1991) did not observe any significant improve-

Table 19.2 Summary of Controlled Exercise Training/Physical Activity Interventions Reported in the Literature

Studies	Dialysis mode	Intervention (n)	Controls (n)	Training mode	Training frequency	Training intensity (%)	Exercise duration (months)	Main outcomes	VO_2peak % Δ	METs
RANDOMIZED CONTROLLED TRIALS										
Greene et al. 1979	HD	6 (5)	6	NR	3/wk	NR	2.5	Blood chemistry, ↔ lipids		
Goldberg et al. 1983	HD	14 (11)	11 (9)	off/w, c	3/wk	60-80% VO_2p	12	TG ↓ 33%, HDL ↑ 16%, GDP ↑ 42%, Hct ↑ 27%, ↓ BP and BDI improved in intervention group; depression anxiety and hostility worsened in Con	21	>1
Akiba et al. 1995	HD	9	6	off/c	3/wk	RPE 12	3		NR	
Kouidi et al. 1997	HD	24 (20)	12 (11)	off/w, c, sw, j	3-4/wk	50-70% VO_2p	6	BDI and QLI improved in exerc	38	2
Deligiannis et al. 1999a	HD	30	30	off/w, c, sw, j	3-4/wk	50-70% VO_2p	6	HRV improved	41	+2/0.8
Deligiannis et al. 1999b	HD	16, 10	12	off/home/w, c, wt	3-4/wk	50-70% VO_2p	6	SV, EF, CO improved in both exerc groups, ↓ BP	42.7/20	+2
Tawney et al. 2000	HD	51 (39)	48 (43)	PA advice, anything they wanted	30 min daily		6	↔ KDQOL-SF, exerc reported ↑ RAND in leisure activities		
Koufaki et al. 2002a	HD, CAPD	26 (18)	22 (15)	on/off, c	3/wk	90% VT	3	↔ in VO_2 kinetics, STS5 ↑ 22%, STS60 ↑ 29%, ↔ in walk	15.8	<1
Konstantinidou et al. 2002	HD	21 (16) 12 (10) 12 (10)	13	off/on/home, c, w, wt, sw	3/wk	50-70% HRmax	6		42/23/17	2/>1/<1
DePaul et al. 2002	HD	20 (15)	18 (14)	on/c, wt	3/wk	RPE 13	3	5RM ↑, ↔ in SF-36, 6-min walk, and KDQ		
NONRANDOMIZED CONTROLLED TRIALS										
Zabetakis et al. 1982	HD	6 (5)	4	off	3/wk	% RPP	2.5		21	>1

Hagberg et al. 1983	HD	6	6	off/c, w, j	3-5/wk	50-85% VO_2p	4–39	BP ↓, med discontinued, Hb ↑	17	<1
Painter et al. 1986b	HD	14 (11)	7	on/c	3/wk	65-85% VO_2p	6	SBP ↓, med discontinued, ↔ Hb	23	<1
Carney et al. 1987	HD	11 (10)	10 (7)	off/w, c, j	3/wk	50-80% VO_2p	6	BDI improved in intervention group and depression anxiety and hostility worsened in Con	20	>1
Stephens et al. 1991	HD	30 (10)	NR	home/sw, w, c		RPE	8	↔ chol, ↔ Hb		
Ota et al. 1996	HD	27 (13)	6 (5)	off/ stretching, w	3-5/wk	NA	12	Grip strength ↑ 16%, flexibility ↑	–	
Moore et al. 1993c	HD	23 (10)	x-over	on/c	3/wk	NR	3	No change in CO, SV, $(a\text{-}v)O_2$, muscle biopsy	13.5	<1
Lo et al. 1998	CAPD	16 (13)	7	off/w, c	3/wk	70-85% HRmax	3	Glucose ↓, ↔ lipids, ↑ BP and MAP, PF of KDQOL and disease burden ↑, BP ↔	16.2	<1
Painter et al. 2000	HD	?	?	home/on	3-4/wk	RPE	2/2	Gait speed, SF-36 (results not clear)		
Mercer et al. 2002	HD, CAPD	12 (7)	9 (7)	off/c, body weight exerc	2/wk	RPE vs. W from VO_2p	3	Walk +15, stair climb +22, stair descend +18		
Headley et al 2002	HD	16 (10)	x-over	off and home, wt	3/wk	RPE	3	↔ Grip strength, ↑ peak torque 12.7%, 6-min walk ↑ 26 m, STS10 improved 13.6%, normal gait speed was similar		
Miller et al. 2002	HD	40 (24)	32	on/c	3/wk	NR	6	BP medication and cost ↓		

Δ refers to positive changes unless otherwise indicated by the preceding sign. ↑ = increase; ↓ = decrease; ↔ = no change; $(a\text{-}v)O_2$ = arteriovenous oxygen difference; BDI = Beck Depression Inventory; BP = blood pressure; c = cycling; CAPD = continuous ambulatory peritoneal dialysis; CO = cardiac output; con = number of control subjects; EF = ejection fraction; EPQ = Eysenck personality questionnaire; exerc = number of exercising patients (in parentheses n left at the end of intervention); GDP = glucose disappearance rate; HD = hemodialysis; HRV = heart rate variability; j = jogging; KDQOL-SF = kidney disease quality of life short form; MAP = mean arterial pressure phrase; NR = not reported; off = off-dialysis day; on = during dialysis; QLI = quality of life index; RAND = physical activity questionnaire; RM = repetition maximum; STS = sit-to-stand; SV = stroke volume; sw = swimming; TG = triglycerides; w = walking; wt = weight training. Data are presented as means.

ments in the lipoprotein profiles of their subjects. The variability in findings reported by these investigators likely reflects substantial differences in the exercise prescriptions employed (12 months vs. 2.5 months for Green et al. 1979; 3 months for Lo et al. 1998). Rate of glucose disappearance and fasting plasma glucose were seen to improve following exercise training in the study by Goldberg et al. (1983), but only in a subgroup of patients with fasting hyperinsulinemia. Lo and colleagues (1998) years later also reported a small but significant reduction in fasting blood glucose in their exercise training group.

Hypertension is prevalent among dialysis patients and constitutes an important and independent risk marker for the development of life-threatening complications. Mean group resting BPs were reported to be significantly reduced from a group average of 147/85 to 137/78 mmHg following exercise training, with some patients able to reduce or discontinue BP medication (Deligiannis et al. 1999b; Goldberg et al. 1983; Hagberg et al. 1983; Painter et al. 1986b). The reductions in systolic and diastolic BP were more pronounced in those patients with initially higher systolic or diastolic BP (Goldberg et al. 1983; Hagberg et al. 1983). Deligiannis et al. (1999b) described significant reductions in resting systolic and diastolic BP (from 145/87 to 136/79 mmHg), but only for the group that performed outpatient supervised exercise. No changes were observed for the home exercise group. On the other hand, Lo et al. (1998) reported a significant increase in whole-day systolic BP (from 142 to 157 mmHg) and mean arterial pressure (from 101 to 110 mmHg) as measured using 24-hr ambulatory BP monitoring. Recently Miller and colleagues (2002) reported the effects of exercise training on BP and use of antihypertensive medications. Out of a group of 24 hypertensive patients who completed six months of cycle ergometer exercise, 54% were able to reduce their antihypertensive medication (either required frequency or dose or both) in contrast to 12.5% of the nonexercising control patients. The authors reported that exercise training resulted in a 36% reduction in overall medication use. Cost analysis revealed savings of $653 per exercising patient per year in contrast to an increase of $232 per control patient per year.

In summary, based on the limited information available, generated by small-size trials employing a variety of methodological and assessment procedures, it seems that long-term exercise rehabilitation may have the potential to positively affect lipid metabolism and BP control in patients with ESRD. The limited quantity and quality of published data make it more difficult to evaluate the effects of exercise training on more overt indices of cardiac function.

Muscle Morphology and Metabolism

Preservation of muscle mass and function is considered to be of paramount importance in the treatment of patients with renal disease (Beddhu et al. 2003; Johansen et al. 2003). Measures of muscle mass and function have been shown to be the strongest predictors of functional and exercise capacity (Diesel et al. 1990; Johansen et al. 2003) and, more recently, survival (Beddhu et al. 2003) in patients with ESRD. This is also supported by reports that the most common complaints among patients during exercise testing relate to severe muscle fatigue, weakness, and pain (Painter et al. 1986b; Moore et al. 1993c; Koufaki et al. 2002a). In addition, in comparison to age-, gender-, and physical activity-matched non-uremic control subjects, dialysis patients were found to be significantly more impaired in relation to strength/power-related tasks such as chair rise, stair ascent, and stair descent times, with deficits ranging from 20% to 120% in elderly dialysis patients (Naish et al. 2000). Continued loss of muscle mass, the inability to preserve muscle mass, or the two in combination are hallmark characteristics of ESRD and are greatly implicated in the progression of malnutrition and renal cachexia, both of which are major determinants of morbidity and mortality (Beddhu et al. 2003; Kopple 1999).

To date, only three published clinical trials have directly assessed the effects of exercise training on muscle morphology and histochemistry in patients with ESRD using muscle biopsy techniques (Kouidi et al. 1998; Moore et al. 1993; Sakkas et al. 2003a). Using a gastrocnemius muscle model, Sakkas et al. (2003a) found increases of 32%, 54%, and 36% in the cross-sectional area (CSA) of type I, type IIa, and type IIx fibers, respectively, with an increase in the mean weighted CSA of 46% following six months of moderate-intensity cycle ergometer exercise. Kouidi et al. (1998) reported a significant increase of 24% in vastus lateralis muscle fiber CSA following six months of training. In contrast, Moore et al. (1993c) were unable to demonstrate a significant increase in CSA of the rectus femoris after three months of moderate-intensity cycle ergometer exercise training. Significant reductions in the percentage of atrophic muscle fibers present (especially in type II fibers) following exercise training were also reported by Sakkas et al. (2003b) and Kouidi and colleagues (1998). Sakkas observed that after training, the proportion of atrophic fibers was significantly decreased in type I, IIa, and IIx fiber populations (from 51% to 15%, 58% to 21%, and 62% to 32%, respectively). Moreover, in contrast to the observations of Moore and colleagues (1993c), Sakkas et al. (2003b) reported a significant 24% increase in capillary contacts per fiber.

The variability of responses reported may possibly be explained by the different volume and patterns of exercise training experienced by the subjects in these studies. While Moore and colleagues (1993c) restricted their subjects to exercise training during HD sessions for a period of three months only, Kouidi et al. (1998) implemented a cycle ergometer training regime of six months' duration that progressed to incorporate sport-related activity and muscle conditioning exercise. Taken together, the studies of Sakkas et al. (2003b) and Kouidi et al. (1998) indicate that the skeletal muscles of ESRD patients retain their capacity to adapt to endurance training, at least in terms of CSA.

Muscle Metabolism

There is no clear consensus regarding the altered muscle energy production observed in ESRD patients. Some investigators have suggested that there is no significant impairment in the intrinsic muscle oxidative capacity of patients with ESRD, but rather that a defect in O_2 supply mechanisms exists (Bradley et al. 1990; Moore et al. 1993c). In contrast, Kemp et al. (2004) have recently reported the existence of abnormal mitochondrial function in HD patients following a magnetic resonance spectroscopy investigation. In addition, previous investigators have presented evidence to suggest that abnormalities are likely present in the whole spectrum of muscle energy metabolism, including aerobic and anaerobic energy production and energy transport and utilization (Brautbar 1983). The available information on the effects of exercise training on muscle metabolism in ESRD patients (Moore et al. 1993c; Sakkas et al. 2003b) seems to suggest that moderate-intensity aerobic exercise does not significantly alter the activity of anaerobic (phosphofructokinase), aerobic (succinate dehydrogenase), or respiratory chain (cytochrome c oxidase) enzymes. Taken together, these limited observations may possibly indicate the absence of any significant preexisting abnormalities but equally may simply reflect the small sample sizes involved, the diversity of muscles sampled, and possibly the dialysis vintage of the patients.

A recent development in trials of exercise training in patients with renal disease has been toward examination of the potential role of exercise as a modulator of muscle wasting and improvements in nutritional state. Recent reports have shown subtle improvements in overall nutritional status in response to weight training in predialysis renal failure patients (Castaneda et al. 2001). Relatively few studies have directly assessed the effects of exercise training on nutritional status in patients on dialysis (Cappy et al. 1999; Koufaki et al. 2002a, 2002b). In a randomly allocated control trial of thrice weekly cycle ergometer aerobic exercise training, nutritional status (assessed using the 7-point subjective global assessment method [SGA]) was seen to significantly improve from 5.7 ± 1.4 to 6.4 ± 1.0 for the exercise group. This observation reflected a modest, but consistent, increase in the SGA score corresponding to change of group mean nutritional status from borderline malnourished (SGA B+ rating) to well nourished (SGA A, A– ratings). However, more studies will definitely be needed to further explore/confirm mechanisms of adaptations to exercise training in regard to the aforementioned areas.

Functional Capacity and Muscle Strength

Virtually none of the early controlled exercise training studies of dialysis patients included objective functional capacity (chair rise, walk speed, stair climb) or muscle strength measures in their outcomes. Since 1996 the range of objective functional capacity and strength-related assessments used to assess exercise training effectiveness in patients with ESRD has expanded (DePaul et al. 2002; Gleeson et al. 2002; Headley et al. 2002; Koufaki et al. 2002a; Mercer et al. 1998, 2002; Ota et al. 1996; Painter et al. 2000).

Only one controlled study demonstrated an improvement in walking ability, indicating a 15% improvement following 12 weeks of low-volume (two intermittent exercise sessions per week) exercise rehabilitation (Mercer et al. 2002). Although Headley et al. (2002) reported a statistically significant increase of 26 m for 6-min walk test performance after training, this improvement did not achieve the level of clinical significance. The type of exercise modality (specificity) employed and other training characteristics, such as duration and intensity of exercise, may partly explain the relatively small, or complete absence of, improvement in walking performance recorded in many studies (see table 19.1). The majority of training programs that had walking capacity as an outcome consisted mainly of cycling exercise alone. Exercises specific to walking muscles may be required to yield substantial improvements. It is also noteworthy that walking is a daily activity that the majority of patients are accustomed to and therefore longer or more intense training may be required to provoke changes.

Functional capacity assessments such as climbing and descending stairs, chair rise performance (also known as sit-to-stand tests, as quickly as possible [STS-5 and STS-10] and as many times as possible within a set time period [STS-60]), grip strength, 1- and 5-repetition maximum (RM) strength, and leg peak torque have been shown to be sufficiently responsive to allow detection of training adaptations across a variety of rehabilitation programs (see table 19.2). Group mean improvements in the aforementioned parameters ranged

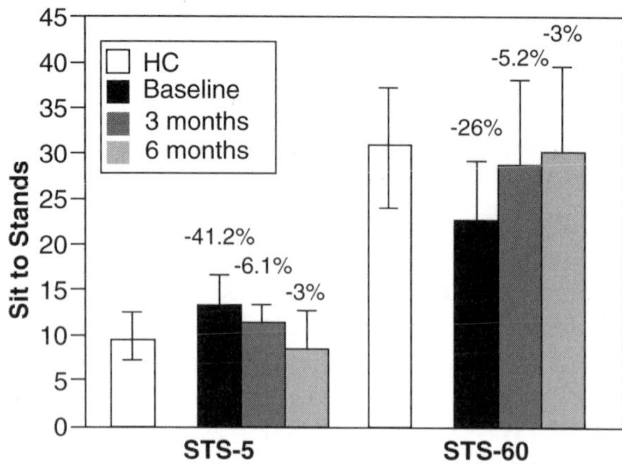

Figure 19.5 Near "normalization" of sit-to-stand performance of end-stage renal disease patients after six months of exercise training.

Reprinted, by permission, from P. Koufaki, 2001, *The effect of erythropoietin therapy and exercise rehabilitation on the cardiorespiratory performance of patients with end stage renal disease.* PhD thesis. The Manchester Metropolitan University.

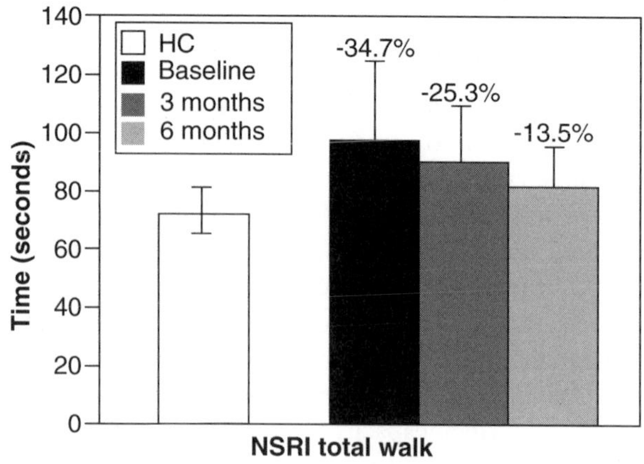

Figure 19.6 Improvement of walking–stair climbing performance of end-stage renal disease patients after six months of exercise training.

Reprinted, by permission, from P. Koufaki, 2001, *The effect of erythropoietin therapy and exercise rehabilitation on the cardiorespiratory performance of patients with end stage renal disease. PhD thesis.* The Manchester Metropolitan University.

from 13.5% to 29% (DePaul et al. 2002; Headley et al. 2002; Koufaki et al. 2002a; Ota et al. 1996). In direct comparison with age-, gender-, and physical activity-matched healthy control subjects, dialysis patients were found to have significantly impaired levels of functional performance in chair rise (STS-5, STS-60) and walk times ranging from 26% to 40% (Koufaki 2001; see figures 19.5 and 19.6). Exercise training for six months virtually "normalized" STS function and significantly narrowed the gap in walking impairment between people on dialysis and asymptomatic control subjects (figures 19.5 and 19.6; Koufaki 2001). Taken together, these results indicate that improvements in functional capacity are possible following exercise rehabilitation. Normalization of functional ability can be achieved, especially if activity-specific training imitating actions of daily living is employed.

Quality of Life

Evaluation of QOL is becoming one of the most important outcomes in clinical research trials. Quality of life assessment is performed by requesting patients to respond to a variety of questions concerning their ability to perform physical tasks, their mental health, social interactions, psychological state, financial state, employment, and so on. It is evident that QOL evaluation is very subjective and open to numerous influences. As a consequence its true responsiveness to therapeutic interventions is more difficult to assess than other measures.

In general, compared to age-matched healthy counterparts, patients with ESRD score very low in overall QOL evaluations (Blake et al. 2000; Diaz-Buxo et al. 2000; Evans et al. 1985). The areas that seem to be more affected reflect their ability to perform ADL and self-care, lack of energy and ease of fatigability, employment and financial state, emotional disturbances, depression, lack of social life and holidays, burden of dialysis therapy and frequent hospitalizations, and insecurity about the future (Blake et al. 2000; Diaz-Buxo et al. 2000; Evans et al. 1985; Kouidi et al. 1998).

The effects of exercise rehabilitation in modifying QOL have received considerable attention even from the very earliest clinical exercise trials (see table 19.2). Significant improvements in the physical functioning component of QOL evaluation, as assessed by a variety of tools, have been reported following supervised exercise rehabilitation (Kouidi et al. 1997; Lo et al. 1998; Painter et al. 2000). The change noted was related to improvements in the patient's ability to perform ADL, such as walking and climbing stairs, and to perform more leisure activities. Some earlier studies (Goldberg et al. 1983; Carney et al. 1987; Kouidi et al. 1997) also reported distinct psychosocial benefits and lower levels of depression, anxiety, and hostility compared to the control group. On the other hand, Painter et al. (2000), DePaul et al. (2002), and Tawney et al. (2000) found no significant differences between exercisers and controls in the majority of subcategories (mental, social, physical function, physical, emotional role, bodily pain, vitality, general health) of the Short Form-36 questionnaire.

The inconsistency of these results may reflect a variety of confounding factors ranging from exercise prescription characteristics to clinical and demographic characteristics of the patients, sample sizes, and methodological issues concerning the assessment protocols—and may even be affected by the psychological state of the patient at the time of questionnaire administration.

Summary

To date, as evidenced by data reported in the English language literature, 409 patients receiving dialysis treatment have participated in the exercise arms of controlled studies conducted across the world. Out of the 409 patients beginning exercise training, around 285 patients actually completed the prescribed exercise programs (see table 19.1). The dropout rate was calculated to be ~31%, with the reasons for prematurely terminating an exercise program ranging from loss of interest to death (unrelated to the exercise training participation). High levels of interstudy variability in exercise training prescription, length of time of the intervention, methodological and assessment procedures, and research outcomes all combine to limit the strength of conclusions to be drawn about the effectiveness of exercise rehabilitation for ESRD patients. Based on the evidence presented, however, there are some conclusions and recommendations that can be made with some degree of confidence, as follows.

Conclusions

Exercise training is feasible and extremely safe for patients with ESRD. Patients can safely engage in exercise during their HD sessions or on non-dialysis days. Improvements in peak exercise capacity have been reported in response to supervised on- and off-dialysis training and even following unsupervised home-based exercise.

Most patients can achieve some benefits from exercise training. This outcome typically is seen as improvements in one or more of the following: (i) peak exercise tolerance (VO_2peak or W peak); (ii) submaximal exercise tolerance (delayed onset of fatigue during submaximal exertion [VT/LT]); (iii) ability to perform activities of daily living (ADL-related functional capacity); and (iv) BP control and reduction of hypertensive medication.

Recommendations

Greater efforts should be made to promote exercise training during HD sessions, as this may

- enhance the frequency of both exercise adoption and compliance and
- provide an opportunity for patients to more actively engage with certain aspects of their health care.

Finally, in order to address the effectiveness of exercise rehabilitation for patients with ESRD, there is a need for more studies to be conducted with significantly larger numbers of subjects and for much longer durations (longer than one year) than have been previously reported. This will probably be achievable only through multicenter collaborative trials. However, only when such trials are conducted will we be able to meaningfully address the potential efficacy of exercise training as a means of influencing the survival and QOL of people with ESRD.

PART IV

Specific Patient Populations

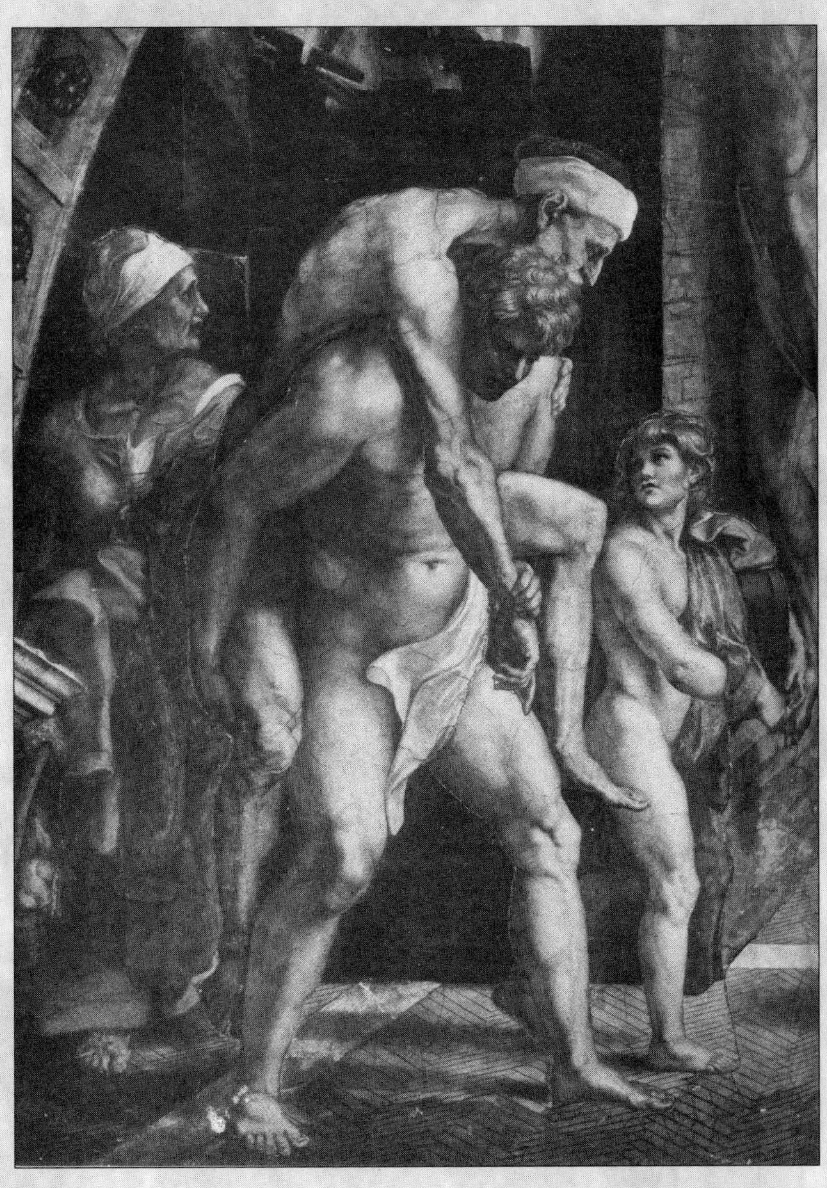

From Uffizi Gallery.

CHAPTER 20

Aging, Function, and Exercise

Jonathan F. Bean, MD, MS; and Charles T. Pu, MD

Unlike the preceding chapters, this one deals not with a pathologic condition, but rather with a process—the process of aging. As defined by Miller, "Aging is a process that converts healthy adults into frail ones, with diminished reserves in most physiologic systems and an exponentially increasing vulnerability to most diseases and to death" (Miller 1994, p. 3). No other condition or single category of illness comes close to approaching the impact that aging has on health and well-being. Perhaps most significantly, the process of aging brings dramatic declines in function that lead to physical impairment, disability, and loss of independence. One of the supreme goals of care for the elderly, therefore, is to prevent or reduce disability and maximize independence. This goal defines the primary objectives of both rehabilitation and geriatric medicine. In fact, a rehabilitative philosophy lies at the very heart of geriatrics.

Health care providers increasingly look to physical activity and to exercise, in particular, as an intervention that may maximize physical capacities, minimize declines, or even restore function in this population. This chapter explores the rationale for this interest. We first describe the significance of this topic from a demographic perspective. Secondly, we describe the aging process from a functional perspective, specifically, that of disablement, and characterize major forces associated with aging that contribute to disablement. We review the primary modes of exercise, as well as their specific effects on physiological and functional performance on older adults. Finally, we offer practical recommendations for exercising older adults.

The International Demographics of Aging

The single most significant demographic trend in the United States is the aging of its population. This trend has been both relative and absolute. In the decade between 1980 and 1990, the population over age 65 quietly grew from 11.2% to 12.5% of the total population (Campion 1994). This rate of growth proved greater than that of any other group—more than double the growth rate of the total population. Barring major societal changes, the U.S. elderly population will continue its dramatic expansion. When the "baby boom" generation begins to turn 65 around the year 2011, the demographic face of the United States will change even more dramatically. By 2030 the percentage of the population over age 65 will double, and one out of every five Americans will be elderly (Centers for Disease Control and Prevention 2003).

Buried within these numbers is a disproportionate growth in the group over age 85, the "oldest-old," who in 1990 numbered 3.3 million. Conservative estimates of the oldest-old from the Census Bureau, beginning in the year 2000, project growth from 4.9 million to a range of 8 to 13 million by the year 2030—as much as a 160% increase in that 30-year period alone (Campion 1994). More optimistic projections, in light of expected improvements in disease prevention and treatment, estimate that the number of Americans 85 years and older in 2030 will be as high as 24 million (390% increase over the number in 2000) or even higher (Suzman et al. 1992). Increasing life expectancy has been one of the driving forces behind these changes. Americans live longer now than ever before (Liao et al. 2001). Thirty years ago, average life expectancy at age 65 was about 15 years. Average life expectancy today at age 65 years approaches 18 years (Liao et al. 2001).

Few changes in the coming century will affect America's health care system so profoundly as these demographic trends. On one hand, this extension in longevity is expected to bring heavy burdens of illness and disability, as health care needs shift from acute disease processes to chronic disorders. Some experts worry that these trends will stress the current health care system beyond its capacities. In 2001, U.S. Medicare expenditures on benefits for 40 million elderly and disabled people were estimated at $237 billion, accounting for 12% of the total federal budget, or 2.3% of gross domestic product. By 2011, Medicare will likely more than double—reaching $490 billion, reflecting an average increase of 7.7% per year and far exceeding that of inflation. At that rate, and assuming no changes in current tax and spending policies, Medicare spending in 2011 will constitute 19% of the federal budget, accounting for the single largest projected increase (36%) in federal spending by the end of this decade (Crippen 2001). On the other hand, the relatively long periods of remaining life after age 65 offer ample opportunity for efforts at risk reduction and health promotion to produce meaningful benefits. At present, one of the few viable solutions to this demographic pressure lies with strategies to prevent or delay age-related morbidity. Interventions that focus on reducing morbidity and disability have great potential to influence future health care resource utilization.

The changing demographic landscape facing Americans and the challenge to develop preventive interventions apply globally as well. Today, persons over the age of 60 make up 10% of the world's population, totaling 629 million people worldwide. By 2050, experts project that one in every five persons will be 60 or older, totaling 2 billion; at this point, the population of older persons will outnumber children younger than 14 years. Similar to the situation with U.S. demographics, individuals 80 years or older (the oldest-old) represent the fastest growing segment of the older population. Currently making up 12% of the population over 60, the ranks of the oldest-old are projected to increase to 19% by the year 2050 (United Nations 2002).

The world has experienced dramatic improvements in life expectancy at birth, which has climbed about 20 years since 1950 to its current level of 66 years. Men or women who survive to age 60 can expect to live another 17 or 20 years, respectively. Global inequalities in mortality, however, exist between developed and developing countries. Individuals living in developed countries show longer average life spans than those in developing countries. In the least developed countries, people reaching age 60 can expect only 15 more years of life for men and 16 more years for women, whereas in developed countries the same groups can expect an additional 18 to 23 years of life (United Nations 2002). The significance of global aging is increasingly evident in the old-age dependency ratio, which represents the number of working-age persons (ages 15-64 years) per older person (65 years or older). Used as an indicator of the "dependency burden" on potential workers, the old-age dependency ratio from now until 2050 will double in more developed regions and will triple in less developed regions. The potential socioeconomic impact on society that may result from this swelling old-age dependency ratio is an area of growing concern, posing serious challenges for health care professionals across the world (Centers for Disease Control and Prevention 2003; Liao et al. 2001).

A Functional Perspective

From a rehabilitation perspective, though it is important to understand the many physiologic changes that occur with aging, clinical experience tells us that it is functional problems that most commonly lead patients to seek rehabilitative care.

The Disablement Paradigm

Surveys reveal that the elderly fear dying less than they fear becoming physically dependent, as evidenced by their strong desire to remain independent (Buchner et al. 1992). Forty-one percent of the "young-old" (64-74 years) fear dependency, a number that climbs to over 60% in the "old-old" (85 and older). Of the elderly who live alone, more than 75% fear becoming dependent on others. Eighty-six percent of this population cling toward remaining in their own homes even when faced with significant functional limitations (Commonwealth Fund Commission 1988).

Although many older persons maintain highly engaged and functionally intact lives into very late years, the rate of disability in the population increases markedly with age (Tinetti and Speechley 1989). It has been estimated that almost 20% of men and 25% of women experience mobility problems (Liao et al. 2001). Over 15% of older adults are unable to perform one activity of daily living (ADL) (Liao et al. 2001). Prospectively following noninstitutionalized men and women aged 55 to 84, the Framingham Disability Study showed that the risk of physical disability increased with advancing age as a greater percentage of elderly adults were unable to perform some of the most basic physical tasks (Jette and Branch 1981). One-fourth of the people in this study over age 65 stated that they were able neither to lift 10 lb nor walk a half-mile. Fifteen percent reported inability to climb stairs, and 7% were unable to walk across a small room. By age 85, the percentage of women unable to lift 10 lb increased to 66%.

Approximately one in five persons among the old-old is institutionalized, compared to only 1.4% of those 65 to 74 years of age. Of the noninstitutionalized old-old, many are either close to being institutionalized or need increased social and medical support to remain independent. Although fewer than 5% of older adults over the age of 65 live in nursing homes at any given time, the lifetime risk of admission to a nursing home for this population is about 45% for women and 28% for men (Kemper and Murtaugh 1991). Finally, death in old age is usually preceded by 8 to 10 years with some disability and about a year of near-total to total dependency (Guralnik et al. 1991). When it is considered that by 2030 the U.S. population of adults 65 years or older will exceed 71 million, representing over 20% of the total population, the functional concerns of older adults take on even greater importance (Centers for Disease Control and Prevention 2003).

The interrelationship between physiologic changes, functional decline, and disability are best understood through the concepts of disablement first described by Nagi (1965) and later expanded upon by Jette (1997) (figure 20.1). In this context physiologic changes are manifested as impairments, which can lead to functional limitations and result in disability. Jette (1997) defines these terms as follows:

- Impairments represent dysfunction or abnormalities in body systems.
- Functional limitations are restrictions in basic physical actions.
- Disability refers to difficulties in doing activities of daily life (ADL).

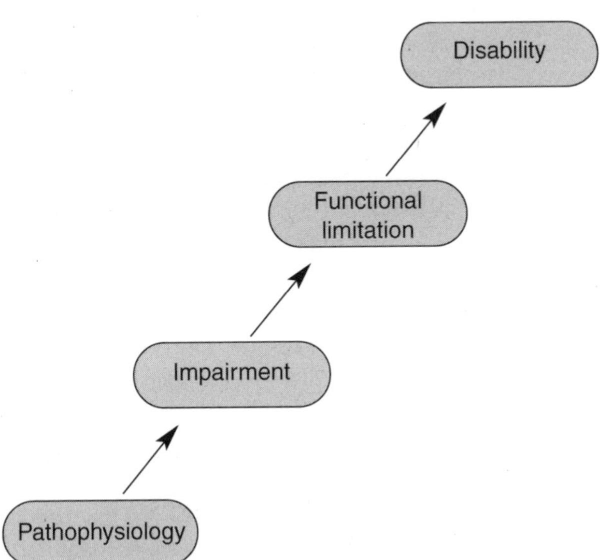

Figure 20.1 The disablement spectrum is characterized as a progression from pathophysiologic changes to impairments to functional limitations which lead to disability. This can be conceived as age-related changes in muscle, which lead to weakness. The weakness may alter the performance of observable tasks such as walking. This is considered a functional limitation. When an individual's walking limitations are so significant that they cannot function normally in their environment, they have become disabled.

In the past, though using similar terminology, this paradigm differed from that advocated by the classical ICIDH classification system (International Classification of Impairments, Disabilities and Handicaps), leading to the potential for conceptual confusion (Jette 1997). Interestingly, the revised ICIDH-2, though it uses different terminology, is more consistent with the concepts advocated by Nagi and Jette (Haley et al. 2002; Jette et al. 2002).

This disablement paradigm has more than just conceptual relevance. As demonstrated through population-based longitudinal studies evaluating both healthy and disabled older adults, limitations in function are predictive of subsequent disability (Gill et al. 1995). In fact, risk for ensuing disability, mortality, and morbidity can actually be stratified by the severity of mobility limitations (Guralnik et al. 1995, 2000). This suggests that a simple mobility evaluation may be a useful clinical tool for both prognostication and therapeutic purposes (Morley 2003; Studenski et al. 2003). For example, Guralnik et al. (2000) have published formulas that calculate four-year mobility and ADL disability based on a mobility performance score, giving added relevance to functional improvements derived from therapeutic exercise. Additionally, modifiable physiologic impairments, such as deficits in strength, power, and balance, have all been demonstrated to be strong predictors of mobility performance, providing important foci for exercise prescription (Bean et al. 2003b; Rantanen et al. 1999). Therefore, for the remainder of our discussion we will use the disablement paradigm to discuss the benefits of rehabilitative exercise for older adults.

FACTORS INFLUENCING DISABLEMENT IN OLDER ADULTS

In older adults, three common factors influencing the disablement process are (1) the physiologic aging process, (2) the accumulation of chronic diseases, and (3) levels of physical activity. Although all three factors are discussed here, we devote the major focus of this chapter to the multisystem physiologic changes associated with aging.

PHYSIOLOGIC AGING PROCESSES THAT CONTRIBUTE TO DISABILITY

The typical aging process is characterized by physiologic restriction or homeostenosis in a wide range of organ systems as summarized in table 20.1. Although there is no current "unifying theory of aging," these near-ubiquitous physiologic decrements average on the order of 2% per year per organ system (Harman 2001). Fortunately, most declines in the absence of significant pathology and under resting conditions impose few restrictions on daily function. The older adult's vulnerability, however, is usually exposed in the face of an acute stress such as illness or significant disuse. This perturbation of homeostatic equilibrium often causes dramatic functional declines, such that previously simple tasks become major ones and require near-maximal effort. The following is a brief review of the physiologic changes associated with aging that have most relevance to function.

Table 20.1 A Comparison of Physiologic Changes Occurring With Aging, Physical Inactivity, and Exercise

Physiologic variable	Aging	Physical inactivity	Exercise
AEROBIC CAPACITY			
Maximal	↓	↓	↑
Submaximal	↓	↓	↑
CARDIOVASCULAR			
Maximal heart rate	↓	↔	↔
Maximal cardiac output	↓	↓	↑
Maximal stroke volume	↓	↓	↑
Resting blood pressure	↑	↑	↓
BODY COMPOSITION			
Fat mass	↑	↑	↓
Lean mass	↓	↓	↑
Bone mass	↓	↓	↑
SKELETAL MUSCLE			
Muscle strength	↓	↓	↑
Muscle fiber number	↓	↔	↔
Muscle fiber area	↓	↓	↑
Muscle oxidative capacity	?	↓	↑
NEUROLOGIC			
Nerve conduction velocity	↓	↔	?
Motor unit function	↓	↓	↑

EFFECTS OF AGING ON CARDIOVASCULAR FUNCTION

Numerous alterations in cardiac structure and function that occur with advancing age result in an overall "stiffening" of the cardiovascular system (Lakatta 1990; Limacher 1994). Microscopic changes in the heart include increased fat, collagen, amyloid content, and lipofuscin. Myocyte numbers decrease, whereas myocyte size increases. Grossly, although overall cardiac size does not change, left ventricular mass and wall thickness tend to increase. Finally, the aorta loses elasticity as a result of increased collagen, calcification, and other degenerative processes. These cardiac alterations typically have minimal effects on individuals at rest, but are unmasked during physical exertion.

The most significant and consistent change that impairs cardiac output is the decrease in maximal achievable heart rate (Ogawa et al. 1992; Seals et al. 1984). Attributed to an age-related decline in sensitivity to myocardial sympathetic stimulation, this phenomenon occurs in all aging human populations, including those who are maximally conditioned such as elite athletes (Pimentel et al. 2003; Pollock et al. 1987).

The effects of age on other cardiac parameters such as stroke volume and cardiac output are more varied, and depend on the population studied. In an older population free of underlying coronary artery disease or hypertension, resting stroke volume and cardiac output are maintained throughout one's life (Rodeheffer et al. 1984; Stratton et al. 1992). During peak exertion, cardiac output, although reduced, can still achieve high levels. In response to exercise, peak exercise stroke volume, in fact, increases more in older than in younger adults, thus preserving some peak cardiac output with advancing age. To compensate for the inability to increase peak heart rate, aged hearts seem to maintain cardiac output during exercise by a greater dependence on the Frank-Starling mechanism via increased end-diastolic volume. There may be a cost to this age-related dependence upon the Frank-Starling mechanism, however, since the myocardium must function at a larger volume, implying greater wall tension stress and therefore greater energy demand (Stratton et al. 1994).

The standard physiologic measure used to determine one's overall ability to perform physical work is oxygen consumption or VO_2. Cross-sectional studies consistently demonstrate that peak VO_2 declines at a rate of approximately 10% per decade (1% per year) after the third decade of life in healthy, sedentary individuals (Anderson and Hermansen 1965; Grimby and Saltin 1966). On average, therefore, the peak VO_2 of a typical 70-year-old is 40% lower than that of a typical sedentary 30-year-old. The rate of decline for older individuals, however, can vary greatly depending on lifestyle factors such as physical activity status, disease processes such as underlying coronary artery disease, or changes in body composition such as increased body fat (Spina 1999).

Cross-sectional and longitudinal data have shown that VO_2 not only starts higher but declines more slowly (up to a twofold difference) in habitually active or regularly exercising populations compared to sedentary adults (Hagberg 1987; Heath et al. 1981; Rogers et al. 1990). Recently, however, Pimental et al. (2003) have challenged this traditional view and demonstrated that although endurance-trained men have much higher VO_2 levels than their age-matched sedentary peers, they had a greater rate of decline in $\dot{V}O_2max$. Although declining VO_2 appears inevitable even in older master athletes, for men in the 50- to 59-year range this difference theoretically translates into a 10-year difference between physiologic and chronologic aging.

These studies and more recent prospective evidence clearly highlight the fact that men and women even into older age (60-75) retain the ability to adapt physiologically to exercise (Spina 1999). Some investigators have estimated the energy requirements of a broad range of physical tasks and compared them to the average $\dot{V}O_2max$ of sedentary 75- to 80-year-old men and women as portrayed in figure 20.2 (Evans 1995). Theoretically, an individual has difficulty performing tasks which require movement energy expenditure. For example, a typical sedentary older woman with a $\dot{V}O_2max$ of 17 ml · kg^{-1} · min^{-1} (low) may have difficulty walking faster than 2.5 miles per hour for a sustained period of time and usually cannot climb more than 20 steps per minute. As these tasks of daily living represent an increasing percentage of the individual's maximal aerobic capacity, it becomes obvious why many older adults increasingly choose to avoid them altogether, thereby further exacerbating their declines (Grembowski et al. 1993). Cunningham et al. (1982) have shown that aerobic capacity is an independent predictor of functional performance such as gait speed, which in older adults has been independently associated with risk of falling and with functional status.

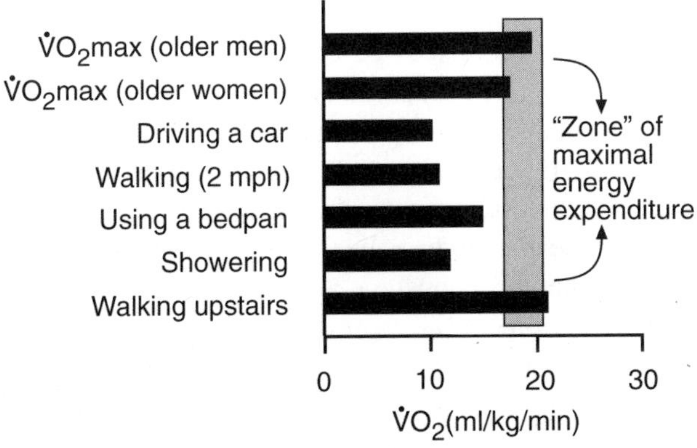

Figure 20.2 The average $\dot{V}O_2max$ values of a typical sedentary 75- to 80-year-old man or woman, compared to the oxygen cost of activities of daily living. In the elderly, many of these activities require near-maximal efforts, with some requiring even supermaximal efforts.

Adapted from Evans 1995.

Effects of Aging on Musculoskeletal Function

Declining motor ability is one of the most obvious results of the aging process that contribute to disability. This decline is mediated by alterations in body composition that lead to losses in both muscle mass and performance, a condition commonly referred to now as sarcopenia. Disease effects aside, musculoskeletal performance, which encompasses strength, power, endurance, is determined mostly by the quantity and quality of muscle mass contracting, and to a lesser extent by other factors such as the surrounding connective tissue around a joint or neuronal conduction velocity.

With advancing age, significant and steady changes in body composition occur such that fat mass increases and, to a lesser degree, lean body or fat-free mass (FFM) decreases (Cohn et al. 1980; Forbes 1999; Kehayias et al. 1997; Parizkova 1974). Both cross-sectional and longitudinal studies show that individuals can lose between 30% and 40% of muscle mass over their life spans, percentages similar in magnitude to losses in muscle strength (Borkan and Norris 1977; Evans 1995; Evans and Campbell 1993; Hughes et al. 2002). Furthermore, FFM appears to decline primarily at the expense of skeletal muscle mass (Cohn et al. 1980). Forbes has estimated that an average sedentary adult can expect to gain about 1 lb of fat and lose approximately one-half pound of muscle every year between the third and sixth decade of life. This shift in body composition, which can be masked by relative weight stability, is equivalent to a 15-lb loss of muscle mass and a 30-lb gain in body fat over an adult's life (Gallagher et al. 2000).

In addition to declines in muscle mass (quantity), the aging process is associated with alterations in muscle quality (Marcell 2003; Yarasheski et al. 2003). Morphologic studies of aging muscle demonstrate both loss and atrophy of type II, fast-twitch fibers, those recruited for actions requiring rapid or high-intensity muscle contractions. Lexell and colleagues (1983a) found that limb muscles of older men and women were 25% to 35% smaller, and had significantly more fat and connective tissue, than tissues from younger adults. Comparative muscle biopsies revealed that the preferential reduction in number and size of type II, fast-twitch fibers was mainly responsible for the gross muscle atrophy noted in the older adult.

The end physiologic result of sarcopenia, whatever the cause, is loss of muscle strength, power, and endurance. This decline in muscle performance is well documented in numerous cross-sectional and longitudinal studies (Aniansson et al. 1980; Bassey et al. 1992; Frontera et al. 1991; Larsson et al. 1979). Examining muscle strength and mass measured by computerized tomographic (CT) imaging in 200 healthy 45- to 78-year-old men and women, Frontera and colleagues concluded that muscle mass and not intrinsic muscle quality is the major determinant of age- and gender-related differences in strength (Frontera et al. 1991). More recently, however, this same group reported that when muscle performance is studied at the single-fiber level, there indeed seems to be an age-related reduction in intrinsic muscle fiber quality (Frontera et al. 2000).

Most importantly to the older adult, decreases in muscle mass and strength directly affect functional ability (Ory et al. 1993; Posner et al. 1995; Wolfson et al. 1995). Lower extremity muscle performance, for example, is a critical component of selected ADL such as walking speed, balance, stair climbing ability, and getting up from a seated position (Alexander et al. 1991; Bassey et al. 1992; Brown et al. 1995; Buchner et al. 1992; Judge et al. 1992). Finally, reduced lower extremity strength independently contributes to an increased risk of falling (Whipple et al. 1987), as well as predicting nursing home placement (Guralnik et al. 1994; Hubert et al. 1993) and mortality after bone fractures (Rantanen et al. 2002).

As with most age-related physiologic changes, there is great heterogeneity in musculoskeletal alterations with advancing age. Rather than being an inevitable part of the aging process, loss of muscle mass and strength may be more related to changes in habitual activity patterns. Klitgaard et al. (1990) reported that musculoskeletal strength and mass in older men (mean age 69 years) who had been strength training for 12 to 17 years were far greater than in age-matched swimmers or runners, and no different from values in young sedentary controls in their 30s. Furthermore, the muscle mass and strength of the older strength-trained men (but not the runners or swimmers) were indistinguishable from values in men 40 to 50 years younger than they.

Changes in Bone Density

As reviewed elsewhere, sedentary adults over the age of 40 typically lose approximately 1% of bone density per year (Dalsky et al. 1988; Layne and Nelson 1999; South-Paul 2001). Osteoporosis results in compromised bone that is susceptible to fragility fractures. Although the connection between bone density and physical function needs further study, osteoporosis and its consequences contribute significantly to physical frailty. Increasing the risk for disabling and fatal injury, osteoporosis carries tremendous personal, economic, and societal costs.

Exercise attenuates the risks for osteoporotic fractures in the elderly. Wolff's law states that remodeling of bone is directly related to the mechanical loads placed on it. One can therefore hypothesize that strength training could stimulate increases in bone density. Cross-sectional studies, indeed, have shown a relationship between muscle strength and bone density (Bevier et al. 1989; Pocock et al. 1989). Furthermore, controlled trials suggest that strength training can modify the physiologic declines in bone density associated with aging (Nelson et al. 1994; Dalsky et al. 1988; Layne and Nelson 1999; South-Paul 2001).

Accumulation of Chronic Diseases

In addition to diminishing physiologic reserves associated with typical aging, the elderly are the population with the greatest risk of developing chronic diseases that accelerate these declines, contribute to frailty, and lead to compromised function. Important examples are cardiovascular diseases such as coronary artery disease, congestive heart failure, and hypertension; diabetes mellitus; chronic obstructive pulmonary disease; arthritis; obesity; and neurological disorders such as Parkinson's disease, stroke, sensory deficits, or dementia. A review of each of these areas is beyond the scope of this chapter; but they are discussed elsewhere in this book. In elderly people, moreover, disease processes do not exist by themselves as is often the case in their younger counterparts, but accumulate and subsist as multiple, coexistent entities or comorbidities.

Because the elderly bear the greatest burden of disease, they also consume a disproportionate amount of medication and are prone to more adverse side effects than other groups. Although less appreciated than drug-drug interactions, drug-exercise interactions may assume increasing importance as exercise is prescribed for a wider range of the geriatric population. Many diuretics commonly prescribed for hypertension and fluid-overload conditions cause intracellular depletion of potassium and magnesium, which may lead to fatigue, muscle weakness, or arrhythmias (Dorup et al. 1988) and reduced exercise performance. Psychoactive medications such as antidepressants, antipsychotics, and sedatives can depress central nervous system function, which, in addition to increasing potential for falls, can lead to even more immobility and deconditioning. Beta-blockers, including ophthalmic drops for glaucoma, can diminish cardiac output by blunting the heart rate response to exercise. Finally, glucocorticoids used in chronic inflammatory conditions can induce their own form of myopathy and osteopenia.

Lifestyle Factors—Physical Inactivity

Because many physiologic changes associated with typical aging—such as sarcopenia—bear a remarkable resemblance to changes seen with bed rest (the most extreme example of physical inactivity) (Harper and Lyles 1988; Muller 1970), a sedentary lifestyle is increasingly recognized as a major problem in the elderly. Bed rest can lead to dramatic losses of strength and aerobic capacity—as high as 1% to 5% per day. Unfortunately, both cross-sectional and longitudinal studies of diverse populations show that individuals become less physically active with advancing age (Dishman 1994). This problem achieved recognition on a national level with the 1996 Surgeon General's report on physical activity and health (U.S. Department of Health and Human Services [USDHHS] 1996). These observations give rise to two critical implications:

- First, because disuse syndromes closely resemble age-related changes in many organ systems, it becomes difficult to separate "usual" or typical aging from declines that result from chronic disuse or deconditioning. As we have seen, this point is supported by the fact that the long-term maintenance of high physical activity levels, as in the case of master athletes, often leads to an apparent separation of chronologic and physiologic aging (Rogers et al. 1990).
- Second, the resumption of activity at any point in one's life, even after a lifetime of sedentariness, may reverse certain deficits in physiologic structure and function previously regarded as the inevitable consequence of the aging process. Table 20.1 (p. 314) summarizes some of the important physiologic similarities observed between typical aging and disuse as well as the potential ability for exercise to reverse these deficits. Despite the theoretical arguments for maintaining physical activity with age, most older adults are sedentary. Only about 22% of older adults engage in regular, sustained exercise (Dishman 1989; USDHHS 1996).

Chronic inactivity also contributes to subclinical disorders such as intra-abdominal obesity, glucose intolerance, osteopenia, hypertension, dyslipidemia, and coronary artery disease (Shephard 1990). The vicious downward spiral of further inactivity is further enhanced by the accumulation of overt disease and the medications used as treatment. Bortz (1989) introduced the concept that aging may be little more than a chronic disuse/inactivity syndrome. He emphasizes the possible role that physical activity, as reflected by active energy flow, may play in mitigating the age-related drift toward entropic decay.

In summary, the triad of

1. typical physiologic aging and
2. the accumulative effects of chronic diseases and of medications used to treat these conditions, along with
3. a typically sedentary lifestyle

often places the older person on a path hurtling toward disability. The myriad of possible dependent interrelationships among these forces, however, makes it difficult if not impossible to ascribe specific causality for the typical loss of physical vigor or function in many cases. On the other hand, the striking similarities between disuse syndromes and the typical aging process, as well as the variability of these effects in the elderly, suggest that exercise, or more generally the preservation or restoration of physical activity, can modify some aging effects.

Effects of Exercise on Physiologic Aging

The typical aging process as described is associated with physiologic reductions in cardiovascular and skeletal muscle performance that contribute to impairments, which ultimately lead to disability. In the remaining sections, we summarize some of the major exercise modalities and their effectiveness in counteracting aging processes.

Aerobic (Endurance) Training

Aerobic exercise, also known as cardiovascular conditioning or endurance training, is characterized by many repetitive contractions of large muscle groups without significant overloading of those muscles. Examples of endurance training include walking, jogging, cycling, climbing stairs, and rowing. It is important when reviewing training studies to remember the components of an aerobic training program: intensity, frequency, duration, and length. Training intensity is usually measured as a percentage of maximal heart rate (HR) or heart rate reserve (HRR), both of which are attempts to reflect a percentage of $\dot{V}O_2max$. Frequency of exercise sessions is typically measured in number of sessions per week, with duration ranging from 30 min to 1 hr. The length of training ranges from weeks to years.

An improved aerobic capacity is the fundamental specific physiologic response to aerobic exercise training (Green and Crouse 1995). Aerobic exercise training studies in the elderly demonstrate that healthy older adults adapt physiologically to moderate- to high-intensity training similarly to younger adults (Kohrt et al. 1991). Depending on training intensity, improvements in VO_2 range from 7% to 35% for healthy older adults. Based on these studies, training at moderate intensity levels, defined as approximately 60% of heart rate reserve or maximal exercise capacity, seems sufficient to achieve most health outcomes. Other aerobic training effects are improved stroke volume and cardiac output mediated by augmentation of diastolic function via the Frank-Starling mechanism (Levy et al. 1993; Schocken et al. 1983). Finally, skeletal muscle adaptations such as improved oxidative capacity and reduced systemic vascular resistance in response to aerobic training are also seen (Cartee 1994; Meredith et al. 1989; Orlander and Aniansson 1980; Souminen et al. 1977).

In highlighting the physiologic specificity of exercise training modalities, it is important to emphasize that although aerobic training clearly induces oxidative improvements in skeletal muscle, it is less clear whether aerobic training can slow down or reverse sarcopenic processes. Although the majority of studies demonstrate that aerobic training results in little or no improvement in age-related muscle mass or strength loss (Harridge et al. 1997; Meredith et al. 1989; Klitgaard et al. 1990), a recent cross-sectional study suggests that chronic endurance training can delay the onset of sarcopenia up to age 70 years (Tarpenning et al. 2004). It is generally accepted, however, that resistance training in which the overloading of muscle is accomplished with weightlifting exercises is the most effective exercise modality to mitigate sarcopenia of aging. Nevertheless, the physiologic adaptations attributed to aerobic training theoretically allow the trained older adult to better tolerate submaximal workloads such as those encountered during day-to-day functional activities.

Resistance (Strength) Training

Resistance, strength, or weightlifting exercises represent the other major training modality. In progressive strength training, the resistance against which a muscle generates force is progressively increased over time. The effects of weightlifting exercises on younger adult athletes such as bodybuilders are well known to the public. Recently investigators have applied progressive resistance training techniques in older populations as a means to counteract the sarcopenia of aging (Fiatarone et al. 1990, 1994; Frontera et al. 1988).

The basic physiologic response to strength training even into old age is an increase in muscle strength measured by maximal voluntary contraction (MVC). As with aerobic exercise, strength training effects depend on intensity, duration, frequency, and length. Training intensity is typically characterized as a percentage of maximal strength measured as a single MVC, also known as a single repetition maximum (1RM). Training at higher intensities apparently leads to greater increases in strength (Buchner 1993). While studies involving low intensities in older adults have shown modest strength increases of approximately 20% (Fisher et al. 1991; Larsson 1982), high-intensity training protocols have resulted in increases of up to 227% (Fiatarone et al. 1990; Frontera et al. 1988). These controlled trials strongly suggest that, if engaged in training of sufficiently high intensity, older men and women can attain strength gains at least similar to those of their younger counterparts. Depending on training intensity and subject characteristics, most progressive resistance exercise programs of three to six months' duration are able to increase muscle strength by 40% to 150% in older adults between 65 and 90 years (Latham et al. 2004). Muscle strength gains, however, have been the greatest when training is at moderate to high intensities, defined as 60% to 80% of the 1RM, with progression of 5% to 10% per week (Evans 1995; MacDougall 1986).

Most studies have utilized a training frequency of three times per week, which has been adopted by many recent consensus guidelines (American College of Sports Medicine 1998; National Institute on Aging 1999). In one notable study evaluating training frequency, Taaffe and colleagues reported significant improvements in strength and functional performance with high-intensity progressive resistance training conducted either three times, two times, or even once per week, suggesting that less frequent training of a sufficient intensity may still be beneficial (Taaffe et al. 1999).

In addition to increasing muscle strength, strength training improves submaximal muscle performance (muscle endurance) in older adults, defined as the number of repetitions that can be completed at a fixed resistance (typically a percentage of pretraining 1RM). These increases in submaximal muscle performance range in magnitude between 100% and 300% (Brown et al. 1990; Pu et al. 2001). This adaptation theoretically could improve an individual's ability to perform activities requiring sustained submaximal effort (e.g., climbing a flight of stairs) rather than a single maximal effort (lifting objects whose weight is at the limit of the person's ability).

The benefits of strength training in the elderly can extend to other physiologic outcomes, including overall exercise capacity (Frontera et al. 1990; Grimby 1992;

Pu et al. 2001), balance (Nelson et al. 1994), and flexibility (Beniamini et al. 1999). Additionally, other modes of resistance training, in which concentric actions are performed at higher velocities, have gained increased attention as a means of enhancing muscle power. This topic is addressed directly in subsequent sections of this chapter.

Finally, only resistance training has the ability to attenuate the dramatic losses of muscle mass associated with advancing age. Typical strength training programs of three to six months and moderate intensity can increase total body lean mass by 1 to 3 kg or muscle fiber size by 10% to 30% (Cartee 1994; Castaneda et al. 2001; Hopp 1993; Pu et al. 2001; Skelton et al. 1995; Welle et al. 1996). Klitgaard and colleagues found that older men who had been weightlifting for 12 to 17 years had muscle quality far superior to that of their sedentary peers. In fact, the skeletal muscle of these older weightlifters was indistinguishable from that of healthy men up to 50 years younger. In contrast, elderly men with high cardiovascular fitness who engaged regularly in aerobic exercises such as running and swimming had measures of muscle size and strength that were similar to those of their sedentary peers (Klitgaard et al. 1990).

In summary, it is clear that habitual exercise training has the potential to mitigate two of the most dramatic physiologic aspects of aging: overall exercise capacity and muscle strength. Furthermore there is evidence that other modalities not described in detail here, such as balance and flexibility training, induce favorable adaptations as well (American College of Sports Medicine 1998; Wolf et al. 1996; Wolfson et al. 1996).

Effects of Exercise on Function and Disability

Initial exercise studies in older adults focused primarily on physiologic outcomes and impairments, and it has been more recently that the appropriate measurement of more distal outcomes has been emphasized. For example, in 1988, Frontera et al. published an important early study applying progressive resistance training (PRT) to older adults. This study was the first to show improvements in leg strength and thigh muscle cross-sectional area after 12 weeks of exercise training. Much of this early work was done from a physiologic perspective, under the presumption that improvements in strength would lead to changes in function and disability, the more distal disablement outcomes. Fiatarone et al. (1990) applied these exercise methods to frail elders, demonstrating dramatic improvements in strength. Additionally, the 1990 study utilized functional performance measures, demonstrating a 48% improvement in mean tandem gait speed after eight weeks of PRT. Interestingly, neither of these seminal studies possessed a control group, reflecting the immaturity of this field of inquiry at that time. They did, however, lay the groundwork for exercise research within the fields of aging and rehabilitation, leading to subsequent studies utilizing broader outcomes and more rigorous research methods.

Randomized Controlled Studies

With the development and validation of more sophisticated performance measures, a number of subsequent randomized controlled exercise studies utilized functional measures. This interest in part coincided with the epidemiological investigations of Guralnik et al., demonstrating that a physical performance battery was predictive of disability (Guralnik et al. 1995, 1994). This work highlighted the importance of physical performance measures as functional measures that could serve as proximal outcomes predictive of disability. The findings from investigations in healthy elders were reinforced by subsequent investigations among disabled older adults (Guralnik et al. 2000). Building upon the ongoing work of Guralnik and others, researchers are still emphasizing the importance of performance-based measures of functioning (Morley 2003).

Though some studies showed robust changes in functioning with exercise, early work utilizing physical performance measures demonstrated disparate findings. For example, Judge and colleagues published two investigations, one with residents of a life care community and the other with community-dwelling older adults (Judge et al. 1993, 1994). Interestingly, though exercises among the respective intervention arms of these different studies were similar and augmented strength was seen in both, improvements in functioning (walking) were seen among the "frailer" life care community residents and not among the relatively "healthier" community dwellers. Similarly, in her subsequent study of nursing home residents, along with robust improvements in strength, Fiatarone et al. (1994) reported 12% improvements in gait speed. However, other investigations utilizing resistance training in community-dwelling older adults did not show improved functional performance despite improvements in strength (Buchner et al. 1997; Skelton et al. 1995).

Review of these different investigations does show variations in intensity of training in some cases; for example, Skelton et al. (1995) used a relatively low-intensity training as compared to that provided by Fiatarone and colleagues. Nevertheless, training methodology does not fully account for the variations among these findings. Investigators realized that they did not fully understand the relationship between changes in impairment and changes in function among older adults.

Curvilinear Relationship Between Impairment and Function

In a seminal paper by Buchner and de Lateur (1991), the concept of a curvilinear relationship between impairment and function was introduced. The authors demonstrated that disablement relationships are not always linear, and that among older adults with varying baseline functioning, the impairment-function relationship is, in fact, curvilinear. More specifically, incremental improvements in impairments (i.e., strength) lead to significant functional improvements for frailer, more functionally limited older adults and, at best, modest functional improvements for healthier, less limited individuals. As seen in figure 20.3, it is highlighted that for older adults who have significant functional limitations, strength improvements can lead to large changes in function. In contrast, for healthier individuals with minimal functional compromise, similar strength improvements lead to minimal additional functional improvement—but on the positive side, do add a physiologic reserve preserving functional capacity.

When viewed from an alternative perspective, a curvilinear relationship implies that there is a threshold of impairment after which further decline leads to significant functional compromise. This nonlinear relationship between impairment and function was subsequently demonstrated for impairments in balance, muscle strength, and muscle power (Bean et al. 2003a, 2004). It accounts for many of the variations seen among functional outcomes within the exercise literature. Most importantly, it suggests that a successful rehabilitative exercise program will progress individuals to a level above the threshold at which function can be easily compromised.

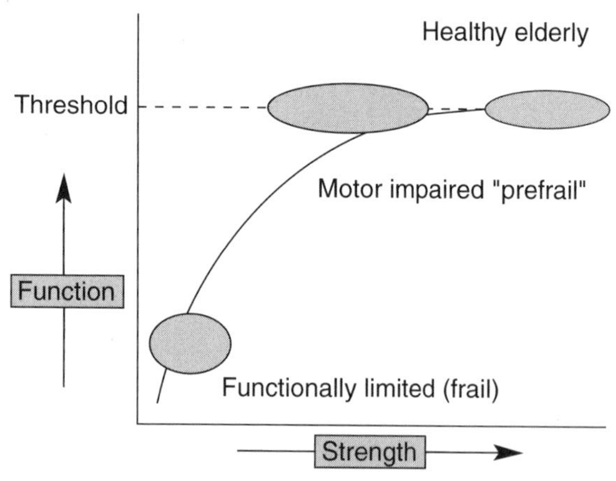

Figure 20.3 The curvilinear relationship between impairments (i.e., reduced strength) and function. At low levels, small increases in strength lead to large increases in function. In contrast, for healthy individuals at or above the functional threshold, improvements in strength have diminishing effects on function, but add to reserves of strength, augmenting resistance to functional decline.

Adapted, by permission, from J.F. Bean, A. Vora, and W.R. Frontera, 2004, "The benefits of exercise for community-dwelling older adults," *Archives of Physical Medicine and Rehabilitation* 85(7 Suppl 3):S31-S42.

Resistance Training

The term *resistance training* refers to the performance of exercise in which muscular movements are conducted against an external resistance. In contrast to aerobic training, resistance training emphasizes muscular force production. Training technique can be modified to emphasize enhancement of strength versus power through modification of movement speed. Also, training mode can emphasize isolation of selected muscles as seen with classical progressive resistance training or in contrast emphasize more generalized functional movements, as seen with task-specific training.

Resistance Training Versus Aerobic Training

When viewed in terms of the mode of training, the overwhelming evidence suggests that PRT is the most robust means of enhancing functioning and that the influence of aerobic exercise on this outcome is, at best, limited. Though many studies have combined aerobic and resistance training, review of the literature reveals few reports demonstrating improved functioning when aerobic exercise is the sole mode of training. In the three investigations that did yield positive findings, an aerobic walking program was conducted for a relatively long duration, ranging between 10 and 15 months (Ettinger et al. 1997; Minor et al. 1989; Rooks et al. 1997). Two of these studies were conducted in older adults with osteoarthritis of the knee (Ettinger et al. 1997; Minor et al. 1989). The study by Ettinger et al. (1997) is worth mentioning as it directly compared resistance training, aerobic training, and an attention control among community-dwelling older adults with radiographically evident knee osteoarthritis. Both the walking program and the resistance training programs demonstrated improvements in functioning as compared to the control groups; however, the authors specifically noted that the low intensity of training in both groups may have dampened differences between the two interventions.

In two separate studies comparing three day per week walking programs to novel modes of resistance training, the walking groups demonstrated improvements in functioning from baseline; but training effects, when compared to those from the resistance training, were less generalized (Bean et al. 2002a; Rooks et al. 1997). Therefore, given the large number of studies demonstrating functional improvements with exercise (Keysor and Jette 2001), it can be concluded that aerobic exercise is not optimal as a sole mode of exercise for addressing functional compromise in older adults. Aerobic exercise is acknowledged, however, for its benefits to both morbidity and mortality, necessitating its inclusion in generalized exercise recommendations (Bean et al. 2004).

The Effect of Resistance Training on Functioning

In contrast to aerobic exercise, among healthy and frail older adults, resistance training regardless of mode can serve as a vigorous stimulus augmenting functioning. Improvements in functioning have been reported within randomized controlled trials using solely PRT techniques in long-term care residents (Fiatarone et al. 1994; Lazowski et al. 1999), community-dwelling older adults (Chandler et al. 1998; Ettinger et al. 1997; Sayers et al. 2003), and also in combination with other modes of exercise (Cress et al. 1999; Lord et al. 1995; Minor et al. 1989; Rubenstein et al. 2000). Studies featuring less rigorous intensity or progression of resistance training programs have not always been as successful in producing augmented functional performance (King et al. 2000; McMurdo and Johnstone 1995; Skelton et al. 1995); however, a common theme among those achieving success may be a duration of six months or longer (Jette et al. 1999; Rooks et al. 1997). In recognition of these benefits, in 1999 a consensus panel from the National Institute on Aging (1999) published guidelines for exercise that were primarily structured around PRT with free weights.

Muscle Power Resistance Training

Since the publication of the National Institute on Aging guidelines, alternative forms of resistance training have gained greater attention. One specific area of focus has been the importance of muscle power and the development of suitable means of muscle power training (Evans 2000). Muscle power, defined as the rate of muscular work per unit time, is an attribute related to, but separate from, muscular strength. Though long acknowledged as an essential component of athletic performance, the importance of muscle power to older adults has not received attention until recently. Whereas strength generally refers to a measurement of muscular force production, power refers to the product of force and velocity of movement (power = force × velocity). Muscular power declines in late life more precipitously than strength does (Metter et al. 1997). Impairments in lower extremity muscle power production have been linked to falls (Skelton et al. 1994; Whipple et al. 1987), limitations in mobility (Bean et al. 2002b, 2003b; Suzuki et al. 2001), and self-reported disability (Foldvari et al. 2000).

Important investigations evaluating impairments underlying mobility performance have directly compared strength and power. In these studies, muscle power consistently had an influence on mobility performance equal to or greater than that of strength. (Bean et al. 2002b, 2003b; Suzuki et al. 2001). In a large population-based study evaluating factors underlying mobility limitations, impairments in leg power were found to impart a two- to threefold greater likelihood for significant mobility limitations as compared to leg strength (Bean et al. 2002b). Taken together, these findings highlight muscle power as an important attribute that when targeted through exercise interventions may influence the mode and method of exercise training.

Muscle power can be enhanced through resistance training. Enhancements of force production at a given velocity will increase muscle power. For example, when PRT was provided to nursing home residents, along with the >100% improvements in strength, 28% improvements in stair climb power were seen (Fiatarone et al. 1994). More recently, in a study evaluating healthy older adults, improvements of 20% to 40% in muscle power were demonstrated with PRT (Jozsi et al. 1999). Interestingly, both of these studies involved exercise at relatively slow velocities and demonstrated greater improvements in strength as compared to power.

Recognizing that velocity may be a key factor determining improvements in muscle power, Fielding et al. (2002) conducted a direct comparison of PRT conducted at slow and fast velocities. In this study of older women with self-reported mobility problems, subjects were randomized to one group in which the eccentric and concentric components of each repetition were conducted over 2 sec (slow velocity), or a second group in which subjects performed identical exercises on the same equipment except that the concentric component of each repetition was conducted as quickly as possible (high velocity). Though strength improvements between the groups were not significantly different, the high-velocity group had an almost twofold greater improvement in muscle power than the slow-velocity group. Importantly, other studies incorporating methods that emphasize higher speed of repetitions have shown improvements in muscle power utilizing exercise machines (Earles et al. 2001; Hakkinen et al. 2001; Miszko et al. 2003) and also with the use of simpler forms of exercise (Bean et al. 2002, 2004; Shaw and Snow 1998). Review of these studies suggests that this means of training appears to be safe, with no disproportionate frequency of injuries being reported.

The effect on functioning of resistance training programs designed to enhance muscle power has yet to be fully investigated. Initial studies evaluating muscle power training did not demonstrate meaningful improvements in functioning despite improvements in leg power (Earles et al. 2001; Skelton et al. 1995). The relatively high functional level of study participants at baseline and the relatively low intensity of training may explain these findings in part. Supporting this suggestion, pilot studies conducted with mobility-limited older adults evaluating alternative forms of power training have shown both improvements in leg power and functional improvements from baseline (Bean et al. 2002, 2004).

In the two studies directly comparing "strength" and "power" training regimens, findings are contrasting. Analysis of Fielding's study reported overall improvements in functioning (dynamic balance, stair climbing) with resistance training independent of whether it was conducted at high velocity or low velocity, with no added benefit of either regimen (Sayers et al. 2003). Nevertheless, limitations in regard to sample size, functional diversity of the cohort, and outcome measurements used may have influenced the results. More recently, Miszko et al. (2003) conducted a randomized controlled trial with an attention control group and power and strength training groups similar to those of Fielding et al. Using a broader functional performance measure designed for older adults, they reported significantly greater improvement within the power training group as compared to the strength training group, though both groups had augmented functioning relative to controls. Taken together, these studies suggest that the optimal mode of exercise for functional enhancement is not yet known. Training regimens that emphasize muscle power production may provide added functional benefits in comparison to more classical PRT. Direct comparisons within larger-scale studies are currently under way.

Task-Specific Training

The fact that the higher-velocity mode of training can produce greater improvements in muscle power underscores a fundamental concept of athletic rehabilitation, known as specificity of training. Essentially, this refers to the fact that optimal training for a given sport will involve tasks very closely related (specific) to that sport. If one considered living independently the "sport" of older adults, then it would follow that exercises should be very similar to the functional tasks that enable independence. Therapies based on task-specific training methods have been utilized successfully in older adults with chronic hemiplegia due to stroke (Dean and Shepherd 1997; Dean et al. 2000; Monger et al. 2002). Schnelle et al. have reported successful management of both mobility and incontinence problems among nursing home residents utilizing an exercise program based on specific functional tasks (Schnelle et al. 1995, 2002). Using a similar approach, Alexander et al. (1991) reported improvements in chair and bed rise capabilities among congregate housing residents. Task-specific training has also been applied to community-dwelling older adults (Bean et al. 2002, 2004).

The potential for task-specific activity to provide an effective training stimulus is nicely illustrated by two additional examples. In the first case, it is beneficial to review the meta-analysis from the Frailty and Injuries: Cooperative Studies of Intervention Techniques (FICSIT trials). The FICSIT trials comprised seven separate randomized controlled intervention studies in which at least one study arm of each site included some form of exercise training (Province et al. 1995). Though training techniques varied among the sites, review of the respective studies suggests that the treatment arm containing the exercises highest in specificity was in the Atlanta site, where one group of study subjects performed tai chi (Wolf et al. 1996). Interestingly, among all of the 13 treatment arms included within the meta-analysis, the greatest effect in reducing falls was seen within these subjects. Though there may be other means by which tai chi exercise imparts benefits to balance and falls reduction, it can be concluded that one main mechanism is through specificity of exercise (Wolf et al. 1997).

A second example of the importance of training specificity comes from a recently published pilot study (Bean et al. 2004). This study in mobility-limited older women utilized a training protocol based on principles of PRT, enhancement of muscle power, and specificity of training. The control exercise group performed open chain, low-resistance flexion/extension exercises at a relatively slow velocity in which body weight served as resistance. Included within this group's exercise program were three sets of 10 chair rises. The intervention group, wearing a weighted vest, performed functional progressive resistance exercises in which a component of each repetition was performed as quickly as possible. This group performed exercises with greater functional specificity, such as rising from a chair, stepping up on a platform, climbing stairs, and reaching activities. At the end of 12 weeks of training, both groups demonstrated significant improvements in chair rise performance from baseline; however, there was a significantly greater improvement in chair rise performance among the vest exercise group. This suggests that the added components in the intervention group, which included a greater magnitude of specificity through "high-velocity" training, mediated greater improvements in functioning (Bean et al. 2003).

EXERCISE EFFECT ON DISABILITY UPDATED

Though the optimal means of exercise to enhance functioning is being explored, the benefit of exercise on disability is only beginning to be clarified. In 2000, basing their work on disablement concepts, Keysor and Jette (2001) reviewed the randomized controlled trials to date in order to ascertain the benefits of late-life exercise on disability. Of 31 studies meeting inclusion criteria, only 25% included an attempt to evaluate changes in physical disability, and five demonstrated positive effects. Of these five studies, three were in subjects with arthritis. In their assessment of the literature and of the weaknesses of the previous studies, Keysor and Jette did not deny that exercise could influence late-life disability, but laid out recommendations for future investigations. They cautioned investigators to carefully consider the target sample, type and duration of the exercise intervention, statistical power needed to detect disability outcomes, and the specific disability outcomes to be tested as well as how they will be assessed to maximize the likelihood of detecting any positive effects. Lastly, the authors emphasized that interventions should be theoretically driven by cognitive-behavioral concepts of disablement (see "The Role of Self-Efficacy").

Since publication of Keysor and Jette's review, three additional publications have shown changes in disability with interventions involving exercise (Gill et al. 2002; Morris et al. 1999; Penninx et al. 2001). All three adhere to many of Keysor and Jette's recommendations and highlight an additional concept surrounding the influence of exercise on disability—whether exercise prevents or ameliorates disability, or does both:

- Penninx and colleagues (Penninx et al. 2001) reported a multicenter randomized controlled trial among 250 community-dwelling older adults with arthritis. They demonstrated that after 18 months of exercise, both aerobic and resistance training programs reduced the incidence of disability as compared to that in a control group. Risk was reduced 60% within the resistance group and 53% within the aerobic exercise groups, for a combined 57% reduced risk of developing ADL disability.
- Morris and colleagues (Morris et al. 1999) evaluated high-intensity PRT, a nursing behavioral intervention, and normal care among six matched nursing homes. After 10 months, the exercise intervention and the nursing intervention slowed progression of both functional and ADL loss among the 392 nursing home residents.
- In a study among 188 frail community-dwelling older adults, Gill and colleagues (Gill et al. 2002) also demonstrated slowed progression of ADL loss after 12 months. In a multifaceted intervention that the authors named "prehabilitation," participants underwent home-based physical therapy evaluations and received, among other treatments, a tailored exercise program that is best characterized as progressive, low resistance, and specific toward many functional needs (Gill et al. 2003).

The latter two investigations demonstrated that exercise could slow progression of disability.

In considering these studies it should be acknowledged that all three utilized large sample sizes, long durations of exercise, and measures sensitive to change and that all were designed with an understanding of cognitive and behavioral factors influencing exercise and disability. Taken together, these studies evaluating the benefit of exercise on both function and disability demonstrate that exercise can indeed enhance functioning and prevent as well as ameliorate disability. Table 20.2 summarizes the randomized controlled trials (and studies of similar scientific rigor) to date that have addressed disablement outcomes in older adults. In comparison to aerobic exercise, there is broader support for resistance training, in its various forms, as the best treatment for enhancing function and delaying disability. The exception may be among individuals with osteoarthritis, in whom the benefits of aerobic exercise toward both disablement outcomes have been reported.

At this point, however, questions remain unanswered. For example, the optimal mode(s), frequency, and intensity of training for functional enhancement need to be defined. Full understanding of how exercise programs should be designed to prevent and ameliorate disability has yet to be established. As is the case for osteoarthritis, further investigation is necessary to understand how exercise can be used to prevent and treat disability associated with the most common chronic diseases and conditions of older age.

THE ROLE OF SELF-EFFICACY

Embedded within the cognitive-behavioral concepts to which Keysor and Jette alluded are some important influential factors mediating the relationship between exercise and disability (Rejeski et al. 2000). Perhaps the most fully developed factor is self-efficacy. Self-efficacy is defined as an individual's belief that he or she can complete any given task(s). Tinetti et al. (1990) have reported that self-efficacy to avoid falls, independent of injury or actual falls, is an important factor influencing activity restrictions in older adults.

It was also reported that self-efficacy was an independent predictor of physical performance among individuals with osteoarthritis (Rejeski and Focht 2002; Rejeski et al. 2001). Additionally, in a prospective study among

Table 20.2 Randomized Controlled Trials Evaluating the Effect of Exercise on Disablement Outcomes in Older Adults

Study	Study design	Exercise program	Impairment	Function	Disability
Ades et al. 1996	RCT (n = 24) Healthy community-dwelling elderly persons Age range: 65-79 Mean age: 70	IG: Strength training 3 ×/wk for 12 wk	Strength: PE among women Aerobic capacity: NE Body composition: NE	Walking: PE among men	
Bean et al. 2002a	RCT (n = 45) Mobility-limited community dwellers Age range: 65+ Mean age: 73	IG: Progressive stair climbing with weighted vests CG: Progressive walking program 3 ×/wk for 12 wk	Leg power: PE IG Aerobic capacity: PE for both from baseline CG = IG	Mobility: PE IG Stair climb: PE IG, CG Gait: PE CG	
Bean et al. 2004	RCT (n = 21) Mobility-limited community-dwelling women Age: 70+ Mean age: 78	IG: PRT with weighted vests, performing functional exercises with high-velocity component CG: body weight-resisted slow-velocity exercises 3 ×/wk for 12 wk	Power: PE among IG from baseline and vs. CG	Mobility: PE for IG, CG Chair rise: PE for IG, CG and IG > CG	
Buchner et al. 1997	RCT (n = 105) HMO enrollees with impaired balance and strength Age range: 68-85 Mean age: 75	IG1: Strength training IG2: Endurance training IG3: Strength and endurance training IGs: 3 ×/wk for 6 mo	Strength: PE IG1 and IG3 Aerobic capacity: PE IG2 and IG3	Walking: NE Stair climbing: NE Balance: NE	Physical disability: NE
Chandler et al. 1998	RCT (n = 100) Community-dwelling adults who were functionally impaired Age range: 66-97 Mean age: 78	IG: In-home strength training 3 ×/wk for 10 wk	Strength: PE	Walking: PE Chair rise: PE among more impaired participants Mobility skills: PE Balance: NE	Physical disability: NE
Cress et al. 1999	RCT (n = 49) Adults living independently in retirement community or apartment Age: 70+ Mean age: 76	IG: Aerobic and strength training 3 ×/wk for 6 mo	Strength: PE Range of motion (ROM)/flexibility: PE Neuromuscular control: NE	Walking: NE Mobility: PE Balance: PE	Physical disability: NE Emotional disability: NE Social disability: NE Overall disability: NE

Damush and Damush 1999	RCT (n = 71) Women living in retirement residential communities Age: 55+ Mean age: 68	IG: Strength training 2 ×/wk for 8 wk CG: Participant attended the exercise session but did not participate in exercise	Strength: PE		Physical disability: NE Emotional disability: NE
Ettinger et al. 1997	RCT (n = 439) Community-dwelling adults radiographic known osteoarthritis, pain, and self-reported disability Age: 60+ Mean age: 69	IG1: Walking program IG2: Strengthening program Both IGs: 3-mo facility-based program followed by a 15-mo home-based program CG: Health education program	Strength: PE both IGs Aerobic capacity: PE in IG1 Symptoms: pain decreased IG1 and IG2	Walking: PE IG1 and IG2 Sit/stand: PE IG1 and IG2 Stair ascent and descent: PE IG1 Weighted lift task: PE both IG1 and IG2	Physical disability: PE IG1
Fiatarone et al. 1994	RCT (n = 100) Frail nursing home residents Age range: 72-98 Mean age: 87	IG: Resistance training 3 ×/wk for 10 wk CG: Social activity 3 ×/wk for 10 wk	Strength: PE Body composition: PE (muscle mass)	Walking: PE Stair climb: PE	
Fielding et al. 2002	RCT (n = 30) Community-dwelling women with self-reported disability Age: 65+ Mean age: 73	IG1: High-velocity resistance training IG2: Slow-velocity resistance training 3 ×/wk for 16 wk	Strength: PE both groups IG1 = IG2 Power: PE both groups and IG1 > IG2		
Gill et al. 2002	RCT (n = 188) Frail community-dwelling older adults Age: 75+ Mean age: 83	IG: Multifaceted home-based intervention including progressive low-resistance functional exercises CG: Educational program Both 6-mo programs			Physical disability: PE IG1
Jette et al. 1996	RCT (n = 102) Community-dwelling nondisabled adults Age range: 66-87 Mean age: 72	IG: In-home strengthening program; one visit by a health professional to establish the program, followed by a phone call on the next day and then follow-up phone calls periodically over 11 wk; adherence goal for participants was 3 ×/wk for 12-15 wk	Strength: PE among younger participants		Physical disability: NE Social disability: PE among older participants Emotional disability: PE "vigor" improved in IG among men

(continued)

Table 20.2 *(continued)*

Study	Study design	Exercise program	Impairment	Function	Disability
Jette et al. 1999	RCT (n = 215) Community-dwelling adults, functionally impaired Age: 60+ Mean age: 75	IG: Theoretically driven cognitive-behavioral resistance training program; two visits by a health professional to establish exercise and behavior change program; telephone follow-up for support and to monitor progress; incentives sent when participants adhered to intervention program for 6 mo	Strength: PE	Sit/stand with walk: PE Balance: PE	Physical disability: PE Emotional disability: NE Overall disability: PE
Judge et al. 1993	RCT (n = 34) Residents of two life care communities Age range: 71-97 Mean age: 82	IG: Flexibility, resistance, and balance training 3 ×/wk for 12 wk CG: Sitting ROM exercise 1 ×/wk for 12 wk	Strength: PE	Walking: PE	
Judge et al. 1994	RCT (n = 110) Community-dwelling adults on a voter registration list who were able to walk 8 m without an assisted device and who had a Folstein Mini-Mental Status score >24 Age: 75+ Mean age: 80	IG1: Floor and computer balance training IG2: Strength training IG3: Balance and resistance IG All IGs participated in the intervention program 3 ×/wk for 3 mo IGs and CG participated in five educational sessions	Strength: PE in resistance training group	Walking: NE Chair rise: NE	
King et al. 2000	RCT (n = 103) Inactive community-dwelling adults Age: 65+ Mean age: 70	IG: Theoretically driven aerobic and strengthening program to enhance behavior changes; class sessions 2 ×/wk, home exercise encouraged 2×/wk for 12 mo CG: Stretch and relaxation program with similar group and home program	Flexibility/ROM: PE Aerobic capacity: PE IG symptoms: NE	Walking: NE Sit/stand: NE Weight lift: PE	Physical disability: NE Emotional disability: NE
Kovar et al. 1992	RCT (n = 102) Patients with known osteoarthritis Age range: 40-89 Mean age: 69	IG: Theoretically driven supervised walking and education program to enhance behavior change 3 ×/wk for 8 wk	Symptoms: PE (pain decreased)	Walking: PE	Physical disability: PE
Lazowski et al. 1999	RCT (n = 96) Long-term care residents Mean age: 80	IG: Strength training, balance, flexibility, and walking program 3 ×/wk for 16 wk CG: ROM exercise program	Strength: PE ROM/flexibility: PE	Walking: NE Sit/stand with walk: PE Stair climbing: NE Balance: PE	

Lord et al. 1995	RCT (n = 197) Community-dwelling women Age: 60+ Mean age: 72	IG: Aerobic, flexibility, and strengthening program 2 ×/wk for 12 mo	Strength: PE Reaction time: PE Neuromuscular control: PE	Balance: PE	
Lord et al. 1996a	RCT (n = 160) Community-dwelling women Age range: 60-83 Mean age: 71	IG: Aerobic, flexibility, and strengthening program 2 ×/wk for 22 wk	Strength: PE	Walking: PE Balance: PE	
McMurdo and Johnstone 1995	RCT (n = 86) Adults with physical disability who lived in local authority and private sheltered housing Age: 75+ Mean age: 82	IG1: In-home flexibility and strengthening exercises; exercise program established by a health professional with monthly follow-up visits for 6 mo IG2: Flexibility exercise program same as IG1 CG: Monthly health education sessions delivered in the home	Strength: NE ROM/flexibility: NE	Sit/stand with and without walk: NE (trend)	Physical disability: NE Emotional disability: NE
Minor et al. 1989	RCT (n = 120) Adults with osteoarthritis or rheumatoid arthritis Age range: 21-83 Mean age: 61 Outcomes assessed at 3 and 12 mo (reported outcomes are 12 mo)	IG1: Walking, flexibility, and strengthening 3 ×/wk for 12 wk IG2: Water aerobics, flexibility, and strengthening 3 ×/wk for 12 wk CG: ROM exercises	Strength: PE IGs ROM/flexibility: NE Aerobic capacity: PE IGs Joint count: NE Morning stiffness: PE Pain: NE	Walking: PE	Physical disability: PE Social disability: NE Emotional disability: PE
Morris et al. 1999	Quasi-experimental control (n = 468) Nursing home residents from 6 separate facilities	IG1: Resistance training IG2: Nursing intervention CG: Usual care	Endurance: IG1		Physical disability: PE IG1 and IG2
Penninx et al. 2001	Multicenter RCT (n = 250) Adults with osteoarthritis who were disability free Age: 60+ Mean age: 69	IG1: Resistance training IG2: Aerobic training Both IGs: 3-mo facility-based program followed by a 15-mo home-based program CG: Attention control			Physical disability: PE IG1 and IG2

(continued)

Table 20.2 *(continued)*

Study	Study design	Exercise program	Impairment	Function	Disability
Rooks et al. 1997	RCT (n = 131) Community-dwelling adults, independent Age range: 65-95 Mean age: 74	IG1: Strength training 3 ×/wk for 10 mo IG2: Walking group 3 ×/wk for 10 mo	Strength: PE in IG Reaction time (foot): PE IG1	Mobility: PE IG1 (pen pickup from floor) Stairs: PE both IGs Balance: PE both IGs	
Rubenstein et al. 2000	RCT (n = 59) Community-dwelling men at risk of falling Age: 70+ Mean age: 75	IG: Strength, endurance, and balance training 3 ×/wk for 12 wk	Strength: PE	Walking: PE Sit/stand: NE (trend) Mobility: NE (indoor obstacle course) Balance: NE	Physical disability: NE (trend)
Sayers et al. 2003	Same as for Fielding et al.			Stair climb: PE Balance: PE IG1= IG2	Physical disability: PE IG1= IG2
Sherrington and Lord 1997	RCT (n = 42) Adults 7 mo post-fall-related hip fracture Age range: 64-91 Mean age: 80	IG: Home-based, weight-bearing exercise daily for 1 mo (one visit by a health professional to establish program and one follow-up visit during intervention)	Strength: PE	Walking: PE Weight-bearing step test: PE Balance: NE	
Skelton et al. 1995	RCT (n = 52) Community-dwelling women Age range: 75-93 Mean age: 79.5	IG: Strengthening program, 12 wk	Strength: PE Body composition: NE	Walking: NE Sit/stand: NE Floor/stand: NE Stair climbing: NE Kneel rise time: PE Weighted lift task: NE Balance: NE	
Wolfson et al. 1996	RCT (n = 110) Community-dwelling adults who were registered to vote Aged: 75+ Mean age: 80	Same intervention as for Judge et al. 1994 Intervention duration for all IGs: 3 mo; all subjects then received 6 mo weekly tai chi (results reported here are at 3-mo follow-up)	Strength: PE IG2 and IG3	Gait: NE Balance: PE IG1 and IG3	

RCT = randomized controlled trial; IG = intervention group; CG = control group; PE = positive treatment effect; NE = no treatment effect.

older adults with knee pain, Rejeski et al. (2001) demonstrated that low self-efficacy—especially when coupled with leg weakness—was a major factor predicting disability progression. Consistent with Keysor and Jette's results, these findings have led Rajeski and Focht to argue that in order for exercise programs to be effective in modifying disability, provision of exercise only is not sufficient. Counseling at the group or individual level (or both) that addresses self-efficacy beliefs is essential to effectively enhance function and ameliorate disability (Rejeski and Focht 2002).

PRACTICAL RECOMMENDATIONS

We present here only general guidelines, since detailed guidelines are beyond the scope of this chapter and are found elsewhere (Fiatarone-Singh 2002; Bean et al. 2004; Dishman 1994; Pollock et al. 1994; Frontera and Bean 2004). The key point is that age by itself should not be a deterrent to exercise but, in fact, should be one of the most important indications to begin or to continue exercising.

SETTING GOALS

Older adults have widely differing goals, reflecting the heterogeneity of their population. On one end of the spectrum are the robust, nonfrail, healthy elderly who may have been exercising for many years. Goals for these individuals include preserving vitality, function, and independence for as long as possible. These older adults should be challenged to extend themselves by increasing intensity or including other modalities such as resistance training. On the other end of the functional spectrum are the frail elderly who, by living at the limits of their physiologic and functional capacity, struggle with normal ADL. Within this frail elderly group are some who are physically dependent and others who may still be independent, albeit marginally. The goals here should be to improve or restore functional capacity so that ADL may be easier. Between these two extremes are the majority of older adults: the typically aging, sedentary elderly, who are at mild to moderate risk for disability. While most of the elderly people in this group have had minimal if any experience with exercise, it is they who have the most to gain by altering their sedentary ways. Reversing and preventing the downward functional spiral associated with the typical sedentary aging process should be the primary goal for this group.

THE TRAINING PROGRAM

The ideal exercise program should be tailored to the older adult, using a combination of aerobic, resistance, stretching, and balance training. However, whereas programs for younger adults usually emphasize aerobic training, we agree with Fiatarone-Singh (2002) and believe that resistive exercises may be the most beneficial form of exercise, at least initially, for the frail elderly. An effective program will use all exercise modalities and will target large muscle groups of the upper and lower body such as the legs, arms, shoulders, calves, and back. As with younger adults, the elderly should train aerobically three to five days a week, 5 to 60 min/session. Strength training, on two to three nonconsecutive days per week, should include two to three sets of 8 to 12 repetitions for each muscle group, with short rests between sets.

Although studies show that the elderly can train safely at and respond to high-intensity exercise sessions, it is probably wise to begin at lower intensities (according to self-perception, or 30%-50% 1RM, or 40%-50% HRmax) and gradually work up to higher intensity levels. Frequent use of an exercise intensity scale such as Borg's rating of perceived exertion scale is strongly recommended (Borg 1998; figure 20.4).

Finally, an exercise program for the elderly should be progressive, although the rate of progression may need to be more gradual than with younger individuals. An improvement in physiologic capacity (strength or aerobic capacity) may occur just through increase in muscle repetitions or aerobic duration; however, most older people reach a limit where further physiologic gains are not possible without increased resistance or aerobic training intensity. On the other hand, intensity

6	No exertion at all
7	Extremely light
8	
9	Very light
10	
11	Light
12	
13	Somewhat hard
14	
15	Hard (heavy)
16	
17	Very hard
18	
19	Extremely hard
20	Maximal exertion

Borg RPE scale

Figure 20.4 Borg's rating of perceived exertion scale.

Reprinted, by permission, from G. Borg, 1998, *Borg's perceived exertion and pain scales*. (Champaign, IL: Human Kinetics), 47.

is not necessarily as important as participation for most elderly participants. No exercise program is effective unless the individual continues with the program. The highest priority in regulating training intensity is to enhance exercise compliance. A reasonable intensity goal for older adults is one that feels "somewhat hard" to "hard" on the Borg scale. Another guideline is the "talk test," whereby people know they are exercising excessively when they cannot carry on a conversation during the activity. A few missed exercise sessions are insignificant when the goals are long-term, and should not discourage the older participant from continuing.

Special Considerations

Although the same general principles of exercise employed for younger adults (e.g., intensity, training regimen, and frequency) apply also to the elderly, unique characteristics of the older adult require some special considerations.

"Start Low, Go Slow"

Reduced physiologic reserve, and therefore longer recoveries from injury, make the geriatric axiom "Start low, go slow" perhaps the most important guideline for older individuals who begin exercising. Close supervision and attention to proper form are very important, given the risk for musculoskeletal injury. Pollock et al. (1991) have reported rates of soft tissue injury up to 57% among elderly participants in training programs that included a jogging component. Warm-up and cool-down calisthenics involving large muscle groups should begin and end each exercise session. Older adults must avoid breath holding, which can cause increases in blood pressure, especially during strengthening exercises in which the Valsalva maneuver tends to occur naturally. Proper technique typically involves inhaling before the lift or during the eccentric contraction and exhaling during the lift (concentric contraction), and avoiding ballistic movements during stretching or lifting weights. Depending on a person's baseline physical state and past experience with exercise, training programs for the elderly may begin with flexibility training, then progress to resistance exercises, and then to aerobic and balance exercises.

Pre-Exercise Evaluation

Most experts recommend a pre-exercise assessment, including a complete history and physical examination. There are few absolute contraindications for exercising. The most common contraindication is any acute or unstable medical condition; and even this contraindication is often temporary. In fact, aerobic and resistance exercise are now even being used as adjunctive treatment in severe but stable cardiopulmonary disease (Beniamini et al. 1997; Ghilarducci et al. 1989). The elderly are also the greatest consumers of medications. Anyone prescribing or overseeing exercise therapy for older people must have a clear understanding of their medications, and of the cardiovascular and neurologic effects of those medications, and should instruct patients to report all changes in their medications. Close monitoring of pulse, blood pressure, and symptoms is crucial at the beginning of an exercise program and whenever the program is changed.

It is not clear whether a monitored, graded exercise stress test is warranted for every older adult about to embark on an exercise program. The substantial costs of such across-the-board evaluations would decrease the chances that local governments will adopt exercise as a public health measure; they would also limit the participation of many older individuals with limited financial means. Many older individuals on their own have probably participated safely in community-based exercise programs without formal screening. It is our belief that the certain risks of continued chronic inactivity outweigh the possible risks of exercise.

Cardiac stress testing, however, may be appropriate for individuals with a known or suggestive cardiac history, even for the very old. On the other hand, stress testing protocols may not be feasible or even necessary in the frail elderly for whom the test would present an overwhelming physical or even emotional challenge. For such individuals, close supervision during the exercise activity, with monitoring of blood pressure and pulse, may be sufficient to predict the risks of the proposed program.

Behavioral Issues Motivating the Elderly to Exercise

Young and old individuals generally share similar attitudes about exercise and physical activity, with some exceptions (Dishman 1994). Although both groups have a positive attitude toward exercise, the elderly feel less confident and have more fear of hurting themselves. Another major difference between adults under and over age 65 is that physically inactive older persons usually have no intention of becoming active. A third difference is that despite the positive attitudes toward physical activity, most elderly people consider it a low priority for leisure time. The unfortunate fact is that most older adults have been sedentary for most of their adult lives. Although it need not be so, beginning an exercise program often represents a major change. The first step usually involves transforming an older person's belief system. Behavioral modification programs developed for and successfully applied to smoking cessation may be increasingly applied to exercise programs as well.

For those who do begin to exercise, adherence is usually poor on the first try. More than 50% of individuals drop out of exercise programs within six months (Borg 1998). Adding counseling, education, or behavior modification, or changing the amount of exercise prescribed, may only modestly increase participation (Dishman 1994). Middle-aged adults are less likely to begin and continue a vigorous exercise program designed for cardiovascular fitness than one involving less intense activities such as walking or gardening (Dishman 1989). The most successful programs include some combination of ongoing supervision and efforts to monitor and promote compliance.

Unfortunately, there are few guidelines available to help health care professionals increase participation in or adherence to exercise programs by older individuals. It is important to remember that training goals for the elderly often differ from those of younger persons. Rather than focusing on traditional exercise measures such as intensity, workload, or percent of maximal heart rate, programs for the elderly should target ease of mobility, maintenance of flexibility, and strength. It is these outcomes that maximize individuals' function and social integration. Creative, varied programs leading to sustained continuous involvement in exercise may be far more important than the specifics of the exercise regimen. Clearly, more research is needed in this area if we are to achieve the physical activity objectives set for older adults for the coming millennium.

SUMMARY

The aging process presents challenges to health care systems throughout the world, centered mainly around problems of physical frailty and declining function. This property of function allows the geriatric and psychiatric disciplines to intersect. The current aging paradigm attributes age-related declines to a combination of genetics, physiologic aging, chronic illness, medications, and lifestyle, although the degree to which each component contributes to frailty needs much further clarification. Exercise as an intervention, however, produces numerous physiologic changes that appear to counteract effects of the typical aging process. The extent to which these physiologic benefits do and potentially might mitigate functional disability requires further study.

While these and other issues are being clarified, there is little question that exercise is the single most effective way to preserve or even improve function in old age. As stated by Dr. Robert Butler, former director of the National Institute on Aging, "If exercise could be put in a bottle, it would be the strongest medicine money could buy." With a few exceptions, the general guidelines for exercising apply equally to younger and to older individuals. Exercise programs should focus on long-term goals; and they should be individualized, to address the functional heterogeneity of the aging population. Also, rehabilitation specialists should not be afraid to "push" their patients to higher levels so long as this is done gradually and carefully. Studies have clearly demonstrated that older adults respond positively to progressive exercise training. Finally, while closely monitoring patients, therapists must exercise clear knowledge of both medication-exercise interactions and comorbid conditions. Ultimately, regardless of age or level of frailty, nearly all elderly persons can derive some physiologic, functional, or quality of life benefit from initiating an exercise program.

CHAPTER 21

Elite Athletes With Impairments

Rory A. Cooper, PhD; Michael L. Boninger, MD; Ian Rice, MS, OTR/L; Sean D. Shimada, PhD; and Rosemarie Cooper, MPT, ATP

Sport and recreation have changed the way in which people with disabilities perceive themselves and the way in which society as a whole perceives them (Cook and Webster 1982; Cooper et al. 1992; Wade 1993). The concept that someone with a disability can be athletic and compete at high levels of sport has helped remove the stigma of being sick that was long associated with a physical impairment (Galvin and Scherer 1996; Loverock 1980; Rick Hansen Centre 1988; Snell 1992). Sport continues to be an important tool for social change as well as for individual rehabilitation. There is a growing trend toward integrated activities, in which people with and without physical impairments can participate in sports and recreational activities side by side. People with disabilities participate in nearly every recreational activity that exists, in some cases using specialized equipment, in others using standard equipment (Asato et al. 1992; Cooper and Bedi 1990; Skinner and Effeney 1985). Figure 21.1 shows specialized equipment used by individuals for snow skiing. Recreation is an important aspect of people's lives, and good recreation habits can lead to a fuller and healthier life. People participate in a variety of recreational activities ranging from gardening to skydiving. Recreational activities change over the life span as well. It is important for people with disabilities to learn healthy recreational activities during rehabilitation.

From Patient to Athlete

Shortly after World War II, Sir Ludwig Guttmann and his colleagues at Stoke Mandeville Hospital in England needed exercise and recreational outlets for the large number of young people recently injured in the war. Out of this need came wheelchair sports as a rehabilitation tool (Cooper 1990). News of Dr. Guttmann's success in rehabilitating his patients through sport spread through Europe and to the United States. In 1948, he organized "Games" for British veterans with disabilities. In 1952, the Games developed into the first international wheelchair sporting competition for people with physical disabilities, with participants from the Netherlands, the Federal Republic of Germany, Sweden, Norway, and Israel. During this event, the International Stoke Mandeville Games Federation (ISMGF) was formed to govern and develop wheelchair sporting competitions. The ISMGF established ties to the International Olympic Committee (IOC), thus expanding the scope of wheelchair sports.

As the international sport movement for people with disabilities grew, and international multidisability events multiplied, the ISMGF expanded to include all wheelchair sporting events, renaming itself the International Stoke Mandeville Wheelchair Sports Federation (ISMWSF). The first international games for the disabled held in conjunction with the Olympic Games took place in 1960 in Rome. The name "Paralympics" was coined during the 1964 Tokyo Games, and this competition still occurs every four years under that name (Cooper 1990).

In the early years of wheelchair racing, participants used bulky depot-type wheelchairs and did not compete in events with distances over 200 m (Cooper 1989a, 1989b, 1989c, 1990, 1992a; Cooper et al. 1992). In the 1970s, athletes began to modify their wheelchairs for specific sports and started to take an

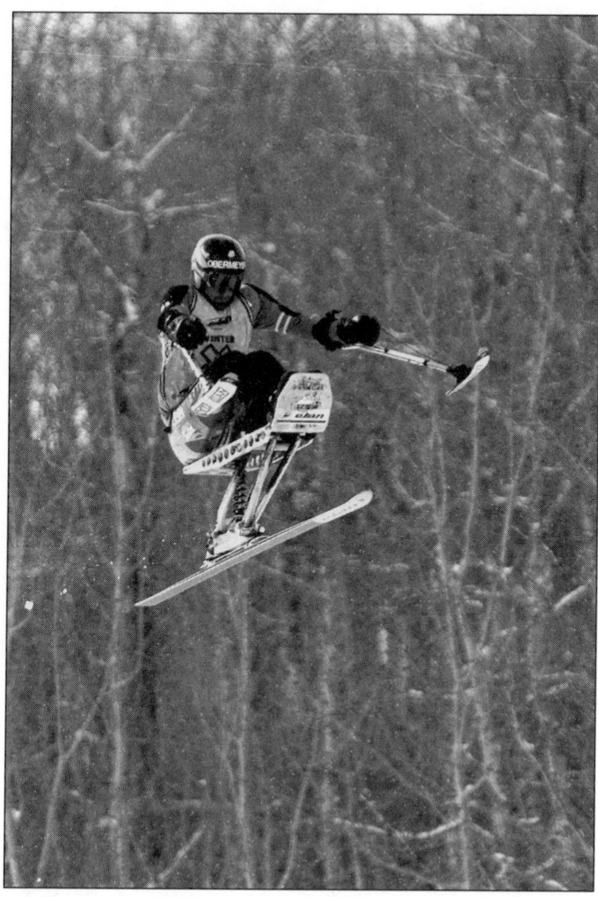

Figure 21.1 Using specialized equipment to ski.
Tony Donaldson/Icon SMI.

interest in road racing. In 1975, Bobby Hall, a young man with paraplegia, became the first person to compete in the Boston Athletic Association Marathon in a wheelchair. This opened the door for many future road racers, prompting Dr. Caibre McCann, a leading physician for the ISMGF, to say, "Running is natural, but propelling yourself in a wheelchair is an unnatural phenomenon. People never realize what a wheelchair athlete is capable of. This is a breakthrough in man's limits" (Cooper 1990). Wheelchair racers competing in the world's premier marathons have proven how capable they are. Many of these racers have set themselves apart not only as the finest wheelchair athletes in the world, but also as some of the most dedicated, well-conditioned athletes in the world. Ernst Van Dyk of South Africa holds the course record in the wheelchair marathon with a time of 1:18:27; Jean Driscoll of the United States holds the women's record of 1:34:22. It is interesting to note that the able-bodied course record times for males and females are 2:07:15 and 2:20:43, respectively.

It has taken many years for wheelchair racers to achieve this level of success, however. In the early years of racing, several recognized U.S. road races initiated wheelchair divisions, and more people with disabilities than ever anticipated began to train for these races (Cooper 1990). In 1976, the ISMGF started to coordinate with other international sport organizations to launch a unified international sport movement for people with disabilities (Cooper 1990). Racing wheelchairs began to evolve as special-purpose pieces of equipment easily distinguishable from everyday wheelchairs (Cooper 1992b; MacLeish et al. 1993). Distances on the track were extended to include races up to 1500 m, and during this time the mile record dropped below five minutes.

The early 1980s saw the development of more sophisticated racing wheelchairs and training techniques (Cooper 1989c, 1992a; MacLeish et al. 1993). By 1985, most racing wheelchairs had no components in common with everyday wheelchairs (which had also improved dramatically), and George Murray became the first wheelchair racer to break the four-minute mile. In the years that followed, wheelchair racing continued to progress with improved equipment, training, and nutrition; consequently, world records were continually falling. Wheelchair racing began the path toward recognition as a legitimate Olympic sport in 1984, when the Olympic Games in Los Angeles included as demonstration events the men's 1500-m and the women's 800-m wheelchair races. Wheelchair racing continued to be an exhibition event at every Olympiad since 1988. Athletes and organizers continue to work for further integration of wheelchair sports into the Olympic movement. Each year the International Paralympic Committee (IPC) works with the International Olympic Committee to improve access to elite sport venues and to work for greater recognition of people with disabilities who are elite athletes. Sports for individuals with disabilities, with few exceptions, are technical sports. As equipment improves and as coaches and athletes learn how to improve the fit between the athlete and equipment, performances improve. An interesting phenomenon is that as sports mature and equipment becomes widely available, performances become more dependent on the athlete and records fall with decreasing frequency.

ORGANIZATIONAL STRUCTURE OF SPORTS FOR PEOPLE WITH DISABILITIES

In the United States there are numerous sporting organizations for people with disabilities, five of which participate in the Paralympics. Figure 21.2 lists these organizations, with the exception of the Special Olympics. Special Olympic athletes participate in a

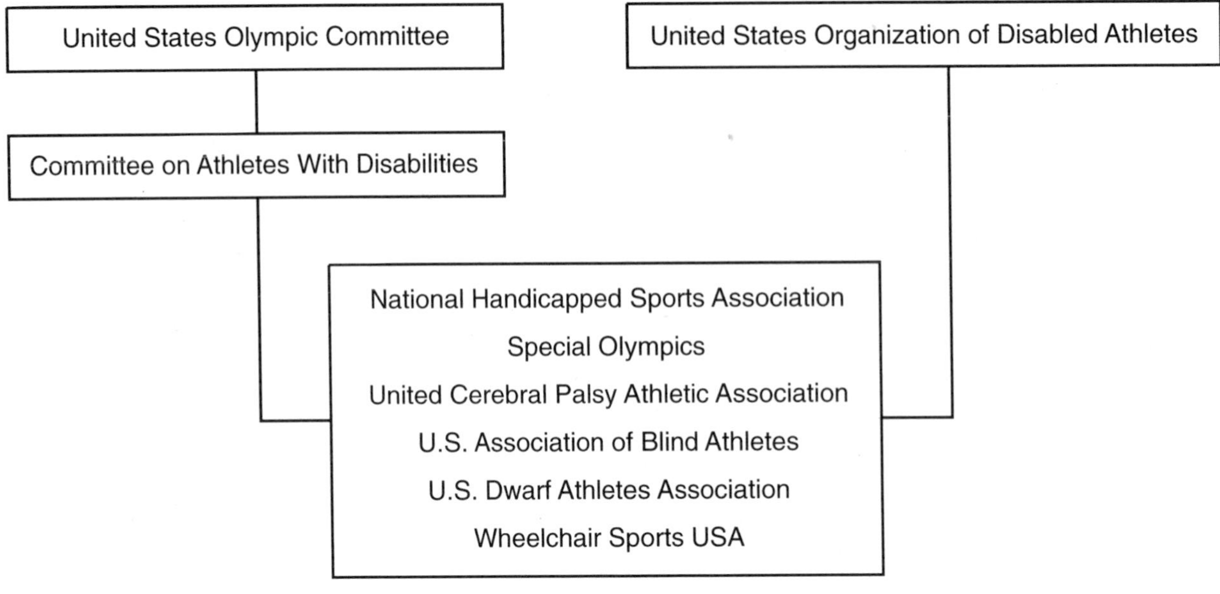

Figure 21.2 Structure of Paralympic sports within the United States.

separate international competition organized by Special Olympics International. The Paralympics and Special Olympics grew out of two separate sport movements for people with disabilities. Special Olympics is focused on athletes with cognitive impairments, although participants may have multiple disabilities. The five U.S. Paralympic sport organizations are loosely linked through the United States Organization of Disabled Athletes (USODA). Formed after U.S. athletes and organizers experienced severe difficulties in raising funds for the 1984 Paralympic Games, USODA aims primarily to raise funds—it exercises no administrative power over the member organizations. The strength of USODA lies in its abilities to represent a large number of athletes and to speak with a unified voice.

The six organizations of athletes with disabilities presented in figure 21.2 also receive support from the United States Olympic Committee (USOC), via the Committee on Athletes With Disabilities (CAD) and through grant programs. The CAD distributes funds based on number of members, participation in international events, and number of elite athletes. These funds can be used for core support of organizations. Grants are also available from the USOC to support training camps, employ athletes, and support teams at Paralympic Games. Each of the sport organizations whose athletes participate in the Paralympics chooses its own teams and works directly with the international governing bodies.

Figure 21.3 illustrates the international structure of sport for athletes with disabilities. The IOC selects the sites of Olympic Games. Since Paralympic Games coordinate with the Olympic Games, the IOC and International Paralympic Committee (IPC) work together for the benefit of both. The IPC selects the sites for the Paralympics, determines the number of athletes, and approves the local organizing committee. The international governing bodies (IGBs) implement the decisions of the IPC, determining how many athletes from each organization and from each sport will compete. The IGBs also set the performance standards that athletes must meet in order to be eligible to compete. The IGBs also organize and sanction international events. The IGBs must work closely with the national governing bodies (NGBs) of each member country. The NGBs choose their team members, organize teams, and participate in the governance of the IGBs.

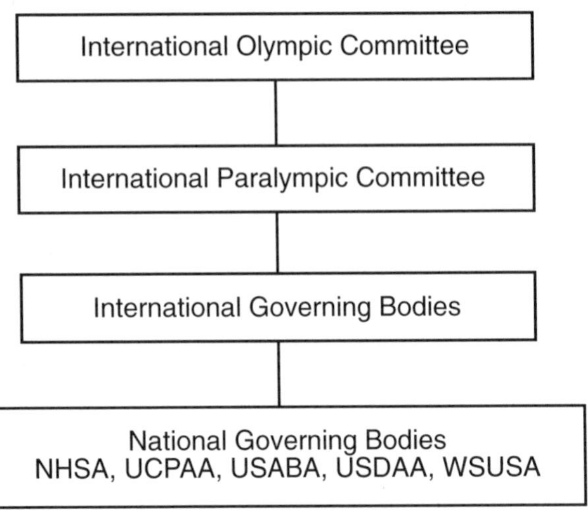

Figure 21.3 Structure of International Paralympic sports.

SPORTS EQUIPMENT TECHNOLOGY AND USE

A growing number of people participate in some form of wheelchair exercise or sport, including swimming, track and field events, basketball, rugby, and more. Along with expansion of the types of sports and exercise engaged in by individuals with a disability, there is a growth in assistive technology that helps these individuals participate safely in sports and exercise. There are so many different sports that people compete in at an elite level that an entire book could be dedicated to the topic. Therefore, we have chosen to focus on a few of the most popular and established sports. We have specifically focused on aerobic sports competed in the Summer Paralympics. There are of course, a large number of sports competed in the Winter Paralympics as well.

RACING WHEELCHAIR TECHNOLOGY

The rules of wheelchair racing allow a wide variety of designs, the major concerns being safety, equity, and speed; however, most racing wheelchairs have some common characteristics.

BASIC CONSTRUCTION

Racing wheelchairs are propelled by arm power only, and steered by the hands and/or arms. The frames are stiff and lightweight, typical frames weighing less than five pounds excluding the wheels. Athletes sit near rear axle height. Four-wheeled chairs commonly employ a rectangular main frame with a cross-member immediately fore and aft of the seat. Three-wheeled chairs are similar, but with a triangular main frame (as viewed from above). The rear wheels attach rigidly to the frame by a threaded insert welded either through the side frame tubes or into a cross-member. The rear wheel inserts are aligned with 2-15 degrees of wheel camber, and no toe in/out (misalignment of the rear wheels), making the chair more stable and allowing the athlete to reach the bottom of the pushrims without hitting the top of the wheels or pushrim. Toe in/out causes problems for wheelchair racers: it can cause a significant increase in rolling resistance if not aligned properly, and may change with use (some manufacturers incorporate an alignment mechanism into the frame). Pushrims on racing chairs are smaller than those used on standard chairs, and they may be coated—usually with a tire or high-density foam—to achieve higher friction with the athlete's gloves. In addition, many wheelchair racers, particularly those competing at an elite level have made a shift from using traditional spoke wheels to using carbon fiber disc wheels. Disc wheels tend to be light, rigid and have low inertia in rotation.

Some elite racers use racing wheelchairs that incorporate seat and leg supports as an integral unit. Since they are more accustomed to racing wheelchairs, elite athletes usually prefer tighter fitting seat cages than do novice athletes. Seat and leg supports should hold the athletes solidly, so they can focus their energy on propelling the wheelchair rather than maintaining balance. Seat cages also offer greater chair control than conventional seats and provide some protection in the event of an upset. Seat cages have side panels to provide support and to prevent the athlete's arms from rubbing against the wheels. Well-designed side panels follow the curvature of the wheel and allow the athlete a large range of motion fore and aft. Most seat upholstery is made of nylon or cotton canvas slung from the seat cage. Some racing chairs use plastic or fiberglass seats. Athletes typically use low-profile foam or air-floatation cushions.

The frame and seat cage are made to fit each individual, and for different disability etiologies and levels. Both experience and disability etiology determine the location of rear axles with respect to the seat cage. While experienced athletes with paraplegia prefer 15-25 cm from the seat back to the rear axles inserts, those with tetraplegia prefer 5-20 cm. Novice athletes generally choose more stable configurations. The seat cage upholstery adjustment and rear axle positions must be such that athletes can position their shoulders over the front edge of the pushrims and be able to reach the bottom of the pushrims with both arms.

PERFORMANCE AND SAFETY FEATURES

Many racing wheelchairs have features that contribute to performance or safety—for example, computers that aid in pacing and training; water bottles for fluid replacement; and caliper brakes (to help control the tremendous speeds attainable on some downhill sections). Brakes make training safer, and many races require their use. It is important that athletes be able to reach brakes from a comfortable position; and the brake levers must be long enough and at the proper angle so that the athlete can apply sufficient leverage to stop the racing chair. This is a critical issue for people with tetraplegia. Helmets have improved the safety of wheelchair racing, and most road and track races require them. Athletes should purchase helmets when they purchase their racing wheelchairs. Helmets should meet national safety standards, provide good airflow over the head (which is a primary area for cooling the body), and fit snugly. Many helmets are adjustable. Aerodynamic helmets can enhance speed compared with that of someone wearing no helmet.

CUSTOMIZING THE RACING WHEELCHAIR

It is important that a racing chair fit the user properly. The match between the user and equipment is among the most difficult to achieve of all sports for individuals with disabilities. Racing chairs are similar to shoes, in that a poorly fitted chair can be uncomfortable and awkward (Cooper 1989a, 1989b, 1989c, 1992a, 1992b; Cooper et al. 1992). They should fit as closely as possible without causing discomfort or pressure sores. Most manufacturers ask for a number of anatomical measurements when a chair is ordered (Cooper 1990): most commonly hip width, chest width, thigh length, arm length, trunk length, height, and weight. It is important for the manufacturer to know of the athlete's special needs, such as asymmetry or limited range of motion. Knowing a rider's disability etiology and racing ability will help a manufacturer properly fit a racing chair to its rider for maximum performance with least risk of injury.

Because racing wheelchairs are very user-specific, and athletes vary greatly in their abilities, it is impossible to design a chair that is effective for every athlete. Racing wheelchairs often are handcrafted for individuals based on their specific needs. Getting into a racing wheelchair should be like slipping on a glove. Many new athletes make the mistake of getting a loose-fitting wheelchair. Top athletes can fit into their racers only when wearing racing/training tights. To push properly, athletes must sit properly. If they are flexible enough and feel comfortable leaning on their knees, they generally find kneeling to be the fastest position. If kneeling remains uncomfortable after a trial period, or if the athlete has very good trunk control, then a more upright posture is best. When seated in the chair and kneeling, or lying upon their knees, athletes should be able to touch the ground with both hands, and be able to reach all the way around both pushrims. The center of each shoulder should line up with the front of each pushrim in the fully down position. The athletes should move their arms, simulating stroking, and test how difficult it is to breathe. They will need to synchronize breathing with stroking; but if it seems difficult to breathe, they should raise their knees.

Athletes with paraplegia, tetraplegia, or amputated limbs have different preferences, and each person has unique abilities and anatomical structure. There are three basic seats to consider: kneeling bucket, kneeling cage, and upright cage. The kneeling position is very aerodynamic and has allowed paraplegic and quadriplegic athletes to make tremendous improvements in their performance. The kneeling bucket helps decrease the racing wheelchair weight. Athletes inexperienced with the kneeling position should use a kneeling cage, which affords them the option of sitting upright or kneeling and permits some adjustment of body position. Upright cage seats work well for athletes with lower limb amputations, and for athletes with low levels of paraplegia (i.e., those who have the trunk control to adjust their body position while racing). Athletes with contractures should order a cage seat, unless they have substantial experience. Athletes are held in their racing chairs with straps and webbing. Additional padding or extra width can be requested to reduce the risk of developing pressure sores for people who are prone to skin breakdown. Although many competitors do not use a seat cushion in their racing chairs, the danger of skin breakdown makes use of a cushion advisable.

RACING IN A WHEELCHAIR

The wheelchair racing stroke has two primary phases: propulsion and recovery. **Propulsion** is when the arms are applying force, and **recovery** is when they are off the pushrims getting ready for the next stroke. Wheelchair racing is a particularly challenging sport. It readily takes a year or more to develop proficiency in wheelchair racing techniques before even a talented athlete can be minimally competitive. In order to effectively push a racing wheelchair, the upper body must rapidly apply a large force to the pushrims. Although athletes theoretically can achieve the greatest velocity by applying a large force over a long time period, it is difficult for them to effectively apply a large force during the entire propulsion phase. Ordinarily, athletes would tend to use the triceps and biceps muscles; by consciously learning and training to use the deltoids and pectoralis muscles, they can develop greater force over the propulsion cycle by using more of the upper body. The resulting larger force value and longer time of application create greater momentum. The price for this higher mechanical energy, however, is a higher consumption of metabolic energy.

Figure 21.4 illustrates the five phases of a racing wheelchair stroke:

1. Pushrim contact (a)
2. Pushing through to the bottom of the pushrims (b)-(d)
3. Push-off or follow-through (e)
4. Elbow drive to the top (f)-(h)
5. Drive forward and downward (i)-(j)

During the entire stroke the head should remain in line with the trunk, with head movement kept to a minimum. Elbow height before the drive forward and downward is critical to generating propulsion force. Maximal elbow height requires strength and flexibility. Optimal force transfer from the body to the pushrim requires properly fitted and designed gloves and a nonslip pushrim coating. The hand should be in line with the forearm at contact (i.e., wrist in the neutral position) to transfer maximum energy. The athlete must push continuously from contact through to the bottom of the pushrims. If the propulsion phase is done properly, the hand will push

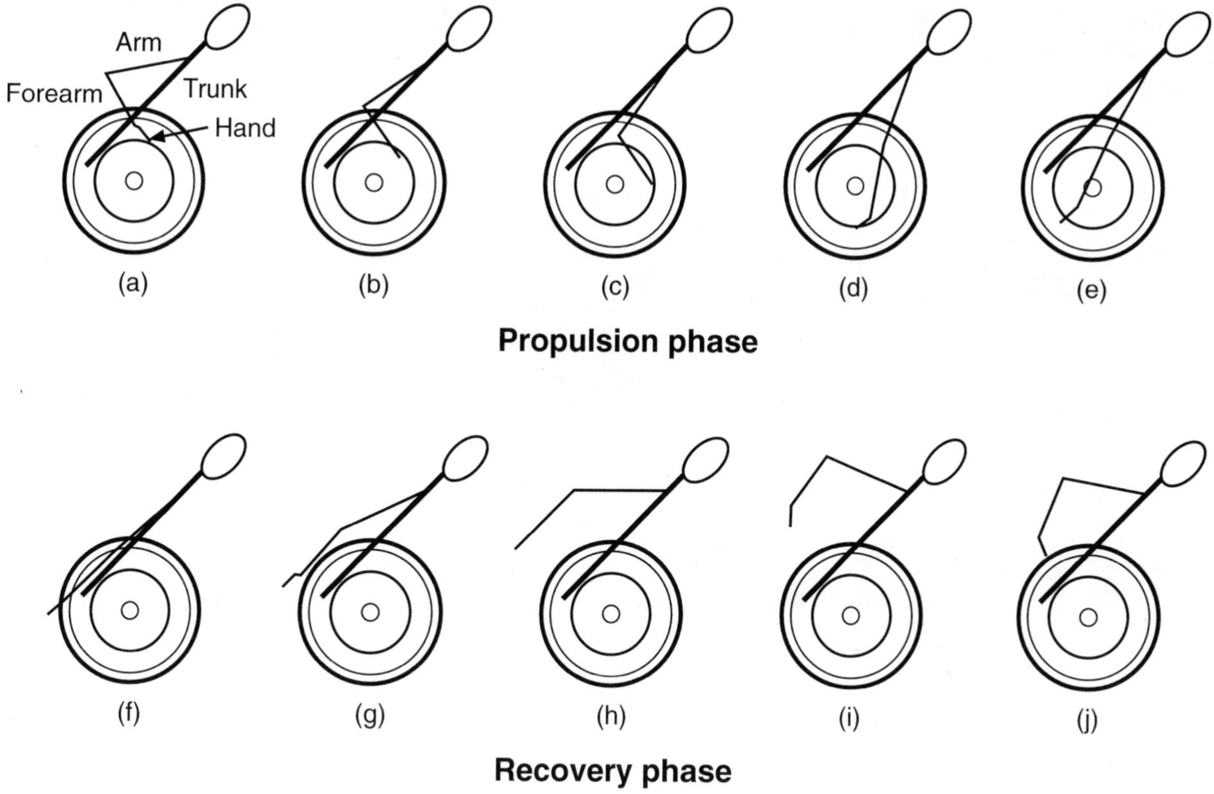

Figure 21.4 Schematic illustrating the phases of an efficient racing wheelchair stroke.

off the pushrim with a flick. The momentum of the arms is used to carry the elbows upward. When the elbows are at their peaks, the athlete should contract chest, shoulder, and arm muscles to punch the pushrims.

BICYCLES AND TRICYCLES

Hand cycles are the bicycle of people with mobility impairments (figure 21.5). Handcycling is the most rapidly growing sport for people with disabilities worldwide. This is likely due to the ability of the technology to accommodate a much wider variety of impairments and body types than most wheelchair-dependent sports. Handcycling can also be practiced as an integrated sport. For example, handcyclists can train alongside friends on bicycles. Furthermore, handcycling is easy to learn while remaining challenging to master. The large and growing popularity of this sport has raised competition to the ranks of the Paralympics. The enormous popularity has reduced the number of participants in other sports, and has drawn elite competitors from wheelchair racing over to handcycling.

People with mobility impairments want alternatives for recreational activities. Some people are interested in physically demanding sports such as marathons or triathlons. Others enjoy touring and prefer the increased efficiency of levers and gears (Cooper 1989d; Janssen et al. 2001). Alternatives to wheelchair locomotion have been in development for a number of years (Engel and Seeliger 1986), but the commercial availability of arm-crank recreational equipment was delayed because

- people with mobility impairments lacked awareness of the equipment,
- insurance carriers have not been willing to purchase such devices,
- low-volume production of adaptive recreation equipment carried high liability risks for manufacturers (since appropriate liability insurance was very expensive), and
- building arm-powered vehicles at home was very complex.

Currently there are only a few restrictions on arm-powered vehicles for use in competitions: they can use no motors or external energy sources and may have no structures that serve the sole purpose of reducing air/wind resistance.

The present generation of hand cycles use from 18 to 27 gears. Whether going downhill or uphill, the rider searches for the gear ratio that best permits low effort and high pedal turnover with cadences between 80 and 100 revolutions per minute to minimize both energy consumption and the risk of musculoskeletal injury. Before riding independently, people must consider

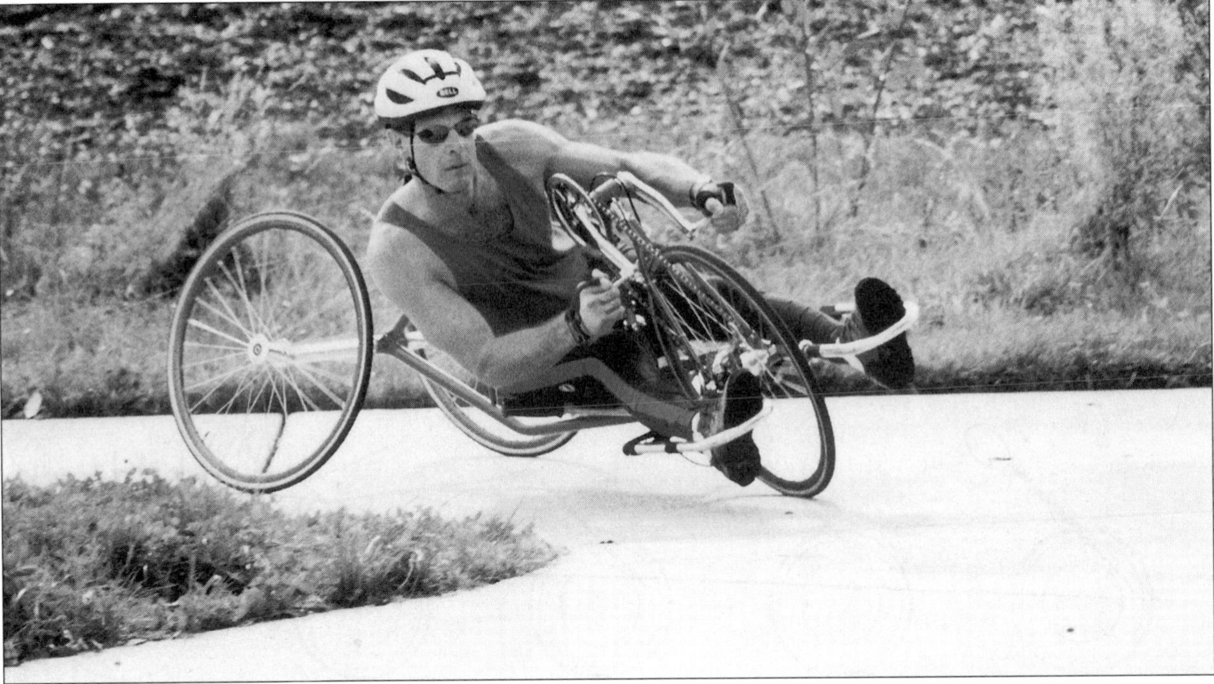

Figure 21.5 Handcycling can be a fun and exciting sport.
Photo courtesy of Freedom Ryder.

several questions:

- Where will I do most of my riding (beach, neighborhood, country, city)?
- What kind of riding will I do (recreational, racing, touring)?
- Is the hand cycle appropriate to my abilities (disability etiology, physical function)?
- When the pedal(s) are fully extended (hands on the pedals, back against the backrest), are my elbows slightly bent?

Basic Construction

Arm-powered vehicles should efficiently convert the user's energy into motion while permitting good control over the vehicle on normal surface streets. Ideally, arm-powered vehicles use as many standard bicycle components as possible and fit into a van without requiring disassembly. The vehicle frames are typically steel alloy (SAE 4130) or aluminum (SAE 6061) tubing, with milled ends for best fit and stronger joints. Frames may be either brass-welded (simple and inexpensive) or tungsten inert gas-welded.

Balance Factors

A limitation of most arm-powered bicycles is the balance of the pilot. Accustomed to the support and positioning provided by an everyday wheelchair, a bicycle, by virtue of its design, poses a distinct contrast in the sitting position, balance, and steering. The kinesthetic and neuromuscular control techniques an individual with paraplegia has learned through years of manual wheelchair use do not directly translate to the bicycle. The position of the trunk and lower limbs often increases the difficulty of balancing a bicycle. A bucket seat as used on a racing wheelchair is effective in ameliorating these challenges for some people. In order to assure that the cranks clear the lower legs, some positions require placing the crank center farther away from the rider than is otherwise desirable. The result is a suboptimal center position and more difficulty steering at the front end of the crank cycle. Some bicycles position the rider low enough to the ground that riders may place their hands on the ground when starting or stopping. Some people prefer fully retractable side wheels. Riders power the bicycles through a combination of leaning and turning the crank about the steering axis. Side wheels may limit the rider's ability to lean the bicycle; when used, however, they must not interfere with normal lean steering. Since the height of the center of gravity, the user's balance, and the vehicle's steering geometry all interact, anyone designing an arm-powered vehicle must consider all these factors in order to make the device safe and efficient.

Most handcycles use three wheels to provide a stable base for the rider. Typically, the front wheel is driven through a series of gears, cranks, and a chain. Three-wheeled handcycles are readily available commercially and dominate competitions. The ability to focus on propulsion provides a significant advantage of three-wheel designs over two wheels. Also, three-wheel designs can accommodate a wide variety of body types and impairment levels. Three-wheeled racing handcycles typically place the rider in a posterior recumbent position. This helps to reduce wind resistance (i.e., reduces the frontal area) and allows the user to pull as well as push on the cranks (significant advantage when using a symmetrical crank setup).

STEERING

Since the steering and drive train are interconnected in many arm-powered vehicles, a primary design consideration is how the rider will both power the vehicle and maintain directional control. Arm-powered bicycles and tricycles generally use direct arm steering because they require fine steering control to maintain balance. Some designers of arm-powered tricycles, however, have had moderate success in decoupling steering from the drive train by using the tilt (from side to side like a skateboard) of the seat for steering. These vehicles have a large turning radius for their size.

CRANK-ARM POSITIONING, GEARS, AND BRAKES

Crank arms may be adjacent (symmetrical) or opposed. Asymmetrical cranks whose lever arms are situated 180 degrees apart provide greater mechanical efficiency. But because they create a moment about the head-set (the bearing housing that permits crank rotation), causing the front wheel(s) to turn from side to side as the rider cranks, the rider must waste energy in order to dampen the moment. A friction (nylon bushings in the head-set) or a viscous dampener can minimize the undesired turning moment. Most hand-cycles are tricycles, and the athletes use symmetrical crank positions. This allows the athlete to push and pull symmetrically applying more power as s/he does not need to exert as much effort trying to control direction. Bicycles and tricycles require different steering techniques: one initiates a turn on a bicycle by leaning with the front wheel turned opposite to the desired direction; the front wheels of tricycles go in the direction of the turn, and the rider does not lean.

Arm-powered vehicles must have a wide range of gear ratios, since the power output of the arms can be quite limited and fine increments are required to achieve optimal pedaling rates. Shift levers should be of the indexing type and should be easily reachable. Chain guards are necessary to help keep fingers out of the sprockets and to protect the rider in the event of an accident. Index shifting works best and is used by nearly all elite handcycle racers. Index shifting allows the racers to change gears accurately without looking. Twist shifters mounted on the handles of the crank are probably the most popular and efficient form of shifting. They allow the user to shift gears while both hands remain on the handles. The ability to crank with both hands and shift can have a significant competitive advantage and is especially important for hill climbing.

Standard bicycle brakes are acceptable, but with levers positioned so they can be grasped with one hand or both hands. Some brakes are mounted to the frame in order to avoid having the cables become entangled in the drive train, for these systems the rider steers with one hand and brakes with the other. More frequently, the brake levers are mounted to the crank handles allowing braking with both hands without removing the hands from the cranks. Some arm-powered vehicles use a cam-activated brake, which is engaged by reversing the crank direction. This simplifies braking but prohibits back pedaling for balance at low speeds and when attempting to maximize leverage on inclines. Recently, hydraulic disk brakes have become more popular because they offer consistent controlled braking.

A variety of handles are available to match a user's grip strength, hand size, and personal preference. It is best to try a variety of handles and to find a pair that is comfortable. Bicycle gloves can also help to increase the comfort of the handles, and the padded palms can help to reduce some of the road vibration on the hands transmitted through the frame.

ALTERNATIVE ARM-POWERED VEHICLES

Arm-powered vehicles do not exclude wheelchairs: **add-on units** can convert a wheelchair into an arm-crank vehicle. These devices are useful for introducing people to the sport of hand cycling because a unit owned by a club or clinic can be used on multiple wheelchairs, eliminating the need to customize the device. Once a person demonstrates interest and/or talent, they can transition to a recumbent-style hand cycle for racing. Some of these devices incorporate quick-release mechanisms that attach a self-contained front wheel-gear-crank system. Other devices which may also be quick-release attach cranks to each of the rear drive wheels. The clear advantage of quick-release units is that users can easily remove them in order to use their wheelchairs in the usual fashion. Add-on units are often easier to transport in an automobile. Although add-on units usually trade performance for convenience, they are relatively inexpensive and quite functional for recreational riders.

Tandems permit an ambulatory rider to use a leg crank while the other rider uses an arm crank. Tandems may be two- or three-wheeled, with the ambulatory rider sitting either in front or in back. When in the rear, ambulatory riders can sit higher and see over the other rider, providing both a clear view. With the ambulatory rider sitting forward, the wheelchair rider can use a carriage that permits cranking from the wheelchair. The ambulatory rider often does the steering and the shifting, in order to decouple cranking and gear changing from steering. Drive trains of tandems are most efficient when each rider can pedal at his/her own pace and coast independently.

Equipment for Field Events

The field events in which people in wheelchairs most often participate are the club, shot put, discus, and javelin. Only the most severely involved people (e.g., those with C4-C5 tetraplegia) compete in the club, in which individuals place the grip of the club (shaped like a bowling pin) between their fingers and then throw it.

Field event wheelchairs are not required to have wheels. Prior to the 1989 international athletics season, however, wheels were required. At that time most field athletes used old depot-type chairs that were as heavy as possible, since the weight made them stiffer and less likely to move while the athlete threw an implement (e.g., shot, discus, javelin). The rules describing the throwing chair were changed in order to modernize and revitalize the sport, leading to some interesting new features.

Field event chairs provide a rigid base of support. The chair is strapped to the ground within a 1.5-m throwing circle. Straps secure the chair to steel stakes that have been pounded into the ground. Although the thrower generally has the option of having the stakes moved, in many competitions the stakes are in a fixed location to expedite setup. Throwing chairs include a means of leveling the seat, to help the thrower obtain the proper angle at release (40-50 degrees from horizontal). The seat of a throwing wheelchair usually has less than 1 cm of padding, because throwers desire maximum sitting height and the cushion is counted in the seat height. As throwers are not in the chair for very long, risk of pressure sores is minimal (but throwers should be cautious during extended training sessions). Figure

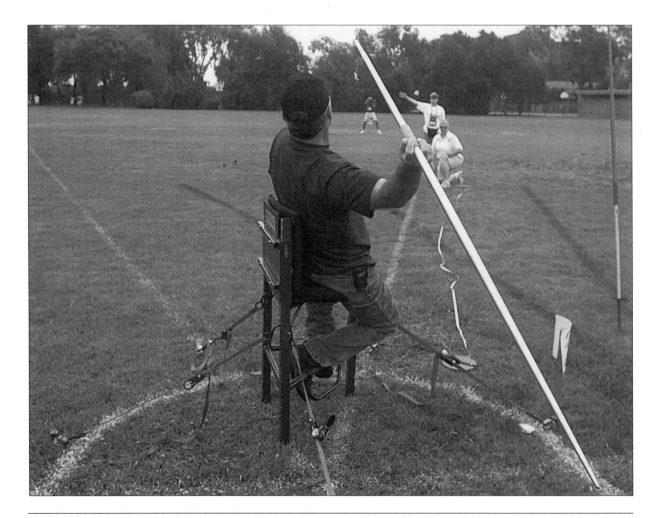

Figure 21.6 An athlete using a new style throwing chair during javelin competition.

21.6 illustrates one type of throwing chair used for the javelin competition.

A large footplate supports the feet, permitting them to move as the thrower changes body positions. Some throwers use the frame and straps of the throwing chair to restrict foot movement. In order for a throw to be legal, no part of the body may extend outside the throwing area until the judge signals. Rails guide the motion of the upper body through the throwing sequence, their shape customized to the size and abilities of the user. Those with lower impairments and high skills use the least restrictive rails to guide the trunk, whereas the rails are more restrictive (providing greater support) for people who are more severely impaired or less skilled. The rails are padded to protect the thrower's body from the impact received while moving through the throwing motion.

Since during major competitions the thrower and coach must move the chair into the throwing circle and secure it within a three- to five-minute period, most athletes add quick release wheels to the throwing frame for transport. This requirement has also led to simple attachment points and leveling mechanisms.

EQUIPMENT FOR COURT SPORTS

Court sports wheelchairs are similar to ultralight wheelchairs designed for daily use, but with distinguishing features that make them more effective for use in specific sports (Coutts 1991; Golbranson and Wirta 1982). Court sports wheelchairs often display extreme camber in their rear wheels and small roller blade-type front casters. They use rigid frames. Many current features of lightweight wheelchairs were originally developed for wheelchair basketball and wheelchair racing. Figure 21.7 shows a version of the court chair that is used for floor hockey.

BASKETBALL

Basketball wheelchairs must be lightweight so that players can accelerate and brake rapidly. Although basketball is not a contact sport, some incidental contact is inevitable. For this reason, spoke guards cover the rear wheel spokes. Exposed spokes can be broken during a game; sometimes, in fact, opponents may (illegally) try to disrupt play by ramming exposed spokes with parts of their chairs. Made of high-impact plastic, spoke guards provide several added benefits: they make it easier for players to pick up the ball from the floor by pushing it against the spoke guard and rolling it onto their lap; they protect hands and fingers when players are struggling for the ball; and they provide a convenient space to identify team affiliations.

Basketball wheelchairs are required to have forward anti-tip rollers or forward skids (commonly mounted to the footrests), both of which reduce the risk of forward falls and minimize damage to the basketball court.

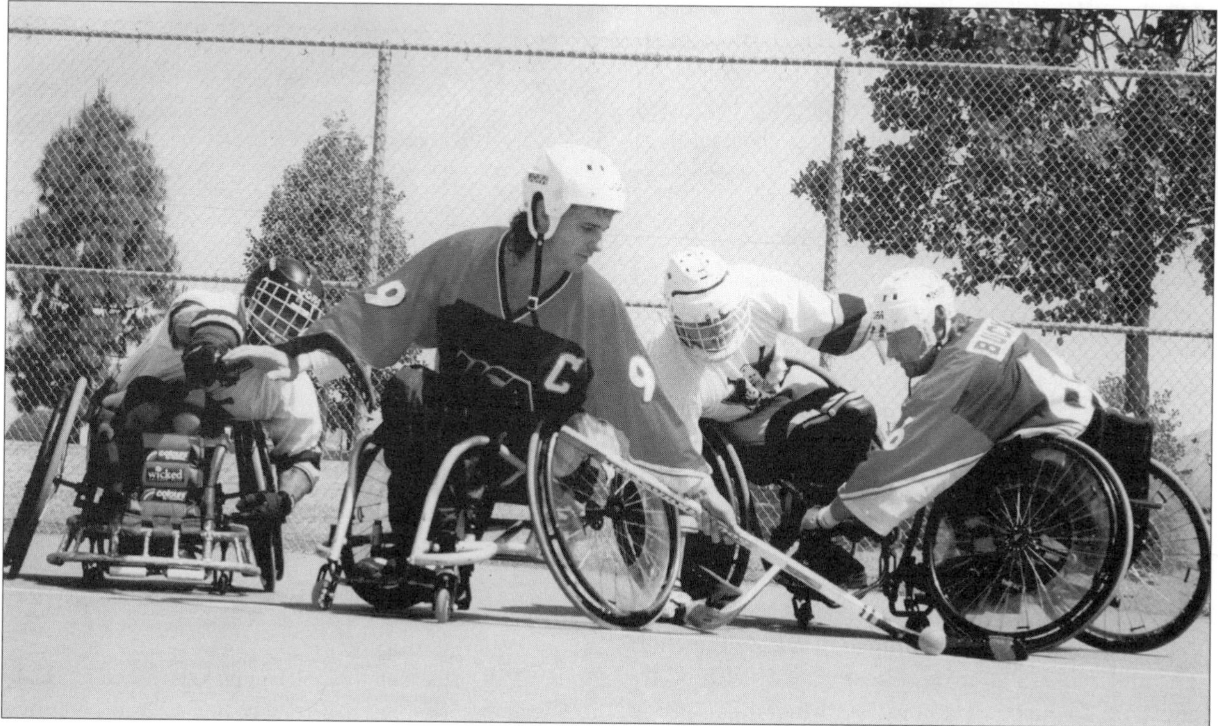

Figure 21.7 Athletes using court wheelchairs to play floor hockey on an outdoor court.
Courtesy of Sports 'N Spokes/Paralyzed Veterans of America.

Some players use rear anti-tip casters, which help keep the wheelchair from falling over backward (especially important for people with higher levels of impairment), but which can make it more difficult to accelerate the wheelchair by having the anti-tip wheels contacting the ground as a player pushes. Basketball wheelchairs have four wheels: two large wheels in the rear, used to push the chair, and two casters in the front for steering. The front casters are nearly always polyurethane with precision roller bearings, 5 cm (2 in.) in diameter. The rear wheels are commonly 61 cm (24 in.) or 66 cm (26 in.) in diameter and typically use high-pressure tires with no or very low-profile tread. High-pressure (120 to 200 psi) tires make it easier to push the wheelchair, and help to make it faster on the court.

Camber is an important feature of basketball wheelchairs, as it makes them more responsive during turns. Camber also protects players' hands when two wheelchairs collide from the sides, by limiting the collision to the bottom of the wheels and leaving a gap at the top to protect the hands.

Basketball wheelchairs seats typically slope backward about 5-15 degrees. Since the rules of basketball limit the maximum height of any portion of the seat, athletes usually try to make their seats as high as possible. Guards are an exception, as lower seat heights and greater seat angles can make chairs faster and more maneuverable for ball handling. Basketball wheelchairs often include loops for strapping the player into the chair. Strapping (the use of nylon or elastic straps) can be used to position a player in his wheelchair to improve performance. In fact, positioning has been used so effectively by some players that it has changed their functional classification.

Tennis

Tennis is a very fast sport despite the two-bounce rule applied for wheelchair players. The wheelchair player must be able to cover the entire court. Many players focus on the baseline and move forward as necessary to make a shot. Winning play requires quickness, speed, maneuverability, and agility. For these reasons, tennis wheelchairs have evolved to include several specialized features: they use three wheels, the rear wheels typically being 61 cm (24 in.) or 66 cm (26 in.) in diameter; they use high-pressure tires (120-200 psi) to lower rolling resistance on the court and to increase speed; a single front caster, 5 cm (2 in.) in diameter, makes the chair light and more maneuverable; the rear wheels are cambered to increase lateral stability during side shots and to make the chair turn faster (figure 21.8). Neither front nor rear anti-tip casters are common on tennis wheelchairs.

Tennis players introduced the concept of radical seat angle: a steep seat angle, or dump helps keep players against the seat backs, giving them greater control over the wheelchair and providing greater balance. The knees are flexed, with the feet on the footrest behind the player's knees. With the body in a relatively compact position, the combined inertia of rider and wheelchair is reduced (similar to figure skaters bringing their arms in to spin faster), making the chair more maneuverable. Tennis wheelchairs commonly use a rigid footrest so that the feet remain in place and do not touch the ground. Most players strap their feet to the footrests. Handles incorporated into the front of the seat help the player balance while leaning forward or to the side to hit the ball; the handles also help keep the knees in place.

Wheelchair Rugby

Wheelchair rugby was developed by people with tetraplegia who can propel a manual wheelchair but who are not competitive at basketball. Because the rules

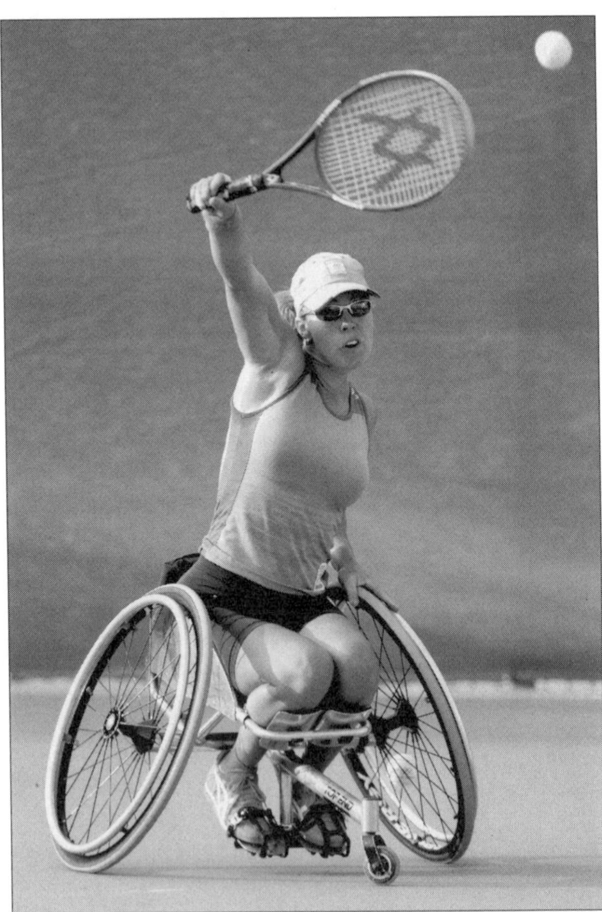

Figure 21.8 The tennis wheelchair includes several specialized features. Here, the Netherlands' Sonja Peters competes in a women's singles quarterfinals match at the 2004 Paralympics in Athens, Greece.

Mark Cowan/Icon SMI.

of wheelchair basketball favor people who are not as severely involved (many of the top players do not even use a wheelchair as their primary source of mobility), people with low-level tetraplegia effectively had no team sporting opportunities prior to wheelchair rugby. Wheelchair rugby is a combination of team handball and rugby. Contact is permitted, and teams must carry the ball across their goal line to score. The ball may be passed or carried. In terms of player qualification, most of the players have sustained cervical level spinal injuries and have some type of tetraplegia as a result. Players are given a classification number from one of seven classifications ranging from 0.5 to 3.5. The 0.5 player has the greatest impairment and is comparable to a C5 quadriplegic. Of those eligible to participate, the 3.5 player has the least impairment and is similar to a C7-8 incomplete quadriplegic. Both males and females are encouraged to play, and because of the classification process gender advantages don't exist.

There is tremendous interest in wheelchair rugby, whose rapid growth has led to the development of specialized four-wheeled chairs. The rear wheels are typically 61 cm (24 in.) in diameter, and the front casters 5 cm (2 in.) in diameter with precision roller bearings. The rear wheels are radically cambered to around 15 degrees, and protective framing is used around the wheels and the base of the chair (figure 21.9). This helps to protect the players from side impacts and glancing blows, and makes the chair turn faster. Guards wrap around the bottom front of the chair, from one rear wheel to another, and protect feet and legs against injury from other players' front casters. The guards also make it more difficult to hook the wheelchair—if a chair can be hooked, the player can be stopped and the opposing team gains an advantage.

In common with tennis wheelchairs, wheelchair rugby wheelchairs use a radical seat angle—up to 20 degrees—that helps players maintain balance and maneuver more effectively. A highly stable seating position, with knees flexed and the feet behind the knees, provides the user good control over the chair. Because the rules for wheelchair rugby restrict team members to wheelchair users who are more physically impaired, they require front and rear anti-tip casters that not only provide some protection from forward and rearward falls but also help protect the court during impacts. Wheelchair rugby chairs are a hybrid of basketball and tennis wheelchairs; however, elite athletes are more frequently using titanium frames for their light weight and increased strength.

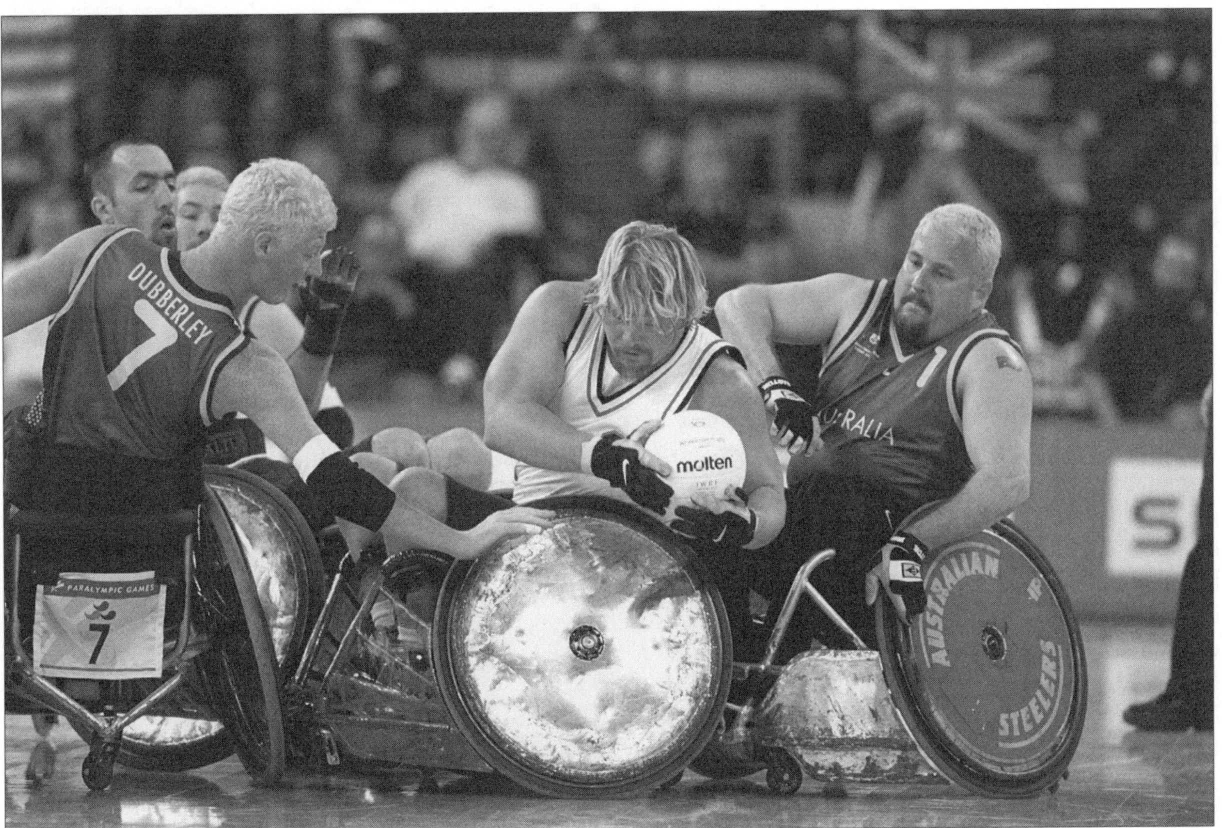

Figure 21.9 Note the protective framing around the wheels and base of the rugby chair.

Prostheses

The major concern of people who undergo a lower limb amputation is whether they will be able to regain their previous level of physical activity (Czerniecki et al. 1991; Flowers et al. 1990; Gage and Ounpuu 1989; Gottschalk et al. 1985; James 1991). Prosthetic technology allows many individuals to achieve functional recovery nearly equal to preamputation potential (Krouskop et al. 1985; Krouskop et al. 1987; McDonnell et al. 1989; Michael 1989). People with amputations not only can participate in life's activities, but in many cases can participate with nondisabled people. Legro et al. (2001) surveyed 92 persons with lower limb amputations, who regularly used prostheses, to determine their preferred recreational and sport activities. Up to 88% of the respondents indicated that they could perform the sports and recreational activities that were of high importance to them. Activities that require a high energy level were often more problematic to perform. The respondents reported participating in a very wide variety of sports and recreational activities.

Foot Amputation Prostheses

Custom padding or inserts within conventional shoes often can treat partial foot amputation. Flexible shanks may prevent shoes from bending sharply at the end of the foot (Schneider et al. 1993; Suzuki 1972). Plastic laminate prostheses can provide functional ambulation for people with Syme amputations. With the aid of energy-storing feet—possibly the greatest advance in prosthetic design—people with lower limb amputation are able to move quickly and to run with a foot-over-foot gait (Wirta et al. 1991). These devices store energy via a flexible keel, which provides nonlinear spring action similar to the push-off phase of walking or running (Walker et al. 1985; Wirta et al. 1990).

The stationary attachment flexible endoskeletal (SAFE) foot is considered the first modern energy-storing prosthetic foot design (Wirta et al. 1991). Since the introduction of SAFE, a number of other energy-storing feet have become commercially available. Energy-storing feet may be customized for an individual or may be semi-customized. There are lightweight prosthetic feet with totally flexible keels to provide the appropriate dynamic elastic response for walking on uneven terrain. Lightweight graphite feet provide a strong push at toe-off for activities like running. Feet that provide a strong push-off are referred to as superdynamic elastic response prosthetic feet (Torburn et al. 1990). These devices must have proper alignment for the leg to roll smoothly from heel-strike to toe-off (Nissan 1991; Wirta et al. 1991). This type of foot requires time to adjust to the spring action. A multiaxis foot provides motion in dorsiflexion, inversion, and eversion as well as plantar flexion. These features help to accommodate uneven terrain by having the foot conform to the terrain (Pinzur et al. 1991). Multiaxis feet can also store energy.

Swimming With Amputations

For a person with an amputation, swimming can be an important form of exercise because it is not traumatic to the residual limb. Although most people can enjoy swimming without a prosthesis, some choose to swim with one because it provides balance in the water (figure 21.10). Both exoskeletal and endoskeletal prostheses can be used for swimming. Some prostheses are buoyant and may require the addition of weights. There are several types of swim legs: waterproofed walking prostheses, peg legs, stubbies, and hollow-chambered legs. Standard feet that are molded without an external heel cushion are less susceptible to becoming water-soaked. Any foot or standard prosthesis used in the water should be treated with a waterproof coating (e.g., New Skin, foot paint). Swimmers can add fins to stubbies or feet for added speed and control.

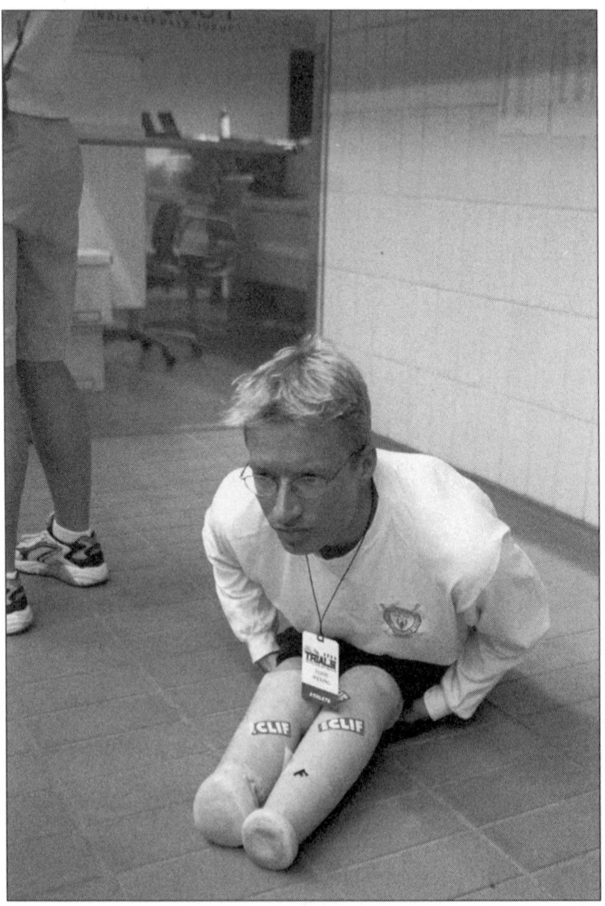

Figure 21.10 This athlete stretches in preparation for swimming with a custom molded prosthesis.

FACTORS TO CONSIDER IN CHOOSING LEG PROSTHESES

The conventional patellar tendon-bearing (PTB) socket is adequate for activities of daily living but not for active sports; it does not evenly distribute the impact impulse generated by active people. It is also uncomfortable to run with a prominent patellar bar. In contrast, a total surface-bearing socket provides for full contact and dampens impact loading. Side joints and a thigh lacer can also reduce the forces on the residual limb by transferring some weight to the thigh.

Latex rubber suspension sleeves provide suction cup-type suspension and help reduce pistoning for people with below-knee (BK) amputation. They may be used without additional support. A waist belt attached to a cuff suspension socket can provide additional suspension within the socket to prevent pistoning. Neoprene suspension sleeves can also provide atmospheric suspension. A silicone-suction socket (3S) can provide good suspension properties and a socket interface that reduces shear forces. A simple Muley strap just above the femoral condyles, connected to smaller flexible straps pointing downward and backward along the medial and lateral aspects and connected via a pivot to the shank, is effective for some people.

Computer-aided design and manufacturing (CAD-CAM) systems in prosthetics provide alternatives to traditional methods of producing positive molds used to make sockets. Several commercial CAD-CAM systems produce prosthetic sockets. Measurement intervals of 1.0 to 2.5 mm are satisfactory (Torres-Moreno et al. 1992).

Hydraulic knees allow stance and swing control, providing stability during single-limb support (Popovic et al. 1991). Hyperextension of the hydraulic knee allows it to lock; otherwise, the knee provides hydraulic resistance to flexion. Force above a threshold at the prosthesis forefoot can be used to unlock the knee. Many hydraulic knees incorporate a manual lock for activities requiring maximum stability (e.g., driving an automobile, standing on a bus, standing at a work cell), and a release that allows maximum flexibility. Hydraulic knees typically incorporate a piston in a cylinder perforated with roughened holes that allow fluid to flow from one side of the cylinder to the other as the piston moves. Distribution of the holes within the cylinder determines the amount of dampening. Fewer holes are placed near the ends of the cylinder to provide terminal deceleration. The distribution of holes is asymmetrical. A consequence of using hydraulic knees is that some of the body's energy is dissipated through the hydraulic piston and cylinder.

Many knees incorporate several degrees of freedom. Flexible, or bouncy, knees can reduce impact and provide knee stability. Friction and elastic components can be adjusted for an individual. However, fixed friction and elastic components of the knee are optimal only for the walking speed for which they are adjusted. Increases in gait speed may cause excessive heel rise and premature locking of the knee, while decreases in speed may result in toe stubbing due to inadequate knee flexion. Allowing friction adjustment by the user helps to alleviate these problems for some people. Computer-controlled knees have provided for the friction and dampening properties to vary during the gait cycle. Also, programs can be optimized for the activity. For example, one program can be used for daily activities and another for the sport of the individual's choosing. Computer-controlled knees provide more options for tuning, and have the potential for higher performance. The proper selection of the socket, knee, and foot can make possible such activities as heel-toe running for people with bilateral below-knee amputations.

Walking and running with a prosthetic limb varies substantially with surface inclination, side-slope, and roughness. Prosthetics designers must be familiar with all aspects of gait in people with lower limb amputations, as well as with the biomechanics of periodic events like stumbling, slipping, and falling. They must design prosthetics to minimize the occurrence and risk of injury associated with these events, while providing functional and efficient gait.

Biomechanical assessment techniques are not standard tools in most clinical settings. Most research has focused on level, steady-state walking; yet simple and easily measurable parameters related to various pathologies or misalignments are needed. People can achieve normal prosthetic gait kinetics and kinematics using a variety of active muscles and neuromuscular control schemes; therefore, level, steady-state gait analysis can miss many pathologies, prosthetic misalignments, or discomforts for which individuals compensate or which they hide.

CLASSIFICATION

Classification of disabled athletes helps level the playing field for competitors with different disabilities or different degrees of the same disability. Competitions for athletes without disabilities use classification schemes for the same purpose (e.g., male and female competitions in marathons, and the senior PGA tour). The idea is that individuals with similar physical attributes compete against each other, allowing in the end for greater overall competition. The task of classifying athletes with disabilities is very complex because of the diversity of the populations.

An ideal classification system would

- be inclusive, including as many types of disabilities as possible;
- be fair, with no individual having an edge based solely on classification;
- enhance competition;
- enable individuals with different disabilities to compete on the same field;
- be easy to understand and apply.

Clearly no system can meet all the above criteria. Because there is no perfect system, there is also no uniformly accepted system. Each group representing a certain disability tends to have its own classification scheme. One example is the classification used by the United States Cerebral Palsy Association (USCPA), listed in table 21.1. This classification system is used in all individual sports, including track and field, swimming, cycling, and cross-country, where athletes compete only against athletes with their same classification. In the remaining sports, athletes are grouped in divisions according to classification as described in the Web site www.uscpaa.org. Unfortunately, it is difficult to use this type of classification scheme to allow individuals with cerebral palsy to compete with other athletes with disabilities.

The Paralympics, the largest sports competition for individuals with a variety of disabilities, several different classification schemes have governed competition. In earlier years, classification was based solely on type of disability such as blindness, spinal cord injury, amputation, and other orthopedic conditions. As the competition evolved, increasingly complex classification schemes resulted in a greater number of events which, unfortunately, decreased competition by reducing the number of competitors (Paralympic Spirit 1996). To assure that competition remains intense, the Paralympics have strict performance standards that must be met in order to qualify.

The Paralympics have moved toward a functional classification system based on the athlete's ability to perform in a certain event. Wheelchair basketball, in which the wheelchair acts as an equalizer, is a leader in this movement: skills in the wheelchair determine competition level (Malone et al. 2002). Classifiers observe a player's functions during competitions and assign classifications based on their observations. Observed trunk movement and stability during actual basketball participation, rather than one's medical diagnosis or muscle function on an examining table, form the basis for a player's classification. Players are assigned a point value based on their classification. These points are summed during basketball play, with teams allowed only a predetermined maximum number of points on the floor.

Unfortunately, functional classification in basketball has made it harder for individuals with tetraplegia to compete. This situation led, in part, to the development of wheelchair rugby. Moreover, functional classification cannot work for all sports: in many sports, complex medical examinations are still needed to determine class. As in wheelchair basketball, many believe that the use of prosthetics or adaptive equipment may make it easier to combine individuals with different disabilities. The current classification scheme used by the International Paralympic Committee is too complex to detail in this text. The full scheme is on the Web at the official site of the International Paralympic Committee (www.paralympic.org) and is available from the IPC Headquarters:

International Paralympic Committee
Adenauerallee 212 53113
BONN Germany
Telephone: +49 228 209 7200
Fax: +49 228 209 7209

Despite controversy over classification systems, each Paralympic game has been more inclusive and more successful than its predecessor. In addition, the Paralympics includes exhibit events that are open and have no classification system. It is anticipated that classification systems will continue to evolve with time, leading to systems that most closely meet the ideal.

Exercise Science and the Athlete With Impairments

Because the number of individuals participating in wheelchair sports and exercise is increasing, the need for research in this area is also increasing. Individuals with disabilities may have unique physiological adaptations to exercising or participating in sports activities. We need to investigate these physiological differences in order to help these individuals participate and succeed in their exercise and sport endeavors. Good research should lead to decreased injuries and health problems that stem from exercise or sports participation. If individuals with a disability can improve their health and fitness levels through exercise, they may be able to decrease their health care costs.

Physiological Studies

The bulk of exercise physiology research since the late 1920s has focused on the unimpaired population. Research on special populations has developed at a much slower pace. Several recent investigators,

Table 21.1 Classifications Used by the USCPA

Class	Challenge
1	Severe involvement in all four limbs. Limited trunk control. Unable to grasp a softball. Poor functional strength in upper extremities, often necessitating the use of an electric wheelchair for independence.
2	Severe to moderate quadriplegic normally able to propel a wheelchair very slowly with arms or by pushing with feet. Poor functional strength and severe control problems in the upper extremities.
3	Moderate quadriplegic, fair functional strength and moderate control problems in upper extremities and torso. Uses wheelchair.
4	Lower limbs have moderate to severe involvement. Good functional strength and minimal control problems in upper extremities and torso. Uses wheelchair.
5	Good functional strength and minimal control problems in upper extremities. May walk with or without assistive devices for ambulatory support.
6	Moderate to severe hemiplegic. Ambulates without walking aids. Less coordination. Balance problems when running or throwing. Has greater upper extremity involvement.
7	Moderate to minimal hemiplegic. Good functional ability in nonaffected side. Walks/runs with noted limp.
8	Minimally affected. May have minimal coordination problems. Able to run and jump freely. Has good balance.

however, are doing significant work in exercise physiology research on physically impaired populations (Cooper et al. 2003, 1992, 1993; Glaser 1989; Glaser et al. 1980; Janssen et al. 1994; Langbein and Maki 1995; Rodgers et al. 1994). The early stages of research focused on developing specialized exercise testing and training techniques for people with disabilities. Janssen et al. (2001) examined physical capacity of male handcycle users and demonstrated that peak power output, maximal rate of oxygen consumption, and gross mechanical efficiency were associated with 10K race performance.

Several groups have studied the kinematics of racing wheelchair propulsion and its relationship to efficiency. Cooper and Bedi (1990) report that racing wheelchair propulsion has a gross mechanical efficiency over 30%, while Cooper et al. (1992) reported that 10K wheelchair racers have a maximum gross efficiency of 35%. Other investigators have studied physiological variables such as oxygen consumption, ventilation, and heart rate in elite wheelchair racers (Cooper et al. 1999b; Langbein and Maki 1995; Langbein et al. 1994; van der Woude et al. 1988). Studies have shown that regular aerobic exercise and strength training is important for all sports at the elite level (Cooper et al. 1999a). The physiological response of wheelchair racers has been shown to be influenced by the type of protocol employed (Cooper et al. 2001). A common goal of exercise research today is to better understand the physiological responses of wheelchair athletes who seek to prevent or reduce secondary medical complications.

How Disability Affects Physiologic Control

Both the somatic and the autonomic nervous systems regulate the body during exercise. The somatic nervous system innervates and controls voluntary movements such as throwing a ball or propelling a wheelchair. The **autonomic nervous system** has two divisions. The **sympathetic nervous system** mediates the body's response to stress. It increases heart rate and blood pressure, mobilizes energy stores, and prepares to fight or flee. In contrast, the **parasympathetic nervous system** works to restore homeostasis—it slows heart rate, reduces blood pressure, and prepares the body for rest. The somatic, sympathetic, and parasympathetic nervous systems together are a finely tuned network that prepares the body for every physiological need.

Physical impairments, however, significantly alter this finely tuned system. A traumatic spinal cord injury, for example, interrupts the **efferent** (motor) and **afferent** (sensory) pathways, so that communication between brain and the pathways below the level of injury generally does not occur. Damage to efferent pathways paralyzes the muscle fibers innervated by the damaged nerve: injury to the thoracic and/or lumbar region of the spine, for example, generally results in lower limb paralysis. Partial paralysis of the trunk muscles often occurs, depending on the level of the lesion. An injury to the cervical region typically results in both upper and lower limb paralysis, along with impairment to the trunk musculature. Injury to afferent pathways hinders communication to the brain regarding skin stimuli, muscle tension, muscle length, limb position, and rate of movement.

Skeletal muscle paralysis ultimately results in muscle atrophy. Atrophy of the skeletal muscles reduces functional capacity for voluntary exercise, especially since the primary movers below the level of injury, such as the leg and/or arm muscles, cannot be used for exercise. Many people, moreover, fail to consider how paralysis of the intercostal and abdominal muscles also diminishes physiological capacity. Because these muscles assist with ventilation, paralysis reduces one's ability to forcefully ventilate during exercise. The paralysis of primary movers and ventilatory musculature can greatly hinder athletic performance.

Injury to the sympathetic nervous system also hampers athletic performance. The sympathetic system strongly influences performance because it supports the fight or flight reflex. An impaired sympathetic system decreases the cardiovascular response to exercise, the effect during exercise varying with the level of injury. Impaired sympathetic systems influence athletic performance primarily by affecting smooth muscle regulation (for example, by impairing the ability to increase blood pressure) and by diminishing the capacity of the heart rate to increase during vigorous activity in particular, individuals with high thoracic or cervical spinal cord injuries no longer have the capability of increasing the heart rate. This greatly hinders performance, since stroke volume and cardiac output cannot increase during exercise to meet the higher oxygen demands.

Spinal cord injury can also end sympathetic control of blood vessels. Injuries to the thoracic region have various effects on the sympathetic system, depending on the level of the injury. Individuals with cervical injuries lose the ability to constrict and dilate blood vessels—and the inability of arteries, arterioles, veins, and venules to dilate deprives active skeletal muscles of oxygen during exercise. Furthermore, the vessels can no longer shunt blood away from inactive organs and tissues (e.g., kidneys, stomach, intestines) to active skeletal muscles, further depriving them of oxygenated blood. These processes together greatly decrease one's ability to perform intense exercise.

Biomechanical Studies

Athletes with physical impairments who participate in a variety of sports ranging from road racing to table tennis constantly look for new ways to improve performance. But biomechanical studies of wheelchair sports are limited, as are studies of the biomechanics of tennis, rugby, basketball, field events, table tennis, weightlifting, rifle and pistol, archery, bowling, and swimming.

An exception is racing wheelchair propulsion. In order to increase athletic performance, investigators (Alexander 1989; Davis and Ferrara 1988; van der Woude et al. 1988) have extensively examined the biomechanics of this activity, especially such measures as segment angular and linear displacements, velocities, and accelerations. More specifically, they have studied the kinematics of the upper extremity during wheelchair propulsion in order to identify the most effective arm stroke pattern. O'Connor et al. (1998) showed that increased efficiency was related to minimizing head motion, a lower trunk angle, a larger push angle, and higher peak elbow height during recovery. Spectral analysis has shown that the frequency of the wrist (i.e., the most distal and hence fast-moving segment) increases with speed and that a filter frequency of 6 Hz suffices for low speed (e.g., less than 15 km/hr) but may need to increase to 10 Hz at higher speeds (e.g., 25 km/hr) (DiGiovine et al. 2000). Cooper et al. (2003) showed there was a maximal economy (i.e., steady-state oxygen consumption) for wheelchair athletes that was associated with efficient biomechanics and level of fitness.

Training Techniques for Elite Athletes With Disabilities

The key to becoming an elite athlete is to attain peak performance at the appropriate time. Athletes cannot expect to be in peak condition during the entire season. It is best to focus on one event during the season, but this does not mean athletes should compete in only one event. In many instances, athletes must participate in preliminary events in order to qualify for larger events (e.g., Boston Marathon). In these cases, athletes should use the preceding events to train for the most important event, rather than attempting to win them. Because every game is important in team sports, however, such athletes should plan to peak immediately prior to the season and strive to maintain high levels of performance for the remainder of the season. They can do this by implementing a training technique called periodization.

Periodization is the technique of dividing the year into training intervals. Using team sports as an example, the year is divided into a preseason, in-season, main-season, and end-season. Even when training for one event, teams can use similar divisions: precompetition, initial competition, main competition, and postcompetition. Athletes should implement the following five training regimens into their periodization program: endurance, speed, skill, strength, and flexibility.

Because each athlete and sport has different needs, time should not be allocated equally to each training program; implementing all five training regimens to some extent, however, will facilitate peak performance.

Endurance Training

Endurance training typically involves training for a particular event; a road racer would prepare for a 5K or 10K event, for example, by performing the event at least three days a week. Some athletes may train more frequently, others less, depending on their capabilities and levels of ambition. Training for a 6K event is a good way to prepare for an actual 5K event; the extra 1000 m prepares the athlete for every weather condition and terrain, and also creates a psychological condition wherein the athlete, knowing he/she can easily complete a 6K, will push even harder during the competition.

Athletes should do interval training on days when they do not endurance train. During interval training, the athlete

- sprints a given distance,
- reduces his/her speed dramatically for a shorter distance, then
- performs the interval over again.

For example, a 400-m sprinter would sprint for 200 m, coast or lightly propel for 100 m, then start the entire process over again, performing the intervals 5 to 10 times (depending on the distance of the intervals). As the athlete approaches competition, the sprinting portion of the intervals should increase while the rest interval decreases. This type of training stresses the cardiovascular and neuromuscular systems, preparing the body for competition.

Athletes who compete in endurance events should not focus solely on these two training regimens. They also should include training in speed, skill, strength, and flexibility in order to approach the highest possible physical condition. The following sections will discuss these training techniques.

SPEED TRAINING

Every periodization program should include speed training. Athletes who participate in sports such as basketball, rugby, track and field events, swimming, and weight training will benefit from speed training. Speed training increases reaction time: a fundamental element that separates first from second place.

Performing short sprinting intervals is the best method to train for speed. For an athlete who competes in 100-m events, a single training session would be separated into four different distances. The following is a typical training day for a 100-m athlete:

Distance (m)	Repetitions
80	3
90	3
100	3
110	3

The last set of repetitions is 10% longer than the event itself, so that the athlete will sprint for the entire 110 m, which means he/she will drive through the entire 100 m during competition. As athletes often slow down during the last portion of their workouts, this method assures that they will push through the entire event.

Another aspect of speed training is a technique called plyometrics. Plyometric exercise integrates strength and power into a single training session, resulting in explosive power. **Plyometrics** utilizes an external force to store energy within the musculature. The stored energy is immediately followed by an equal and opposite reaction, utilizing the natural elastic tendencies of the muscles to produce energy. Wheelchair sprinters can utilize a medicine ball or plyoball to perform upper body plyometrics. The athlete performs plyometrics by quickly catching and explosively passing the ball to a partner for multiple repetitions. The goal of plyometric exercises is to minimize the time the body has to recover from the external force (e.g., the thrown ball), thereby optimizing the amount of energy stored within the muscle. Because plyometric exercise is a very intense training technique, athletes should consult a certified trainer before performing these exercises.

The University of Illinois, a leader in applied wheelchair sport science, has experimented with numerous training programs for wheelchair athletes (University of Illinois at Urbana-Champaign n.d.). One program in particular was designed specifically to improve explosive upper-body power through use of the Engineering Marketing Associates Inertial Training System (ITS). This ITS system was used by World Boxing Champion, Evander Holyfield, to enhance punching power and quickness; it is now used by basketball players to improve power and quickness in ball handling. Wheelchair racers have adopted the system as well to improve speed and quickness in propulsion. More information can be found on the ITS training system on the Web at www.impulsepower.com.

SKILL TRAINING

Skill training in the context of this book is essentially equivalent to specificity training, which many athletes overlook because they think it encompasses only the competitive event. This is not entirely true. Although performing from a macroscopic standpoint is important, athletes should regularly examine events microscopically. For example, wheelchair sprinters should break down their stroking techniques into distinct phases: preparatory, propulsion, and recovery phase, with each phase examined for proper form and execution. This is the primary purpose for specificity training: proper form and execution of particular events will increase an athlete's performance. This chapter cannot cover every sport individually. Athletes should review relevant literature and consult coaches for training in specific activities. It is important for athletes to find third-party sources to consult rather than relying on themselves, since athletes almost universally find it difficult to criticize themselves.

STRENGTH TRAINING

Strength training typically refers to resistance training, which most commonly employs weight training. While noting that plyometric exercise and overspeed training (training at shorter distances with higher speeds) are often classified as resistance training, we have chosen to focus on weight training. Previous sections covered plyometric exercise, while overspeed training techniques have not been widely used by athletes with physical impairments because of the lack of available commercial equipment. More information on strength training and people with disabilities can be found in Kumar (2003).

FREE WEIGHTS VERSUS MACHINES

Weight training can employ free weights or machines (e.g., Universal, Cybex, Nautilus). There are numerous advantages to using free weights:

- They permit small increments of weight.
- They teach coordination and balance.
- They allow creation of specific exercises for specific sports.

The primary disadvantage of free weights is that they require a spotter at all times. The advantage of machines is that they control the direction of movement, they do not allow for extraneous movements that can contribute to injury. A disadvantage is that coordination and balance are minimized: an athlete can push entirely with one arm on a typical chest press machine, and the weight stack will still move. This is not true with free weights. Another disadvantage to machines is that they cannot be modified to become sport-specific, since they are usually created to perform one basic exercise. Resistance training should not focus solely on free weights or machines: it is best rather to use both methods in order to provide a comprehensive workout.

POPULAR TRAINING REGIMENS

Opinions differ regarding optimal weight-training regimens. There is no one program that will suit every athlete. Athletes must consider their age, sex, weight, position, and particular sport when conditioning for the upcoming season. It is best initially to change training routines every few weeks in order to get an idea of what training program works best for an individual's particular needs—this should be done in the early preseason so that the athlete's training program will be established before the preseason is well underway, allowing the athlete to train hard for the greater part of the preseason.

Athletes use four common training routines. The first consists of training the entire body in one day: athletes perform fundamental exercises that train every major muscle of the body. A comprehensive weight-training program can include exercises such as the bench press, overhead/military press, seated rows, lat-pulls, squats, and standing calf-raises. To prevent overtraining, at least one day should be spaced between each workout of this type, with athletes devoting off days to training regimens for skill, flexibility, endurance, or speed.

The second training program consists of dividing the body into upper and lower portions. The individual dedicates one day to an upper body workout, with the second day focused on the lower body. Although this training program focuses on the fundamental exercises previously mentioned, it employs a more intense workout since only one-half of the body is exercised per workout. The higher intensity occurs via use of heavier weights or by performing more sets or repetitions (a later section will elaborate on the topic of sets and repetitions). The training program should include at least one off day to allow the body to recover from the more intense workout.

The third (and least commonly used) weight training program consists of exercising only one body part per day. This type of program allows the athlete to focus his/her training routine on a single body part. A sample chest workout would include exercises such as bench press, incline press, decline press, and/or close-grip chest press, thus overloading the chest musculature in order to facilitate strengthening. The remaining days should be dedicated to the back, arm, shoulder, and leg musculature. Although this type of workout is very taxing to the body, it allows each body part to rest for at least three or four days, allowing for proper recuperation of the muscles. This program is useful not only for novice weightlifters; because of its taxing nature, well-conditioned athletes also should use it when they are concentrating on building their strength.

The last (and very popular) program is commonly referred to as the push-pull workout. The push-pull workout divides the training program into three primary training days. The first day focuses on the chest and triceps area (the push day). The second day focuses on the back and biceps musculature (the pull day). The last day exercises the leg and shoulder musculature. This program permits very intense workouts, because each body part has at least three days to recuperate, yet even with three days of muscle recuperation, individuals should dedicate at least one day to other training regimens after the last day of the entire push-pull routine.

SETS AND REPETITIONS

The number of sets and repetitions per exercise depends on the purpose of the training program. Sets generally should remain between 2-5 per exercise, while repetitions should be between 6-15 per set. A general conditioning program should entail 3 sets per exercise, with 10-12 repetitions. The weight allocated to each set should be moderate. For more intense strength training purposes, the repetitions should be reduced to 6 per set. The repetitions are reduced so higher weights can be used. Sets should typically be on the higher side (5), in order to properly overload the muscle. Endurance athletes should focus on lighter weights with higher repetitions (12-15), with the number of sets remaining around 3-4. It is important to remember that these are general recommendations. Each athlete should determine through experience the optimal number of sets and repetitions. It is best to begin a weight-training program by implementing a general conditioning program, moving to a more strenuous program only after general conditioning is completed. Most importantly, athletes should implement weight-training programs that complement their athletic events.

FLEXIBILITY TRAINING

Flexibility training should be an integral part of any athlete's daily workout. Everyone should stretch before and after every workout, with static stretches held for at least 30 seconds. Everyone should avoid ballistic stretching, which can injure muscles.

Before each training session begins, the athlete should complete a warm-up session. This can consist of lightly pushing around the track a few times, or performing high-repetition/low-weight sets in a weight room. After the warm-up session, the athlete should perform a number of upper- and lower-extremity stretches, especially those specific to the competitive activity.

After every training session, athletes should cool down and stretch. Cool-downs can be similar to the exercises used to warm up, and can help alleviate muscle tightness and prepare the body for stretching. Stretching sessions after a workout should be comprehensive: both the upper and lower body require stretching after workouts. To ensure that all muscles are properly stretched, a post-exercise stretching session should last at least 20 minutes.

INJURIES EXPERIENCED BY ATHLETES WITH DISABILITIES

Since the inception of wheelchair athletics, health care providers have expressed great concern for the well-being of athletes with disabilities. Some early researchers argued against competition, stating that it could be harmful for the athletes. Yet Curtis et al. (1996), comparing two groups of individuals with spinal cord injuries, found that wheelchair athletes had fewer physician visits, and a trend toward fewer medical complications and fewer re-hospitalizations, when compared with nonathletes. Sports participation did not lead to increased risk of medical complications and did not limit available time for vocational pursuits.

As in all sports, wheelchair athletes can be prone to acute injuries as well as repetitive strain type injuries. According to Ferrara et al. (1992), a wheelchair athlete is at no greater risk for acute injuries than any other athlete is. The most common acute injuries related to wheelchair sports are soft tissue injuries such as sprains, strains, muscle pulls, tendinitis, and bursitis (Curtis and Dillon 1985). The next two most common injuries are blisters and lacerations.

Treatment of these types of injuries is similar to that in the unimpaired population. The most common treatments are ice, nonsteroidal anti-inflammatory drugs, and relative rest. Relative rest is more difficult to achieve than in the general population, because wheelchair athletes use their arms for mobility and for all activities of daily living. For this reason, *prevention* of soft-tissue injuries is the best form of treatment. Selective strengthening and stretching, as well as appropriate warm-up exercises, are the mainstays of preventing injury.

Of special consideration for wheelchair athletes are the problems of hypothermia and hyperthermia, to which wheelchair athletes are more prone because temperature regulation is disordered below the level of a spinal cord injury. In addition, typical treatments for these conditions may not be as effective in individuals with spinal cord injury as in the general population. Standard techniques used to heat nondisabled athletes with hypothermia are ineffective: foil blankets commonly used after marathons do not work, because athletes do not shiver to generate the body heat necessary to rewarm inside a blanket. For this reason, it is important to remove wet clothing and use active methods to heat athletes, such as warm-water compresses. Unfortunately, clinicians who staff injury tents at the ends of marathons do not always know this information.

Athletes with spinal cord injuries bear increased risk of hyperthermia because of a decreased ability to perspire below the level of the injury. One way to check for hyperthermia in a distressed athlete is to feel beneath the arm (Bloomquist 1986): if it is hot, one should employ cooling techniques such as spraying water on extremities and removing layers of clothing. Adequate hydration is critical to preventing both hyperthermia and hypothermia.

As in acute injuries, research has shown that most wheelchair athletes are no more prone to repetitive-strain injuries than nonathletes. Boninger et al. (1996) and Burnham and Steadward (1994) found that neither elite wheelchair racers nor wheelchair basketball players had a higher incidence of carpal tunnel syndrome than that reported in the nonathletic disabled population. Wheelchair setup and body mass management appear to be two of the most critical factors for prevention of repetitive strain injuries (Boninger et al. 2003, 2001, 2000, 1999). One exception may be weightlifters: all five competitive weightlifters whom Landsmeer (1961) tested (using nerve conduction studies) had carpal tunnel syndrome, and most also had ulnar nerve injuries at the wrists. In light of this finding, it is prudent to monitor weightlifters for signs and symptoms of nerve entrapments.

Wheelchair athletes are by far the most studied group of athletes with disabilities. It is difficult to find studies assessing the risk to injury for athletes with dwarfism, visual impairment, or amputations. Although there is literature that shows increased risk to the contralateral limb in individuals with unilateral amputation, most researchers have studied individuals with dysvascular amputations. The pathology for the majority of athletes with amputations is traumatic or congenital; yet it is wise for athletes with amputation who participate in running sports to follow common-sense precautions in order to protect the contralateral limb from overuse injuries. Precautions include performing adequate stretching and strengthening exercises and choosing appropriate footwear. Many injuries occur when athletes are fatigued; appropriate conditioning training can prevent many of these injuries, reducing the likelihood of acquiring a secondary disability. Athletes should pay considerable attention to pain, as pain is often an indicator of injury or overtraining.

SUMMARY

People with disabilities who are athletes, especially elite athletes, are members of a worldwide social movement for the recognition and integration of people with disabilities. Even countries that do not officially recognize the existence of people with disabilities (for example several countries report no people with disabilities in their reports to the World Health Organization) participate in the Paralympic Games and other international sporting events for people with disabilities and often prize their athletes more than those in supposedly more enlightened countries. The sports movement for people with disabilities has helped to create access to sports and recreation facilities, all the way to elite venues like the Olympic Games. Sporting events for people with disabilities have been televised worldwide, and nearly everyone admires the talent and dedication that it takes to propel a wheelchair over 1500 m in three minutes and change, to make multiple 3 point shots in a row in basketball from a wheelchair, or to run a 100 m sprint in less than 11 seconds using prosthetic limbs. These are athletic accomplishments that most people without a physical impairment will never achieve. By demonstrating their talents in the athletic arena, people with disabilities have shown that they can compete in many aspects of life given appropriate opportunities and accommodations (figure 21.11).

Advancements in the quality of emergency medical services, technology, and diagnostic tools have helped individuals with a disability to survive the initial accidents or illnesses and live longer lives. Individuals with a disability try to work themselves back into the general population, including all common aspects of life: work, everyday living activities, sports, and exercise.

Individuals with a disability are challenging many areas in regard to their participation in sports and exercise. Each individual can require different assis-

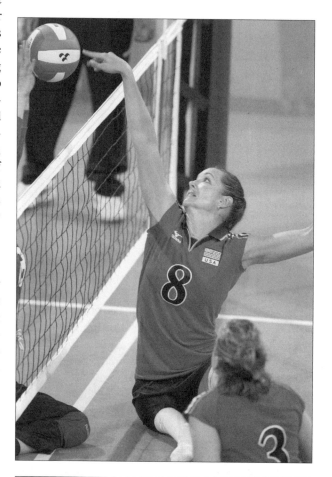

Figure 21.11 The USA's Allison Ahlfeldt tips a shot over the net at a 2004 Athens Paralympics women's sitting volleyball match.

Mark Cowan/Icon SMI.

tive technology in order for to participate in a given sport or exercise and to obtain some success therein. Individuals need to achieve a certain level of success in order to maintain motivation to continue with sports and/or exercise.

Participation in sport and exercise leads to healthier and more fulfilling lifestyles. Advances in assistive technologies have enabled individuals with disabilities to participate increasingly in sports and exercise. There is need for much more research in this area, to help individuals with a disability to achieve their sport and exercise goals. Improvement in individuals health and fitness levels may decrease their future health care costs.

REFERENCES

PREFACE

DeLisa J., G. Martin, and D. Carrie. 1998. Rehabilitation medicine: Past, present, and future. In *Rehabilitation medicine: Principles and practice,* ed. J. DeLisa and B. Grans, 3. Philadelphia: Lippincott.

CHAPTER 1

American College of Sports Medicine. 1995. *ACSM's guidelines for exercise testing and prescription.* 5th ed. Media, PA: Williams & Wilkins.

Andersen, P. 1975. Capillary density in skeletal muscle of man. *Acta Physiol Scand* 95: 203-205.

Arvill, A. 1967. Relationship between the effects of contraction and insulin on the metabolism of the isolated levator ani muscle of the rat. *Acta Endocr* 56(Suppl. 122): 27.

Åstrand, I. 1960. Aerobic work capacity in men and women with special reference to age. *J Appl Physiol* 169: 1-92.

Åstrand, P.O., T.E. Cuddy, B. Saltin, and J. Stenberg. 1964. Cardiac output during maximal and submaximal work. *Acta Physiol Scand* 19: 268-272.

Atkins, J.M., O.A. Matthews, C.G. Blomquist, and C.B. Mullins. 1976. Incidence of arrhythmias induced by isometric and dynamic exercise. *Br Heart J* 38: 465-471.

Berger, M., S. Hagg, M.N. Goodman, and N.B. Ruderman. 1976. Glucose metabolism in perfused skeletal muscle: Effects of starvation, diabetes, fatty acids, acetoacetate, insulin, and exercise on glucose uptake and disposition. *Biochem J* 158: 191-202.

Bergstrom, J., L. Hermansen, E. Hultman, and B. Saltin. 1967. Diet, muscle glycogen and physical performance. *Acta Physiol Scand* 71: 140-150.

Blackmon, J.R., L.B. Rowell, J.W. Kennedy, R.D. Twiss, and R.D. Conn. 1967. Physiological significance of maximal oxygen uptake in "pure" mitral stenosis. *Circulation* 36: 497-510.

Blair, S.N., H.W. Kohl, R.S. Paffenbarger, D.G. Clark, K.H. Cooper, and L.W. Gibbons. 1989. Physical fitness and all-cause mortality: A prospective study of healthy men and women. *JAMA* 262: 2395-2401.

Blomqvist, C.G., and B. Saltin. 1983. Cardiovascular adaptations to physical training. *Ann Rev Physiol* 45: 169-189.

Bloomfield, S.A. 1997. Changes in musculoskeletal structure and function with prolonged bed rest. *Med Sci Sports Exerc* 29: 197-206.

Buck, J.A., L.R. Amundsen, and D.H. Nielsen. 1980. Systolic blood pressure responses during isometric contractions of large and small muscle groups. *Med Sci Sports Exerc* 12: 145-147.

Center for Functional Assessment Research. 1996. *Guide for uniform data set for medical rehabilitation,* Version 5. Buffalo: School of Medicine and Biomedical Sciences, State University of New York at Buffalo.

Convertino, V.A. 1997. Cardiovascular consequences of bed rest: Effect on maximal oxygen uptake. *Med Sci Sports Exerc* 29: 191-196.

Convertino, V.A., S.A. Bloomfield, and J.E. Greenleaf. 1997. An overview of the issues: Physiological effects of bed rest and restricted physical activity. *Med Sci Sports Exerc* 29: 187-190.

Coote, J.H., S.M. Hilton, and J.F. Perez-Gonzalez. 1971. The reflex nature of the pressor response to muscular exercise. *J Physiol* 215: 789-804.

Costill, D.L., W.J. Fink, M. Hargreaves, D.S. King, R. Thomas, and R.A. Fielding. 1985. Metabolic characteristics of skeletal muscle during detraining from competitive swimming. *Med Sci Sports Exerc* 17: 339-343.

Coyle, E.F., A.R. Coggan, M.K. Hemmert, and J.L. Ivy. 1986. Muscle glycogen utilization during prolonged exercise when fed carbohydrate. *J Appl Physiol* 61: 165-172.

Coyle, E.F., J.M. Hagberg, B.F. Hurley, W.H. Martin, A.H. Ehsani, and J.O. Holloszy. 1983. Carbohydrate feeding during prolonged strenuous exercise can delay fatigue. *J Appl Physiol* 55: 230-235.

Crawford, M.H., M.A. Petru, and C. Rabinowitz. 1985. Effect of isotonic exercise training on left ventricular volume during upright exercise. *Circulation* 72: 1237-1243.

DeLisa, J.A. 1993. *Rehabilitation medicine: Principles and practice.* 2nd ed. Philadelphia: J.P. Lippincott.

Dempsey, J.A., and R.F. Fregosi. 1985. Adaptability of the pulmonary system to changing metabolic requirements. *Am J Cardiol* 55: 55D-59D.

Dempsey, J.A., B.D. Johnson, and K.W. Saupe. 1990. Adaptations and limitations in the pulmonary system during exercise. *Chest* 97: 81S-87S.

Dempsey, J.A., A.W. Sheel, H.C. Haverkamp, M.A. Babcock, and C.A. Harms. 2003. The John Sutton Lecture: CSEP, 2002. Pulmonary system limitations to exercise in health. *Can J Appl Physiol* 28(Suppl.): S2-24.

Dempsey, J.A., E.H. Vidruk, and G.S. Mitchell. 1985. Pulmonary control systems in exercise: Update. *Fed Proc* 44: 2260-2270.

DiTunno, J.F., and C.S. Formal. 1994. Chronic spinal cord injury. *New Engl J Med* 330: 550-556.

Dohm, G.L. 2002. Invited review: Regulation of skeletal muscle GLUT-4 expression by exercise. *J Appl Physiol* 93: 782-787.

Donald, K.W., A.R. Lind, and G.W. McNichol. 1967. Cardiovascular response to sustained [static] contractions. *Circ Res* XX-XXI (Suppl.): 1: 15-32.

Dowell, R.T. 1983. Cardiac adaptations to exercise. *Exerc Sport Sci Rev* 11: 99-117.

Drinkwater, B.L. 1984. Women and exercise: Physiologic aspects. *Exerc Sport Sci Rev* 12: 12-51.

Ekelund, L.G., and A. Holmgren. 1967. Central hemodynamics during exercise. *Circ Res* (Suppl.): 20: 33-43.

Felig, P., A. Cherif, A. Minigawa, and J. Wahren. 1982. Hypoglycemia during prolonged exercise in normal men. *N Engl J Med* 302: 895-900.

Felig, P., and J. Wahren. 1975. Fuel homeostasis in exercise. *N Engl J Med* 293: 1078-1084.

Fielding, R.A., D.L. Costill, W.J. Fink, D.S. King, J.E. Kovaleski, and J.P. Kirwan. 1986. Effect of pre-exercise carbohydrate feedings on muscle glycogen use during exercise in well-trained runners. *Eur J Appl Physiol* 56: 225-229.

Figoni, S.F., R.M. Glaser, M.M. Rodgers, S.P. Hooker, B.N. Ezenwa, S.R. Collins, T. Matthews, A.G. Suryaprasad, and S.C. Gupta. 1991. Acute hemodynamic responses of spinal cord injured individuals to functional neuromuscular stimulation-induced knee extension exercise. *J Rehab Research* 28: 9-18.

Galbo, H. 1983. *Hormonal and metabolic adaptations to exercise*. New York: Thieme Verlag.

Galbo, H., E. Richter, J. Hilsted, J. Holst, N. Christensen, and J. Henrickson. 1977. Hormonal regulation during prolonged exercise. *Ann NY Acad Sci* 301: 72-80.

Giacca, A.M., J. Davidson, and H. Lickley. 1991. Exercise and stress in diabetes mellitus. In *Clinical diabetes mellitus: A problem oriented approach*, ed. J. Davidson. New York: Thieme-Stratton, Inc.

Glaser, R.M. 1989. Arm exercise training for wheelchair users. *Med Sci Sports Exerc* 21: S147-S149.

Goldberg, L.I., J. White, and K.B. Pandolf. 1982. Cardiovascular and perceptual responses to isometric exercise. *Arch Phys Med Rehabil* 63: 211-216.

Graves, J.E., M.L. Pollock, A.E. Jones, A.B. Colvin, and S.H. Leggett. 1989. Specificity of limited range of motion variable resistance training. *Med Sci Sports Exerc* 21: 84-89.

Greer, M., S. Dimick, and S. Burns. 1984. Heart rate and blood pressure response to several methods of strength training. *Phys Ther* 64: 179-183.

Guyton, A.C. 1991. *Textbook of medical physiology*. 8th ed. Philadelphia: W.B. Saunders.

Helmreich, E., and C.F. Cori. 1957. The distribution of pentoses between plasma and muscle. *J Biol Chem* 224: 663.

Henriksson, J., and J.S. Reitman. 1977. Time course of changes in human skeletal muscle succinate dehydrogenase and cytochrome oxidase activities and maximal oxygen uptake with physical activity and inactivity. *Acta Physiol Scand* 99: 91-97.

Hermansen, L., and K.L. Anderson. 1965. Aerobic work capacity in young Norwegian men and women. *J Appl Physiol* 20: 425-431.

Hermansen, L., B. Ekblom, and B. Saltin. 1970. Cardiac output during submaximal and maximal treadmill and bicycle exercise. *J Appl Physiol* 29: 82-86.

Hermansen, L., E. Hultman, and B. Saltin. 1967. Muscle glycogen during prolonged severe exercise. *Acta Physiol Scand* 71: 129-137.

Hermansen, L., and M. Wachlova. 1971. Capillary density of skeletal muscle in well-trained and untrained men. *J Appl Physiol* 30: 860-863.

Hespel, P., and E.A. Richter. 1990. Glucose uptake and transport in contracting, perfused rat muscle with different pre-contraction glycogen concentrations. *J Physiol* 427: 347-359.

Hill, A.V., and H. Lupton. 1923. Muscular exercise, lactic acid, and the supply and utilization of oxygen. *Q J Med* 16: 135-171.

Hilsted, J. 1982. Pathophysiology in diabetic autonomic neuropathy: Cardiovascular, hormonal, and metabolic studies. *Diabetes* 31 (August): 730-737.

Holloszy, J.O. 1967. Biochemical adaptations in muscle. Effects of exercise on mitochondrial oxygen uptake and respiratory enzyme activity in skeletal muscle. *J Biol Chem* 242: 2278-2282.

Holloszy, J.O., and E.F. Coyle. 1984. Adaptations of skeletal muscle to endurance exercise and their metabolic consequences. *J Appl Physiol* 56: 831-838.

Hurley, B.F., P.M. Nemeth, W.H. Martin, J.M. Hagberg, G.P. Dalsky, and J.O. Holloszy. 1986. Muscle triglyceride utilization during exercise: Effect of training. *J Appl Physiol* 60: 562-657.

Ivy, J.L., J.C. Young, J.A. McLane, R.D. Fell, and J.O. Holloszy. 1983. Exercise training and glucose uptake by skeletal muscle in rats. *J Appl Physiol* 55: 1393-1396.

Jacobs, I. 1980. Lactate concentrations after short maximal exercise at various glycogen levels. *Acta Physiol Scand* 111: 465-469.

Katz, A., S. Broberg, K. Sahlin, and J. Wahren. 1986. Leg glucose uptake during maximal dynamic exercise in humans. *Am J Physiol* 251: E65-E70.

Katzmarzyk, P.T., T.S. Church, and S.N. Blair. 2004. Cardiorespiratory fitness attenuates the effects of the metabolic syndrome on all-cause and cardiovascular disease mortality in men. *Arch Intern Med* 164: 1092-1097.

Kawamori, R., and M. Vranic. 1977. Mechanism of exercise-induced hypoglycemia in depancreatized dogs maintained on long-acting insulin. *J Clin Invest* 59: 331-337.

Kemmer, F., and M. Berger. 1986. Therapy and better quality of life: The dichotomous role of exercise in diabetes mellitus. *Diabetes Metab Rev* 2(1-2): 53-68.

King, M.L., S.W. Lichtman, J.T. Pellicone, R.J. Close, and P. Lisanti. 1994. Exertional hypotension in spinal cord injury. *Chest* 106: 1166-1171.

Klein, S., E.F. Coyle, and R.R. Wolfe. 1994. Fat metabolism during low-intensity exercise in endurance-trained and untrained men. *Am J Physiol* 267: E934-E940.

Krip, B., N. Gledhill, V. Jamnik, D. Warburton. 1997. Effect of alterations in blood volume on cardiac function during maximal exercise. *Med Sci Sports Exerc* 29: 1469-76.

Lasko-McCarthey, P., and J.A. Davis. 1991. Protocol dependency of VO_2max during arm cycle ergometry in males with quadriplegia. *Med Sci Sports Exerc* 23: 1097-1101.

Lee, I.M., R.S. Paffenbarger, and C.C. Hsieh. 1992. Physical activity and risk of prostatic cancer among college alumni. *Am J Epidemiol* 135: 169-179.

Maughan, R.J., and D.C. Poole. 1981. The effects of a glycogen loading regimen on the capacity to perform anaerobic exercise. *Eur J Appl Physiol* 46: 211-219.

McGuire, D.K., B.D. Levine, J.W. Williamson, P.G. Snell, G. Bloomqvist, B. Saltin, and J.H. Mitchell. 2001. A 30-year follow-up of the Dallas Bedrest and Training Study: I. Effect of age on the cardiovascular response to exercise. *Circulation* 104: 1350-1357.

Meredith, C.N., M.J. Zackin, W.R. Frontera, and W.J. Evans. 1989. Dietary protein requirements and body protein metabolism in endurance-trained men. *J Appl Physiol* 66: 2850-2856.

Newsholme, E.A., and A.R. Leech. 1983. Biochemistry for the medical sciences. In *Biochemistry for the medical sciences*. New York: Wiley.

Newsholme, E.A., and C. Start. 1973. Regulation in metabolism. In *Regulation in metabolism*. New York: Wiley.

O'Connor, P.J., G.A. Sforzo, and P. Frye. 1989. Effect of breathing instruction on blood pressure responses during isometric exercise. *Phys Ther* 69: 757-761.

Olefsky, J.M., W.T. Garvey, R.R. Henry, D. Brillon, S. Matthaei, and G.R. Freidenberg. 1988. Cellular mechanisms of insulin resistance in non-insulin dependent (type II) diabetes. *Am J Med* 85: 86-105.

Paffenbarger, R.S., R.T. Hyde, A.L. Wing, and C.-C. Hsieh. 1986. Physical activity, all-cause mortality and longevity of college alumni. *N Engl J Med* 314: 605-613.

Polinar, L.R., G.J. Dehmer, S.E. Lewis, R.W. Parkey, C.G. Blomquist, and J.T. Willerson. 1980. Left ventricular performance in normal subjects: A comparison of the responses to exercise in the upright and supine positions. *Circulation* 62: 528-534.

Pollack, M.L. 1973. Quantification of endurance training programs. *Exerc Sport Sci Rev* 1: 155-188.

Rennie, M.J., R.H.T. Edwards, S. Krywawych, C.T.M. Davies, D. Halliday, J.C. Waterlow, and D.J. Milward. 1981. Effect of exercise on protein turnover in man. *Clin Sci* 62: 627-639.

Richter, E.A., and H. Galbo. 1986. High glycogen levels enhance glycogen breakdown in isolated contracting skeletal muscle. *J Appl Physiol* 61: 827-831.

Richter, E.A., L. Turcotte, P. Hespel, and B. Kiens. 1992. Metabolic responses to exercise: Effects of endurance training and implications for diabetes. *Diabetes Care* 15: 1767-1776.

Rodgers, M.M., R.M. Glaser, S.F. Figoni, S.P. Hooker, B.N. Ezenwa, S.R. Collins, T. Matthews, A.G. Suryaprasad, and S.C. Gupta. 1991. Musculoskeletal responses of spinal cord injured individuals to functional neuromuscular stimulation-induced knee extension exercise training. *J Rehab Research* 28: 19-26.

Rowell, L.B. 1974. Human cardiovascular adjustments to exercise and thermal stress. *Physiol Rev* 54: 75-159.

Rowell, L.B. 1986. *Human circulation: Regulation during physical stress*. New York: Oxford University Press.

Rowland, T., B. Popowski, and L. Ferrone. 1997. Cardiac responses to maximal upright cycle exercise in healthy boys and men. *Med Sci Sports Exerc* 29: 1146-1151.

Sakamoto, K., and L.J. Goodyear. 2002. Invited review: Intracellular signaling in contracting skeletal muscle. *J Appl Physiol* 93: 369-383.

Saltin, B. 1985. Hemodynamic adaptations to exercise. *Am J Cardiol* 55: 42D-47D.

Saltin, B., G. Blomqvist, J.H. Mitchell, R.L. Johnson, K. Wildenthal, and C.B. Chapman. 1968. Response to exercise after bed rest and after training: A longitudinal study of adaptive changes in oxygen transport and body composition. *Circulation* 38(5 Suppl.): VII1-VII78.

Saltin, B., and L.B. Rowell. 1980. Functional adaptations to physical activity and inactivity. *Fed Proc* 39: 1506-1513.

Saltin, B., and S. Strange. 1992. Maximal oxygen uptake: "Old" and "new" arguments for a cardiovascular limitation. *Med Sci Sports Exerc* 24: 30-37.

Sawka, M.N., W.A. Latzka, and K.B. Pandolf. 1989. Temperature regulation during upper body exercise: Able-bodied and spinal cord injured. *Med Sci Sports Exerc* 21: 132S-140S.

Seals, D.R., R.G. Victor, and A.L. Mark. 1988. Plasma norepinephrine and muscle sympathetic discharge during rhythmic exercise in humans. *J Appl Physiol* 65: 940-944.

Shephard, R.J. 1990. The scientific basis of exercise prescribing for the very old. *J Am Ger Soc* 38: 62-69.

Smith, S.A., S.J. Montain, G.P. Zientara, and R.A. Fielding. 2004. Use of phosphocreatine kinetics to determine the influence of creatine on muscle mitochondrial respiration: An in vivo 31P-MRS study of oral creatine ingestion. *J Appl Physiol* 96: 2288-2292.

Sorrentino, E., D. Stump, B.J. Potter, R.B. Robinson, R. White, C. Kiang, and P.D. Berk. 1988. Oleate uptake by cardiac myocytes is carrier mediated and involves a 40-kD plasma membrane fatty acid binding protein similar to that of liver, adipose tissue, and gut. *J Clin Invest* 82: 928-935.

Stone, H.L., K.J. Dormer, R.D. Foreman, R. Thies, and R.W. Blair. 1985. Neural regulation of the cardiovascular system during exercise. *Fed Proc* 44: 2271-2278.

Stremmel, W. 1988. Fatty acid uptake by isolated rat heart myocytes represents a carrier-mediated transport process. *J Clin Invest* 81: 844-852.

Tarnopolsky, M.A., S.A. Atkinson, J.D. MacDougall, A. Chesley, S. Phillips, and H.P. Schwarcz. 1992. Evaluation of protein requirements for trained strength athletes. *J Appl Physiol* 73: 1986-1995.

Taylor, H.L., E. Buskirk, and A. Henschel. 1955. Maximal oxygen uptake as an objective measure of cardiorespiratory performance. *Am J Physiol* 8: 73-80.

Turcotte, L.P. 1992. Increased plasma FFA uptake and oxidation during prolonged exercise in humans. *Am J Physiol* 262: E791-E799.

Veves, A., R. Saouaf, V.M. Donaghue, C.A. Mullooly, J.A. Kistler, J.M. Giurini, E.S. Horton, and R.A. Fielding. 1997. Aerobic exercise capacity remains normal despite impaired endothelial function in the micro- and macrocirculation of physically active IDDM patients. *Diabetes* 46: 1846-1852.

Vitug, A., S. Schneider, and N. Ruderman. 1988. Exercise and type I diabetes mellitus. *Exerc Sport Sci Rev* 16: 285-304.

Vranic, M., R. Kawamori, S. Pek, N. Kovacevic, and G.A. Wrenshall. 1976. The essentiality of insulin and the role of glucagon in regulating glucose utilization and production during strenuous exercise in dogs. *J Clin Invest* 57: 245-255.

Vranic, M., D. Wasserman, and L. Bukowiecki. 1990. Metabolic implications of exercise and physical fitness in physiology and diabetes. In *Diabetes mellitus: Theory and practice*, ed. H. P. Rifkin, Jr. New York: Elsevier Science.

Vranic, M., and G. Wrenshall. 1969. Exercise, insulin and glucose turnover in dogs. *Endocrinology* 85: 165-171.

Wahren, J., Y. Sato, J. Ostman, L. Hagenfeldt, and P. Felig. 1984. Turnover and splanchnic metabolism of free fatty acids and ketones in insulin deficient diabetes at rest and in response to exercise. *J Clin Invest* 73: 1367-1376.

Wallberg-Henriksson, H. 1987. Glucose transport into skeletal muscle. Influence of contractile activity, insulin, catecholamines on diabetes mellitus. *Acta Physiol Scand* 131: 1-80.

Wasserman, D.H. 1995. Control of glucose fluxes in the post-absorptive state. *Ann Rev Physiol* 57: 191-218.

Wasserman, D., and B. Zinman. 1995. Fuel homeostasis. In *Health professionals' guide to diabetes and exercise*, ed. N. Ruderman and J. Devlin. Alexandria, VA: American Diabetes Association.

Wiley, R.L., C.L. Dunn, R.H. Cox, N.A. Hueppchen, and M.S. Scott. 1992. Isometric exercise training lowers resting blood pressure. *Med Sci Sports Exerc* 24: 749-754.

Winder, W.W., and D.G. Hardie. 1999. AMP-activated protein kinase, a metabolic master switch: Possible roles in type 2 diabetes. *Am J Physiol* 277: E1-10.

Zinman, B., F. Murray, M. Vranic, A. Albisser, B. Leibel, P. McClean, and E. Marliss. 1977. Glucoregulation during moderate exercise in insulin treated diabetics. *J Clin Endocrinol* 45: 641-652.

Zinman, B., S. Zuniga-Guajardo, and D. Kelly. 1984. Comparison of the acute and long term effects of exercise on glucose control in type I diabetes. *Diabetes Care* 7: 515-519.

CHAPTER 2

Aloia, J., S. Cohn, J. Ostuni, R. Cane, and K. Ellis. 1987. Prevention of involutional bone loss by exercise. *Ann Intern Med* 89: 356-358.

American College of Sports Medicine. 1998. ACSM position stand on the recommended quantity and quality of exercise for developing and maintaining cardiorespiratory and muscular fitness, and flexibility in healthy adults. *Med Sci Sports Exerc* 30: 975-991.

Åstrand, I. 1960. Aerobic work capacity in men and women with special reference to age. *Acta Physiol Scand (Suppl)* 169: 1-92.

Åstrand, P.-O., and K. Rodahl. 1986. *Textbook of work physiology: Physiological bases of exercise*. 3rd ed. New York: McGraw-Hill.

Baldwin, K.M., W.W. Winder, R.L. Terjung, and J.O. Holloszy. 1973. Glycolytic enzymes in different types of skeletal muscle: Adaptation to exercise. *Am J Physiol* 225: 962-966.

Barnes, D.E., K. Yaffe, W.A. Satariano, and I.B. Tager. 2003. A longitudinal study of cardiorespiratory fitness and cognitive function in healthy older adults. *J Am Geriatr Soc* 51(4): 459-465.

Bigland-Ritchie, B. 1990. Discussion: Nervous system and sensory adaptations. In *Exercise, fitness, and health,* ed. C. Bouchard, R.J. Shephard, T. Stephens, J.R. Sutton, and B.D. McPherson, 377-383. Champaign, IL: Human Kinetics.

Blake, M.J., E.A. Stein, and A.J. Vomachka. 1984. Effects of exercise training on brain opioid *Peptides* and serum LH in female rats. *Peptides* 5: 953-958.

Bloom, S.R., R.H. Johnson, D.M. Park, M.J. Rennie, and W.R. Sulaiman. 1976. Differences in the metabolic and hormonal responses to exercise between racing cyclists and untrained individuals. *J Appl Physiol* 48: 1-18.

Blumenthal, J.A., M. Fredrikson, C.M. Kuhn, R.L. Ulmer, M. Walsh-Riddle, and M. Appelbaum. 1990. Aerobic exercise reduces levels of cardiovascular and sympathoadrenal responses to mental stress in subjects without prior evidence of myocardial ischemia. *Am J Cardiol* 65: 93-98.

Borg, G. 1970. Perceived exertion as an indicator of somatic stress. *Scand J Rehabil Med* 2-3: 92-98.

Borghouts, L.B., and H.A. Keizer. 2000. Exercise and insulin sensitivity: A review. *Int J Sports Med* 21: 1-12.

Bortz, W.M. IV, and W.M. Bortz II. 1996. How fast do we age? Exercise performance over time as a biomarker. *J Gerontol A Biol Sci Med Sci* 51A: M223-M225.

Bouchard, C., P. An, T. Rice, J.S. Skinner, J.H. Wilmore, J. Gagnon, L. Perusse, A.S. Leon, and D.C. Rao. 1999. Familial aggregation of VO_2max response to exercise training: Results from the HERITAGE Family Study. *J Appl Physiol* 87: 1003-1008.

Bouchard, C., E.W. Daw, T. Rice, L. Perusse, J. Gagnon, M.A. Province, A.S. Leon, D.C. Rao, J.S. Skinner, and J.H. Wilmore. 1998. Familial resemblance for VO_2max in the sedentary state: The HERITAGE Family Study. *Med Sci Sports Exerc* 30: 252-258.

Bouchard, C., F.T. Dionne, J.-A. Simoneau, and M.R. Boulay. 1992. Genetics of aerobic and anaerobic performances. *Exerc Sport Sci Rev* 20: 27-58.

Bouchard, C., R. Lesage, G. Lortie, J.A. Simoneau, P. Hamel, M.R. Boulay, L. Perusse, G. Theriault, and C. Leblanc. 1986. Aerobic performance in brothers, dizygotic and monozygotic twins. *Med Sci Sports Exerc* 18: 639-646.

Brisson, G.R., M.A. Volle, D. DeCarufel, M. Desharnais, and M. Tanaka. 1980. Exercise-induced dissociation of the blood prolactin response in young women according to their sports habits. *Horm Metab Res* 12: 201-205.

Busch, A., C.L. Schachter, P.M. Peloso, and C. Bombardier. 2002. Exercise for treating fibromyalgia syndrome. (Cochrane Review). In *The Cochrane Library,* Issue 3. Oxford: Update Software.

Buskirk, E.R., and J.L. Hodgson. 1987. Age and aerobic power: The rate of change in men and women. *Federation Proc* 46: 1824-1829.

Cann, C.E., M.C. Martin, H.K. Genant, and R.B. Jaffe. 1984. Decreased spinal mineral content in amenorrheic women. *JAMA* 251: 626-629.

Carr, D.B., B.A. Bullen, G.S. Skrinar, M.A. Arnold, M. Rosenblatt, I.Z. Beitins, J.B. Martin, and J.W. McArthur. 1981. Physical conditioning facilitates the exercise-induced secretion of beta-endorphin and beta-lipotropin in women. *N Engl J Med* 305: 560-563.

Carter, L.B., E.W. Banister, and A.P. Blaber. 2003. Effect of endurance exercise on autonomic control of heart rate. *Sports Med* 33(1): 33-46.

Casaburi, R., T.W. Storer, and K. Wasserman. 1987. Mediation of reduced ventilatory response to exercise after endurance training. *J Appl Physiol* 63: 1533-1538.

Cavanagh, P.R., and R. Kram. 1985. The efficiency of human movement: A statement of the problem. *Med Sci Sports Exerc* 17: 304-308.

Chi, M.M., C.S. Hintz, E.F. Coyle, W.H. Martin III, J.L. Ivy, P.M. Nemeth, J.O. Holloszy, and O.H. Lowry. 1983. Effects of detraining on enzymes of energy metabolism in individual human muscle fibers. *Am J Physiol* 244: C276-C287.

Christie, M.J., and G.B. Chesher. 1983. [^{3}H]Leu-enkephalin binding following chronic swim-stress in mice. *Neurosci Lett* 36: 323-328.

Clanton, T., G.F. Dixon, J. Drake, and J.E. Gadek. 1987. Effects of swim training on lung volumes and inspiratory muscle conditioning. *J Appl Physiol* 62: 39-46.

Clausen, J.P. 1977. Effect of physical training on cardiovascular adjustments to exercise in man. *Physiol Rev* 57: 779-815.

Clausen, J.P., K. Klausen, B. Rasmussen, and J. Trap-Jensen. 1973. Central and peripheral circulatory changes after training of the arms or legs. *Am J Physiol* 225: 675-682.

Clausen, J.P., and J. Trap-Jensen. 1976. Heart rate and arterial blood pressure during exercise in patients with angina pectoris. Effects of training and of nitroglycerin. *Circulation* 53: 436-442.

Clausen, J.P., J. Trap-Jensen, and N.A. Lassen. 1970. The effects of training on the heart rate during arm and leg exercise. *Scand J Clin Lab Invest* 26: 295-301.

Convertino, V.A., L.C. Keil, E.M. Bernauer, and J.E. Greenleaf. 1981. Plasma volume, osmolality, vasopressin, and renin activity during graded exercise in man. *J Appl Physiol* 50: 123-128.

Convertino, V.A., L.C. Keil, and J.E. Greenleaf. 1983. Plasma volume, renin, and vasopressin responses to graded exercise after training. *J Appl Physiol* 54: 508-514.

Cronan, T.L., and E.T. Howley. 1974. The effect of training on epinephrine and norepinephrine excretion. *Med Sci Sports* 6: 122-125.

Cureton, K., P. Bishop, P. Hutchinson, H. Newland, S. Vickery, and L. Zwiren. 1986. Sex differences in maximal oxygen uptake: Effect of equating haemoglobin concentration. *Eur J Appl Physiol* 54: 656-660.

Cureton, K.L., and P.B. Sparling. 1980. Distance running performance and metabolic responses to running in men and women with excess weight experimentally equated. *Med Sci Sports Exerc* 12: 288-294.

Da Costa, D., N. Rippen, M. Dritsa, and A. Ring. 2003. Self-reported leisure-time physical activity during pregnancy and relationship to psychological well-being. *J Psychosom Obstet Gynecol* 24: 111-119.

Dela, F., K.J. Mikines, and H. Galbo. 1987. Arginine stimulated insulin response in trained and untrained man. *Diabetologia* 30: 513A.

Delp, M.D. 1995. Effects of exercise training on endothelium-dependent peripheral vascular responsiveness. *Med Sci Sports Exerc* 27: 1152-1157.

deVries, H.A. 1968. Immediate and long-term effects of exercise upon resting muscle action potential. *J Sports Med* 8: 1-11.

Drinkwater, B.L., K. Nilson, C.H. Chestnut, III, W. Bremmer, S. Shainholtz, and M. Southworth. 1984. Bone mineral content of amenorrheic and eumenorrheic athletes. *N Engl J Med* 311: 277-281.

Droste, C., M.W. Greenlee, M. Schreck, and H. Roskamm. 1991. Experimental pain thresholds and plasma beta-endorphin levels during exercise. *Med Sci Sports Exerc* 23: 334-342.

Dudley, G.A., W.M. Abraham, and R.L. Terjung. 1982. Influence of exercise intensity and duration on biochemical adaptations in skeletal muscle. *J Appl Physiol* 53: 844-850.

Ehsani, A.A., T. Ogawa, T.R. Miller, R.J. Spina, and S.M. Jilka. 1991. Exercise training improves left ventricular systolic function in older men. *Circulation* 83: 96-103.

Ekblom, B. 1969. Effect of physical training on oxygen transport system in man. *Acta Physiol Scand (Suppl.)* 328: 1-45.

Fagard, R., E. Bielen, and A. Amery. 1991. Heritability of aerobic power and anaerobic energy generation during exercise. *J Appl Physiol* 70: 357-362.

Farrell, P.A., A.B. Gustafson, W.P. Morgan, C.B. Pert. 1987. Enkephalins, catecholamines, and psychological mood alterations: Effects of prolonged exercise. *Med Sci Sports Exerc* 19: 347-353.

Farrell, P.A., M. Kjaer, F.W. Bach, and H. Galbo. 1987. Beta endorphin and adrenocorticotropin responses to supramaximal treadmill exercise in trained and untrained males. *Acta Physiol Scand* 130: 619-625.

Farrell, P.A., J.H. Wilmore, E.F. Coyle, J.E. Billings, and D.L. Costill. 1979. Plasma lactate accumulation and distance running performance. *Med Sci Sports* 11: 338-344.

Fentem, P.H. 1992. Exercise in prevention of disease. *Br Med Bull* 48: 630-650.

Ferketich, A.K., T.E. Kirby, and S.E. Always. 1998. Cardiovascular and muscular adaptations to combined endurance and strength training in elderly women. *Acta Physiol Scand* 164: 259-267.

Fitts, R.H., and J.J. Widrick. 1996. Muscle mechanics: Adaptations with exercise-training. *Exerc Sport Sci Rev* 24: 427-273.

Fries, J.F. 1996. Physical activity, the compression of morbidity, and the health of the elderly. *J R Soc Med* 89: 64-68.

Fries, J.F., G. Singh, D. Morfeld, H.B. Hubert, N.E. Lane, B.W. Brown Jr. 1994. Running and the development of disability with age. *Ann Intern Med* 121: 502-509.

Galbo, H., J.J. Holst, and N.J. Christensen. 1975. Glucagon and plasma catecholamine responses to graded and prolonged exercise in man. *J Appl Physiol* 38: 70-76.

Galbo, H., E.A. Richter, J. Hilsted, J.J. Holst, N.J. Christensen, and J. Henriksson. 1977. Hormonal regulation during prolonged exercise. *Ann NY Acad Sci* 301: 72-80.

Glaser, R.M., M.N. Sawka, R.J. Durbin, D.M. Foley, and A.G. Suryaprasad. 1981. Exercise program for wheelchair activity. *Am J Phys Med* 60: 67-75.

Gleeson, P.B., E.J. Protas, A. Leblanc, V.S. Schneider, and H.J. Evans. 1990. Effects of weight lifting on bone mineral density in premenopausal women. *J Bone Miner Res* 5: 153-158.

Goldman, J.A. 1991. Hypermobility and deconditioning: Important links to fibromyalgia/fibrositis. *South Med J* 84: 1192-1196.

Gollnick, P.D., R.B. Armstrong, C.W. Saubert, K. Piehl, and B. Saltin. 1972. Enzyme activity and fiber composition in skeletal muscle of untrained and trained men. *J Appl Physiol* 33: 312-319.

Hackney, A.C. 1996. The male reproductive system and endurance exercise. *Med Sci Sports Exerc* 28: 180-189.

Hagberg, J.M., J.E. Graves, M. Limacher, D.R. Woods, S.H. Leggett, C. Cononie, J.J. Gruber, and M.L. Pollock. 1989. Cardiovascular responses of 70- to 79-yr-old men and women to exercise training. *J Appl Physiol* 66: 2589-2594.

Hambrecht, R., A. Wolf, S. Gielen, A. Linke, J. Hofer, S. Erbs, N. Schoene, and G. Schuler. 2000. Effect of exercise on coronary endothelial function in patients with coronary heart disease. *N Engl J Med* 342(7): 454-460.

Hartley, H.L. 1975. Growth hormone and catecholamine response to exercise in relation to physical training. *Med Sci Sports Exerc* 7: 34-36.

Hartley, L.H., J.W. Mason, R.P. Hogan, L.G. Jones, T.A. Kotchen, E.H. Mougey, F.E. Wherry, L.L. Pennington, and P.T. Ricketts. 1972a. Multiple hormonal responses to graded exercise in relation to physical training. *J Appl Physiol* 33: 602-606.

Hartley, L.H., J.W. Mason, R.P. Hogan, L.G. Jones, T.A. Kotchen, E.H. Mougey, F.E. Wherry, L.L. Pennington, and P.T. Ricketts. 1972b. Multiple hormonal responses to prolonged exercise in relation to physical training. *J Appl Physiol* 33: 607-610.

Hawkins, H.L., A.F. Kramer, D. Capaldi. 1992. Aging, exercise, and attention. *Psychol Aging* 7(4): 643-53.

Hawley, J.A. 2002. Adaptations of skeletal muscle to prolonged, intense endurance training. *Clin Exp Pharmacol Physiol* 29(3): 218-222.

Heath, G., J. Hagberg, A.A. Ehsani, and J.O. Holloszy. 1981. Physical comparison of young and old endurance athletes. *J Appl Physiol* 51: 634-640.

Henriksson, J. 1977. Training induced adaptations of skeletal muscle and metabolism during submaximal exercise. *J Physiol* (Lond) 270: 661-675.

Hermansen, L., E. Hultmen, and B. Saltin. 1967. Muscle glycogen during prolonged severe exercise. *Acta Physiol Scand* 71: 129-139.

Hiatt, W.R., E.E. Wolfel, R.H. Meier, and J.G. Regensteiner. 1994. Superiority of treadmill walking exercise versus strength training for patients with peripheral arterial disease. Implications for the mechanism of the training response. *Circulation* 90: 1866-1874.

Hickson, R.C., B.A. Dvorak, E.M. Gorostiaga, T.T. Kurowski, and C. Foster. 1988. Potential for strength and endurance training to amplify endurance performance. *J Appl Physiol* 65: 2285-2290.

Hickson, R.C., J.M. Hagberg, A.A. Ehsani, and J.O. Holloszy. 1981. Time course of the adaptive responses of aerobic power and heart rate to training. *Med Sci Sports Exerc* 13: 17-20.

Hoffman, M.D. 1986. Cardiorespiratory fitness and training in quadriplegics and paraplegics. *Sports Med* 3: 312-330.

Hoffman, M.D., K.M. Kassay, A.I. Zeni, and P.S. Clifford. 1996. Does the amount of exercising muscle alter the aerobic demand of dynamic exercise? *Eur J Appl Physiol* 74: 541-547.

Hoffman, M.D., M.A. Shepanski, S.B. Ruble, J.B. Buckwalter, and P.S. Clifford. 2004. Intensity and duration threshold for aerobic exercise-induced analgesia to pressure pain. *Arch Phys Med Rehabil* 85(7): 1183-1187.

Hoffmann, P., L. Terenius, and P. Thoren. 1990. Cerebrospinal fluid immunoreactive beta-endorphin concentration is increased by voluntary exercise in the spontaneously hypertensive rat. *Regul Pept* 28: 233-239.

Holloszy, J.O. 1973. Biochemical adaptations to exercise: Aerobic metabolism. *Exerc Sport Sci Rev* 1: 45-71.

Holloszy, J.O., and E.F. Coyle. 1984. Adaptations of skeletal muscle to endurance exercise and their metabolic consequences. *J Appl Physiol* 56: 831-838.

Hosobuchi, Y., and C.H. Li. 1978. The analgesic activity of human beta-endorphin in man (1,2,3). *Commun Psychopharmacol* 2: 33-37.

Hurley, B.F., J.M. Hagberg, W.K. Allen, D.R. Seals, J.C. Young, R.W. Cuddihee, and J.O. Holloszy. 1984. Effect of training on blood lactate levels during submaximal exercise. *J Appl Physiol* 56: 1260-1264.

Janal, M.N., E.W.D. Colt, W.C. Clark, and M. Glusman. 1984. Pain sensitivity, mood and plasma endocrine levels in man following long-distance running: Effects of naloxone. *Pain* 19: 13-25.

Jansson, E., and L. Kaijser. 1977. Muscle adaptation to extreme endurance training in man. *Acta Physiol Scand* 100: 315-324.

Juel, C. 1997. Lactate-proton cotransport in skeletal muscle. *Physiol Rev* 77: 321-358.

Karlsson, J., L.-O. Nordesjo, L. Jorfeldt, and B. Saltin. 1972. Muscle lactate, ATP, and CP levels during exercise after physical training in man. *J Appl Physiol* 33: 199-203.

Kasch, F.W., J.L. Boyer, S.P. Van Camp, L.S. Verity, and J.P. Wallace. 1990. The effect of physical activity and inactivity on aerobic power in older men (a longitudinal study). *Physician Sportsmed* 18(4): 73-83.

Keizer H.A., H. Kuipers, J. de Haan, G.M. Janssen, E. Beckers, L. Habets, G. van Kranenburg, and P. Geurten. 1987. Effect of a 3-month endurance training program on metabolic and multiple hormonal responses to exercise. *Int J Sports Med* 8;Suppl 3: 154-60.

Kemppainen, P., P. Paalasmaa, A. Pertovaara, A. Alila, and G. Johansson. 1990. Desamethasone attenuates exercise-induced dental analgesia in man. *Brain Res* 519: 329-332.

Kemppainen, P., A. Pertovaara, T. Huopaniemi, G. Johansson, and S.L. Karonen. 1985. Modification of dental pain and cutaneous thermal sensitivity by physical exercise in man. *Brain Res* 360: 33-44.

Kjaer, M., P.A. Farrell, N.J. Christensen, and H. Galbo. 1986. Increased epinephrine response and inaccurate glucoregulation in exercising athletes. *J Appl Physiol* 61: 1693-1700.

Kohrt, W.M., M.T. Malley, A.R. Coggan, R.J. Spina, T. Ogawa, A.A. Ehsani, R.E. Bourey, W.H. Martin III, and J.O. Holloszy. 1991. Effects of gender, age and fitness level on response of VO_2max to training in 60-71 yr olds. *J Appl Physiol* 71: 2004-2011.

Kohrt, W.M., D.B. Snead, E. Slatopolsky, and S.J. Birge, Jr. 1995. Additive effects of weight-bearing exercise and estrogen on bone mineral density in older women. *J Bone Miner Res* 10: 1303-1311.

Koltyn, K.F., A.W. Garvin, R.L. Gardiner, and T.F. Nelson. 1996. Perception of pain following aerobic exercise. *Med Sci Sports Exerc* 28: 1418-1421.

Kramer, A.F., S. Hahn, N.J. Cohen, M.T. Banich, E. McAuley, C.R. Harrison, J. Chason, E. Vakil, L. Bardell, R.A. Boileau, and A. Colcombe. 1999. Ageing, fitness and neurocognitive function. *Nature* 400(6743): 418-419.

LaFontaine, T.P., B.R. Londeree, and W.K. Spath. 1981. The maximal steady state versus selected running events. *Med Sci Sports Exerc* 13: 190-192.

Landry, F., C. Bouchard, and J. Dumesnil. 1985. Cardiac dimension changes with endurance training. *JAMA* 254: 77-80.

Lavie, C.J., and R.V. Milani. 1995. Effects of cardiac rehabilitation program on exercise capacity, coronary risk factors, behavioral characteristics, and quality of life in a large elderly cohort. *Am J Cardiol* 76: 177-179.

Lavie, C.J., R.V. Milani, and A.B. Littman. 1993. Benefits of cardiac rehabilitation and exercise training in secondary coronary prevention in the elderly. *J Am Coll Cardiol* 22: 678-683.

Londeree, B.R. 1997. Effects of training on lactate/ventilatory thresholds: A meta-analysis. *Med Sci Sports Exerc* 29: 837-843.

Lucia, A., J. Hoyos, J. Pardo, and J.L.Chicharro. 2000. Metabolic and neuromuscular adaptations to endurance training in professional cyclists: A longitudinal study. *Jpn J Physiol* 50(3): 381-388.

MacLean, P.S., D. Zheng, and G.L. Dohm. 2000. Muscle glucose transporter (GLUT4) gene expression during exercise. *Exerc Sport Sci Rev* 28: 148-152.

Maes, H.H., G.P. Beunen, R.F. Vlietinck, M.C. Neale, M. Thomis, B. Vanden Eynde, R. Lysens, J. Simons, C. Derom, and R. Derom. 1996. Inheritance of physical fitness in 10-yr-old twins and their parents. *Med Sci Sports Exerc* 28: 1479-1491.

Magel, J.R., G.F. Foglia, W.D. McArdle, B. Gutin, G.S. Pechar, and F.I. Katch. 1975. Specificity of swim training on maximal oxygen uptake. *J Appl Physiol* 38: 151-155.

Magel, J.R., W.D. McArdle, M. Toner, and D.J. Delio. 1978. Metabolic and cardiovascular adjustment to arm training. *J Appl Physiol* 45: 75-79.

Makrides, L., G.J.F. Heigenhauser, and N.L. Jones. 1990. High-intensity endurance training in 20- to 30- and 60- to 70-yr-old healthy men. *J Appl Physiol* 69: 1792-1798.

Margulies, J.Y., A. Simkin, I. Leichter, A. Bivas, R. Steinberg, M. Giladi, M. Stein, H. Kashtan, and C. Milgrom. 1986. Effect of intense physical activity on the bone-mineral content in the lower limbs of young adults. *J Bone Joint Surg Am* 68: 1090-1093.

Markoff, R.A., P. Ryan, and T. Young. 1982. Endorphins and mood changes in long-distance running. *Med Sci Sports Exerc* 14: 11-15.

Martin, B.J., K.E. Sparks, C.W. Zwillich, and J.V. Weil. 1979. Low exercise ventilation in endurance athletes. *Med Sci Sports* 11: 181-185.

McArdle, W.D., F.I Katch, and V.L. Katch. 2001. *Exercise physiology: Energy, nutrition, and human performance*. 5th ed. Philadelphia: Lippincott Williams & Wilkins.

McCain, G.A., D.A. Bell, F.M. Mai, and P.D. Halliday. 1988. A controlled study of the effects of a supervised cardiovascular fitness training program on the manifestations of primary fibromyalgia. *Arthritis Rheum* 31: 1135-1141.

McCann, L., and D.S. Holmes. 1984. Influence of aerobic exercise on depression. *J Pers Soc Psychol* 46: 1142-1147.

McGuire, D.K., B.D. Levine, J.W. Williamson, P.G. Snell, G. Blumqvist, B. Saltin, and J.H. Mitchell. 2001. A 30-year follow-up of the Dallas bed rest and training study. II. Effect of age on cardiovascular adaptation to exercise training. *Circulation* 104: 1358-1366.

Melin, B., J.P. Eclache, G. Geelen, G. Annat, A.M. Allevard, E. Jarsaillon, A. Zebidi, J.J. Legros, and C. Gharib. 1980. Plasma AVP, neurophysin, renin activity, and aldosterone during submaximal exercise performed until exhaustion in trained and untrained men. *Eur J Appl Physiol* 44: 141-151.

Meredith, C.N., W.R. Frontera, E.C. Fisher, V.A. Hughes, J.C. Herland, J. Edwards, and W.J. Evans. 1989. Peripheral effects of endurance training in young and old subjects. *J Appl Physiol* 66: 2844-2849.

Metzger, J.M., and E.A. Stein. 1984. Beta-endorphin and sprint training. *Life Sci* 34: 1541-1547.

Meyer, T., and A. Broocks. 2000. Therapeutic impact of exercise on psychiatric diseases: Guidelines for exercise testing and prescription. *Sports Med* 30(4): 269-79.

Mikines, K.J., F. Dela, B. Sonne, P.A. Farrell, E.A. Richter, and H. Galbo. 1987. Insulin action and secretion in man. Effects of different levels of physical activity. *Can J Sport Sci* 12 (Suppl. 1): 113-116.

Mikines, K.J., B. Sonne, P.A. Farrell, B. Tronier, and H. Galbo. 1988. Effect of physical exercise on sensitivity and responsiveness to insulin in man. *Am J Physiol* 17: E248-E259.

Mitchell, J.H., C. Tate, P. Raven, F. Cobb, W. Kraus, R. Moreadith, M. O'Toole, B. Saltin, and N. Wenger. 1992. Acute responses and chronic adaptations to exercise in women. *Med Sci Sports Exerc* 24: S258-S265.

Miyachi, M., H. Tanaka, K. Yamamoto, A. Yoshioka, K. Takahashi, and S. Onodera. 2001. Effects of one-legged endurance training on femoral arterial and venous size in healthy humans. *J Appl Physiol* 90: 2439-2444.

Moldofsky, H., and P. Scarisbrick. 1976. Induction of neurasthetic musculoskeletal pain syndrome by selective sleep stage deprivation. *Psychosom Med* 38: 35-44.

Mole, P.A., L.B. Oscai, and J.O. Holloszy. 1971. Adaptation of muscle to exercise. Increase in levels of palmityl CoA synthetase, carnitine palmityltransferase, and palmityl CoA dehydrogenase, and in the capacity to oxidize fatty acids. *J Clin Invest* 50: 2323-2330.

Morgan, W.P. 1979. Anxiety reduction following acute physical activity. *Psychiatr Ann* 9: 36-45.

Morrison, D.A., T.W. Boyden, R.W. Pamenter, B.J. Freund, W.A. Stini, R. Harrington, and J.H. Wilmore. 1986. Effects of aerobic training on exercise tolerance and echocardiographic dimensions in untrained postmenopausal women. *Am Heart J* 112: 561-567.

Mougin, C., A. Baulay, M.T. Henriet, D. Haton, M.C. Jacquier, D. Turnill, S. Berthelay, and R.C. Gaillard. 1987. Assessment of plasma opioid *Peptides*, beta-endorphin and met-enkephalin, at the end of an international Nordic ski race. *Eur J Appl Physiol* 56: 281-286.

Nadel, E.R., K.B. Pandolf, M.F. Roberts, and J.A.J. Stolwijk. 1974. Mechanisms of thermal acclimatization to exercise and heat. *J Appl Physiol* 37: 515-520.

Nichols, D.S., and T.M. Glenn. 1994. Effects of aerobic exercise on pain perception, affect, and level of disability in individuals with fibromyalgia. *Phys Ther* 74: 327-332.

NIH Consensus Development Panel on Physical Activity and Cardiovascular Health. 1996. Physical activity and cardiovascular health. *JAMA* 276: 241-246.

O'Connor, P.J., and S.D. Youngstedt. 1995. Influence of exercise on human sleep. *Exerc Sport Sci Rev* 23: 105-134.

Olausson, B., E. Eriksson, L. Ellmarker, B. Rydenhag, B.-C. Shyu, and S.A. Anderson. 1986. Effects of naloxone on dental pain threshold following muscle exercise and low frequency transcutaneous nerve stimulation: A comparative study in man. *Acta Physiol Scand* 126: 299-305.

Pandolf, K.B., B.S. Cadarette, M.N. Sawka, A.J. Young, and R.P. Francesconi. 1988. Thermoregulatory responses of middle-aged men and young men during dry heat acclimation. *J Appl Physiol* 65: 65-71.

Panenic, R., and P.F. Gardiner. 1998. The case for adaptability of the neuromuscular junction to endurance exercise training. *Can J Appl Physiol* 23: 339-360.

Peronnet, F., J. Cleroux, H. Perrault, D. Cousineau, J. de Champlain, and R. Nadeau. 1981. Plasma norepinephrine responses to exercise before and after training in humans. *J Appl Physiol* 51: 812-815.

Pertovaara, A., T. Huopaniemi, A. Virtanen, and G. Johansson. 1984. The influence of exercise on dental pain thresholds and the release of stress hormones. *Physiol Behav* 33: 923-926.

Pérusse, L., J. Gagnon, M.A. Province, D.C. Rao, J.H. Wilmore, A.S. Leon, C. Bouchard, and J.S. Skinner. 2001. Familial aggregation of submaximal aerobic performance in the HERITAGE family study. *Med Sci Sports Exerc* 33: 597-604.

Pérusse, L., T. Rankinen, R. Rauramaa, M.A. Rivera, B. Wolfarth, and C. Bouchard. 2003. The human gene map for performance and health-related fitness phenotypes: The 2002 update. *Med Sci Sports Exerc* 35: 1248-1264.

Pierce, E.F.A., A. Weltman, R.L. Seip, and D. Snead. 1990. Effects of training specificity on the lactate threshold and O_2 peak. *Int J Sports Med* 11: 267-272.

Poehlman, E.T., C.L. Melby, and M.I. Goran. 1991. The impact of exercise and diet restrictions on daily energy expenditure. *Sports Med* 11: 78-101.

Pollock, M.L. 1977. Submaximal and maximal working capacity of elite distance runners. Part I: Cardiorespiratory aspects. *Ann NY Acad Sci* 301: 310-322.

Pollock, M.L., H.S. Miller, A.C. Linnerud, E. Laughridge, E. Coleman, and E. Alexander. 1974. Arm pedaling as an endurance training regimen for the disabled. *Arch Phys Med Rehabil* 55: 418-424.

Powers, S.K., and E.T. Howley. 1997. *Exercise physiology: Theory and application to fitness and performance*. 3rd ed. Madison, WI: Brown and Benchmark Publishers.

Prior, J.C., L. Jensen, B.H. Yuen, H. Higgins, and L. Brownlie. 1981. Prolactin changes with exercise vary with breast motion: Analysis of running versus cycling. *Fertil Steril* 36: 268.

Prior, B.M., P.G. Lloyd, H.T. Yang, and R. L. Terjung. 2003. Exercise-induced vascular remodeling. *Exerc Sport Sci Rev* 31(1): 26-33.

Prud'Homme, D., C. Bouchard, C. Leblanc, L.F. Landry, and E. Fontaine. 1984. Sensitivity of maximal aerobic power to training is genotype-dependent. *Med Sci Sports Exerc* 16: 489-493.

Reeves, T.J., and L.T. Sheffield. 1971. The influence of age and athletic training on maximal heart rate during exercise. In *Coronary heart disease and physical fitness,* ed. O. Andree-Larsen and R.O. Malmborg, 209-216. Copenhagen: Munksgaard.

Rerych, S.K., P.M. Scholz, D.C. Sabiston Jr., and R.H. Jones. 1980. Effects of exercise training on left ventricular function in normal subjects: A longitudinal study by radionuclide angiography. *Am J Cardiol* 45: 244-252.

Rogers, M.A., J. Hagberg, S.H. Martin, A.A. Eksani, and J.O. Holloszy. 1990. Decline in $\dot{V}O_2$max with aging in masters athletes and sedentary men. *J Appl Physiol* 68: 2195-2199.

Rowell, L.B. 1974. Human cardiovascular adjustments to exercise and thermal stress. *Physiol Rev* 54: 75-159.

Rowell, L.B. 1986. *Human circulation-regulation during physical stress*. New York: Oxford University Press.

Sale, D.G. 1987. Influence of exercise and training on motor units activation. *Exerc Sport Sci Rev* 15: 95-151.

Saltin, B. 1969. Physiological effects of physical conditioning. *Med Sci Sports* 1: 50-56.

Saltin, B., and P.-O. Åstrand. 1967. Maximal oxygen uptake in athletes. *J Appl Physiol* 23: 353-358.

Saltin, B., L.H. Hartley, A. Kilbom, and I. Åstrand. 1969. Physical training in sedentary middle-aged and older men. II. Oxygen uptake, heart rate, and blood lactate concentration at submaximal and maximal exercise. *Scand J Clin Lab Invest* 24: 323-334.

Saltin, B., K. Nazar, D.L. Costill, E. Stein, E. Jansson, B. Essen, and P.D. Gollnick. 1976. The nature of the training response: Peripheral and central adaptations to one-legged exercise. *Acta Physiol Scand* 96: 289-305.

Sawka, M.N., V.A. Convertino, E.R. Eichner, S.M. Schnieder, and A.J. Young. 2000. Blood volume: Importance and adaptations to exercise training, environmental stresses, and trauma/sickness. *Med Sci Sports Exerc* 32: 332-348.

Schantz, P., J. Henriksson, and E. Jansson. 1983. Adaptations of human skeletal muscle to endurance training of long duration. *Clin Physiol* 3: 141-151.

Seals, D.R., J.M. Hagberg, B.F. Hurley, A.A. Ehsani, and J.O. Holloszy. 1984. Endurance training in older men and women. I. Cardiovascular responses to exercise. *J Appl Physiol* 57: 1024-1029.

Sforzo, G.A., T.F. Seeger, C.B. Pert, A. Pert, and C.O. Cotson. 1986. In vivo opioid receptor occupation in the rat brain following exercise. *Med Sci Sports Exerc* 18: 380-384.

Sharkey, B.J. 1970. Intensity and duration of training and the development of cardiorespiratory endurance. *Med Sci Sports* 2: 197-202.

Sheldahl, L.M., F.E. Tristani, J.E. Hastings, R.B. Wenzler, and S.G. Levandoski. 1993. Comparison of adaptations and compliance to exercise training between middle-aged and older men. *J Am Geriatr Soc* 41: 795-801.

Shephard, R.J. 1968. Intensity, duration, and frequency of exercise as determinants of the response to a training regime. *Int Z Angew Physiol* 26: 272-278.

Shephard, R.J. 1991. Benefits of sport and physical activity for the disabled: Implications for the individual and for society. *Scand J Rehab Med* 23: 51-59.

Shephard, R.J. 1993. Exercise and aging: Extending independence in older adults. *Geriatrics* 48(5): 61-64.

Shephard, R.J., and K.H. Sidney. 1975. Effects of physical exertion on plasma GH and cortisol levels in human subjects. *Exerc Sport Sci Rev* 3: 1-30.

Simons, A., C.R. McGowan, L.H. Epstein, D.J. Kuper, and R.J. Robertson. 1985. Exercise as a treatment for depression: An update. *Clin Psychol Rev* 5: 553-568.

Sjodin, B., and I. Jacobs. 1981. Onset of blood lactate accumulation and marathon running performance. *Int J Sports Med* 2: 23-26.

Sonstroem, R.J. 1984. Exercise and self-esteem. *Exerc Sport Sci Rev* 12: 123-155.

Spina, R.J. 1999. Cardiovascular adaptations to endurance exercise training in older men and women. *Exerc Sport Sci Rev* 27: 317-332.

Spriet, L.L. 2002. Regulation of skeletal muscle fat oxidation during exercise in humans. *Med Sci Sports Exerc* 34: 1477-1484.

Strawbridge, W.J., R.D. Cohen, S.J. Shema, and G.A. Kaplan. 1996. Successful aging: Predictors and associated activities. *Am J Epidemiol* 144: 135-141.

Sundet, J.M., P. Magnus, and K. Tambs. 1994. The heritability of maximal aerobic power: A study of Norwegian twins. *Scand J Med Sci Sports* 4: 181-185.

Surgeon General of the Public Health Service. 1996. *Surgeon General's report on physical activity and health* (S/N 017-023-00196-5).

Sutton, J.R. 1978. Hormonal and metabolic responses to exercise in subjects of high and low work capacities. *Med Sci Sports Exerc* 10: 1-6.

Sutton, J.R., J.D. Young, L. Lazarus, J.B. Hickie, and J. Maksvytis. 1969. The hormonal response to physical exercise. *Aust Ann Med* 18: 84-90.

Terrados, N., and R.J. Maughan. 1995. Exercise in the heat: Strategies to minimize the adverse effects on performance. *J Sports Sci* 13: S55-S62.

Tipton, C.M., R.D. Matthes, J.A. Maynard, and R.A. Carey. 1975. The influence of physical activity on ligaments and tendons. *Med Sci Sports* 7: 165-175.

Ulrich, C.M., C.C. Georgiou, C.M. Snow-Harter, and D.E. Gillis. 1996. Bone mineral density in mother-daughter pairs: Relations to lifetime exercise, lifetime milk consumption, and calcium supplements. *Am J Clin Nutr* 63: 72-79.

van Boxtel, M.P., F.G. Paas, P.J. Houx, J.J. Adam, J.C. Teeken, and J. Jolles. 1997. Aerobic capacity and cognitive performance in a cross-sectional aging study. *Med Sci Sports Exerc* 29(10): 1357-65.

Vander, A.J., J.H. Sherman, and D.S. Luciano. 1985. *Human physiology: The mechanisms of body function*. 4th ed. New York: McGraw-Hill.

Vokac, Z., and K. Rodahl. 1977. Maximal aerobic power and circulatory strain in Eskimo hunters in Greenland. *Nordic Council for Arctic Medical Research Report* no. 1.

Washburn, R.A., and D.R. Seals. 1984. Peak oxygen uptake during arm cranking for men and women. *J Appl Physiol* 56: 954-957.

Williams, J.A., J. Wagner, R. Wasnich, and L. Heilbrun. 1984. The effect of long distance running upon appendicular bone mineral content. *Med Sci Sports Exerc* 16: 223-227.

Wilmore, J.H., and D.L. Costill. 1999. *Physiology of sport and exercise*. 2nd ed. Champaign: Human Kinetics.

Winder, W.W., R.C. Hickson, J.M. Hagberg, A.A. Ehsani, and J.A. McLane. 1979. Training-induced changes in hormonal and metabolic responses to submaximal exercise. *J Appl Physiol* 46: 766-771.

Wyndham, C.H. 1973. The physiology of exercise under heat stress. *Annu Rev Physiol* 35: 193-220.

Young, D.R., K.H. Masaki, and J.D. Curb. 1995. Associations of physical activity with performance-based and self-reported physical functioning in older men: The Honolulu Heart Program. *J Am Geriatr Soc* 43: 845-854.

Zavorsky, G.S. 2000. Evidence and possible mechanism of altered maximum heart rate with endurance training and tapering. *Sports Med* 29(1): 13-26.

Zeni, A.I., M.D. Hoffman, and P.S. Clifford. 1996. Energy expenditure with indoor exercise machines. *JAMA* 275: 1424-1427.

Zhang, L.-F., J. Zheng, S.-Y. Wang, Z.-Y. Zhang, and C. Liu. 1999. Effect of aerobic training on orthostatic tolerance, circulatory response, and heart rate dynamics. *Aviat Space Environ Med* 70: 975-982.

CHAPTER 3

Ades, P.A., P.D. Savage, E.M. Cress, M. Brochu, M.N. Lee, and E.T. Poehlman. 2003. Resistance training of physical performance in disabled older cardiac patients. *Med Sci Sports Exerc* 35: 1265-1270.

Akeson, W.H., D. Amiel, G.L. Mechanic, S.L. Woo, F.L. Harwood, and M.L. Hamer. 1977. Collagen cross linking adhesions in joint contractures: Changes in the reducible cross-links in periarticular connective tissue collagen after nine weeks of immobilization. *Connective Tissue Res* 5: 15-19.

Akima, H., Y. Kawakami, K. Kubo, C. Sekiguchi, H. Ohshima, A. Miyamoto, and T. Fukunaga. 2000. Effect of short-duration spaceflight on thigh and leg muscle volume. *Med Sci Sports Exerc* 32: 1743-1747.

Alfredson H., T. Peitila, P. Jonsson, and R. Lorentzon. 1998. Heavy-load eccentric calf muscle training for the treatment of chronic Achilles tendinosis. *Am J Sports Med* 26(3): 360-366.

Alway, S.E., P.K. Winchester, M.E. Davis, and W.J. Gonyea. 1989. Regionalized adaptations and muscle fiber proliferation in stretch-induced enlargement. *J Appl Physiol* 66: 771-781.

Antonio, J., and W.J. Gonyea. 1993. Skeletal muscle fiber hyperplasia. *Med Sci Sports Exerc* 25: 1333-1345.

Åstrand, P-O., K. Rodahl, H.A. Dahl, and S.B. Stromme. 2003. *Textbook of work physiology: Physiological bases of exercise*, chapters 3 and 8. Champaign, IL: Human Kinetics.

Ayalon, J., A. Simkin, I. Leichter, and S. Raifmann. 1987. Dynamic bone loading exercises for postmenopausal women: Effect on density of distal radius. *Arch Phys Med Rehabil* 68: 280-283.

Baldwin, K.M., T.P. White, S.B. Arnaud, V.R. Edgerton, W.J. Kraemer, R. Kram, D. Raab-Cullen, and C.M. Snow. 1996. Musculoskeletal adaptations to weightlessness and development of counter measures. *Med Sci Sports Exerc* 10: 1247-1253.

Bean, J., S. Herman, D.K. Kiely, D. Callahan, K. Mizer, W. Frontera, and R.A. Fielding. 2002. Weighted stair climbing in mobility-limited older people: A pilot study. *J Am Geriatr Soc* 50: 663-670.

Berg, H.E., L. Larsson, and P.A. Tesch. 1997. Lower limb skeletal muscle function after 6 wk of bed rest. *J Appl Physiol* 82: 182-188.

Bloomfield, S.A. 1997. Changes in musculoskeletal structure and function with prolonged bed rest. *Med Sci Sports Exerc* 29: 197-206.

Booth, S.W. 1977. Time course of muscular atrophy during immobilization of hind limbs of rats. *J Appl Physiol* 43: 656-661.

Buckwalter, J.A., S.L. Woo, V. Goldberg, E.C. Hadley, F. Booth, T.R. Oegema, and D.R. Eyre. 1993. Current concepts review: Soft-tissue aging and musculoskeletal function. *J Bone Joint Surg* 75A: 1533-1547.

Caiozzo, V.J., and S. Green. 2002. Breakout session: Muscle mechanics. *Clin Orthop* 1(403) Suppl.: S77-S80.

Clarkson, P.M., and M.E. Dedrick. 1988. Exercise-induced muscle damage, repair, and adaptation in old and young subjects. *J Gerontol* 43: M91-96.

Convertino, V.A., S.A. Bloomfield, and J.E. Greenleaf. 1997. An overview of the issues: Physiological effects of bed rest and restricted physical activity. *Med Sci Sports Exerc* 29: 187-190.

Cook J.L., K.M. Khan, N. Maffulli, and C. Purdam. 2000. Overuse tendinosis, not tendonitis: Part 2: Applying the new approach to patellar tendinopathy. *Phys Sportsmed* 28: 31-46.

Crowthers, G.J., and R.K. Gronka. 2002. Fiber recruitment affects oxidative recovery measurements of human muscle in vivo. *Med Sci Sports Exerc* 34: 1733-1737.

Darr, K.C., and E. Schultz. 1987. Exercise-induced satellite cell activation in growing and mature skeletal muscle. *J Appl Physiol* 63: 1816-1821.

Delitto, A., and A.J. Robinson. 1989. Electrical stimulation of muscle: Techniques and applications. In *Clinical electrophysiology: Electrotherapy and electrophysiologic testing,* ed. L. Snyder-Mackler and A.J. Robinson, 95-135. Baltimore: Williams & Wilkins.

DeLorme, T.L., and A.L. Watkins. 1951. *Progressive resistance exercise.* New York: Appleton-Century-Croft.

Deschenes, M.R., C.M. Maresh, J.F. Crivello, I.E. Armstrong, W.J. Kraemer, and J. Covault. 1993. The effects of exercise training of different intensities on neuromuscular junction morphology. *J Neurocytol* 22: 603-615.

Dishman, R.K. 1988. *Exercise adherence: Its impact on public health.* Champaign, IL: Human Kinetics.

Dook, J.E., C. James, N.K. Henderson, and R.I. Price. 1997. Exercise and bone mineral density in mature female athletes. *Med Sci Sports Exerc* 29: 291-296.

Edstrom, L., and L. Larsson. 1987. Effects of age on contractile and enzyme-histochemical properties of fast- and slow-twitch single motor units in the rat. *J Physiol (Lond)* 392: 129-145.

Enoka, R.M. 1994. Chronic Adaptations. In *Neuromechanical basis of kinesiology.* 2nd ed., ed. R.M. Enoka, 303-349. Champaign, IL: Human Kinetics.

Ettinger, W.H., R. Burns, S.P. Messier. W. Applegate, W.J. Rejeski, T. Morgan, S. Shumaker, M.J. O'Toole, J. Monu, and T. Craven. 1997. A randomized trial comparing aerobic exercise and resistance exercise with a health education program in older adults with knee osteoarthritis. The Fitness Arthritis and Seniors Trials (FAST). *JAMA* 277: 25-31.

Evans, W.J. 1995. Effects of exercise on body composition and functional capacity of the elderly. *J Gerontol A Biol Sci Med Sci* 50A (Special issue): 147-150.

Fahrer, H., H.U. Rentsch, N.J. Gerber, C. Beyeler, C.W. Hess, and B. Grunig. 1988. Knee effusion and reflex inhibition of the quadriceps. *J Bone Joint Surg (Br)* 70B: 635-638.

Falkel, J.E., and D.J. Cipriani. 1996. Physiologic principles of resistance training and rehabilitation. In *Athletic injuries and rehabilitation,* ed. J.E. Zachazewski, D.J. Magee, and W.S. Quillen, 206-226. Philadelphia: W.B. Saunders.

Fiatarone, M.A., N.D. Ryan, K.M. Clements, G.R. Solares, M.E. Nelson, S.B. Roberts, J.J. Kehayias, L.A. Lipsitz, and W.J. Evans. 1994. Exercise training and nutritional supplementation for physical frailty in very elderly people. *N Engl J Med* 330: 1769-1775.

Gonyea, W. 1980. Role of exercise in inducing increases in skeletal muscle fiber number. *J Appl Physiol* 48: 421-426.

Gossman, M.E., S.A. Sahrmann, and S.J. Rose. 1982. Review of length associated changes in muscle: Experimental evidence and clinical implications. *Phys Ther* 62: 1799-1808.

Haggmark, T., E. Jansson, and E. Erikson. 1981. Fibre type area, metabolic potential of the thigh muscle in man after knee surgery and immobilization in man. *Int J Sports Med* 2: 12-17.

Hakkinen, K., and P.V. Komi. 1983. Electromyographic changes during strength training and detraining. *Med Sci Sports Exerc* 15: 455-460.

Hall-Craggs, E.C.B. 1970. The longitudinal division of fibres in overloaded rat skeletal muscle. *J Anat* 107: 459-470.

Hardy, M.A. 1989. The biology of scar formation. *Phys Ther* 69: 1014-1024.

Harris, B.A., and M.P. Watkins. 1993. Muscle performance: Principles and general theory. In *Muscle strength,* ed. K. Harms-Ringdahl, 5-18. Edinburgh: Churchill Livingstone.

Heinonen, A., P. Kannus, H. Sievanen, P. Oja, M. Pasanen, M. Rinne, K. Uusi-Rafi, and I. Vuori. 1996. Randomized controlled trial of effect of high impact exercise on selected risk factors for osteoporotic fractures. *Lancet* 348: 1343-1347.

Henneman, E., and C.B. Olson. 1965. Relations between structure and function in the design of skeletal muscle. *J Neurophysiol* 28: 581-598.

Henneman, E., G. Somjen, and D.O. Carpenter. 1965. Functional significance of cell size in spinal motoneurons. *J Neurophysiol* 28: 560-598.

Holmich, P., P. Uhrskou, L. Ulnits, I.L. Kanstrup, M.B. Nielsen, A.M. Bjerg, and K. Krogsgaard. 1999. Effectiveness of active physical training as treatment for long-standing adductor-related groin pain in athletes: Randomized trial. *Lancet* 353(9151): 439-443.

Hopp, J.F. 1993. Effects of age and resistance training on skeletal muscle: A review. *Phys Ther* 73: 361-373.

Jette, A.M., B.A. Harris, L. Sleeper, M.E. Lachman, D. Heislein, M. Giorgetti, and C. Levenson. 1996. A home-based exercise program for nondisabled older adults. *J Am Geriatr Soc* 44: 644-649.

Jette, A.M., M. Lachman, M.M. Giorgetti, S.F. Assmann, B.A. Harris, C. Levenson, M. Wernick, and D. Krebs. 1999. Exercise—it's never too late: The strong-for-life program. *Am J Public Health* 89(1): 66-72.

Jones, K.D., S.R. Clark, and R.M. Bennett. 2002. Prescribing exercise for people with fibromyalgia. *AACN Clin Issues* 13: 277-293.

Khan, K.M., J.L. Cook, J.E. Taunton, and F. Bonar. 2000. Overuse tendinosis, not tendonitis. Part 1: A new paradigm for a difficult clinical problem. *Phys Sportsmed* 28: 38-48.

King, A.C., R.F. Oman, G.S. Brassington, D.L. Bliwise, and W.L. Haskell. 1997. Moderate-intensity exercise and self-rated quality of sleep in older adults. *JAMA* 277: 32-37.

Knuttgen, H.G., ed. 1976. *Neuromuscular mechanisms for therapeutic and conditioning exercise,* 97-118. Baltimore: University Park Press.

Komi, P.V. 1986. Training of muscle strength and power: Interaction of neuromotoric, hypertrophic and mechanical factors. *Int J Sports Med* 7(Suppl.): 10-15.

Kraemer, W.J., S.J. Fleck, and W.J. Evans. 1996. Strength and power training: Physiologic mechanisms of adaptation. *Exerc Sport Sci* 46: 363-397.

Krebs, D.E. 1990. Biofeedback in therapeutic exercise. In *Therapeutic exercise,* ed. J.V. Basmajian and S. L. Wolfe, 109-124. Baltimore: Williams & Wilkins.

LaPierre, A., G. Ironson, M.H. Antoni, N. Schneiderman, N. Klimas, and M.A. Fletcher. 1994. Exercise and psychoneuroimmunology. *Med Sci Sports Exerc* 26: 182-190.

Leon, A.S. 1985. Physical activities and coronary heart disease. *Med Clin N Am* 69: 3-17.

Lord, S.R., and S. Castell. 1994. Physical activity program for older persons: Effect on balance, strength, neuromuscular control and reaction time. *Arch Phys Med Rehabil* 75: 648-652.

Martin, W.H. 1996. Effects of acute and chronic exercise on fat metabolism. *Exerc Sport Sci Rev* 24: 203-231.

Nelson, M.E., M.A. Fiatarone, C.M. Morganti, I. Trice, R.A. Greenberg, and W.J. Evans. 1994. Effects of high intensity strength training on multiple risk factors for osteoporotic fractures: A randomized controlled trial. *JAMA* 272: 1909-1914.

Newham, D. F. 1993. Eccentric muscle activity in theory and practice. In *Muscle strength*, ed. K. Harms-Ringdahl, 61-81. Edinburgh: Churchill Livingstone.

Nichols, J.F., D.K. Omizo, K.K. Peterson, and K.P. Nelson. 1993. Efficacy of heavy-resistance training for active women over sixty: Muscular strength, body composition and program adherence. *J Am Geriatr Soc* 41: 205-210.

Oatis, C.A. 2004. Biomechanics of skeletal muscle. In *Kinesiology: The mechanics and pathomechanics of human movement,* ed. C.A. Oatis, 44-65. Philadelphia: Lippincott Williams & Wilkins.

Rose, D.L., S.F. Radzyminski, and R.R. Beatty. 1957. Effect of brief maximal exercise on the strength of the quadriceps femoris. *Arch Phys Med Rehabil* 33: 157-164.

Rowbottom, D.G., and K.J. Green. 2000. Acute exercise effects on the immune system. *Med Sci Sports Exerc* 32: S396-S405.

Sale, D.G. 1988. Neural adaptation to resistance training. *Med Sci Sports Exerc* 20: S135-145.

Saltin, B., J. Henriksson, and E. Nygaard. 1977. Fibre types and metabolic potentials in sedentary man and endurance runners. *Ann NY Acad Sci* 301: 3-29.

Sargeant, A.J., C.T. Davies, and R.H. Edwards. 1977. Structural and functional changes after disuse of human muscle. *Clin Sci Mol Med* 52: 337-342.

Shoepe, T.C., J.E. Stelzer, D.P. Garner, and J.J. Widrick. 2003. Functional adaptability of muscle fibers to long-term resistance exercise. *Med Sci Sports Exerc* 35: 944-951.

Smith, R., and O.M. Rutherford. 1993. Spine and total body bone mineral density and serum testosterone levels in male athletes. *Eur J Appl Physiol* 67: 330-334.

Spector, S.A., C.P. Simard, and M. Fournier. 1982. Architectural alterations of the rat hind-limb skeletal muscles immobilized at different lengths. *Exp Neurol* 76: 94-110.

Spencer, J.D., K.C. Hayes, and I.J. Alexander. 1984. Knee joint effusion and quadriceps reflex inhibition in man. *Arch Phys Med Rehabil* 65: 171-177.

Starkey, D.B., M.L. Pollock, Y. Ishida, M.A. Welch, W.F. Brechue, J.E. Graves, and M.S. Feigenbaum. 1996. Effect of resistance training volume on strength and muscle thickness. *Med Sci Sports Exerc* 28: 1311-1320.

Staron, R.S., D.L. Karapondo, W.J. Kraemer, A.C. Fry, S.E. Gordon, J.E. Falkel, F.C. Hagerman, and R.S. Hikida. 1994. Skeletal muscle adaptations during the early phase of heavy resistance training in men and women. *J Appl Physiol* 76: 1247-1255.

Stevens, J.E., R.L. Mizner, and L. Snyder-Mackler. 2003. Quadriceps strength and volitional activation before and after total knee arthroplasty for osteoarthritis. *J Orthop Res* 21: 775-779.

Stone, M.H. 1988. Implications for connective tissue and bone alterations resulting from resistance exercise training. *Med Sci Sports Exerc* 20(Suppl.): 162-168.

St. Pierre, D., and P.F. Gardner. 1987. The effect of immobilization and exercise on muscle function: A review. *Physiotherapy Canada* 39: 24-35.

Sullivan, P.E., and P.D. Markos. 1995. *Clinical decision making in therapeutic exercise*. Norwalk, CT: Appleton & Lange.

Taaffe, D.R., C. Duret, S. Wheeler, and R. Marcus. 1999. Once-weekly resistance exercise improves muscle strength and neuromuscular performance in older adults. *J Am Geriatr Soc* 47: 1208-1214.

Tardieu, C., J.C. Tabary, C. Tabary, and G. Tardieu. 1982. Adaptation of connective tissue length to immobilization in the lengthened and shortened positions in the cat soleus muscle. *J Physiol Paris* 78: 214-220.

Tardieu, C., J.C. Tabary, and G. Tardieu. 1980. Adaptation of sarcomere number to the length imposed on the muscle. *Advances in Physiologic Science* 24: 99-114.

Tesch, P.A., and L. Larsson. 1982. Muscle hypertrophy in bodybuilders. *Eur J Appl Physiol* 49: 301-306.

Thompson, L.V. 1994. Effects of age and training on skeletal muscle physiology and performance. *Phys Ther* 74: 71-84.

Thompson, L.V. 2002. Skeletal muscle adaptations with age, inactivity and therapeutic exercise. *J Orthop Sports Phys Ther* 32: 44-57.

Thorstensson, A., G. Grimby, and J. Karlsson. 1976. Force-velocity relations and fibre composition in human extensor muscles. *J Appl Physiol* 40: 12-16.

Treuth, M.S., G.R. Hunter, T. Kekes-Szabo, R.L. Weinsier, M.I. Goran, and L. Berland. 1995. Reduction in intra-abdominal adipose tissue after strength training in older women. *J Appl Physiol* 78: 1425-1431.

Wenger, H.A., P.F. McFadyen, and R.A. McFadyen. 1996. Physiological principles of conditioning. In *Athletic injuries in rehabilitation,* eds. J.E. Zachazewski, D.J. Magee, and W.S. Quillen. Philadelphia: W.B. Saunders 189-205.

Williams, P., and G. Goldspink. 1984. Connective tissue changes in immobilized muscle. *J Anat* 138: 343-350.

Young, A., M. Stokes, and J. Iles. 1987. Effects of joint pathology on muscle. *Clin Orthop* 219: 21-27.

Zinovieff, A.N. 1951. Heavy resistance exercise: The "Oxford technique". *Br J Phys Med* 14: 129-132.

CHAPTER 4

Al-Rawi, Z.S., A.J. Al-Aszawi, and T. Al-Chalabi. 1985. Joint mobility among university students in Iraq. *Br J Rheumatol* 24: 326-331.

Bandy, W.D., and J.M. Irion. 1994. The effect of time of static stretch on the flexibility of hamstring muscles. *Phys Ther* 74: 845-852.

Barbosa, A.R., J.M. Santarém, W.J. Filho, and M. de F.N. Marucci. 2002. Effects of resistance training on the sit-and-reach test in elderly women. *J Strength Cond Res* 16(1): 14-18.

Barnekow-Bergkvist, M., G. Hedberg, U. Janlert, and E. Jansson. 1996. Development of muscular endurance and strength from adolescence to adulthood and level of physical capacity in men and women at the age of 34 years. *Scand J Med Sci Sports* 6: 145-155.

Baumhauer, J.F., D.M. Alosa, A.F. Renstrom, S. Trevino, and B. Beynnon. 1995. A prospective study of ankle injury risk factors. *Am J Sports Med* 23: 564-570.

Beighton, P., L. Solomon, and C.L. Soskolone. 1973. Articular mobility in an African population. *Ann Rheum Dis* 32: 413-418.

Buroker, K.C., and J.A. Schwane. 1989. Does postexercise static stretching alleviate delayed muscle soreness? Physician *Sports Med* 17: 65-83.

Carter, C., and J. Wilkinson. 1964. Persistent joint laxity and congenital dislocation of the hip. *J Bone Joint Surg (Br)* 46: 40-45.

Cavagna, G.A., F.P. Saibene, and R. Margaria. 1964. Mechanical work in running. *J Appl Physiol* 19: 249-256.

Church, J.B., M.S. Wiggins, F.M. Moode, and R. Crist. 2001. Effect of warm-up and flexibility treatments on vertical jump performance. *J Strength Cond Res* 15(3): 332-336.

Cornu, C., O. Maietti, and I. Ledoux. 2003. Muscle elastic properties during wrist flexion and extension in healthy sedentary subjects and volleyball players. *Int J Sports Med* 24: 277-284.

Cornwell, A., A.G. Nelson, and B. Sidway. 2002. Acute effects of stretching on the neuromechanical properties of the triceps surae muscle complex. *Eur J Appl Physiol* 86: 428-434.

Craib, M.W., V.A. Mitchell, K.B. Fields, T.R. Cooper, R. Hopewell, and D.W. Morgan. 1996. The association between flexibility and running economy in sub-elite male distance runners. *Med Sci Sports Exerc* 28: 737-743.

DeLateur, B.J. 1994. Flexibility. *Phys Med Rehabil Clin* 5: 295-307.

DeVries, H.A. 1962. Evaluation of static stretching procedures for improvement of flexibility. *Res Q* 33(2): 222-229.

DeVries, H.A. 1963. The "looseness" factor in speed and O_2 consumption of an anaerobic 100 yard dash. *Res Q* 34: 305-312.

Diaz, M.A., E.C. Estevez, and P.S. Guijo. 1993. Joint hyperlaxity and musculoligamentous lesions: Study of a population of homogeneous age, sex and physical exertion. *Br J Rheumatol* 32: 120-122.

Eldred, E., D.E. Linsley, and J.S. Buchwald. 1960. The effect of cooling on mammalian muscle spindles. *Exp Neurol* 2: 144-157.

Etnyre, B.R., and E.J. Lee. 1988. Chronic and acute flexibility of men and women using three different stretching techniques. *Res Q* 59: 222-228.

Fatouros, I.G., K. Taxildaris, S.P. Tokmakidis, V. Kalapotharakos, N. Aggelousis, S. Athanasopoulos, I. Zeeris, and I. Katrabasas. 2002. The effect of strength training, cardiovascular training and their combination on flexibility of inactive older adults. *Int J Sports Med* 23: 112-119.

Friden, J., and R.L. Lieber. 2003. Spastic muscle cells are shorter and stiffer than normal cells. *Muscle Nerve* 26: 157-164.

Friden, J., M. Sjostrom, and B. Ekblom. 1983. Myofibrillar damage following intense eccentric exercise in man. *Int J Sports Med* 4: 170-176.

Fukashiro, S., T. Abe, A. Shibayama, and W.F. Brechue. 2002. Comparison of viscoelastic characteristics in triceps surae between black and white athletes. *Acta Physiol Scand* 175: 183-187.

Funk, D.C., A.M. Swank, B.M. Mikla, T.A. Fagan, and B.K. Farr. 2003. Impact of prior exercise on hamstring flexibility: A comparison of proprioceptive neuromuscular facilitation and static stretching. *J Strength Cond Res* 17(3): 489-492.

Gajdosik, R.L. 1995. Flexibility or muscle length? *Phys Ther* 75: 238-239.

Gajdosik, R.L., and R.W. Bohannon. 1987. Clinical measurement of range of motion: Review of goniometry emphasizing reliability and validity. *Phys Ther* 67: 1867-1872.

Gehlsen, G.M., and M.H. Whaley. 1990. Falls in the elderly: Part II. Balance, strength, and flexibility. *Arch Phys Med Rehabil* 71: 739-741.

Gersten, J.W. 1955. Effect of ultrasound on tendon extensibility. *Am J Phys Med Rehabil* 34: 362-369.

Girouard, C.K., and B.H. Hurley. 1995. Does strength training inhibit gains in range of motion from flexibility training in older adults? *Med Sci Sports Exerc* 27: 1444-1449.

Gleim, G.W., and M.P. McHugh. 1997. Flexibility and its effects on sports injury and performance. *Sports Med* 24: 289-299.

Gleim, G.W., N.S. Stachenfeld, and J.A Nicholas. 1990. The influence of flexibility on the economy of walking and jogging. *J Orthop Res* 8: 814-823.

Godges, J.J., H.M. MacRae, C. Longdon, C. Tinberg, and P. MacRae. 1989. The effects of two stretching procedures on hip range of motion and gait economy. *J Orthop Sports Phys Ther* 10: 350-357.

Godshall, R.W. 1975. The prediction of athletic injury: An eight year study. *J Sports Med* 3: 50-54.

Gottlieb, G.L. 1996. Muscle compliance: Implications for control of movement. In *Exerc Sports Sci Rev* 24: 1-34, ed. J.O. Holloszy. Philadelphia: Williams & Wilkins.

Grady, J.F., and A. Saxena. 1991. Effects of stretching the gastrocnemius muscle. *J Foot Surg* 30: 465-469.

Grana, W.A., and J.A. Moretz. 1978. Ligamentous laxity in secondary school athletes. *JAMA* 240: 1975-1976.

Halbertsma, J.P.K., and N.H. Goeken. 1994. Stretching exercises: Effect on passive extensibility and stiffness in short hamstrings of healthy subjects. *Arch Phys Med Rehabil* 75: 976-982.

Halbertsma, J.P.K., A.I. van Bolhius, and L.N.H. Goeken. 1996. Sport stretching: Effect on passive muscle stiffness of short hamstrings. *Arch Phys Med Rehabil* 77: 688-692.

Hartig, D.E., and J. Henderson. 1999. Increasing hamstring flexibility decreases lower extremity overuse injuries in military basic trainees. *Am J Sports Med* 27: 173-176.

Harvey, L.A., J. Batty, J. Crosbie, S. Poulter, and R.D. Herbert. 2000. A randomized trial assessing the effects of 4 weeks of daily stretching on ankle mobility in patients with spinal cord injuries. *Arch Phys Med Rehabil* 81: 1340-1347.

Harvey, L.A., and R.D. Herbert. 2002. Muscle stretching for treatment and prevention of contracture in people with spinal cord injury. *Spinal Cord* 40: 1-9.

Herbert, R.D., A.M. Moseley, J.E. Butler, and S.C. Gandevia. 2002. Change in length of relaxed muscle fascicles and tendons with knee and ankle movement in humans. *J Physiol* 539(2): 637-645.

High, D.M., E.T. Howley, and B.D. Franks. 1989. The effects of static stretching and warm-up on prevention of delayed-onset muscle soreness. *Res Q* 60(4): 357-361.

Hilyer, J.C., K.C. Brown, A.T. Sirles, and L. Peoples. 1990. A flexibility intervention to reduce the incidence and severity of joint injuries in municipal firefighters. *J Occup Med* 32: 631-637.

Hortobagyi, T., J. Faludi, J. Tihanyi, and B. Merkely. 1985. Effects of intense "stretching"—flexibility training on the mechanical profile of the knee extensors and on the range of motion of the hip joint. *Int J Sports Med* 6: 317-321.

Johansson, P.H., L. Lindstöm, G. Sundelin, and B. Lindstöm. 1999. The effects of preexercise stretching on muscular soreness, tenderness and force loss following heavy eccentric exercise. *Scand J Med Sci Sports* 9: 219-225.

Kalenak, A., and C.A. Morehouse. 1975. Knee stability and knee ligament injuries. *JAMA* 234: 1143-1145.

Kandel, E.R., and J.H. Schwartz. 1991. *Principles of neural science*. Norwalk, CT: Appleton & Lange.

Klemp, P., J.E. Stevens, and S. Isaacs. 1984. A hypermobility study in ballet dancers. *J Ortho Rheumatol* 11: 692-696.

Klinge, K., S.P. Magnusson, E.B. Simonsen, P. Aagaard, K. Klausen, and M. Kjaer. 1997. The effect of strength and flexibility training on skeletal muscle electromyographic activity, stiffness, and viscoelastic stress relaxation response. *Am J Sports Med* 25: 710-716.

Knapik, J.J., C.L. Bauman, B.H. Jones, J.M. Harris, and L. Vaughan. 1991. Preseason strength and flexibility imbalances associated with athletic injuries in female collegiate athletes. *Am J Sports Med* 19: 76-81.

Knott, M., and D.E. Voss. 1968. *Proprioceptive neuromuscular facilitation: Patterns and techniques*. 2nd ed. New York: Harper & Row.

Krabak, B.J., E.R. Laskowski, J. Smith, M.J. Stuart, and G.Y. Wong. 2001. Neurophysiologic influences on hamstring flexibility: A pilot study. *Clin J Sport Med* 11(4): 241-246.

Krivickas, L.S. 1997. Anatomical factors associated with overuse sports injuries. *Sports Med* 24: 132-146.

Krivickas, L.S., and J.H. Feinberg. 1996. Lower extremity injuries in college athletes: Relation between ligamentous laxity and lower extremity muscle tightness. *Arch Phys Med Rehabil* 77: 1139-1143.

Larsson, L., J. Baum, G.S. Mudholkar, and G.D. Kollia. 1993. Benefits and disadvantages of joint hypermobility among musicians. *N Engl J Med* 329: 1079-1082.

Laubach, L.L., and J.T. McConville. 1965. Muscle strength, flexibility and body size of adult males. *Res Q* 37: 384-392.

Laubach, L.L., and J.T. McConville. 1966. Relationship between flexibility, anthropometry, and the somatotype of college men. *Res Q* 37: 241-251.

Lehman, J.F., A.J. Massock, C.G. Warren, and J.N. Koblanski. 1970. Effect of therapeutic temperatures on tendon extensibility. *Arch Phys Med Rehabil* 51: 481-487.

Liebesman, J.L., and E. Cafarelli. 1994. Physiology of range of motion in human joints: A critical review. *Crit Rev Physican Rehabil Med* 6: 131-160.

Lindstedt, S.L., P.C. LaStayo, and T.E. Reich. 2001. When active muscles lengthen: Properties and consequences of eccentric contractions. *News Physiol Sci* 16: 256-261.

Lodish, H., D. Baltimore, and A. Berk et al. 1995. *Molecular cell biology*. New York: Scientific American Books.

Lucas, R., and R. Koslow. 1984. Comparative study of static, dynamic, and proprioceptive neuromuscular facilitation stretching techniques on flexibility. *Percept Mot Skills* 58: 615-618.

Lysens, R.J., M.S. Ostyn, Y.V. Auweele, J. Lefevre, M. Vuylsteke, and L. Renson. 1989. The accident-prone and overuse-prone profiles of the young athlete. *Am J Sports Med* 17: 612-619.

Magnusson, S.P., P. Aagaard, B. Larsson, and M. Kjaer. 2000. Passive energy absorption by human muscle-tendon unit is unaffected by increase in intramuscular temperature. *J Appl Physiol* 88: 1215-1220.

Magnusson, S.P., P. Aagaaard, E. Simonsen, and F. Bojsen-Møller. 1998. A biomechanical evaluation of cyclical and static stretch in human skeletal muscle. *Int J Sports Med* 19: 310-316.

Marshall, J.L., N. Johanson, T.L. Wickiewicz, H.M. Tischler, B.L. Koslin, S. Zeno, and A. Meyers. 1980. Joint looseness:

A function of the person and the joint. *Med Sci Sports Exerc* 12: 189-194.

McGlynn, G.H., N.T. Laughlin, and V. Rowe. 1979. Effect of electromyographic feedback and static stretching on artificially induced muscle soreness. *Am J Phys Med Rehabil* 58: 139-148.

McHugh, M.P., D.A.J. Connolly, R.G. Eston, I.J. Kremenic, S.J. Nicholas, and G.W. Gleim. 1999. The role of passive muscle stiffness in symptoms of exercise induced muscle damage. *Am J Sports Med* 27: 594-599.

McHugh, M.P., I.J. Kremenic, M.B. Fox, and G.W. Gleim. 1998. The role of mechanical and neural restraints to joint range of motion during passive stretch. *Med Sci Sports Exerc* 30(6): 928-932.

McNair, P.J., E.W. Dombroski, D.J. Hewson, and S.N. Stanley. 2001. Stretching at the ankle joint: Viscoelastic responses to holds and continuous passive motion. *Med Sci Sports Exerc* 33: 354-358.

Mense, S. 1978. Effect of temperature on the discharges of muscle spindles and tendon organs. *Pflugers Arch* 374: 159-166.

Micheli, L.J. 1983. Overuse injuries in children's sports: The growth factor. *Orthop Clin North Am* 14: 337-360.

Miglietta, O. 1973. Action of cold on spasticity. *Am J Phys Med Rehabil* 52: 198-205.

Moore, M.A., and R.S. Hutton. 1980. Electromyographic investigation of muscle stretching techniques. *Med Sci Sports Exerc* 12: 322-329.

Moretz, J.A., R. Walters, and L. Smith. 1982. Flexibility as a predictor of knee injuries in college football players. *Physician Sportsmed* 10: 93-97.

Nicholas, J.A. 1970. Injuries to knee ligaments: Relationship to looseness and tightness in football players. *JAMA* 21: 2236-2239.

Petajan, J.H., and N. Watts. 1962. Effects of cooling on the triceps surae reflex. *Am J Phys Med Rehabil* 41: 240-251.

Pope, R., R. Herbert, and J. Kirwan. 1998. Effects of ankle dorsiflexion range and pre-exercise calf muscle stretching on injury risk in army recruits. *Austr J Physiother* 44: 165-177.

Pope, R.P., R.D. Herbert, J. D. Kirwan, and B.J. Graham. 2000. A randomized trial of preexercise stretching for prevention of lower-limb injury. *Med Sci Sports Exerc* 32: 271-277.

Pratt, M. 1989. Strength, flexibility, and maturity in adolescent athletes. *Am J Dis Child* 143: 560-563.

Proske, U. 1997. The mammalian muscle spindle. *News Physiol Sci* 12: 37-42.

Sady, S.S., M. Wortman, and D. Blanke. 1982. Flexibility training: Ballistic, static or proprioceptive neuromuscular facilitation? *Arch Phys Med Rehabil* 63: 261-263.

Safran, M.R., W.E. Garrett, A.V. Seaber, R.R. Glisson, and B.M. Ribbeck. 1988. The role of warmup in muscular injury prevention. *Am J Sports Med* 16: 123-129.

Schwellnus, M. 2003. Flexibility and joint range of motion. In *Rehabilitation of sports injuries: Scientific basis,* 232-257, ed. W.R. Frontera. Oxford: Blackwell Science.

Shellock, F.G., and W.E. Prentice. 1985. Warming-up and stretching for improved physical performance and prevention of sports-related injuries. *Sports Med* 2: 267-278.

Smith, A.D., L. Stroud, and C. McQueen. 1991. Flexibility and anterior knee pain in adolescent elite figure skaters. *J Pediatr Orthop* 11: 77-82.

Soderman, K., H. Alfredson, T. Pietila, and S. Werner. 2001. Risk factors for leg injuries in female soccer players: A prospective investigation during one out-door season. *Knee Surg Sports Traumatol Arthrosc* 9: 313-321.

Tabary, J.C., C. Tabary, C. Tardieu, G. Tardieu, and G. Goldspink. 1972. Physiological and structural changes in the cat's soleus muscle due to immobilization by plaster casts at different lengths. *J Physiol* 224: 231-244.

Taylor, D.C., J.D. Dalton, A.V. Seaber, and W.E. Garrett. 1990. Viscoelastic properties of muscle-tendon units: The biomechanical effects of stretching. *Am J Sports Med* 18: 300-309.

Trappe, T.A., J.A. Carrithers, F. White, C.P. Lambert, W.E. Evans, and R.A. Dennis. 2002. Titin and nebulin content in human skeletal muscle following eccentric resistance exercise. *Muscle Nerve* 25: 289-292.

Wallin, D., B. Ekblom, R. Grahn, and T. Nordenborg. 1985. Improvement of muscle flexibility: A comparison between two techniques. *Am J Sports Med* 13: 263-268.

Waterman-Storer, C.M. 1991. The cytoskeleton of skeletal muscle: Is it affected by exercise? A brief review. *Med Sci Sports Exerc* 23: 1240-1249.

Wessel, J., and A. Wan. 1994. Effect of stretching on the intensity of delayed-onset muscle soreness. *Clin J Sport Med* 4(2): 83-87.

Willig, T.N., J.R. Bach, M.J. Rouffet, L.S. Krivickas, and C. Maquet. 1995. Correlation of flexion contractures with upper extremity function and pain for spinal muscular atrophy and congenital myopathy patients. *Am J Phys Med Rehabil* 74: 33-39.

Wilson, G.J., A.J. Murphy, and J.F. Pryor. 1994. Musculotendinous stiffness: Its relationship to eccentric, isometric, and concentric performance. *J Appl Physiol* 76: 2714-2719.

Wilson, G.J., G.A. Wood, and B.C. Elliot. 1991. The relationship between stiffness of the musculature and static flexibility: An alternative explanation for the occurrence of muscular injury. *Int J Sports Med* 19: 403-407.

Witvrouw, E., L. Danneels, P. Asselman, T. D'Have, and D. Cambier. 2003. Muscle flexibility as a risk factor for developing muscle injuries in male professional soccer players. *Am J Sports Med* 31(1): 41-46.

Witvrouw, E., R. Lysens, J. Bellemans, D. Cambier, and G. Vanderstraeten. 2000. Intrinsic risk factors for the development of anterior knee pain in an athletic population: A two-year prospective study. *Am J Sports Med* 28(4): 480-489.

Worrell, T.W., T.L. Smith, and J. Winegardner. 1994. Effect of hamstring stretching on hamstring muscle performance. *J Orthop Sports Phys Ther* 20: 154-159.

CHAPTER 5

Agre, J.C., and A.A. Rodriquez. 1990. Neuromuscular function: Comparison of symptomatic and asymptomatic polio subjects to control subjects. *Arch Phys Med Rehabil* 71: 545-551.

Agre, J.C., A.A. Rodriquez, and T.M. Franke. 1997. Muscle strengthening exercise can increase strength, endurance, and work capacity in post-polio subjects. *Arch Phys Med Rehabil* 78: 681-686.

Agre, J.C., A.A. Rodriquez, T.M. Franke, E.R. Swiggum, R.L. Harmon, and J.L. Curt. 1996. Low-intensity, alternate-day exercise improves muscle performance without apparent adverse affect in post-polio patients. *Am J Phys Med Rehabil* 75: 50-58.

Alexander, N.B., A.T. Galecki, L.V. Nyquist, M.R. Hofmeyer, J.C. Grunawalt, M.L. Grenier, and J.L. Medell. 2000. Chair and bed rise performance in ADL-impaired congregate housing residents. *J Am Geriatr Soc* 48: 526-533.

American College of Sports Medicine. 1995. *ACSM's guidelines for exercise testing and prescription*. 5th ed. Baltimore: Williams & Wilkins.

American College of Sports Medicine. 2000. *ACSM's guidelines for exercise testing and prescription*. 6th ed. Baltimore: Lippincott Williams & Wilkins.

Andres, P.L., W. Hedlund, L. Finison, T. Conlon, M. Felmus, and T.L. Munsat. 1986. Quantitative motor assessment in amyotrophic lateral sclerosis. *Neurology* 36: 937-941.

Åstrand, P.-O., and K. Rodahl. 1986. *Textbook of work physiology: Physiological bases of exercise*. 3rd ed. New York: McGraw-Hill.

Åstrand, P.-O., K. Rodahl, H.A. Dahl, and S.B. Stromme. 2003. *Textbook of work physiology: Physiological bases of exercise*. 4th ed. Champaign, IL: Human Kinetics.

Bean, J.F., D.K. Kiely, S. Herman, S.G. Leveille, K. Mizer, W.R. Frontera, and R.A. Fielding. 2002. The relationship between leg power and physical performance in mobility-limited older people. *J Am Geriatr Soc* 50(3): 461-467.

Berlly, M.H., W.W. Strauser, and K.M. Hall. 1991. Fatigue in postpolio syndrome. *Arch Phys Med Rehabil* 72: 115-118.

Bhambhani, Y.N., L.J. Holland, and R.D. Steadward. 1993. Anaerobic threshold in wheelchair athletes with cerebral palsy: Validity and reliability. *Arch Phys Med Rehabil* 74: 305-311.

Borg, G.A.V. 1973. Perceived exertions: A note on "history" and methods. *Med Sci Sports Exerc* 5: 90-93.

Bougenot, M.P., N. Tordi, A.C. Betik, X. Martin, D. Le Foll, B. Parratte, J. Lonsdorfer, and J.D. Rouillon. 2003. Effects of a wheelchair ergometer training programme on spinal cord-injured persons. *Spinal Cord* 41: 451-456.

Buchfuhrer, M.J., J.E. Hansen, T.E. Robinson, D.Y. Sue, K. Wasserman, and B.J. Whipp. 1983. Optimizing the exercise protocol for cardiopulmonary assessment. *J Appl Physiol* 55: 1558-1564.

Buschbacher, R.M., and R.L. Braddom, eds. 1994. *Sports medicine and rehabilitation: A sport-specific approach*. Philadelphia: Hanley & Belfus.

Canadian Society for Exercise Physiology. 2002. *Physical Activity Readiness Questionnaire – PAR-Q, revised 2002*. Ottawa, ON: Canadian Society for Exercise Physiology. Available online at www.csep.ca/pdfs/par-q.pdf. Accessed June 3, 2005.

Clarke, D.H. 1973. Adaptations in strength and muscular endurance resulting from exercise. In *Exercise and sports science reviews*. Vol. 1, ed. J.H. Wilmore. New York: Academic Press.

Clarke, D.H., and H.H. Clarke. 1984. *Research processes in physical education, recreation, and health*. Englewood Cliffs, NJ: Prentice-Hall.

Clarke, H.H. 1952. New objective strength tests of muscle groups by cable tension methods. *Res Q* 23: 136.

Cooper, R.R., F.D. Baldini, M.L. Boninger, and R. Cooper. 2001. Physiological responses to two wheelchair-racing exercise protocols. *Neurorehabil Neural Repair* 15: 191-195.

Davies, G.J. 1987. *A compendium of isokinetics in clinical usage and rehabilitation techniques*. 3rd ed. Onalaska, WI: S&S Publishers.

DeBolt, L.S., and J.A. McCubbin. 2004. The effects of home-based resistance exercise on balance, power, and mobility in adults with multiple sclerosis. *Arch Phys Med Rehabil* 85: 290-297.

de Lateur, B.J. 1996. Therapeutic exercise. In *Physical medicine and rehabilitation,* ed. R.L. Braddom, R.M. Buschbacher, D. Dumitru, E.W. Johnson, D. Matthews, and M. Sinaki, 401-419. Philadelphia: W.B. Saunders.

Einarsson, G., and G. Grimby. 1987. Strengthening exercise program in post-polio subjects. In *Research and clinical aspects of the late effects of poliomyelitis,* ed. L.S. Halstead and D.O. Wiechers, 275-283. White Plains, NY: March of Dimes Birth Defects Foundation.

Eriksson, P., L. Lofstrom, and B. Ekblom. 1988. Aerobic power during maximal exercise in untrained and well-trained persons with quadriplegia and paraplegia. *Scand J Rehabil Med* 20: 141-147.

Feldman, R.M., and C.L. Soskolne. 1987. The use of non-fatiguing strengthening exercises in post-polio syndrome. In *Research and clinical aspects of the late effects of poliomyelitis,* ed. L.S. Halstead and D.O. Wiechers, 335-341. White Plains, NY: March of Dimes Birth Defects Foundation.

Fillyaw, M.J., G.J. Badger, G.D. Goodwin, W.G. Bradley, T.J. Fries, and A. Shukla. 1991. The effects of long-term non-fatiguing resistance exercise in subjects with post-polio syndrome. *Orthopedics* 14: 1253-1256.

Fletcher, G.F., G.J. Balady, E.A. Amsterdam, B. Chaitman, R. Eckel, J. Fleg, V.F. Froelicher, A.S. Leon, I.L. Pina, R. Rodney, D.A. Simons-Morton, M.A. Williams, and T. Bazzarre. 2001. Exercise standards for testing and training: A statement for healthcare professionals from the American Heart Association. *Circulation* 104(14): 1694-1740.

Frontera, W.R., C.N. Meredith, K.P. O'Reilly, H.G. Knuttgen, and W.J. Evans. 1988. Strength conditioning in older men: Skeletal muscle hypertrophy and improved function. *J Appl Physiol* 64: 1038-1044.

Hahn, R.A., S.M. Teutsch, R.S. Paffenbarger, and J.S. Marks. 1990. Excess deaths from nine chronic diseases in the United States, 1986. *JAMA* 264: 2654-2659.

Halstead, L.S., and C.D. Rossi. 1985. New problems in old polio patients: Results of a survey of 539 polio survivors. *Orthopedics* 8: 845-850.

Halstead, L.S., and C.D. Rossi. 1987. Post-polio syndrome: Clinical experience of 132 consecutive outpatients. In *Research and clinical aspects of the late effects of poliomyelitis,* ed. L.S. Halstead and D.O. Wiechers, 13-26. White Plains, NY: March of Dimes Birth Defects Foundation.

Hutzler, Y., Y. Vanlandewijck, and M. Van Vlierberghe. 2000. Anaerobic performance of older female and male wheelchair basketball players on a mobile wheelchair ergometer. *Adapt Phys Activity Q* 17: 450-465.

Janssen, T.W., C.A. van Oers, A.P. Hollander, H.E. Veeger, and L.H. van der Woude. 1993. Isometric strength, sprint power, and aerobic power in individuals with a spinal cord injury. *Med Sci Sports Exerc* 25: 863-870.

Jones, D.R., J. Speier, K. Canine, R. Owen, and A. Stull. 1989. Cardiorespiratory responses to aerobic training by patients with post-poliomyelitis sequelae. *JAMA* 261: 3255-3258.

Kerk, J.K., P.S. Clifford, A.C. Snyder, T.E. Prieto, K.P. O'Hagan, P.K. Schot, J.B. Myklebust, and B.M. Myklebust. 1995. Effect of an abdominal binder during wheelchair exercise. *Med Sci Sports Exerc* 27: 913-919.

Kervio, G., F. Carre, and N.S. Ville. 2003. Reliability and intensity of the six-minute walk test in healthy elderly subjects. *Med Sci Sports Exerc* 35: 169-174.

Knechtle, B., and W. Kopfli. 2001. Treadmill exercise testing with increasing inclination as exercise protocol for wheelchair athletes. *Spinal Cord* 39: 633-636.

Knechtle, B., K. Hardegger, G. Muller, P. Odermatt, P. Eser, and H. Knecht. 2003. Evaluation of sprint exercise testing protocols in wheelchair athletes. *Spinal Cord* 41: 182-186.

Knuttgen, H.G. 1976. Development of muscular strength and endurance. In *Neuromuscular mechanisms for therapeutic and conditioning exercises,* ed. H.G. Knuttgen, 97-118. Baltimore: University Park Press.

Kottke, F.J. 1966. The effects of limitation of activity upon the human body. *JAMA* 196: 825-830.

Kriz, J.L., J.L. Speier, J.K. Canine, R.R. Owen, and R.C. Serfass. 1992. Cardiorespiratory responses to upper extremity aerobic training in postpolio subjects. *Arch Phys Med Rehabil* 73: 49-54.

Langbein, W.E., and K.C. Maki. 1995. Predicting oxygen uptake during counterclockwise arm crank ergometry in men with lower limb disabilities. *Arch Phys Med Rehabil* 76: 642-646.

Leon, A.S., and H. Blackburn. 1977. The relationship of physical activity to coronary artery disease and life expectancy. *Ann NY Acad Sci* 301: 561-578.

Lin, K.H., J.S. Lai, M.J. Kao, and I.N. Lien. 1993. Anaerobic threshold and maximal oxygen consumption during arm cranking exercise in paraplegia. *Arch Phys Med Rehabil* 74: 515-520.

McArdle, W.D., F.I. Katch, and V.L. Katch. 1991. *Exercise physiology energy, nutrition, and human performance*. 3rd ed. Philadelphia: Lea & Febiger.

McPeak, L.A. 1996. Physiatric history and examination. In *Physical medicine and rehabilitation,* ed. R.L. Braddom, R.M. Buschbacher, D. Dumitru, E.W. Johnson, D. Matthews, and M. Sinaki, pp. 3-42. Philadelphia: W.B. Saunders.

Moldover, J.R., and M.N. Bartels. 1996. Cardiac rehabilitation. In *Physical medicine and rehabilitation,* ed. R.L. Braddom, R.M. Buschbacher, D. Dumitru, E.W. Johnson, D. Matthews, and M. Sinaki, 649-670. Philadelphia: W.B. Saunders.

Morris, C.K., J.N. Myers, V.F. Froelicher, T. Kawaguchi, K. Ueshima, and A. Hideg. 1993. Nomogram based on metabolic equivalents and age for assessing aerobic exercise capacity in men. *J Am Coll Cardiol* 22: 175-182.

Mundale, M.O. 1970. The relationship of intermittent isometric exercise to fatigue of handgrip. *Arch Phys Med Rehabil* 51: 532-539.

Myers, J., N. Buchanan, D. Smith, J. Neutel, E. Bowes, D. Walsh, and V.F. Froelicher. 1992. Individualized ramp treadmill: Observations on a new protocol. *Chest* 101: 2305-2315.

Myers, J., N. Buchanan, D. Walsh, M. Kraemer, P. McAuley, M. Hamilton-Wessler, and V.F. Froelicher. 1991. Comparison of the ramp versus standard exercise protocols. *J Am Coll Cardiol* 17: 1334-1342.

Okawa, H., F. Tajima, K. Makino, T. Kawazu, T. Mizushima, K. Monji, and H. Ogata. 1999. Kinetic factors determining wheelchair propulsion in marathon racers with paraplegia. *Spinal Cord* 37: 542-547.

Owen, R.R., and D. Jones. 1985. Polio residuals clinic: Conditioning exercise program. *Orthopedics* 8: 882-883.

Paffenbarger, R.S., and R.T. Hyde. 1984. Exercise in the prevention of coronary heart disease. *Prev Med* 13: 3-22.

Pare, G., L. Noreau, and C. Simard. 1993. Prediction of maximal aerobic power from a submaximal exercise test performed by paraplegics on a wheelchair ergometer. *Paraplegia* 31: 584-592.

Piva, S.R., G.K. Fitzgerald, J.J. Irrgang, F. Bouzubar, and T.W. Starz. 2004. Get Up and Go Test in patients with knee osteoarthritis. *Arch Phys Med Rehabil* 85: 284-289.

Podsiadlo, D., and S. Richardson. 1991. The timed "Up and Go": A test of basic functional mobility for frail elderly persons. *J Am Geriatr Soc* 39: 142-148.

Prentice, W.E. 1994. The healing process and the pathophysiology of musculoskeletal injury. In *Rehabilitation techniques in sports medicine*. 2nd ed., ed. W.E. Prentice, 1-26. St. Louis: Mosby.

Price, D.T., R. Davidoff, and G.J. Balady. 2000. Comparison of cardiovascular adaptations to long-term arm and leg exercise in wheelchair athletes versus long-distance runners. *Am J Cardiol* 15: 996-1001.

Serfass, R.C., and S.G. Gerberich. 1984. Exercise for optimal health: Strategies and motivational considerations. *Prev Med* 13: 79-99.

Simonson, E. 1971. *Recovery and fatigue,* 440-458. Springfield, IL: Charles C Thomas.

Siscovick, D.S., N.S. Weiss, R.H. Fletcher, and T. Lasky. 1984. The incidence of primary cardiac arrest during vigorous exercise. *N Engl J Med* 311: 874-877.

Taylor, H.L., A. Henschel,, J. Brozek, and A. Keys. 1949. Effects of bed rest on cardiovascular function and work performance. *J Appl Physiol* 2: 223-239.

Thomas, S., J. Reading, and R.J. Shephard. 1992. Revision of the Physical Activity Readiness Questionnaire (PAR-Q). *Can J Sport Sci* 17: 338-345.

Thompson, P.D., E.J. Funk, R.A. Carleton, and W.Q. Sturner. 1982. The incidence of death during jogging in Rhode Island from 1975 through 1980. *JAMA* 247: 2535-2538.

Topol, E.J., K. Burek, W.W. O'Neill, D.G. Kewman, N.H. Kander, M.J. Shea, M.A. Schork, J. Kirscht, J.E. Juni, and B. Pitt. 1988. A randomized controlled trial of hospital discharge three days after myocardial infarction in the era of reperfusion. *N Engl J Med* 318: 1083-1088.

Vanlandewijck, Y.C., A.J. Spaepen, and R.J. Lysens. 1994. Wheelchair propulsion efficiency: Movement pattern adaptations to speed changes. *Med Sci Sports Exerc* 26: 1373-1381.

Weber, K.T., J.S. Janicki, and P.A. McElroy. 1987. Determination of aerobic capacity and the severity of chronic cardiac and circulatory failure. *Circulation* (Suppl. VI) 76: 40-46.

Yanagiya, T., H. Kanehisa, M. Tachi, S. Kuno, and T. Fukunaga. 2004. Mechanical power during maximal treadmill walking and running in young and elderly men. *Eur J Appl Physiol* 92: 33-38.

CHAPTER 6

Activity Counseling Trial Research Group. 2001. Effects of physical activity counseling in primary care: The Activity Counseling Trial: A randomized controlled trial. *JAMA* 286: 677-687.

Ajzen, I. 1988. *Attitudes, personality, and behavior.* Chicago: Dorsey Press.

Ajzen, I., and M. Fishbein. 1980. *Understanding attitudes and predicting social behavior.* Englewood Cliffs, NJ: Prentice-Hall.

American Academy of Pediatrics. 1994. Assessing physical activity and fitness in the office setting. *Peds* 93: 686-689.

American College of Sports Medicine. 1998. Position stand on the recommended quantity and quality of exercise for developing and maintaining cardiorespiratory and muscular fitness in healthy adults. *Med Sci Sports Exerc* 30(6): 975-991.

American College of Sports Medicine. 1998. *Resource manual for guidelines for exercise testing and prescription.* 2nd ed. Philadelphia: Lea & Febiger.

American College of Sports Medicine. 2000. *Guidelines for exercise testing and prescription.* 6th ed. Lippincott Williams & Wilkins.

American Heart Association. 2003. Exercise and physical activity in the prevention and treatment of atherosclerotic cardiovascular disease. *Circulation* 107: 3109-3116.

Bandura, A. 1977a. Self-efficacy: Toward a unifying theory of behavioral change. *Psychol Rev* 84: 191-215.

Bandura, A. 1977b. *Social learning theory.* Englewood Cliffs, NJ: Prentice-Hall.

Bandura, A. 1986. *Social foundations of thought and action: A social-cognitive theory.* Englewood Cliffs, NJ: Prentice-Hall.

Barry, H.C., and S.W. Eathorne. 1994. Exercise and aging: Issues for the practitioner. *Med Clin N Am* 78: 357-376.

Bassuk, S.S., and J.E. Manson. 2003. Physical activity and cardiovascular disease prevention in women: How much is good enough? *Exerc Sport Sci Rev* 31(4): 176-181.

Braith, R.W., J.E. Graves, J.L. Pollock, S.L. Leggett, D.M. Carpenter, and A.B. Colvin. 1989. Comparison of 2 vs. 3 days/week of variable resistance training during 10-and 18-week programs. *Int J Sports Med* 10: 450-454.

Cady, L.D., D.P. Bischoff, E.R. O'Connell, P.C. Thomas, and J.H. Allan. 1979. Strength and fitness and subsequent back injuries in firefighters. *J Occup Med* 21: 269-272.

Calfas, K.J., B.J. Long, J.F. Sallis, W.J. Wooten, M. Pratt, and K. Patrick. 1996. A controlled trial of physician counseling to promote the adoption of physical activity. *Prev Med* 25: 225-233.

Calfas, K.J., J.F. Sallis, M.F. Zabinski, D.E. Wilfley, J. Rupp, J.J. Prochaska, S. Thompson, M. Pratt, and K. Patrick. 2002. Preliminary evaluation of a multi-component program for nutrition and physical activity change in primary care: PACE+ for adults. *Prev Med* 34: 153-161.

Caspersen, C.J., K.E. Powell, and G.M. Christenson. 1985. Physical activity, exercise, and physical fitness: Definitions and distinctions for health-related research. *Public Health Rep* 100: 126-131.

Ching, P.L.Y.H., W.C. Willet, E.B. Rimm, G.A. Colditz, S.L. Gortmaker, and M.J. Stampfer. 1996. Activity level and risk of overweight in male health professionals. *Am J Public Health* 86: 25-30.

Dishman, R.K. 1991. Increasing and maintaining exercise and physical activity. *Behavior Therapy* 22: 345-378.

Eden, K.B., T.C. Orleans, C.D. Mulrow, N.J. Pender, and S.M. Teutsch. 2002. Does counseling by clinicians improve physical activity? A summary of the evidence for the U.S. Preventive Services Task Force. *Ann Intern Med* 137(3): E208-E215.

Estabrooks, P.A., R.E. Glasgow, and D.A. Dzewaltowski. 2003. Physical activity promotion through primary care. *JAMA* 289(22): 2913-2916.

Glanz, K., and B.K. Rimer. 1995. *Theory at a glance: A guide for health promotion practice*. Bethesda, MD: U.S. Department of Health and Human Services.

Harris, S.S., C.J. Caspersen, G.H. DeFriese, and E.H. Estes Jr. 1989. Physical activity counseling for healthy adults as a primary prevention intervention in the clinical setting. *JAMA* 261: 3590-3598.

Hassmen, P., R. Ceci, and L. Backman. 1992. Exercise for older women: A training method and its influences on physical and cognitive performance. *Eur J Appl Physiol* 64: 460-466.

Heyward, V.H. 2002. *Advanced fitness assessment and exercise prescription,* 4th ed. Champaign, IL: Human Kinetics.

Hirvensalo, M., E. Heikkinen, T. Lintunen, and T. Rantanen. 2003. The effect of advice by health care professionals on increasing physical activity of older people. *Scan J Med Sci Sports* 13(4): 231-236.

Kampert, J.B., S.N. Blair, C.E. Barlow, and H.W. Kohl III. 1996. Physical activity, physical fitness, and all-cause and cancer mortality: A prospective study of men and women. *Ann Epidemiol* 6: 452-7.

King, A.C., R. Friedman, B. Marcus, C. Castro, L. Forsyth, M. Napolitano, and B. Pinto. 2002. Harnessing motivational forces in the promotion of physical activity: The community health advice by telephone (CHAT) project. Health Education Research. *Behav Change Consort*17(5): 627-636.

King, A.C., W.L. Haskell, C.B. Taylor, H.C. Kraemer, and R.F. DeBusk. 1991. Group- vs. home-based exercise training in healthy older men and women. *JAMA* 266: 1535-1542.

King, A.C., W.L. Haskell, D.R. Young, R.K. Oka, and M.L. Stefanick. 1995. Long-term effects of varying intensities and formats of physical activity on participation rates, fitness, and lipoproteins in men and women aged 50 to 65 years. *Circulation* 91: 2596-2604.

King, A.C., C.B. Taylor, and W.L. Haskell. 1993. Effects of differing intensities and formats of 12 months of exercise training on psychological outcomes in older adults. *Health Psychol* 12: 292-300.

Kriska, A.M., C. Bayles, J.A. Cauley, R.E. LaPorte, R.B. Sandler, and G. Pambianco. 1986. Randomized exercise trial in older women: Increased activity over two years and the factors associated with compliance. *Med Sci Sports Exerc* 18: 557-562.

Lee, I.M., R.S. Paffenbarger, and C.C. Hsieh. 1991. Physical activity and risk of developing colorectal cancer among college alumni. *J Natl Cancer Inst* 83: 1324-1329.

Logsdon, D.N., C.M. Lazaro, and R.V. Meier. 1989. The feasibility of behavioral risk reduction in primary medical care. *Am J Prev Med* 5: 249-256.

Long, B.J., K.J. Calfas, K. Patrick, J.F. Sallis, W.J. Wooten, M. Goldstein, B. Marcus, T. Schwenck, R. Carter, T. Torez, L. Palinkas, and G. Heath. 1996. Acceptability, useability, and practicality of physician counseling for physical activity promotion: Project PACE. *Am J Prev Med* 12: 73-81.

Marcus, B.H., S.W. Banspach, R.C. Lefebvre, J.S. Rossi, R.A. Carleton, and D.B. Abrams. 1992. Using the stages of change model to increase adoption of physical activity among community participants. *American Journal of Health Promotion* 6: 424-429.

Marcus, B.H., B.M. Pinto, L.R. Simkin, J.E. Audrain, and E.R. Taylor. 1994. Application of theoretical models to exercise behavior among employed women. *American Journal of Health Promotion* 9: 49-55.

Marcus, B.H., and A.L. Stanton. 1993. Evaluation of relapse prevention and reinforcement interventions to promote exercise adherence in sedentary females. *Res Q Exerc Sport* 64: 447-452.

Marlatt, G.A., and W.H. George. 1990. Relapse prevention and the maintenance of optimal health. In *The handbook of health behavior change,* ed. S.A. Shumaker, E.B. Schron, and J. Ockene, 44-63. New York: Springer Publishing.

McLeroy, K.R., D. Bibeau, A. Steckler, and K. Glanz. 1988. An ecological perspective on health promotion programs. *Health Educ Q* 15: 351-377.

Paffenbarger, R.S., R.T. Hyde, and A.L. Wing. 1978. Physical activity as an index of heart attack risk in college alumni. *Am J Epidemiol* 108: 161-175.

Passmore, R. 1971. The regulation of body weight in man. *Proc Nutr Soc* 30: 122-127.

Pate, R.R., M. Pratt, S.N. Blair, W.L. Haskell, C.A. Macera, C. Bouchard, D. Buchner, W. Ettinger, G.W. Heath, and A.C. King. 1995. Physical activity and public health: A recommendation from the Centers for Disease Control and Prevention and the American College of Sports Medicine. *JAMA* 273: 402-407.

Patrick, K., J.F. Sallis, B. Long, K.J. Calfas, W. Wooten, G. Heath, and M. Pratt. 1994. A new tool for encouraging activity: Project PACE. *Physician Sportsmed* 22: 45-55.

Pollock, M.L. 1988. Prescribing exercise for fitness and adherence. In *Exercise adherence,* ed. R.K. Dishman. Champaign, IL: Human Kinetics.

President's Council on Physical Fitness and Sports. 1993. *The physician's Rx: Exercise.* Washington, DC: President's Council on Physical Fitness and Sports.

Prochaska, J.O., and C.C. DiClemente. 1984. *The transtheoretical approach: Crossing traditional boundaries of change.* Homewood, IL: Dorsey Press.

Rosenstock, I.M. 1990. The health belief model: Explaining health behavior through expectancies. In *Health behavior and health education: Theory, research, and practice.* San Francisco: Jossey-Bass.

Sallis, J.F., and M.F. Hovell. 1990. Determinants of exercise behavior. *Exerc Sport Sci Rev* 18: 307-330.

Sallis, J.F., M.F. Hovell, and C.R. Hofstetter. 1992. Predictors of adoption and maintenance of vigorous physical activity in men and women. *Prev Med* 21: 237-251.

Sallis, J.F., M.F. Hovell, C.R. Hofstetter, P. Faucher, J.P. Elder, J. Blanchard, C.J. Caspersen, K.E. Powell, and G.M. Christenson. 1989. A multivariate study of determinants of vigorous exercise in a community sample. *Prev Med* 18: 20-34.

Saris, W.H.M., S.N. Blair, M.A. van Baak, S.B. Eaton, P.S.W. Davies, L. DiPietro, M. Fogelholm, A. Rissanen, D. Schoeller, A. Trembley, K.R. Westerterp, and H. Wyatt. 2003. How much physical activity is enough to prevent unhealthy weight gain? Outcome of the IASO 1st Stockholm Conference and consensus statement. *Obesity Rev* 4(2): 101-114.

Shephard, R.J. 1993. Exercise and aging: Extending independence in older adults. *Geriatrics* 48: 61-64.

Shephard, R.J., M. Berridge, and W. Montelpare. 1990. On the generality of the "Sit and Reach" Test: An analysis of flexibility data for an aging population. *Res Q Exerc Sport* 61: 326-330.

Sidney, K.H., R.J. Shephard, and J.E. Harrison. 1977. Endurance training and body composition of the elderly. *Am J Clin Nutr* 30: 326-333.

Smith, D.M., M.R.A Khairi, J. Norton, and C.C. Johnston Jr. 1976. Age and activity effects on rate of bone mineral loss. *J Clin Invest* 58: 716-721.

Stokols, D. 1992. Establishing and maintaining healthy environments: Toward a social ecology of health promotion. *Am Psychol* 47: 6-22.

Tipton, C.H. 1991. Exercise, training, and hypertension: An update. *Exerc Sport Sci Rev* 19: 447-505.

U.S. Department of Health and Human Services. 1996. *Physical activity and health: A report of the Surgeon General.* Atlanta: U.S. Department of Health and Human Services, Centers for Disease Control and Prevention, National Center for Chronic Disease Prevention and Health Promotion.

U.S. Department of Health and Human Services. 1996. Chapter 6: Understanding and promoting physical activity. In *Physical activity and health: A report of the Surgeon General.* Atlanta: U.S. Department of Health and Human Services, Centers for Disease Control and Prevention, National Center for Chronic Disease Prevention and Health Promotion.

U.S. Department of Health and Human Services. 1996. Physiologic responses and long-term adaptations to exercise. In *Physical activity and health: A report of the Surgeon General.* Atlanta: U.S. Department of Health and Human Services, Centers for Disease Control and Prevention, National Center for Chronic Disease Prevention and Health Promotion.

U.S. Department of Health and Human Services, Public Health Service, Centers for Disease Control and Prevention, National Center for Chronic Disease Prevention and Health Promotion, Division of Nutrition and Physical Activity. 1999. *Promoting physical activity: A guide for community action.* Champaign, IL: Human Kinetics.

U.S. Department of Health and Human Services. 2000. *Healthy people 2010*. 2nd ed. *Understanding and improving health* and *Objectives for improving health*. 2 vols. Washington, DC: U.S. Government Printing Office, November. Available online at www.healthypeople.gov/. Accessed May 2, 2005.

Wells, K.B., C.E. Lewis, B. Leake, M.K. Schleiter, and R.H. Brook. 1989. The practices of general and subspecialty internists in counseling about smoking and exercise. *Am J Public Health* 76: 1009-1013.

West Virginia University, Department of Safety and Health Studies and Department of Sports and Exercise Studies. 1988. *Physical fitness and the aging driver: Phase I*. AAA Foundation of Traffic Safety, Washington, DC.

Wood, P.D., M.L. Stefanick, D.M. Dreon, D. Frey-Hewitt, B.C. Garay, P.T. Williams, H.R. Superko, S.P. Fortmann, J.J. Albers, K.M. Vranizan, N.M. Ellworth, R.B. Terry, and W.L. Haskell. 1988. Changes in plasma lipids and lipoproteins in overweight men during weight loss through dieting as compared with exercise. *New Engl J Med* 319: 1173-1179.

Young, D.R., W.L. Haskell, C.B. Taylor, and S.P. Fortmann. 1996. Effect of community health education on physical activity knowledge, attitudes, and behavior: The Stanford Five-City Project. *Am J Epidemiol* 144: 264-274.

CHAPTER 7

Abbot, R.D., B.L. Rodriguez, C.M. Burchfiel, and J.D. Curb. 1994. Physical activity in older middle-aged men and reduced risk of stroke: The Honolulu Heart Program. *Am J Epidemiol* 139: 881-893.

Adams, P.F., G.E. Hendershot, and M.A. Marano 1999. Currents estimates from the National Health Interview Survey, 1996. National Center for Health Statistics. Vital and Health Statistics 10(200). Available online at www.cdc.gov/nchs/data/series/sr_10/sr10_200.pdf. Accessed May 27, 2005.

American Cancer Society. 2004. *The complete guide—nutrition and physical activity* [online]. Available at www.cancer.org/docroot/PED/content/PED_3_2X_Diet_and_Activity_Factors_That_Affect_Risks.asp. Accessed February 8, 2005.

American College of Sports Medicine. 1993. Position stand: Physical activity, physical fitness, and hypertension. *Med Sci Sports Exerc* 25: i-x.

American College of Sports Medicine. 2002. *Selecting and effectively using stationary bicycles* [online]. Available at www.acsm.org/health+fitness/pdf/brochures/0380GNBR_3.pdf. Accessed Feb 8, 2005.

Andersen, L.B., and J. Haraldsdottir. 1995. Coronary heart disease risk factors, physical activity, and fitness in young Danes. *Med Sci Sports Exerc* 27: 158-163.

Andersen, R.E., C.J. Crespo, S.J. Bartlett, L.J. Cheskin, and M. Pratt. 1998. Vigorous physical activity and television watching habits among U.S. children and their relation to body weight and level of fatness. *JAMA* 279: 938-942.

Anderson, R.N., K.D. Kochanek, and S.L. Murphy 1997. *Report of final mortality statistics, 1995. Monthly Vital Statistics Report* 45(11) Supplement 2. Hyattsville, MD: National Center for Health Statistics.

Apter, D. 1996. Hormonal events during female puberty in relation to breast cancer risk. *Eur J Cancer Prev* 5: 476-482.

Arias, E. 2004. United States Life Tables, 2002. *National Vital Statistics Reports* 53: 1-40.

Arias, E., R.N. Anderson, H-C. Kung, S.L. Murphy, K.D. Kochanek, and Division of Vital Statistics. 2003. Deaths: Final data for 2001. *Nat Vit Stat Rep* 52(3): 1-115.

Barnes, P.M., and C.A. Schoenborn. 2003. Physical activity among adults: United States, 2000. Advance data from vital and health statistics; no. 333. Hyattsville, MD: National Center for Health Statistics. Available online at www.cdc.gov/nchs/data/ad/ad333.pdf. Accessed May 27, 2005.

Bassuk, S.S., and J.E. Manson. 2003. Physical activity and cardiovascular disease prevention in women: How much is good enough? *Exerc Sport Sci Rev* 31(4): 176-181.

Berlin, J.A., and G.A. Colditz. 1990. A meta-analysis of physical activity in the prevention of coronary heart disease. *Am J Epidemiol* 132: 612-628.

Bernstein, L., B.E. Henderson, R. Hanisch, J. Sullivan-Halley, and R.K. Ross. 1994. Physical exercise and reduced risk of breast cancer in young women. *J Natl Cancer Inst* 86: 1403-1408.

Bernstein, L., R.K. Ross, R.A. Lobo, R. Hanisch, M.D. Krailo, and B.E. Henderson. 1987. The effects of moderate physical activity on menstrual cycle patterns in adolescence: Implications for breast cancer. *Br J Cancer* 55: 681-685.

Bijnen, F.C.H., E.J.M. Feskens, C.J. Caspersen, S. Giampaoli, A.M. Nissinen, A. Menotti, W.L. Mosterd, and D. Kromhout. 1996. Physical activity and cardiovascular risk factors among elderly men in Finland, Italy, and The Netherlands. *Am J Epidemiol* 143: 553-561.

Blair, S.N., N.N. Goodyear, L.W. Gibbons, and K.H. Cooper. 1984. Physical fitness and incidence of hypertension in healthy normotensive men and women. *JAMA* 252: 487-490.

Blair, S.N., J.B. Kampert, H.W. Kohl III, C.E. Barlow, C.A. Macera, R.S. Paffenbarger Jr., and L.W. Gibbons. 1996. Influences of cardiorespiratory fitness and other precursors on cardiovascular disease and all-cause mortality in men and women. *JAMA* 276: 205-210.

Blair, S.N., H.W. Kohl III, C.E. Barlow, R.S. Paffenbarger Jr., L.W. Gibbons, and C.A. Macera. 1995. Changes in physical fitness and all-cause mortality: A prospective study of healthy and unhealthy men. *JAMA* 273: 1093-1098.

Booth, F.W., S.E. Gordon, C.J. Carlson, and M.T. Hamilton. 2000. Waging war on modern chronic diseases: Primary prevention through exercise biology. *J Appl Phys* 88(2): 774-787.

Bouchard, C. 1993. Heredity and health related fitness. *Physical Activity and Fitness Research Digest*, President's Council on Physical Fitness and Sports, Nov: 1-8.

Bullen, B.A., R.B. Reed, and J. Mayer. 1964. Physical activity of obese and nonobese adolescent girls appraised by motion picture sampling. *Am J Clin Nutr* 14: 211-213.

Butler, R.N., R. Davis, C.B. Lewis, M.E. Nelson, and E. Strauss. 1998. Physical fitness: Benefits of exercise for the older patient. 2. *Geriatrics* 53(10): 61-62.

Camacho, T.C., R.E. Roberts, N.B. Lazarus, G.A. Kaplan, and R.D. Cohen. 1991. Physical activity and depression: Evidence from the Alameda County Study. *Am J Epidemiol* 134: 220-231.

Carter, N.D., P. Kannus, and K.M. Khan. 2001. Exercise in the prevention of falls in older people: A systematic literature review examining the rationale and the evidence. *Sports Med* 31(6): 427-438.

Caspersen, C.J., K.E. Powell, and G.M. Christenson. 1985. Physical activity, exercise, and physical fitness: Definitions and distinctions for health related research. *Public Health Rep* 100: 126-131.

Cassaza, B.A., J.L. Young, and S.A. Herring. 1998. The role of exercise in the prevention and management of acute low back pain. *Occup Med* 13(1): 47-60.

Centers for Disease Control and Prevention. 1994. Prevalence of disabilities and associated health conditions: United States, 1991-1992. *MMWR* 43: 730-739.

Centers for Disease Control and Prevention. 2001. Prevalence of disabilities and associated health conditions among adults: United States, 1999. *MMWR* 50: 120-125. Available online at www.cdc.gov/mmwr/preview/mmwrhtml/mm5007a3.htm. Accessed May 31, 2005.

Centers for Disease Control and Prevention. 2003, Aug 15. Prevalence of physical activity, including lifestyle activities among adults: United States, 2000-2001. *MMWR* 52(32): 764-769.

Centers for Disease Control and Prevention. 2003, Aug 22. Physical activity levels among children aged 9-13 years: United States, 2002. *MMWR* 52(33): 785-788.

Centers for Disease Control and Prevention. 2004, Feb 6. Prevalence of no leisure-time physical activity: 35 States and the District of Columbia, 1988-2002. *MMWR* 53(4): 82-86.

Centers for Disease Control and Prevention. 2005. Disparities in deaths from stroke among persons aged <75 years: United States, 2002. *MMWR* 54: 477-481.

Chen, C.L., E. White, K.E. Malone, and J.R. Daling. 1997. Leisure time physical activity in relation to breast cancer among young women (Washington, United States). *Cancer Causes Control* 8: 77-84.

Chen, J. 2001. Aerobic exercise, gene expression and chronic diseases. *World Rev Nutr Diet* 89: 108-117.

Ching, P.L.Y.H., W.C. Willett, E.B. Rimm, G.A. Colditz, S.L. Gortmaker, and M.J. Stampfer. 1996. Activity level and risk of overweight in male health professionals. *Am J Public Health* 86: 25-30.

Chirico, A.M., and A.J. Stunkard. 1960. Physical activity and human obesity. *N Engl J Med* 263: 935-940.

Chobanian, A.V., G.L. Bakris, H.R. Black, W.C. Cushman, L.A. Green, J.L. Izzo, D.W. Jones, B.J. Matterson, S. Oparil, J.T. Wright, E.J. Roccella, and the National High Blood Pressure Education Program Coordinating Committee. 2003. The seventh report of the Joint National Committee on Prevention, Detection, Evaluation, and Treatment of High Blood Pressure: The JNC 7 report. *JAMA* 289(19): 2560-2572.

Chow, W., M. Dosemeni, W. Zheng, R. Vetter, J.K. McLaughlin, Y. Gao, and W.J. Blot. 1993. Physical activity and occupational risk of colon cancer in Shanghai, China. *Int J Epidemiol* 22: 23-29.

Colditz, G.A. 1999. Economic costs of obesity and inactivity. *Med Sci Sports Exerc* 31(11 Suppl. 1): S663.

Collins, J.G. 1997. Prevalence of selected chronic conditions: United States, 1990-1992. National Center for Health Statistics. *Vital Health Statistics* 10(194).

Conroy, B.P., W.J. Kraemer, C.M. Maresh, S.J. Fleck, M.H. Stone, and A.C. Fry. 1993. Bone mineral density in elite junior Olympic weightlifters. *Med Sci Sports Exerc* 26: 1103-1109.

Cramer, D.W., E. Wilson, R.J. Stillman, M.J. Berger, S. Belisle, I. Schiff, B. Albrecht, M. Gibson, B.V. Stadel, S.C. Schoenbaum. 1986. The relation of endometriosis to menstrual characteristics, smoking, and exercise. *JAMA* 255(14): 1904-1908.

Crespo, C.J., S. Keteyian, G.W. Heath, and C.T. Sempos. 1996. Prevalence of leisure time physical activity among U.S. adults. Results from the National Health and Nutrition Examination Survey. *Arch Intern Med* 156: 93-98.

Crespo, C.J., and E. Roccella. 1997. Increased hypertension among those who are less active in the United States. *Med Sci Sports Exerc* 29 (Suppl. 5): 39.

Crespo, C.J., and J.D. Wright. 1995. Prevalence of overweight among active and inactive U.S. adults from the Third National Health and Nutrition Examination Survey (abstract). *Med Sci Sports Exerc* 27(Suppl. 5): 409.

Crespo, C. J., E. Smit, R.E. Andersen, O. Carter-Pokras, and B.E. Ainsworth. 2000. Race/ethnicity, social class and their relation to physical inactivity during leisure time: Results from the Third National Health and Nutrition Examination Survey, 1988-1994. *Am J Prev Med* 18: 46-53.

Cruz-Vidal, M., R. Costas Jr., M.R. Garcia-Palmieri, P.D. Sorlie, and E. Herzmark. 1979. Factors related to diabetes mellitus in Puerto Rican men. *Diabetologia* 28: 300-307.

Dalsky, G.P., K.S. Stocke, and A.A. Ehsani. 1988. Weight bearing exercise training and lumbar bone mineral content in postmenopausal women. *Ann Intern Med* 108: 824-828.

Daltroy, L.H., M.D. Iversen, M.G. Larson, R. Lew, E. Wright, J. Ryuan, C. Zwerling, A.H. Fossel, and M.H. Liang. 1997. A controlled trial of an educational program to prevent low back injuries. *N Engl J Med* 337: 322-328.

Dhillon, P.K., and V.L. Holt. 2003. Recreational physical activity and endometrioma risk. *Am J Epidemiol* 158(2): 156-164.

Diabetes Data Group. 1995. *Diabetes in America*. 2nd ed. NIH Publication 95-1468. Bethesda, MD: National Institutes of Health.

DiPietro, L. 1995. Physical activity, body weight, and adiposity: An epidemiologic perspective. *Exerc Sport Sci Rev* 23: 275-303.

Dorgan, J.F., C. Brown, M. Barrett, G.L. Splasnky, B.E. Kreger, R.B. D'Agostino, D. Albanes, and A. Schatzkin. 1994. Physical activity and risk of breast cancer in the Framingham Heart Study. *Am J Epidemiol* 139: 662-669.

Dorn, J., J. Vena, J. Brasure, J. Freudenheim, and S. Graham. 2003. Lifetime physical activity and breast cancer risk in pre- and postmenopausal women. *Med Sci Sports Exerc* 35(2): 278-285.

Eaton, C.B., K.L. Lapane, C.E. Garber, A.R. Assaf, T.M. Lasater, and R.A. Carleton. 1995. Physical activity, physical fitness, and coronary heart disease risk factors. *Med Sci Sports Exerc* 27: 340-346.

Erickson, P., R. Wilson, and I. Shannon. 1995. *Years of healthy life. Statistical notes. Healthy People 2000*. Hyattsville, MD: National Center for Health Statistics. 7: 1-16.

Folsom, A.R., D.K. Arnett, R.G. Hutchingson, F. Liao, L.X. Clegg, and L.S. Cooper. 1997. Physical activity and incidence of coronary heart disease in middle-aged women and men. *Med Sci Sports Exerc* 29: 901-909.

Folsom, A.R., R.J. Prineas, S.A. Kaye, and R.G. Munger. 1990. Incidence of hypertension and stroke in relation to body fat distribution and other risk factors in older women. *Stroke* 21: 701-706.

Friedenreich, C.M., S.E. McGregor, K.S. Courneya, S.J. Angyalfi, and F.G. Elliott. 2004. Case-control study of lifetime total physical activity and prostate cancer risk. *Am J Epidemiol* 159: 740-749.

Friedenreich, C.M., and M.R. Orenstein. 2002. Physical activity and cancer prevention: Etiologic evidence and biological mechanisms. *J Nutr* 132(11 Suppl.): 3456S-3464S.

Friedenreich, C.M., and T.E. Rohan. 1995. A review of physical activity and breast cancer. *Epidemiology* 6: 311-317.

Friedenreich, C.M., and I. Thune. 2001. A review of physical activity and prostate cancer risk. *Cancer Causes & Control* 12: 461-475.

Fries, J.F., G. Singh, D. Morfeld, H.B. Hubert, N.E. Lane, and B.W. Brown Jr. 1994. Running and the development of disability with age. *Ann Intern Med* 121(7): 502-509.

Frisch, R.E., G. Wyshak, N.L. Albright, T.E. Albright, I. Schiff, and K.P. Jones. 1985. Lower prevalence of breast cancer and cancers of the reproductive system among former college athletes compared to nonathletes. *Br J Cancer* 52: 885-891.

Gammon, M.D., J.B. Schoenberg, J.A. Britton, J.L. Kelsey, R.J. Coates, D. Brogan, N. Potischman, C.A. Swanson, J.R. Daling, J.L. Stanford, and L.A. Brinton. 1998. Recreational physical activity and breast cancer risk among women under age 45 years. *Am J Epidemiol* 147: 273-280.

Gerhardsson, M., G. Steineck, U. Hagman, A. Rieger, and S.E. Norell. 1990. Physical activity and colon cancer: A case-referent study in Stockholm. *Int J Cancer* 46: 985-989.

Giovannucci, E., A. Ascherio, E.B. Rimm, G.A. Colditz, M. Stampfer, and W.C. Willett. 1995. Physical activity, obesity, and risk of colon cancer and adenoma in men. *Ann Intern Med* 122: 327-334.

Greendale, G.A., E. Barret-Connor, S. Edelstein, S. Ingles, and R. Haile. 1995. Lifetime leisure exercise and osteoporosis. The Rancho Bernardo Study. *Am J Epidemiol* 141: 951-959.

Grimston, S.K., N.D. Willows, and D.A. Hanley. 1993. Mechanical loading regime and its relationship to bone mineral density in children. *Med Sci Sports Exerc* 25: 1203-1210.

Haennel, R.G., and F. Lemire. 2002. Physical activity to prevent cardiovascular disease: How much is enough? *Can Fam Physician* 48: 65-71.

Hara, H., T. Kawase, M. Yamakido, and Y. Nishimoto. 1983. Comparative observation of micro- and macroangiopathies in Japanese diabetics in Japan and U.S.A. In *Diabetic microangiopathy,* ed. H. Abe and M. Hoshi. Basel: Karger.

Haskell, W.L. 1995. Physical activity in the prevention and management of coronary heart disease. *Physical Activity and Fitness Research Digest*, President's Council on Physical Fitness and Sports, March: 1-8.

Hassmen, P., N. Koivula, and A. Uutela. 2000. Physical exercise and psychological well-being: A population study in Finland. *Prev Med* 30(1): 17-25.

Heath, G.W., J. Gavin, J. Hinderlites, J. Hagberg, S. Bloomfield, and J. Holloszy. 1983. Effects of exercise and lack of exercise on glucose tolerance and insulin resistance. *J Appl Physiol* 55: 512-517.

Hedley, A.A., C.L. Ogden, C.L. Johnson, M.D. Carroll, L.R. Curtin, and K.M. Flegal. 2004. Prevalence of overweight and obesity among US children, adolescents, and adults, 1999-2002. *JAMA* 291(23): 2847-2850.

Helmrich, S.P., D.R. Ragland, and R.S. Paffenbarger Jr. 1994. Prevention of non-insulin-dependent diabetes mellitus with physical activity. *Med Sci Sports Exerc* 26: 824-830.

Henderson, N.K., C.P. White, and J.A. Eisman. 1998. The roles of exercise and fall risk reduction in the prevention of osteoporosis. *Endocr & Metab Clin N Am* 27(2): 369-387.

Hertel, K.L., and M.G. Trahiotis. 2001. Exercise in the prevention and treatment of osteoporosis: The role of physical therapy and nursing. *Nurs Clin N Am* 36(3): 441-453.

Hoffman-Goetz, L. 2003. Physical activity and cancer prevention: Animal-tumor models. Med Sci Sports Exerc 35(11): 1828-1833.

Hoffman-Goetz, L., M.E. Reichman, A. McTiernan, M.I. Goran, W. Demark-Wahnefried, and D. Apter. 1998. Possible mechanism mediating an association between physical activity and breast cancer. *J Natl Cancer Inst* 83 (3 Suppl.): 621-628.

Holt, V.L., and N.S. Weiss. 2000. Recommendations for the design of epidemiologic studies of endometriosis. *Epidemiology* 11: 654-659.

Housley, E., G.C. Leng, P.T. Donnan, and F.G. Fowkes. 1993. Physical activity and risk of peripheral arterial disease in the general population: Edinburgh Artery Study. *J Epidemiol Community Health* 47: 475-480.

Hu, G., N.C. Barengo, J. Tuomilehto, T.A. Lakka, A. Nissinen, and P. Jousilahti. 2004. Relationship of physical activity and body mass index to the risk of hypertension: A prospective study in Finland. *Hypertension* 43(1): 25-30.

Institute of Medicine. 2002, Sept. *Report on dietary reference intakes for energy, carbohydrates, fiber, fat, fatty acids, cholesterol, protein and amino acids.* National Academies Press, 500 Fifth Street, NW, Washington, DC 20055. Available at www.nap.edu.

International Agency for Research on Cancer (IARC). 2002. *Handbooks of Cancer Prevention. Weight control and physical activity.* IARC Working group on the evaluation of cancer-preventive agents. Lyon, France: World Health Organization, IARC Press.

Ishikawa-Takata, K., T. Ohta, and H. Tanaka. 2003. How much exercise is required to reduce blood pressure in essential hypertensives: A dose-response study. *Am J Hypertens* 16: 629-633.

Jakicic, J.M. 2002. The role of physical activity in prevention and treatment of body weight gain in adults. *J Nutr* 132(12): 3826S-3829S.

Janz, K. 2002. Physical activity and bone development during childhood and adolescence: Implications for the prevention of osteoporosis. *Minerva Pediatr* 54(2): 93-104.

Jenkins, S., D.L. Olive, and A.F. Haney. 1986. Endometriosis: Pathogenetic implications of the anatomic distribution. *Obstet Gynecol* 67: 335-358.

Judge, J.O., R.H. Whipple, and L.I. Wolfson. 1994. Effects of resistive and balance exercises on isokinetic strength in older persons. *J Am Geriatr Soc* 42: 937-946.

Katzmarzyk, P.T., N. Gledhill, and R.J. Shephard. 2000. The economic burden of physical inactivity in Canada. *CMAJ* 163(11): 1435-1440.

Kawate, R., M. Yamakido, Y. Nishimoto, P.H. Bennett, R.F. Hamman, and W.C. Knowler. 1979. Diabetes mellitus and its vascular complications in Japanese migrants on the island of Hawaii. *Diabetes Care* 2: 161-170.

Kaye, S.A., A.R. Folsom, J.M. Sprafka, R.J. Prineas, and R.B. Wallace. 1991. Increased incidence of diabetes mellitus in relation to abdominal adiposity in older women. *J Clin Epidemiol* 44: 329-334.

Kiely, D.K., P.A. Wolf, L.A. Cuppies, A.S. Beiser, and W.B. Kannel. 1994. Physical activity and stroke risk: The Framingham Study. *Am J Epidemiol* 140: 608-620.

Kiningham, R.B. 1998. Physical activity and the primary prevention of cancer. *Oncology* 25: 515-536.

Kirchner, E.M., R.D. Lewis, and P.J. O'Connor. 1996. Effect of past gymnastics participation on adult bone mass. *J Appl Physiol* 80: 225-232.

Knapick, J., J. Zoltick, H.C. Rottner, J. Phillips, C. Bielenda, B. Jones, and F. Drews. 1993. Relationships between self-reported physical activity and physical fitness in active men. *Am J Prev Med* 9: 203-208.

Kriska, A. 1997. Physical activity and the prevention of type 2 (non-insulin dependent) diabetes. *Research Digest,* President's Council on Physical Fitness and Sports, June: 1-8.

Kriska, A. 2003. Can a physically active lifestyle prevent type 2 diabetes? *Exerc Sport Sci Rev* 31(3): 132-137.

Kruger, H.S., C.S. Venter, H.H. Vorster, and B.M. Margetts. 2002. Physical inactivity is the major determinant of obesity in black women in the North West Province, South Africa: The THUSA study. Transition and health during urbanization of South Africa. *Nutr* 18(5): 422-427.

Kuczmarski, R.J., K.M. Flegal, S.M. Campbell, and C.L. Johnson. 1994. Increasing prevalence of overweight among U.S. adults. The National Health and Nutrition Examination Surveys, 1960-1991. *JAMA* 272: 205-211.

Kujala, U.M., S. Sarna, J. Kaprio, and M. Koskenvuo. 1996. Hospital care in later life among former world-class Finnish athletes. *JAMA* 276: 216-220.

Kurl, S., J.A. Laukanen, R. Rauramaa, T.A. Lakka, J. Sivenius, and J.T. Salonen. 2003. Cardiorespiratory fitness and the risk for stroke in men. *Arch Int Med* 163(14): 1682-1688.

Lahad, A., A.D. Malter, A.O. Berg, and R.A. Deyo. 1994. The effectiveness of four interventions for the prevention of low back pain. *JAMA* 272: 1286-1291.

Lakka, T.A., and J.T. Salonen. 1993. Moderate to high intensity conditioning leisure time physical activity and high cardiorespiratory fitness are associated with reduced plasma fibrinogen in eastern Finnish men. *J Clin Epidemiol* 46: 1119-1127.

Lamaitre, R.N., S.R. Hechbert, B.M. Psaty, and D.S. Siscovick. 1995. Leisure time physical activity and the risk of nonfatal myocardial infarction in postmenopausal women. *Arch Intern Med* 155: 2302-2308.

Lane, N.E. 1995. Exercise: A cause of osteoarthritis. *J Rheumatol* 22 (Suppl. 43): 3-6.

Lane, N.E., D.A. Bloch, P.D. Wood, and J.F. Fried. 1987. Aging, long-distance running, and the development of musculoskeletal disability. *Am J Med* 82: 772-780.

Laughlin, M.H. 1994. Effects of exercise training on coronary circulation: Introduction. *Med Sci Sports Exerc* 26: 1226-1229.

Lee, C.D., A.R. Folsom, and S.N. Blair. 2003. Physical activity and stroke risk: A meta-analysis. *Stroke* 34(10): 2475-2481.

Lee, I.M. 1995. Physical activity and cancer. *Research Digest,* President's Council on Physical Fitness and Sports, June: 1-8.

Lee, I.M. 2003. Physical activity and cancer prevention: Data from epidemiologic studies. *Med Sci Sports Exerc* 35(11): 1823-1827.

Lee, I.M., R.S. Paffenbarger Jr., and C. Hsieh. 1992. Physical activity and risk of prostatic cancer among college alumni. *Am J Epidemiol* 135: 169-179.

Leon, A.S. 1991. Effects of exercise conditioning on physiologic precursors of coronary heart disease. *J Cardiopulm Rehabil* 11: 46-57.

Leon, A.S., and J. Connet for the MRFIT Research Group. 1991. Physical activity and 10.5 year mortality in the multiple risk factor intervention trial (MRFIT). *Int J Epidemiol* 20: 690-697.

Leon, A.S., and J. Norstrom. 1995. Evidence of the role of physical activity and cardiorespiratory fitness in the prevention of coronary heart disease. *Quest* 47: 311-319.

Linsdted, K.D., S. Tonstad, and J.W. Kuzma. 1991. Self-report of physical activity and patterns of mortality in Seventh-Day Adventist men. *J Clin Epidemiol* 44: 355-364.

Lord, S.R., R.D. Clark, and I.W. Webster. 1991. Physiological factors associated with falls in an elderly population. *J Am Geriatr Soc* 39: 1194-1200.

Macera, C.A., J.M. Hootman, and J.E. Sniezek. 2003. Major public health benefits of physical activity. *Arth Rheum* 49(1): 122-128.

Maeda, S., T. Tanabe, T. Miyauchi, T. Otsuki, J. Sugawara, M. Iemitsu, S. Kuno, R. Ajisaka, I. Yamaguchi, and M. Matsuda. 2003. Aerobic exercise training reduces plasma endothelin-1 concentration in older women. *J Appl Physiol* 95: 336-341.

Manson, J.E., P. Greenland, A.Z. LaCroix, M.L. Stefanick, C.P. Mouton, A. Oberman, M.G. Perri, D.S. Sheps, M.B. Pettinger, and D.S. Siscovick. 2002. Walking compared with vigorous exercise for the prevention of cardiovascular events in women. *N Engl J Med* 347: 716-725.

Manson, J.E., D.M. Nathan, A.S. Krolewski, M.J. Stampfer, W.C. Willett, and C.H. Hennekens. 1992. A prospective study of exercise and incidence of diabetes among U.S. male physicians. *JAMA* 268: 63-67.

Manson, J.E., E.B. Rimm, M.J. Stampfer, G.A. Colditz, W.C. Willett, and A.S. Krolewski. 1991. Physical activity and incidence of non-insulin-dependent diabetes mellitus in women. *Lancet* 338: 774-778.

McBride, P., J. Einerson, P. Hanson, and K. Heindel. 1992. Exercise and the primary prevention of coronary heart disease. *Medicine, Exercise, Nutrition, and Health* 1: 5-15.

McKechnie, R., and L. Mosca. 2003. Physical activity and coronary heart disease prevention and effect on risk factors. *Card in Rev* 11(1): 21-25.

McTiernan, A. 2003. Physical activity, exercise, and cancer: Prevention to treatment—symposium overview. *Med Sci Sports Exerc* 35(11): 1821-1822.

McTiernan, A., C. Kooperberg, E. White, S. Wilcox, R. Coates, L.L. Adams-Campbell, N. Woods, and J. Ockene. 2003. Recreational physical activity and the risk of breast cancer in postmenopausal women: The Women's Health Initiative Cohort Study. *JAMA* 290(10): 1331-1336.

Mezzetti, M., C.L. Vecchia, A. Decarli, P. Boyle, R. Talamini, and S. Franceschi. 1998. Population attributable risk for breast cancer: Diet, nutrition, and physical exercise. *J Natl Cancer Inst* 90: 389-394.

Moen, M.H., and B. Schei. 1997. Epidemiology of endometriosis in a Norwegian county. *Acta Obstet Gynecol Scand* 76: 559-562.

Mokdad, A.H., J.S. Marks, D.F. Stroup, and J.L. Gerberding. 2004. Actual causes of death in the United States, 2000. *JAMA* 291(10): 1238-1245.

Moore, L.L., U.-S.D.T. Nguyen, K.J. Rothman, L.A. Cupples, and R.C. Ellison. 1995. Pre-school physical activity and changes in body fatness in young children. *Am J Epidemiol* 142: 982-988.

Morris, J.N. 1994. Exercise in the prevention of coronary heart disease: Today's best buy in public health. *Med Sci Sports Exerc* 26: 817-814.

Morris, J.N., A. Kagan, D.C. Pattison, M.J. Gardness, and P.A.B. Raffle. 1966. Incidence and prediction of ischemic heart disease in London busmen. *Lancet* 2: 553-559.

National Center for Health Statistics. 2004. *Health, United States, 2004 with Chartbook on Trends in the Health of Americans.* Hyattsville, MD: National Center for Health Statistics. Available online at www.cdc.gov/nchs/data/hus/hus04.pdf. Accessed May 31, 2005.

National High Blood Pressure Education Program. 1997. *Sixth report of the joint national committee on detection, evaluation, and treatment of high blood pressure.* NIH Publication No. 98-4080. Bethesda, MD: National Heart, Lung, and Blood Institute.

National Institutes of Health, Consensus Development Conference. 1996. Physical activity and cardiovascular health. *JAMA* 276: 241-246.

National Obesity Education Initiative. 1998. *Clinical guidelines on the identification, evaluation, and treatment of overweight and obesity in adults. The evidence report.* Bethesda, MD: National Institutes of Health, National Heart, Lung, and Blood Institute.

Nichols, D.L., C.F. Sanborn, S.L. Bonnick, V. Ben-Ezra, B. Gench, and N.M. DiMarco. 1994. The effects of gymnastics training on bone mineral density. *Med Sci Sports Exerc* 26: 1220-1225.

Niebauer, J., and J.P. Cooke. 1996. Cardiovascular effects of exercise: Role of endothelial shear stress. *J Am Coll Cardiol* 28: 1652-1660.

Nieman, D.C. 1996. *Fitness and sports medicine. A health related approach.* 3rd ed. Palo Alto, CA: Bulls Publishing.

Nieman, D.C., V.D. Cook, D.A. Henson, J. Suttles, W.J. Rejeski, P.M. Ribist, O.R. Fagoaga, and S.L. Nehlsen-Cannarella. 1995. Moderate exercise training and natural killer cell cytotoxic activity in breast cancer patients. *Int J Sports Med* 16: 334-337.

Nieman, D.C., and S.L. Nehlsen-Cannarella. 1992. Exercise and infection. In *Exercise and disease*, ed. R.R. Watson and M. Eisinger. Boca Raton, FL: CRC Press.

Oliveira, S.A., H.W. Kohl III, D. Trichopoulos, and S.N. Blair. 1996. The association between cardiorespiratory fitness and prostate cancer. *Med Sci Sports Exerc* 28: 97-104.

Paffenbarger, R.S. Jr., I.M. Lee, and R. Leung. 1994. Physical activity and personal characteristics associated with depression and suicide in American college men. *Acta Psychiatr Scand Supp* 377: 16-22.

Paffenbarger, R.S. Jr., A.L. Wing, R.T. Hyde, and D.L. Jung. 1983. Physical activity and incidence of hypertension in college alumni. *Am J Epidemiol* 117: 245-257.

Panush, R.S., C.S. Hanson, J.R. Caldwell, S. Longley, J. Stork, and R. Thoburn. 1995. Is running associated with osteoarthritis? *J Clin Rheumatol* 1: 35-39.

Pate, R.R., M. Pratt, S.N. Blair, W.L. Haskell, C.A. Macera, C. Bouchard, B. Buchner, W. Ettinger, G.W. Heath, A.C. King. A. Kriska, A.S. Leon, B.H. Marcus, J. Morris, R.S. Paffenbarger Jr., K. Patrick, M.L. Pollock, J.M. Rippe, J. Sallis, and J.H. Wilmore. 1995. Physical activity and public health. A recommendation from the Centers for Disease Control and Prevention and the American College of Sports Medicine. *JAMA* 273: 402-407.

Peters, K.D., K.D. Kochanek, and S.L. Murphy. 1998. Deaths: Final data for 1996. *Natl Vital Stat Rep* 47: 1-100.

Powell, K.E., and S.N. Blair. 1994. The public health burdens of sedentary living habits: Theoretical but realistic estimates. *Med Sci Sports Exerc* 26: 851-856.

Province, M.A., E.C. Hadley, M.C. Hornbrook, L.A. Lipsitz, J.P. Miller, and C.D. Mulrow. 1995. The effects of exercise on falls in elderly patients: A preplanned meta-analysis of the FICSIT trials. *JAMA* 273: 1341-1347.

Ravussin, E., P.H. Bennett, M.E. Valencia, L.O. Schulz, and J. Esparza. 1994. Effects of traditional lifestyle on obesity in Pima Indians. *Diabetes Care* 17: 1067-1074.

Rockhill, B., G.A. Colditz, D. Spiegelman, S.E. Hankinson, J.E. Manson, D.J. Hunter, and W.C. Willett. 1998. Physical activity and breast cancer risk in a cohort of young women. *J Natl Cancer Inst* 90: 1155-1160.

Rubin, K., V. Schirduan, P. Gendreau, M. Sarfarazi, R. Mendola, and G. Dalsky. 1993. Predictors of axial and peripheral bone mineral density in healthy children and adolescents, with special attention to the role of puberty. *J Pediatr* 123: 863-870.

Ryan, D.H., and Diabetes Prevention Program Research Group. 2003. Diet and exercise in the prevention of diabetes. *Int J Clin Prac* (Suppl., 134): 28-35.

Sallis, J.F., T.L. McKenzie, J.E. Alcaraz, B. Kolody, N. Faucette, and M.F. Hovell. 1997. The effects of a 2-year physical education program (SPARK) on physical activity and fitness in elementary school students. *Am J Public Health* 87: 1328-1334.

Sandler, R.S., M.L. Pritchard, and S.I. Bangdiwala. 1995. Physical activity and risk of colorectal adenomas. *Epidemiology* 6: 602-606.

Sato, Y., M. Nagasaki, N. Nakai, and T. Fushimi. 2003. Physical exercise improves glucose metabolism in lifestyle-related diseases. *Exp Biol & Med* 228(10): 1208-1212.

Sedgwick, A.W., D.W. Thomas, and M. Davies. 1993. Relationships between change in aerobic fitness and changes in blood pressure and plasma lipids in men and women: The "Adelaide 1000" 4-year follow up. *J Clin Epidemiol* 46: 141-151.

Signorello, L.B., B.L. Harlow, D.W. Cramer, D. Spiegelman, and J.A. Hill. 1997. Epidemiologic determinants of endometriosis: A hospital-based case-control study. *Ann Epidemiol* 7(4): 267-274.

Smutok, M., C. Reece, and P. Kokkinos. 1994. Effects of exercise training modality on glucose tolerance in men with abnormal glucose regulation. *Int J Sports Med* 15: 283-289.

Snelling, A.M., C.J. Crespo, M. Schaeffer, S. Smith, and L. Walbourn. 2001. Modifiable and nonmodifiable factors associated with osteoporosis in postmenopausal women: Results from the Third National Health and Nutrition Examination Survey, 1988-1994. *J Womens Health Gend Based Med* 10: 57-65.

Sothern, M.S., M. Loftin, R.M. Suskind, J.N. Udall, and U. Blecker. 1999. The health benefits of physical activity in children and adolescents: Implications for chronic disease prevention. *Eur J Ped* 158(4): 271-274.

Stear, S. 2003. Health and Fitness Series-1. The importance of physical activity for health. *J Fam Hlth Care* 13(1): 10-13.

Steenland, K., S. Nowlin, and S. Palu. 1995. Cancer incidence in the National Health and Nutrition Survey I. Follow-up data: Diabetes, cholesterol, pulse and physical activity. *Cancer Epidemiol Biomarkers Prev* 4: 807-811.

Steinbeck, K.S. 2001. The importance of physical activity in the prevention of overweight and obesity in childhood: A review and an opinion. *Obes Rev* 2: 117-130.

Taylor, R.J., P.H. Bennett, G. LeGonidec, J. Lacoste, D. Combe, and M. Joffres. 1983. The prevalence of diabetes mellitus in a traditional-living Polynesian population: The Wallis Island survey. *Am J Public Health* 6: 334-340.

Thune, I., and A.S. Furberg. 2001. Physical activity and cancer risk: Dose-response and cancer, all sites and site-specific. *Med Sci Sports Exerc* 33: S530-S550.

U.S. Department of Health and Human Services. 1991. *Osteoporosis research, education, and health promotion.* NIH Publication No. 91-3216. Bethesda, MD: National Institute of Arthritis and Musculoskeletal and Skin Diseases.

U.S. Department of Health and Human Services, Centers for Disease Control and Prevention, National Center for Chronic Disease Prevention and Health Promotion. 1996. *Physical activity and health: A report of the Surgeon General.* Atlanta: Centers for Disease Control and Prevention.

Vainio, H., R. Kaaks, and F. Bianchini. 2002. Weight control and physical activity in cancer prevention: International evaluation of the evidence. *Eur J Canc Prev* 11(Suppl. 2): S94-S100.

Wannamethee, G., and A.G. Shaper. 1992. Physical activity and stroke in British middle aged men. *Br Med J* 304: 597-601.

Wannamethee, G., A.G. Shaper, and P.W. Macfarlane. 1993. Heart rate, physical activity, and mortality from cancer and other non-cardiovascular disease. *Am J Epidemiol* 137: 735-748.

Warren, M.P., and N.E. Perlroth. 2001. The effects of intense exercise on the female reproductive system. *J Endocrinol* 170: 3-11.

Westerlind, K.C. 2003. Physical activity and cancer prevention: Mechanics. *Med Sci Sports Exerc* 35(11): 1834-1840.

Weyerer, S. 1992. Physical inactivity and depression in the community: Evidence from the Upper Bavarian Field Study. *Int J Sports Med* 13: 492-496.

Williams, P.T. 1997. Evidence for the incompatibility of age-neutral overweight and age-neutral physical activity standards from runners. *Am J Clin Nutr* 65: 1391-1396.

Woods, J.A. 1998. Exercise and resistance to neoplasia. *Can J Phys & Pharm* 76(5): 581-588.

CHAPTER 8

Ades, P.A., D. Huang, and S.O. Weaver. 1992. Cardiac rehabilitation and participation predicts lower hospitalization costs. *Am Heart J* 123: 916-921.

Ades, P.A., F.J. Pashkow, and J.R. Nestor. 1997. Cost-effectiveness of cardiac rehabilitation after myocardial infarction. *J Cardiopulm Rehab* 17: 222-231.

American College of Sports Medicine. 1995a. *Guidelines for exercise testing and prescription.* 5th ed. Baltimore: Williams & Wilkins.

American College of Sports Medicine. 1995b. Position Stand. Exercise for patients with coronary artery disease. *Med Sci Sports Exerc* 26: i-v.

American Thoracic Society and American College of Chest Physicians. 2003. ATS/ACCP statement on cardiopulmonary exercise testing. *Am J Respir Crit Care Med* 167: 211-277.

Arnold, J.M.O., J.P. Ribeiro, and W.S. Colucci. 1990. Muscle blood flow during forearm exercise in patients with severe heart failure. *Circulation* 82: 465-472.

Atwood, J.E., S. Kawanishi, J. Myers, and V.F. Froelicher. 1988. Exercise testing in patients with aortic stenosis. *Chest* 93: 1083-1087.

Balas, E.A., F. Jaffrey, G.J. Kuprerman, S.A. Boren, G.D. Brown, F. Pinciroli, and J.A. Mitchell, J.A. 1997. Electronic communication with patients: Evaluation of distance medicine technology. *JAMA* 278: 152-159.

Belardinelli, R., D. Georgiou, L. Ginzton, G. Cianci, and A. Purcaro. 1998. Effect of moderate exercise training on thallium uptake and contractile response to low-dose dobutamine of dysfunctional myocardium in patients with ischemic cardiopmyopathy. *Circulation* 97: 553-561.

Beniamini, Y., J.J. Rubenstein, L.D. Zaichkowsky, and M.C. Crim, M.C. 1997. Effects of high-intensity strength training on quality-of-life parameters in cardiac rehabilitation patients. *Am J Cardiol* 80: 841-846.

Bertagnoli, K., P. Hansons, and A. Ward. 1990. Attenuation of exercise-induced ST depression during combined isometric and dynamic exercise in coronary artery disease. *Am J Cardiol* 65: 314-317.

Billman, G.E., P.J. Schwartz, and H.L. Stone. 1984. The effects of daily exercise on susceptibility to sudden cardiac death. *Circulation* 69: 1182-1189.

Blair, S.N., K.E. Powell, T.L. Bazzarre, J.L. Early, L.H. Epstein, L.W. Green, S.S. Harris, W.L. Haskell, A.C. King, J. Koplan,

B. Marcus, R.S. Paffenbarger, and K.K. Yeager. 1993. Physical inactivity. Workshop V. *Circulation* 88: 1402-1405.

Bloch, A., J.P. Maeder, J.C. Haissly, J. Felix, and H. Blackburn. 1974. Early mobilization after myocardial infarction: A controlled study. *Am J Cardiol* 34: 152-157.

Blumenthal, J.A., W.J. Rejeski, M. Walsh-Riddle, C.F. Emery, H. Miller, S. Roark, P.M. Ribisl, P.B Morris, P. Brubaker, and R.S. Williams. 1988. Comparison of high- and low-intensity exercise training after acute myocardial infarction. *Am J Cardiol* 61: 26-30.

Blumenthal, J.A., A. Sherwood, E.C. Gullette, M. Babyak, R. Waugh, A. Georgiades, L.W. Craighead, D. Tweedy, M. Feinglos, M. Appelbaum, J. Hayano, and A. Hinderliter. 2000. Exercise and weight loss reduce blood pressure in men and women with mild hypertension: Effects on cardiovascular, metabolic, and hemodynamic functioning. *Arch Int Med* 160: 1947-1958.

Bondestam, E., A. Breikss, and M. Hartford. 1995. Effects of early rehabilitation on consumption of medical care during the first year after acute myocardial infarction in patients ≥ 65 years of age. *Am J Cardiol* 75: 767-771.

Borg, G. 1982. Psycho-physical bases of perceived exertion. *Med Sci Sports Exerc* 14: 377-387.

Borg, G. 1998. *Borg's perceived exertion and pain scales,* 47. Champaign, IL: Human Kinetics.

Camacho, T.C., R.E. Roberts, N.B. Lazarus, G.A. Kaplan, and R.D. Cohen. 1991. Physical activity and depression: Evidence from the Alameda County Study. *Am J Epidemiol* 134: 220-231.

Carney, R.M., M.W. Rich, A. Tevelde, J. Saini, K. Clark, and A.S. Jaffe. 1987. Major depressive disorder in coronary artery disease. *Am J Cardiol* 60: 1273-1275.

Cheitlin, M.D., P.S. Douglas, and W.W. Parmley. 1994. 26th Bethesda Conference. Recommendations for determining eligibility for competition in athletes with cardiovascular abnormalities. Task Force 2. Valvular heart disease. *J Am Coll Cardiol* 24: 874-880.

Chiappa, G.R., H. Guths, R. Stein, P. Dall Ago, and J.P. Ribeiro. 2003. Inspiratory muscle training improves periodic breathing during exercise in heart failure. *Circulation* (abstract, Suppl. IV): IV-760.

Coats, A.J.S., S. Adamopoulos, A. Radaelli, A. McCance, T.E. Meyer, L. Bernardi, P.L. Solda, P. Davey, O. Ormerod, C. Forfar, J. Conway, and P. Sleight. 1992. Controlled trial of physical training in chronic heart failure. *Circulation* 85: 2119-2131.

Colucci, W.S., J.P. Ribeiro, M.B. Rocco, R.J. Quigg, M.A. Creager, J.D. Marsh, D.F. Gauthier, and L.H. Hartley. 1989. Impaired chronotropic response to exercise in patients with congestive heart failure. Role of postsynaptic β-adrenergic desensitization. *Circulation* 80: 314-323.

Criteria Committee of the New York Heart Association. 1964. *Nomenclature and criteria for diagnosis of diseases of the heart and great vessels.* Boston: Little, Brown.

Dafoe, W., and P. Huston. 1997. Current trends in cardiac rehabilitation. *Can Med Assoc J* 156: 527-532.

DeBusk, R.F., W.L. Haskell, N.H. Miller, K. Berra, and C.B. Taylor. 1985. Medically directed at-home rehabilitation soon after clinically uncomplicated myocardial infarction: A new model for patient care. *Am J Cardiol* 55: 251-257.

DeBusk, R.F., U. Stenestrand, M. Sheehan, and W.L. Haskell. 1990. Training effects of long versus short bouts of exercise in healthy subjects. *Am J Cardiol* 65: 1010-1013.

Dennis, C., N. Houston-Miller, R.G. Schwartz, D.K. Ahn, H.C. Kraemer, D. Gossard, M. Juneau, C.B. Taylor, and R.F. DeBusk, R.F. 1988. Early return to work after uncomplicated myocardial infarction. Results of a randomized trial. *JAMA* 260: 214-220.

Denollet, J., and D.L. Brutsaert. 1995. Enhancing emotional well-being by comprehensive rehabilitation in patients with coronary heart disease. *Eur Heart J* 16: 1070-1078.

Doerfler, L.A., L. Pbert, and D. DeCosimo. 1997. Self-reported depression in patients with coronary artery disease. *J Cardiopulm Rehab* 17: 163-170.

Donahue, R.P., R.D. Abbott, E. Bloom, D.M. Reed, and K. Yano. 1987. Central obesity and coronary heart disease in men. *Lancet* 1: 821-824.

Douard, H., L. Chevalier, L. Labbe, A. Choussat, and J.P. Broustet. 1997. Physical training improves exercise capacity in patients with mitral stenosis after balloon valvuloplasty. *Eur Heart J* 18: 464-469.

Drexler, H., U. Riede, T. Munzel, H. Konig, E. Funke, and H. Just, H. 1992. Alterations of skeletal muscle in chronic heart failure. *Circulation* 85: 1751-1759.

ExTraMATCH Collaborative. 2004. Exercise training meta-analysis of trials in patients with chronic heart failure (ExTraMATCH). *BMJ* 328: 189-192.

Fleg, J.L., I.L. Piña, G.J. Balady, B.R. Chaitman, B. Fletcher, C. Lavie, M.C. Limacher, R.A. Stein, M. Williams, and T. Bazzarre. 2000. Assessment of functional capacity in clinical and research applications. An advisory from the Committee on Exercise, Rehabilitation, and Prevention, Council on Clinical Cardiology, American Heart Association. *Circulation* 102: 1591-1597.

Fletcher, B.J., A. Lloyd, and G.F. Fletcher. 1988. Outpatient rehabilitative training in patients with cardiovascular disease: Emphasis on training method. *Heart Lung* 17: 199-205.

Fletcher, G.F., G. Balady, S.N. Blair, J. Blumenthal, C. Caspersen, B. Chaitman, S. Epstein, E.S.S. Froelicher, V.F. Froelicher, I.L. Pina, and M.L. Pollock. 1996. Statement on exercise: Benefits and recommendations for physical activity programs for all Americans. A statement for health professionals by the committee on exercise and cardiac rehabilitation of the Council on Clinical Cardiology, American Heart Association. *Circulation* 94: 857-862.

Fletcher, G.F., G. Balady, V.F. Froelicher, L.H. Hartley, W.L. Haskell, and M.L. Pollock. 1995. Exercise Standards. A statement for health professional from the American Heart Association. *Circulation* 91: 580-615.

Franciosa, J.A. 1984. Exercise testing in chronic congestive heart failure. *Am J Cardiol* 53: 1447-1450.

Froelicher, V., D. Jensen, F. Genter, M. Sullivan, M.D. Mckirman, K. Witztum, J. Scharf, M.L. Strong, and W. Ashburn. 1984. A randomized trial of exercise training in patients with coronary heart disease. *JAMA* 252: 1291-1297.

Ghilarducci, L.E., R.G. Holly, and E.A. Amsterdam. 1989. Effects of high resistance training in coronary artery disease. *Am J Cardiol* 64: 866-870.

Gobel, A.J., D.J. Hare, P.S. Macdonald, R.G. Oliver, MA. Reid, and M.D. Worcester. 1991. Effects of early programmes of high and low intensity exercise on physical performance after transmural myocardial infarction. *Brit Heart J* 65: 126-131.

Goldman, L., B. Hashimoto, E.F. Cook, and J.A. Loscalzo. 1981. Comparative reproducibility and validity of systems for assessing cardiovascular functional class: Advantages of a new specific activity scale. *Circulation* 6: 1227-1234.

Gordon, N.F., and W.L. Haskell. 1997. Comprehensive cardiovascular disease risk reduction in a cardiac rehabilitation setting. *Am J Cardiol* 80: 69H-73H.

Guyatt, G.H., M.J. Sullivan, and P.J. Thompson. 1985. The 6 minute walk: A new measure of exercise capacity in patients with chronic heart failure. *Can Med Assoc J* 132: 919-923.

Hagberg, J.M. 1991. Physiologic adaptations to prolonged high-intensity exercise training in patients with coronary artery disease. *Med Sci Sports Exerc* 23: 661-667.

Hambrecht, R., E. Fiehn, C. Weigl, S. Gielen, C. Hamann, R. Kaiser, J. Yu, V. Adams, J. Niebauer, and G. Schuler. 1998. Regular physical exercise corrects endothelial dysfunction and improves exercise capacity in patients with chronic heart failure. *Circulation* 98: 2709-2715.

Hambrecht, R., J. Niebauer, C. Marburger, M. Grunze, B. Kalborer, K. Haner, G. Schlorf, W. Kubler, and G. Schuler. 1993. Various intensities of leisure time physical activity in patients with coronary artery disease. Effects on cardiorespiratory fitness and progression of coronary atherosclerotic lesions. *J Am Coll Cardiol* 22: 468-477.

Hambrecht, R., C. Walther, S. Mobius-Winkler, S. Gielen, A. Linke, K. Conradi, S. Erbs, R. Kluge, K. Kendziorra, O. Sabri, P. Sick, and G. Schuler. 2004. Percutaneous coronary angioplasty compared with exercise training in patients with stable coronary artery disease. A randomized trial. *Circulation* 109: 1371-1378.

Haskell, W.L. 1978. Cardiovascular complications during exercise training of cardiac patients. *Circulation* 57: 920-924.

Helmrich, S.P., D.R. Ragland, R.W. Leung, and R.S. Paffenbarger. 1991. Physical activity and reduced occurrence of non-insulin-dependent diabetes mellitus. *New Engl J Med* 325: 147-52.

Hertzeanu, H.L., J. Shemesh, L.A. Aron, A.L Aron, E. Peleg, T. Rosenthal, M. Motro, and J.J. Kellermann. 1993. Ventricular arrhythmias in rehabilitated and nonrehabilitated post-myocardial infarction patients with left ventricular dysfunction. *Am J Cardiol* 71: 24-27.

Hughes, P.D., M.I. Polkey, M.L. Harris, A.J.S. Coats, J. Moxham, and M. Green. 1999. Diaphragm strength in chronic heart failure. *A J Respir Crit Care Med* 160: 529-534.

Jugdutt, B.I., B.L. Michorowski, and C.T. Kappagoda. 1988. Exercise training after anterior myocardial infarction. Importance of left ventricular function and topography. *J Am Coll Cardiol* 12: 362-372.

Kalapura, T., C.J. Lavie, W. Jaffrani, V. Chilakamarri, and R.V. Milani. 2003. Effects of cardiac rehabilitation and exercise training on indexes of dispersion of ventricular repolarization in patients after acute myocardial infarction. *Am J Cardiol* 92: 292-294.

Kelley, G.A., and K.S. Kelley. 2000. Progressive resistance exercise and resting blood pressure. A meta-analysis of randomized controlled trials. *Hypertension* 35: 838-843.

Kubo, N., N. Ohmura, I. Nakada, T. Yasu, T. Katsuki, M. Fujii, and M. Saito. 2004. Exercise at ventilatory threshold aggravates left ventricular remodeling in patients with extensive anterior acute myocardial infarction. *Am Heart J* 147: 113-120.

Laughlin, M.H., R.M. McAllister, J.L. Jasperse, D.A. Crader, and V.H. Huxley. 1996. Endothelium mediated control of the coronary circulation. Exercise training-induced vascular adaptations. *Sports Med* 22: 228-250.

Lavie, J.C., and R.V. Milani. 1996a. Effects of cardiac rehabilitation and exercise training in obese patients with coronary artery disease. *Chest* 109: 52-56.

Lavie, C.J., and R.V. Milani. 1996b. Effects of nonpharmacologic therapy with cardiac rehabilitation and exercise training in patients with low levels of high-density lipoprotein cholesterol. *Am J Cardiol* 78: 1286-1289.

Lavie, C.J., and R.V. Milani. 1997. Effects of cardiac rehabilitation, exercise training, and weight reduction on exercise capacity, coronary risk factors, behavioral characteristics, and quality of life in obese coronary patients. *Am J Cardiol* 79: 397-401.

Lee, J.Y., B.E. Jensen, A. Oberman, G.F. Fletcher, B.J. Fletcher, J.M., and Raczynski. 1996. Adherence in the training levels comparison trial. *Med Sci Sports Exerc* 28: 47-52.

Lee, T.H., J.B. Shammash, J.P. Ribeiro, L.H. Hartley, J. Sherwood, and L. Goldman, L. 1988. Estimation of maximum oxygen uptake from clinical data: Performance of the Specific Activity Scale. *Am Heart J* 115: 203-204.

Liang, C., D.K. Stewart, T.H. LeJemtel, P.C. Kirlin, K.M. McIntyre, H.T. Robertson, R. Brown, A.W. Moore, K.L. Wellington, L. Cahill, M.N. Galvao, P.A. Woods, C. Garces, and P. Held. 1992. Characteristics of peak aerobic capacity in symptomatic and asymptomatic subjects with left ventricular dysfunction. *Am J Cardio* 69: 1207-1211.

Liao, Y., L.A. Emidy, F.C. Gosch, and J. Stamler. 1987. Cardiovascular responses to exercise of patients in a trial on the primary prevention of hypertension. *J Hypertens* 5: 317-321.

Lim, H.Y., C.W. Lee, S.W. Park, J.J. Kim, J.K. Song, M.K. Hong, Y.S. Jin, and S.J. Park. 1998. Effects of percutaneous balloon mitral valvuloplasty and exercise training on the kinetics of recovery oxygen consumption after exercise in patients with mitral stenosis. *Eur Heart J* 19: 1865-1871.

Lund-Johansen, P. 1967. Hemodynamics in early essential hypertension. *Acta Med Scand* 183(Suppl. 482): 1-105.

Mager, G., C. Reinhardt, M. Kleine, R. Rost, and H.W. Hopp. 2000. Patients with dilated cardiomyopathy and less than 20% ejection fraction increase exercise capacity and have less severe arrhythmia after controlled exercise training. *J Cardiopulm Rehab* 20: 196-198.

Malfatto, G., M. Facchini, R. Bragato, G. Branzi, L. Sala, and G. Leonetti, G. 1996. Short and long term effects of exercise training on the tonic autonomic modulation of heart rate variability after myocardial infarction. *Eur Heart J* 17: 532-538.

Mancini, D.M., H. Eisen, W. Kussmaul, R. Mull, L.H. Edwards, and J.R. Wilson. 1991. Value of peak oxygen consumption for optimal timing of cardiac transplantation in ambulatory patients with heart failure. *Circulation* 83: 778-786.

Mancini, D.M., G. Walter, N. Reichek, R. Lendkinski, K.K. McCully, J.L. Mullen, and J.R. Wilson. 1992. Contribution of skeletal muscle atrophy to exercise intolerance and altered muscle metabolism in heart failure. *Circulation* 85: 1364-1373.

Manson, J.E., H. Tosteson, and P.M. Ridker. 1992. The primary prevention of myocardial infarction. *New Engl J Med* 326: 14-6-1416.

Mayou, R., and B. Bryant. 1993. Quality of life in cardiovascular disease. *Brit Heart J* 69: 460-466.

Mertens, D.J., and T. Kavanagh. 1996. Exercise training for patients with chronic atrial fibrillation. *J Cardiopulm Rehab* 16: 193-196.

Meyer, F.J., M.M. Borst, C. Zugck, A. Kirschke, D. Schellberg, W. Kubler, and M. Haass. 2001. Respiratory muscle dysfunction in congestive heart failure: Clinical correlation and prognostic significance. *Circulation* 103: 2153-2158.

Milani, R.V., C.J. Lavie, and M.M. Cassidy. 1996. Effects of cardiac rehabilitation and exercise training programs on depression in patients after major coronary events. *Am Heart J* 132: 726-732.

Minotti, J.R., I. Christoph, R. Oka, M.W. Weiner, L. Wells, and B.M. Massie. 1991. Impaired skeletal muscle function in patients with congestive heart failure. *J Clin Invest* 88: 2077-2082.

Moreira, W.D., F.D. Fuchs, J.P. Ribeiro, and L.J. Appel. 1999. The effects of two aerobic exercise intensities on ambulatory blood pressure in patients with mild hypertension: Results of a randomized trial. *J Clin Epidemiol* 52: 637-642.

NIH Consensus development panel on physical activity and cardiovascular health. 1996. Physical activity and cardiovascular health. *JAMA* 276: 241-246.

O'Connor, G.T., J.E. Buring, S. Yusuf, S.Z. Goldhaber, E.M. Olmstead, R.S. Paffenbarger, and C.H. Hennekens. 1989. An overview of randomized trials of rehabilitation with exercise after myocardial infarction. *Circulation* 80: 234-244.

Oldridge, N., W. Furlong, D. Feeny, G. Torrance, G. Guyatt, J. Crowe, and N. Jones. 1993. Economic evaluation of cardiac rehabilitation soon after acute myocardial infarction. *Am J Cardiol* 72: 154-161.

Oldridge, N.B., G.H. Guyatt, M.E. Fischer, and A.A. Rimm. 1988. Cardiac rehabilitation after myocardial infarction. Combined experience of randomized clinical trials. *JAMA* 260: 945-950.

Pashkow, P., P.A. Ades, C.F. Emery, D.J. Frid, N.H. Miller, G. Peske, J.Z. Reardon, J.H. Schiffert, D. Southard, and R.L. ZuWallack. 1995. Outcome measurement in cardiac and pulmonary rehabilitation by the AACVPR Outcomes Committee. *J Cardiopulm Rehab* 15: 394-405.

Pashkow, F.J., P.S. Pashkow, and M.N. Schafer. 1988. *Successful cardiac rehabilitation: The complete guide for building cardiac rehab programs*. 1st ed. Loveland: The HeartWatchers Press.

Redwood, D.R., D.R. Rosing, and S.E. Epstein. 1972. Circulatory and symptomatic effects of physical training in patients with coronary-artery disease and angina pectoris. *New Engl J Med* 286: 959-965.

Ribeiro, J.P., L.H. Hartley, and W.S. Colucci. 1985. Effects of acute and chronic pharmacologic interventions on exercise and performance in patients with congestive heart failure. *Heart Failure* 1: 102-111.

Ribeiro, J.P., L.H. Hartley, J. Sherwood, and A. Herd. 1984. The effectiveness of a low lipid diet and exercise in the management of coronary artery disease. *Am Heart J* 108: 1182-1189.

Ribeiro, J.P., A. Knutzen, M.B. Rocco, L.H. Hartley, and W.S. Colucci. 1987. Periodic breathing during exercise in severe heart failure. *Chest* 92: 555-556.

Rice, T., P. An, J. Gagnon, A.S. Leon, J.S. Skinner, J.H. Wilmore, C. Bouchard, and D.C. Rao. 2002. Heritability of HR and BP response to exercise training. *Med Sci Sports Exerc* 34: 972-979.

Roberts, J.M., M. Sullivan, V.F. Froelicher, F. Gender, and J. Myers. 1984. Predicting oxygen uptake from treadmill testing in normal subjects and coronary artery disease patients. *Am Heart J* 108: 1454-1460.

Rovena, F., H.R. Middlekauff, M.U.P.B. Rondon, S.F. Reis, M. Sousa, L. Nastari, A.C. Pereira-Barreto, E.M. Krieger, and C.E. Negrão. 2003. The effects of exercise training on sympathetic neural activation in advanced heart failure. A randomized controlled trial. *J Am Coll Cardiol* 42: 854-860.

Sannerstedt, R. 1966. Hemodynamic response to exercise in patients with arterial hypertension. *Acta Med Scand* 180 (Suppl. 458): 7-101.

Schotte, D.E., and A.J. Stunkard. 1990. The effects of weight reduction on blood pressure in 201 obese patients. *Arch Int Med* 150: 1701-04.

Schuler, G., R. Hambrecht, G. Schlierf, M. Grunze, S. Methfessel, K. Hanet, and W. Kubler. 1992. Myocardial perfusion and regression of coronary artery disease in patients on a regimen of intense physical exercise and low fat diet. *J Am Coll Cardiol* 19: 34-42.

Schuler, G., G. Schlierf, A. Wirth, H.P. Mautner, H. Scheurlen, M. Thumm, H. Roth, F. Scharz, M. Kohlmeier, H.C. Mehmel, and W. Kubler, 1988. Low-fat diet and regular, supervised physical exercise in patients with symptomatic coronary artery disease. Reduction of stress-induced myocardial ischemia. *Circulation* 77: 172-181.

Shephard, R.J., and G.J. Balady. 1999. Exercise as cardiovascular therapy. *Circulation* 99: 963-972.

Shiran, A., S. Kornfeld, S. Zur, A. Laor, Y. Karelitz, A. Militianu, A. Merdler, and B.S. Lewis. 1997. Determinants of improvement in exercise capacity in patients undergoing cardiac rehabilitation. *Cardiology* 88: 207-213.

Smart, N., and T.H. Marwick. 2004. Exercise training for patients with heart failure: A systematic review of factors that improve mortality and morbidity. *Am J Med* 116: 693-706.

Smith, S.C., S.N. Blair, M.H. Criqui, G.F. Fletcher, V. Fuster, B.J. Gersh, A.M. Gotto, L. Gould, P. Greenland, S.M. Grundy, M.N. Hill, M.A. Hlatky, N. Houston-Miller, R.M. Krauss, J. LaRosa, I.S. Ockene, S. Oparil, T.A. Pearson, E. Rapaport, R.D. Starke, for the Secondary Prevention Panel. 1995. Preventing heart attack and death in patients with coronary disease. *Circulation* 92: 2-4.

Sovijarvi, A.R.A., H. Naveri, and H. Leinonen. 1992. Ineffective ventilation during exercise in patients with chronic congestive heart failure. *Clinical Physiology* 12: 399-408.

Stein, R., C.M. Medeiros, G.A. Rosito, L.I. Zimerman, and J.P. Ribeiro. 2002. Intrinsic sinus and atrioventricular node electrophysiologic adaptations in endurance athletes. *J Am Coll Cardiol* 39: 1033-1038.

Stratton, J.R., W.L. Chandler, R.S. Schwartz, M.D. Cerqueira, W.C. Levy, S.E. Kahn, V.G. Larson, K.C. Cain, J.C. Beard, and I.B. Abrass. 1991. Effects of physical conditioning on fibrinolytic variables and fibrinogen in young and old healthy adults. *Circulation* 83: 1692-1697.

Sullivan, M.J., H.J. Green, and F.R. Cobb. 1990. Skeletal muscle biochemistry and histology in ambulatory patients with long-term heart failure. *Circulation* 81: 518-527.

Sullivan, M.J., M.B. Higginbotham, and F.R. Cobb. 1989. Exercise training in patients with chronic heart failure delays ventilatory anaerobic threshold and improves submaximal performance. *Circulation* 79: 324-329.

Taylor, R.S., A. Brown, S. Ebrahim, J. Jolliffe, H. Noorami, K. Rees, B. Skidmore, J. Stone, D.R. Thompson, and N. Oldridge. 2004. Exercise-based rehabilitation for patients with coronary heart disease: Systematic review and meta-analysis of randomized controlled trials. *Am J Med* 116: 682-692.

Testa, M.A., and D.C. Simonson. 1996. Assessment of quality-of-life outcomes. *New Engl J Med* 334: 835-840.

Thompson, D.R., G.S. Bowman, A.L. Kitson, D.P. de Bono, and A. Hopkins. 1996. Cardiac rehabilitation in the United Kingdom. Guidelines and audit standards. *Heart* 75: 89-93.

Tran, Z.V., and A. Weltman. 1985. Differential effects of exercise on serum lipid and lipoprotein levels seen with changes in body weight. A meta-analysis. *JAMA* 254: 919-924.

Van Camp, S.P., and R.A. Peterson. 1986. Cardiovascular complications of cardiac rehabilitation programs. *JAMA* 256: 1160-1163.

Vanhees, L., D. Schepers, J. Defoor, S. Brusselle, N. Tchursh, and R. Fagard. 2000. Exercise performance and training in cardiac patients with atrial fibrillation. *J Cardiopulm Rehab* 20: 346-352.

Vanhees, L., D. Schepers, H. Heidbuchel, J. Defoor, and R. Fagard. 2001. Exercise performance and training in patients with implantable cardioverter-defibrillators and coronary heart disease. *Am J Cardiol* 87: 712-715.

Verrill, D.E. 1998. Resistive exercise training in cardiac rehabilitation. In *Training techniques in cardiac rehabilitation*, ed. P.S. Fardy, B.A. Franklin, J.P. Porcari, and D.E. Verrill, 41-87. Champaign, IL: Human Kinetics.

Verrill, D.E., E. Shoup, G. McElveen, K. Witt, and D. Bergey. 1992. Resistive exercise training in cardiac patients. Recommendations. *Sports Med* 13: 171-193.

Vongvanich, P., M.J. Paul-Labrador, and N.B. Merz. 1996. Safety of medically supervised exercise in a cardiac rehabilitation center. *Am J Cardiol* 77: 1383-1385.

Weber, K., J.S. Janicki, and P.A. McElroy. 1986. Cardio-pulmonary exercise testing in the evaluation of mitral and aortic valve incompetence. *Herz* 11: 88-96.

Weber, K., G. Kinasewitz, J. Janicki, and A. Fishman. 1982. Oxygen utilization and ventilation during exercise in patients with chronic heart failure. *Circulation* 65: 1213-1223.

Weiner, D.A., C.H. McCabe, R.L. Roth, S.S. Cutler, R.L. Berger, and T.J. Ryan. 1981. Serial exercise testing after coronary artery bypass surgery. *Am J Cardiol* 101: 149- 154.

Whelton, S.P., A. Chin, X. Xin, and J. He. 2002. Effect of aerobic exercise on blood pressure: A meta-analysis of randomized, controlled trials. *Ann Int Med* 136: 493-503.

Wilson, J.R., J. Groves, and G. Rayos. 1996. Circulatory status and response to cardiac rehabilitation in patients with heart failure. *Circulation* 94: 1567-1572.

World Health Organization Expert Committee. 1964. *Rehabilitation of patients with cardiovascular disease*. Technical Report Series #270. Geneva: World Health Organization.

Wosornu, D., D. Bedford, and D. Ballantyne. 1996. A comparison of the effects of strength and aerobic exercise training on exercise capacity and lipids after coronary artery bypass surgery. *Eur Heart J* 17: 854-863.

CHAPTER 9

Aldrich, T.K., J.P. Karpel, and R.M. Uhrlass. 1989. Weaning from mechanical ventilation: Adjunctive use of inspiratory muscle resistive training. *Crit Care* 17: 143-147.

Austin, J., and G. Pullin. 1984. Improved respiratory function after lessons in the Alexander technique of musculoskeletal education. *Am Rev Respir Dis* 129: A275.

Banzett, R., G. Topulus, D. Leith, and C. Natios. 1988. Bracing arms increases the capacity for sustained hyperpnea. *Am Rev Respir Dis* 138: 106-109.

Beaumont, A., A. Cockcroft, and A. Guz. 1985. A self-paced treadmill walking test for breathless patients. *Thorax* 40: 459-464.

Bellemare, F., and A. Grassino. 1982. Evaluation of diaphragmatic fatigue. *J Appl Physiol* 53: 1196-1206.

Belman, M.J. 1981. Respiratory failure treated by ventilatory muscle training (VMT): A report of two cases. *Eur J Respir Dis* 62: 391-393.

Belman, M.J., and B.A. Kendregan. 1981. Exercise training fails to increase skeletal muscle enzymes in patients with chronic obstructive pulmonary disease. *Am Rev Respir Dis* 123: 256-261.

Belman, M.J., and C. Mittman. 1980. Ventilatory muscle training improves exercise capacity in chronic obstructive pulmonary disease patients. *Am Rev Respir Dis* 121: 273-280.

Belman, M.J., and R. Shadmehr. 1988. Targeted resistive ventilatory muscle training in chronic obstructive pulmonary disease. *J Appl Physiol* 65: 2726-2735.

Benditt, J., M. Pollock, E. Breslin, and B. Celli. 1990. Comprehensive pulmonary rehabilitation decreases the work of breathing during leg cycle ergometry in patients with severe chronic airflow obstruction (CAO). *Am Rev Respir Dis* 141: A509.

Bendstrup, K.E., J. Ingemann Jensen, S. Holm, and B. Bengtsson. 1997. Out-patient rehabilitation improves activities of daily living, quality of life and exercise tolerance in chronic obstructive pulmonary disease. *Eur Respir J* 10: 2801-2806.

Bjerre-Jempsen, K., N. Secher, and A. Kok-Jensen. 1981. Inspiratory resistance training in severe chronic obstructive pulmonary disease. *Eur J Respir Dis* 62: 405-411.

Bobbert, A.C. 1960. Physiological comparison of three types of ergometry. *J Appl Physiol* 15: 1007-1014.

Casaburi, R., A. Patessio, F. Ioli, S. Zanabouri, C. Donner, and K. Wasserman. 1991. Reductions in exercise lactic acidosis and ventilation as a result of exercise training in patients with obstructive lung disease. *Am Rev Respir Dis* 143: 9-18.

Celli, B., G. Criner, and J. Rassulo. 1988. Ventilatory muscle recruitment during unsupported arm exercise in normal subjects. *J Appl Physiol* 64: 1936-1941.

Celli, B., J. Rassulo, and B. Make. 1986. Dyssynchronous breathing associated with arm but not leg exercise in patients with COPD. *N Engl J Med* 314: 1485-1490.

Chen, H., R. Dukes, and B. Martin. 1985. Inspiratory muscle training in patients with chronic obstructive pulmonary disease. *Thorax* 131: 251-255.

Christie, D. 1968. Physical training in chronic obstructive lung disease. *Br Med J* 2: 150-151.

Clausen, J., K. Clausen, B. Rasmussen, and J. Trap-Jensen. 1973. Central and peripheral circulatory changes after training of the arms or legs. *Am J Physiol* 225: 675-682.

Cockcroft, A., M. Saunders, G. Berry. 1981. Randomized controlled trial of rehabilitation in chronic respiratory disability. *Thorax* 36: 200-203.

Couser, J., F. Martinez, and B. Celli. 1993. Pulmonary rehabilitation that include arm exercise, reduces metabolic and ventilatory requirements for simple arm elevation. *Chest* 103: 37-38.

Criner, G., and B. Celli. 1988. Effect of unsupported arm exercise on ventilatory muscle recruitment in patients with severe chronic airflow obstruction. *Am Rev Respir Dis* 138: 856-867.

Davis, C., and A. Sargeant. 1975. Effects of training on the physiological responses to one and two legged work. *J Appl Physiol* 38: 377-381.

Davis, J., P. Vodak, J. Wilmore, J. Vodak, and P. Kwitz. 1976. Anaerobic threshold and maximal power for three modes of exercise. *J Appl Physiol* 41: 549-550.

Dolmage, T., L. Maestro, M. Avendano, and R. Goldstein. 1993. The ventilatory response to arm elevation of patients with Chronic Obstructive Pulmonary Disease. *Chest* 104: 1097-1100.

Epstein, S., E. Breslin, J. Roa, and B. Celli. 1991. Impact of unsupported arm training (AT) and ventilatory muscle training (VMT) on the metabolic and ventilatory consequences of unsupported arm elevation (UAE) and exercise (UAEx) in patients with chronic airflow obstruction. *Am Rev Respir Dis* 143: 81A.

Epstein, S., B. Celli, F. Martinez, J. Couser, J. Roa, M. Pollock, and J. Benditt. 1997. Arm training reduces the VO_2 and VE cost of unsupported arm exercise and elevation in chronic obstructive pulmonary disease. *J Cardpulm Rehabil* 17: 171-177.

Falk, P., A. Eksen, K. Kolliker, and J.B. Andersen. 1985. Relieving dyspnea with an inexpensive and simple method in patients with severe chronic airflow limitation. *Eur J Respir Dis* 66: 181-186.

Finnerty, J.P., I. Keeping, I. Bullough, and J. Jones. 2001. The effectiveness of outpatient pulmonary rehabilitation in chronic lung disease. A randomized controlled trial. *Chest* 119: 1705-1710.

Gerardi, D.A., L. Lovett, M.L. Benoit-Connors, J.Z. Reardon, and R.L. ZuWallack. 1996. Variables related to increased mortality following out-patient pulmonary rehabilitation. *Eur Respir J* 9: 431-435.

Goldstein, R.S., E. Gort, D. Stubing, M.A. Avendano, and G.H. Guyatt. 1994. Randomized trial of respiratory rehabilitation. *Lancet* 344: 1394-1398.

Griffiths, T.L., M.L. Burr, I.A. Campbell, V. Lewis-Jenkins, J. Mullins, K. Shiels, P.J. Turner-Lawlor, N. Payne, R.G. Newcombe, A.A. Ionescu, J. Thomas, and J. Tunbridge. 2000. Results at 1 year of outpatient multidisciplinary pulmonary rehabilitation: A randomized clinical trial. *Lancet* 355(92010: 362-368.

Harver, A., D. Mahler, and J. Daubenspeck. 1989. Targeted inspiratory muscle training improves respiratory muscle function and reduces dyspnea in patients with chronic obstructive pulmonary disease. *Ann Int Med* 111: 117-124.

Holle, R., D. Williams, J. Vandree, G. Starks, and R. Schoene. 1988. Increased muscle efficiency and sustained benefits in an outpatient community hospital-based pulmonary rehabilitation program. *Chest* 94: 1161-1168.

Holliday, J., and T. Hyers. 1990. The reduction of weaning time from mechanical ventilation using tidal volume and relaxation biofeedback. *Am Rev Respir Dis* 141: 1214-1220.

Horowitz, M., B. Littenberg, and D. Mahler. 1997. Dyspnea ratings for prescribing exercise intensity in patients with COPD. *Chest* 109: 1169-1175.

Hughes, R., and R. Davidson. 1983. Limitations of exercise reconditioning in COPD. *Chest* 83: 241-249.

Jones, D., R. Thomson, and M. Sears. 1985. Physical exercise and resistive breathing training in severe chronic airways obstruction. Are they effective? *Eur J Respir Dis* 67: 159-166.

Keens, T., I. Krastins, E. Wannamaker, H. Levinson, D. Crozier, and A. Bryan. 1977. Ventilatory muscle endurance training in normal subjects and patients with cystic fibrosis. *Am Rev Respir Dis* 116: 853-860.

Lake, F., K. Hendersen, T. Briffa, J. Openshaw, and A.W. Musk. 1990. Upper limb and lower limb exercise training in patients with chronic airflow obstruction. *Chest* 97: 1077-1082.

Larson, J., M. Kim, and J. Sharp. 1988. Inspiratory muscle training with a pressure threshold breathing device in patients with chronic obstructive pulmonary disease. *Am Rev Respir Dis* 138: 689-696.

Lecog, A., L. Delhez, and S. Janssens. 1970. Reentrainement de la fonction motrice ventilatoire chez des insuffisants respiratoire chroniques. *Acta Tuberc Pneumol Belg* 61: 63-69.

Leith, D., and M. Bradley. 1976. Ventilatory muscle strength and endurance training. *J Appl Physiol* 4: 508-516.

Levine, S., P. Weiser, and J. Guillen. 1986. Evaluation of a ventilatory muscle endurance training program in the rehabilitation of patients with chronic obstructive pulmonary disease. *Am Rev Respir Dis* 133: 400-406.

Lisboa, C., V. Munoz, T. Beroiza, A. Leiva, and E. Cruz. 1994. Inspiratory muscle training in chronic airflow limitation: Comparison of two different training loads with a threshold device. *Eur Respir J* 7: 1266-1270.

Maestro, L., T. Dolmage, M. Avendano, and R. Goldstein. 1990. Influence of arm position in ventilation during incremental exercise in healthy individuals. *Chest* 98: 113(S).

Make, B., and R. Buckolz. 1991. Exercise training in COPD patients improves cardiac function. *Am Rev Respir Dis* 143: 80A.

Maltais, F., P. LeBlanc, J. Jobin, C. Berube, J. Bruneau, L. Carrier, M.J. Breton, G. Falardeau, and R. Belleau.. 1997. Intensity of training and physiologic adaptation in patient with chronic obstructive pulmonary disease. *Am J Respir Crit Care Med* 155(2): 555-561.

Maltais, F., P. Leblanc, C. Simard, J. Jobin, C. Berube, J. Bruneau, L. Carrier, and R. Belleau. 1996. Skeletal muscle adaptation to endurance training in patients with chronic obstructive pulmonary disease. *Am J Respir Crit Care Med* 154: 442-447.

Maltais, F., A. Simard, J. Simard, J. Jobin, P. Desgagnes, and P. LeBlanc. 1995. Oxidative capacity of the skeletal muscle and lactic acid kinetics during exercise in normal subjects and in patients with COPD. *Am J Respir Crit Care Med* 153: 288-293.

Martin, T., J. Zeballos, and I. Weisman. 1991. Gas exchange during maximal upper extremity exercise. *Chest* 99: 420-425.

Martinez, F., J. Couser, and B. Celli. 1990. Factors influencing ventilatory muscle recruitment in patients with chronic airflow obstruction. *Am Rev Respir Dis* 142: 276-282.

Martinez, F., P. Vogel, D. DuPont, I. Stanopoulos, A. Gray, and J.F. Beamis. 1993. Supported arm exercise vs. unsupported arm exercise in the rehabilitation of patients with chronic airflow obstruction. *Chest* 103: 1397-2002.

McGavin, C., S. Gupta, and G. McHardy. 1976. Twelve minute walking test for assessing disability in chronic bronchitis. *Br Med J* 1: 822-3.

Mohsenifar, Z., D. Horak, H. Brown, and S. Koerner. 1983. Sensitive indices of improvement in a pulmonary rehabilitation program. *Chest* 83: 189-92.

Moser, K., G. Bokinsky, R. Savage, C. Archibald, and P. Hansen. 1980. Results of comprehensive rehabilitation programs. *Arch Int Med* 140: 1596-601.

Niederman, M., P. Clemente, A. Fein, S. Feinsilver, D. Robinson, J. Ilowite, and M. Bernstein. 1991. Benefits of a multidisciplinary pulmonary rehabilitation program. Improvements are independent of lung function. *Chest* 99: 798-804.

Normandin, E., C. McCusker, M.L. Connors, F. Vale, D. Gerardi, and R. ZuWallack. 2002. An evaluation of two approaches to exercise conditioning in pulmonary rehabilitation. *Chest* 121: 1085-1091.

Noseda, A., J. Carpiaux, and N. Vandeput. 1987. Resistive inspiratory muscle training and exercise performance in COPD patients. A comparative study with conventional breathing retraining. *Bull Eur Physiopathol Respir* 23: 457-463.

O'Donnell, D., K. Webb, and M. McGuire. 1993. Older patients with COPD: Benefits of exercise training. *Geriatrics* 48: 59-66.

Oga, T., K. Nishimura, M. Tsukino, S. Sato, and T. Hajiro. 2003. Analysis of the factors related to mortality in chronic obstructive pulmonary disease: Role of exercise capacity and health status. *Am J Respir Crit Care Med* 167: 544-549.

O'Hara, W., B. Lasachuk, P. Matheson, M. Renahan. D. Schloter, and E. Lilker. 1984. Weight training and backpacking in Chronic Obstructive Pulmonary Disease. *Respir Care* 29: 1202-10.

Paez, P., E. Phillipson, M. Mosangkay, and B. Sproule. 1967. The physiologic basis of training patients with emphysema. *Am Rev Respir Dis* 95: 944-53.

Pardy, R., R. Livingston, and P. Despas. 1981. Inspiratory muscle training compared with physiotherapy in patients with chronic airflow limitation. *Am Rev Respir Dis* 123: 421-5.

Pinto-Plata, V., C.G. Cote, H.J. Cabral, J. Taylor, and B. Celli. 2004. The 6-min walk distance: Change over time and value as predictor of survival in severe COPD. *Eur Respir J* 23: 1-6.

Pollock, M., J. Roa, J. Benditt, and B. Celli. 1993. Stair climbing (SC) predicts maximal oxygen uptake in patients with chronic airflow obstruction. *Chest* 104: 1378-1383.

Puente Maestu, L., J. Sanz, J. Rodriguez, and B.J. Whipp. 2000. Effects of two types of training on pulmonary and cardiac responses to moderate exercise in patients with COPD. *Eur Respir J* 15: 1026-1032.

Reardon, J., E. Awad, E. Normandin, F. Vale, B. Clark, and R. ZuWallack. 1994. The effect of comprehensive outpatient pulmonary rehabilitation on dyspnea. *Chest* 105: 1046-1048.

Reid, W., and C. Warren. 1984. Ventilatory muscle strength and endurance training in elderly subjects and patients with chronic airflow limitation: A pilot study. *Physio Canada* 36: 305-311.

Reybrouck, T., G. Heigenhouser, and J. Faulkner. 1975. Limitations to maximum oxygen uptake in arm, leg and combined arm-leg ergometry. *J Appl Physiol* 38: 774-779.

Ries, A., B. Ellis, and R. Hawkins. 1988. Upper extremity exercise training in chronic obstructive pulmonary disease. *Chest* 93: 688-692.

Ries, A., R. Kaplan, T. Linberg, and L. Prewitt. 1995. Effects of pulmonary rehabilitation on physiologic and psychosocial outcomes in patients with chronic obstructive pulmonary disease. *Ann Int Med* 122: 823-827.

Ries, A., and K. Moser. 1986. Comparison of isocapneic hyperventilation and walking exercise training at home in pulmonary rehabilitation. *Chest* 90: 285-289.

Roa, J., S. Epstein, E. Breslin, T. Shannon, and B. Celli. 1991. Work of breathing and ventilatory muscle recruitment during pursed lip breathing. *Am Rev Respir Dis* 143: A77.

Roussos, C., and P. Macklem. 1982. The respiratory muscles. *N Engl J Med* 307: 786-97.

Saltin, B., G. Blomquist, J. H. Mitchell, R. Johnson Jr., K. Wildenthal, and C. Chapman. 1968. Response to exercise after bed rest and training. *Circulation* 38(5 Suppl): VII1-78.

Scheinhorn, D., and C. Ho. 1991. Avoiding home mechanical ventilation; the regional weaning center. Proceedings of the International Conference on Pulmonary Rehabilitation and Home Mechanical Ventilation 3: A35.

Siegel, W., G. Blonquist, and J. Mitchell. 1970. Effects of a quantitated physical training program on middle-aged sedentary man. *Circulation* 41: 19-29.

Sinclair, D., and C. Ingram. 1980. Controlled trial of supervised exercise training in chronic bronchitis. *Br Med J* 1: 519-521.

Stanescu, D., B. Nemery, C. Veriter, and C. Marechal. 1981. Pattern of breathing and ventilatory response to CO_2 in subjects practicing hatha-yoga. *J Appl Physiol* 51: 1625-1629.

Steinberg, J., P. Astrand, B. Ekblom, J. Royce, and P. Sattin. 1967. Hemodynamic response to work with different muscle groups, sitting and supine. *J Appl Physiol* 22: 61-70.

Strijbos, J.H., D.S. Postma, R. van Altena, F. Gimeno, and G.H. Koeter. 1996. A comparison between an outpatient hospital-based pulmonary rehabilitation program and a home-care pulmonary rehabilitation program in patients with COPD. A follow-up of 18 months. *Chest* 109: 366-372.

Tandon, M. 1980. Adjunct treatment with yoga in chronic severe airways obstruction. *Thorax* 33: 514-517.

Tangri, S., and C. Woolf. 1973. The breathing pattern in chronic obstructive lung disease, during the performance of some common daily activities. *Chest* 63: 126-127.

Wedzicha, J.A., J.C. Bestall, R. Garrod, R. Garnham, E.A. Paul, and P.W. Jones. 1998. Randomized controlled trial of pulmonary rehabilitation in severe chronic obstructive pulmonary disease patients, stratified with the MRC dyspnoea scale. *Eur Respir J* 12: 363-369.

Weiner, P., Y. Azgad, and R. Ganam. 1992. Inspiratory muscle training, combined with general exercise reconditioning in patients with COPD. *Chest* 102: 1351-1356.

Weiner, P., Y. Azgad, R. Ganam, and M. Weiner. 1992. Inspiratory muscle training in asthma. *Chest* 102: 1357-1361.

Wijkstra, P., R. Van Altena, J. Kraan, V. Otten, D. Postma, and G. Koeter. 1994. Quality of life in patients with chronic obstructive pulmonary disease improves after rehabilitation in house. *Eur Respir J* 7: 269-274.

Wijkstra, P.J., T.W. van der Mark, J. Kraan, R. van Altena, G.H. Koeter, and D.S. Postma. 1996. Effects of home rehabilitation on physical performance in patients with chronic obstructive pulmonary disease (COPD). *Eur Respir J* 9: 104-110.

Woolf, C., and J. Suero. 1969. Alterations in lung mechanics and gas exchange following training in chronic obstructive lung disease. *Chest* 55: 37-44.

Zack, M., and A. Palange. 1985. Oxygen supplemented exercise of ventilatory and nonventilatory muscles in pulmonary rehabilitation. *Chest* 88: 669-675.

ZuWallack, R., K. Patel, J. Reardon, B. Clark, and E. Normandin. 1991. Predictors of improvement in the 12-minute walking distance following a six-week outpatient pulmonary rehabilitation program. *Chest* 99: 805-08.

CHAPTER 10

American College of Sports Medicine. 2000. *Guidelines for exercise testing and prescription*. 6th ed., 22-32. Philadelphia: Lippincott Williams & Wilkins.

American Diabetes Association. 2005. Diagnosis and classification of diabetes mellitus. *Diabetes Care* 28: S37-S42.

Amiel, S.A., W.V. Tamborlane, D.C. Simonson, and R.S. Sherwin. 1987. Defective glucose counterregulation after strict control of insulin-dependent diabetes mellitus. *N Engl J Med* 316: 1376-1383.

Berger, M., P. Berchtold, H.-J. Cuppers, H. Drost, H.K. Kley, W.A. Muller, W. Wiegelmann, H. Zimmermann-Telschow, F.A. Gries, H.L. Kruskemper, and H. Zimmerman. 1977. Metabolic and hormonal effects of muscular exercise in juvenile type diabetics. *Diabetologia* 13: 355-365.

Bjorntorp, P., K. de Jounge, L. Sjostrom, and L. Sullivan. 1970. The effect of physical training on insulin production in obesity. *Metabolism* 19: 631-637.

Bjorntorp, P., K. de Jounge, L. Sjostrom, and L. Sullivan. 1973. Physical training in human obesity. II. Effects of plasma insulin in glucose intolerant subjects without marked hyperinsulinemia. *Scand J Clin Lab Invest* 32: 42-45.

Bjorntorp, P., M. Fahlen, G. Grimby, A. Gustafson, J. Holm, P. Renstrom, and T. Schersten. 1972. Carbohydrate and lipid metabolism in middle aged physically well-trained men. *Metabolism* 21: 1037-1042.

Bogardus, C., E. Ravussin, D.C. Robbins, R.R. Wolfe, E.S. Horton, and E.A.H. Sims. 1984. Effects of physical training and diet therapy on carbohydrate metabolism in patients with glucose intolerance and non-insulin dependent diabetes mellitus. *Diabetes* 33: 311-318.

Bogardus, C., P. Thuillez, E. Ravussin, B. Vasquez, M. Narimiga, and S. Azhar. 1983. Effect of muscle glycogen depletion on in vivo in insulin action in man. *J Clin Invest* 72: 1605-1610.

Burstein, R., C. Polychronakos, C.J. Toeus, J.D. MacDougall, H.J. Guyda, and B.I. Posner. 1985. Acute reversal of the enhanced insulin action in trained athletes. *Diabetes* 34: 756-760.

Calles, J., J.J. Cunningham, L. Nelson, N. Brown, E. Nadel, R.S. Sherwin, and P. Felig. 1983. Glucose turnover during recovery from intensive exercise. *Diabetes* 32: 734-738.

Caron, D., P. Poussier, E.B. Marliss, and B. Zinman. 1982. The effect of postprandial exercise on meal-related glucose intolerance in insulin-dependent diabetic individuals. *Diabetes Care* 5: 364-369.

Cruickshanks, K.J., S.E. Moss, R. Klein, and B.E. Klein. 1995. Physical activity and the risk of progression of retinopathy or the development of proliferative retinopathy. *Ophthalmology* 102: 1177-1182.

DeFronzo, R.A., E. Ferranni, and V. Koivisto. 1983. New concepts in the pathogenesis and treatment of non-insulin dependent diabetes mellitus. *Am J Med* 74: 52-81.

Devlin, J.T., and E.S. Horton. 1985. Effects of prior high-intensity exercise on glucose metabolism in normal and insulin-resistant men. *Diabetes* 34: 973-979.

Diabetes Control and Complications Trial Research Group. 1993. The effect of intensive treatment of diabetes on the development and progression of long-term complications in insulin-dependent diabetes mellitus. *N Engl J Med* 329: 977-986.

Diabetes Prevention Program Research Group. 2002. Reduction in the incidence of type 2 diabetes with lifestyle intervention or metformin. *N Eng J Med* 346: 393.

Fernqvist, E., B. Linde, J. Ostman, and R. Gunnarsson. 1986. Effects of physical exercise on insulin absorption in insulin-dependent diabetics. A comparison between human and porcine insulin. *Clin Physiol* 6: 489-498.

Fery, F., V. deMaetalaer, and E.O. Balasse. 1987. Mechanism of the hyperketonemic effect of prolonged exercise in insulin-deprived type 1 (insulin-dependent) diabetic patients. *Diabetologia* 30: 298-304.

Goodyear, L.J., M.F. Hirshman, P.M. Valyou, and E.S. Horton. 1992. Glucose transporter number, function and subcellular distribution in rat skeletal muscle after exercise training. *Diabetes* 41: 1091-1099.

Helmrich, S.P., D.R. Ragland, R.W. Leung, and R.S. Paffenbarger. 1991. Physical activity and reduced occurrence of non-insulin-dependent diabetes mellitus. *N Engl J Med* 325: 147-152.

Hilsted, J.J., H. Galbo, and N.J. Christensen. 1979. Impaired cardiovascular responses to graded exercise in diabetic autonomic neuropathy. *Diabetes* 28: 313-319.

Horton, E.S. 1979. The role of exercise in the treatment of hypertension in obesity. *Int J Obes* 5(Suppl. 1): 89-92.

Horton, E.S. 1986. Exercise and physical training: Effects on insulin sensitivity and glucose metabolism. *Diabetes Metab Rev* 2: 1-17.

Horton, E.S. 1988. Role and management of exercise in diabetes mellitus. *Diabetes Care* 11: 201-211.

Huttunen, J.K., E. Lanisimies, E. Voutilainen, C. Ehnholm, F. Hietanen, I. Pantila, O. Siitonen, and R. Rauramua. 1979. Effect of moderate physical exercise on serum lipoprotein. *Circulation* 60: 1220-1229.

Ishii, T., T. Yamakita, T. Sato, S. Tanaka, and S. Fuji. 1998. Resistance training improves insulin sensitivity in NIDDM subjects without altering maximal oxygen uptake. *Diabetes Care* 21: 1353-1355.

Kahn, J.K., B. Zola, J.E. Juni, and A.I. Vinik. 1986. Decreased exercise heart rate and blood pressure response in diabetic subjects with cardiac autonomic neuropathy. *Diabetes Care* 9: 389-394.

Kannel, W.B. 1990. Diabetes, fibrinogen, and risk of cardiovascular disease: The Framingham experience. *Am Heart J* 120: 672-676.

Kemmer, F.W., P. Berchtold, M. Berger, A. Starke, H.-J. Cuppers, F.A. Gries, and H. Zimmerman. 1979. Exercise-induced fall of blood glucose in insulin-treated diabetics unrelated to alteration of insulin mobilization. *Diabetes* 28: 1131-1137.

Koivisto, V., and P. Felig. 1978. Effects of leg exercise on insulin absorption in diabetic patients. *N Engl J Med* 298: 77-83.

Koskinen, P., M. Manttari, V. Manninen, J.K. Huttunen, O.P. Heinonen, and M.H. Frick. 1992. Coronary heart disease incidence in NIDDM patients in the Helsinki heart study. *Diabetes Care* 15: 820-825.

Kriska, A.M., S.N. Blair, and M.A. Pereira. 1991. The potential role of physical activity in the prevention of non-insulin dependent diabetes mellitus: The epidemiological evidence. *Exerc Sports Sci Rev* 22: 121-143.

Kruszynska, Y.T., and J.M. Olefsky. 1996. Cellular and molecular mechanisms of non-insulin dependent diabetes mellitus. *J Investig Med* 44: 413-428.

LaPorte, R.E., J.S. Dorman, N. Tajima, K.J. Cruickshanks, T.J. Orchard, D.E. Cavender, D.J. Becker, and A.L. Drash. 1986. Pittsburgh insulin-dependent diabetes mellitus morbidity and mortality study: Physical activity and diabetic complications. *Pediatrics* 78: 1027-1033.

Lipman, R.L., P. Raskin, T. Love, J. Triebwasser, F.R. LeCocq, and J.J. Schnure. 1972. Glucose intolerance during decreased physical activity in man. *Diabetes* 21: 101-107.

Lipson, L.C., R.W. Bonow, E. J. Schaefer, H. Brewer, and F.T. Lindren. 1980. Effect of exercise condition on plasma high-density lipoprotein and other lipoproteins. *Atherosclerosis* 37: 529-538.

Lohmann, D., F. Liebold, W. Heilmann, H. Senger, and A. Pohl. 1978. Diminished insulin response in highly trained athletes. *Metabolism* 27: 521-542.

MacDonald, M.J. 1987. Postexercise late-onset hypoglycemia in insulin-dependent diabetic patients. *Diabetes Care* 10: 584-588.

Manson, J.E., D.M. Nathan, A.S. Krolewski, M.J. Stampfer, W.C. Willett, and C.H. Hennekens. 1992. A prospective study of exercise and incidence of diabetes among US male physicians. *JAMA* 268: 63-67.

Manson, J.E., E.B. Rimm, M.J. Stampfer, G.A. Colditz, W.C. Willett, A.S. Krolewski, B. Rosner, C.H. Hennekens, and F.E. Speizer. 1991. Physical activity and incidence of non-insulin dependent diabetes mellitus in women. *Lancet* 338: 774-778.

Margonato, A., P. Gerundini, G. Vicedomini, M.C. Gilardi, G. Pozza, and F. Fazio. 1986. Abnormal cardiovascular response to exercise in a young asymptomatic diabetic patient with retinopathy. *Am Heart J* 112: 554-560.

Marrero, D.G., A.S. Fremion, and M.P. Golden. 1988. Improving compliance with exercise in adolescents with insulin-dependent diabetes mellitus: Results of a self-motivated home exercise program. *Pediatrics* 81: 519-525.

Mikines, K.J., B. Sonne, P.A. Farrell, B. Tronier, and H. Galbo. 1988. Effect of physical exercise on sensitivity and responsiveness to insulin in humans. *Am J Physiol* 254: E248-E259.

Mikines, K.J., B. Sonne, B. Tronier, and H. Galbo. 1989. Effects of acute exercise and detraining on insulin action in trained men. *J Appl Physiol* 66: 704-711.

Mitchell, T.H., G. Abraham, A. Shiffrin, L.A. Leiter, and E.B. Marliss. 1988. Hyperglycemia after intense exercise in IDDM subjects during continuous subcutaneous insulin infusion. *Diabetes Care* 11: 311-317.

Mogensen, C.E., and E. Vittinghu. 1975. Urinary albumin excretion during exercise in juvenile diabetes. *Scan J Clin Lab Invest* 35: 295-300.

Nelson, J.D., P. Poussier, E.B. Marliss, A.M. Albisser, and B. Zinman. 1982. Metabolic response of normal man and insulin-infused diabetics to postprandial exercise. *Am J Physiol* 242: E309-E316.

Ohkubo, Y., H. Kishikawa, E. Araki, T. Miyata, S. Isami, S. Motoyoshi, Y. Kojima, N. Furuyoshi, and M. Shichiri. 1995. Intensive insulin therapy prevents the progression of diabetic microvascular complications in Japanese patients with non-insulin-dependent diabetes mellitus: A randomized prospective 6-year study. *Diabetes Res Clin Pract* 28: 103-117.

Olefsky, J.M. 1989. Pathogenesis of non-insulin-dependent (type 2) diabetes. In *Endocrinology*. 3rd ed., ed. L.J. DeGroot, 1369-88. Philadelphia: Saunders.

Pan, X.R., G.W. Li, Y.H. Hu, J.X. Wang, W.Y. Yang, et al. 1997. Effects of diet and exercise in preventing NIDDM in people with impaired glucose tolerance: The Da Qing IGT and Diabetes Study. *Diabetes Care* 20(4): 537-544.

Rosenthal, M., W.L. Haskell, R. Solomon, A. Widstrom, and G.M. Reaven. 1983. Demonstration of a relationship between level of physical training and insulin-stimulated glucose utilization in normal humans. *Diabetes* 32: 408-411.

Rubler, S. 1981. Asymptomatic diabetic female exercise testing. *N Y State J Med* 81: 1185-91.

Sato, Y., A. Iguchi, and N. Sakamoto. 1984. Biochemical determination of training effects using insulin clamp technique. *Horm Metab Res* 16: 483-486.

Schiffrin, A., S. Parikh, E.B. Marliss, and M.M. Desrosier. 1984. Metabolic response to fasting exercise in adolescent insulin-dependent diabetic subjects treated with continuous subcutaneous insulin infusion and intensive conventional therapy. *Diabetes Care* 7: 255-260.

Schneider, S.H., L.F. Amoroso, A.K. Khachadurian, and N.B. Ruderman. 1984. Studies on the mechanism of improved glucose control during exercise in type 2 (non-insulin-dependent) diabetes. *Diabetologist* 26: 355-360.

Simonson, D.C., W.V. Tamborlane, R.A. DeFronzo, and R.S. Sherwin. 1985. Intensive insulin therapy reduces the counter-regulatory hormone responses to hypoglycemia in patients with type 1 diabetes. *Ann Int Med* 103: 184-190.

Storstein, L., and J. Jervell. 1979. Response to bicycle exercise testing of long standing juvenile diabetics. *Acta Med Scand* 205: 227-230.

Stratton, R., D.P. Wilson, R.K. Endres, and D.E. Goldstein. 1987. Improved glycemic control after supervised 8 week exercise program in insulin-dependent diabetic adolescents. *Diabetes Care* 10: 589-593.

Tuomilehto, J., J. Lindstrom, J. Eriksson, T. Valle, H. Hamalainen, P. Ilanne-Parikka, S. Keinanen-Kiukaanniemi, M. Laakso, A. Louheranta, M. Rasta, V. Salminen, M. Uusitupa, and Finnish Diabetes Prevention Study Group. 2001. Prevention of type 2 diabetes mellitus by changes in lifestyle among subjects with impaired glucose tolerance. *N Engl J Med* 344(18): 1343-1350.

United Kingdom Prospective Diabetes Study Group (UKPDS33). 1998. Intensive blood glucose control with sulfonylureas or insulin compared with conventional treatment and risk of complications in patients with type 2 diabetes. *Lancet* 352: 837-853.

Viberti, G.C., R.J. Jarrett, M. McCartney, and H. Keen. 1978. Increased glomerular permeability to albumin induced by exercise in diabetic subjects. *Diabetologia* 14: 293-300.

Wallberg-Henriksson, H., R. Gunnarsson, S. Rossner, and J. Wahren. 1986. Long-term physical training in female type 1 (insulin-dependent) diabetic patients: Absence of significant effect on glycemic control and lipoprotein levels. *Diabetologia* 29: 53-57.

White, N.H., D. Skor, P.E. Cryer, D.M. Bier, L. Levandoski, and J.V. Santiago. 1983. Identification of type 1 diabetic patients at increased risk for hyperglycemia during intensive therapy. *N Engl J Med* 308: 485-491.

Wood, P.D., and W.L. Haskell. 1979. Effect of exercise on plasma high density lipoproteins. *Lipids* 14: 417-427.

Yki-Jarvinen, H., and V.A. Koivisto. 1983. Effects of body composition on insulin sensitivity. *Diabetes* 32: 965-969.

Zinman, B., F.T. Murray, M. Vranic, A.M. Albisser, B.S. Leibel, P.A. McClean, and E.B. Marliss. 1977. Glucoregulation during moderate exercise in insulin treated diabetics. *J Clin Endocrinol Metab* 45: 641-652.

CHAPTER 11

Alexanderson, H., C.H. Stenstrom, G. Jenner, and I. Lundberg. 2000. The safety of a resistive home exercise program in patients with recent onset active polymyositis or dermatomyositis. *Scand J Rheumatol* 29 (5): 295-301.

Alexanderson, H., C.H. Stenstrom, and I. Lundberg. 1999. Safety of a home exercise programme in patients with polymyositis and dermatomyositis: A pilot study. *Rheumatology (Oxford)* 38 (7): 608-611.

Aloia, J.F., S.H. Cohn, J.A. Ostuni, R. Cane, and K. Ellis. 1978. Prevention of involutional bone loss by exercise. *Ann Intern Med* 89 (3): 356-358.

American College of Rheumatology. 2000. Recommendations for the medical management of osteoarthritis of the hip and knee: 2000 update. American College of Rheumatology Subcommittee on Osteoarthritis Guidelines. *Arthritis Rheum* 43 (9): 1905-1915.

American College of Sports Medicine. 1986. *Guidelines for exercise testing and prescription.* 3rd ed. Philadelphia: Lea & Febiger.

Åstrand, P.O. 1986. Why exercise? An evolutionary approach. *Acta Med Scand Suppl* 711: 241-242.

Baker, K.R., M.E. Nelson, D.T. Felson, J.E. Layne, R. Sarno, and R. Roubenoff. 2001. The efficacy of home based progressive strength training in older adults with knee osteoarthritis: A randomized controlled trial. *J Rheumatol* 28 (7): 1655-1665.

Barrett, D.S., A G. Cobb, and G. Bentley. 1991. Joint proprioception in normal, osteoarthritic and replaced knees. *J Bone Joint Surg Br* 73 (1): 53-56.

Baslund, B., K. Lyngberg, V. Andersen, J. Halkjaer Kristensen, M. Hansen, M. Klokker, and B. K. Pedersen. 1993. Effect of 8 wk of bicycle training on the immune system of patients with rheumatoid arthritis. *J Appl Physiol* 75 (4): 1691-1695.

Bautch, J.C., D.G. Malone, and A.C. Vailas. 1997. Effects of exercise on knee joints with osteoarthritis: A pilot study of biologic markers. *Arthritis Care Res* 10 (1): 48-55.

Blom-Bulow, B., B. Jonson, and K. Bauer. 1983. Factors limiting exercise performance in progressive systemic sclerosis. *Semin Arthritis Rheum* 13 (2): 174-181.

Bolen, J., C.G. Helmick, J.J. Sacks, G. Langmaid, Division of Adult and Community Health, National Center for Chronic Disease Prevention and Health Promotion, and Centers for Disease Control and Prevention. 2002. Prevalence of self-reported arthritis or chronic joint symptoms among adults—United States, 2001. *Morbidity and Mortality Weekly Report* 51 (42): 948-950. Available online at www.cdc.gov/mmwr/preview/mmwrhtml/mm5142a2.htm. Accessed May 12, 2005.

Borg, G. A. 1982. Psychophysical bases of perceived exertion. *Med Sci Sports Exerc* 14 (5): 377-381.

Borjesson, M., E. Robertson, L. Weidenhielm, E. Mattsson, and E. Olsson. 1996. Physiotherapy in knee osteoarthrosis: Effect on pain and walking. *Physiother Res Int* 1 (2): 89-97.

Bostrom, C., K. Harms-Ringdahl, H. Karreskog, and R. Nordemar. 1998. Effects of static and dynamic shoulder rotator exercises in women with rheumatoid arthritis: A randomised comparison of impairment, disability, handicap, and health. *Scand J Rheumatol* 27 (4): 281-290.

Bradley, L.A. 1989. Adherence with treatment regimens among adult rheumatoid arthritis patients: Current status and future directions. *Arthritis Care Res* 2 (3): S33-S39.

Brandt, K.D., D.K. Heilman, C. Slemenda, B.P. Katz, S. Mazzuca, E.M. Braunstein, and D. Byrd. 2000. A comparison of lower extremity muscle strength, obesity, and depression scores in elderly subjects with knee pain with and without radiographic evidence of knee osteoarthritis. *J Rheumatol* 27 (8): 1937-1946.

Brighton, S.W., J.E. Lubbe, and C.A. van der Merwe. 1993. The effect of a long-term exercise programme on the rheumatoid hand. *Br J Rheumatol* 32 (5): 392-395.

Byers, P.H. 1985. Effect of exercise on morning stiffness and mobility in patients with rheumatoid arthritis. *Res Nurs Health* 8 (3): 275-281.

Callaghan, J.J., J.A. Oldham, and J. Hunt. 1995. An evaluation of exercise regimes for patients with osteoarthritis: A single blind randomized controlled trial. *Clin Rehabil* 9: 213-218.

Callaghan, J.J., D.R. Pedersen, J.P. Olejniczak, D.D. Goetz, and R.C. Johnston. 1995. Radiographic measurement of wear in 5 cohorts of patients observed for 5 to 22 years. *Clin Orthop* 317: 14-18.

Carter, R., P. Riantawan, S.W. Banham, and R.D. Sturrock. 1999. An investigation of factors limiting aerobic capacity in patients with ankylosing spondylitis. *Respir Med* 93 (10): 700-708.

Casale, R., M. Buonocore, and M. Matucci-Cerinic. 1997. Systemic sclerosis (scleroderma): An integrated challenge in rehabilitation. [comment]. *Arch Phys Med Rehabil* 78 (7): 767-73.

Chamberlain, M.A., G. Care, and B. Harfield. 1982. Physiotherapy in osteoarthrosis of the knees. A controlled trial of hospital versus home exercises. *Int Rehabil Med* 4 (2): 101-106.

Cialdini, R.B. 1993. *Influence: The psychology of persuasion*. rev. ed. New York: Morrow.

Crowe, J., and J. Henderson. 2003. Pre-arthroplasty rehabilitation is effective in reducing hospital stay. *Can J Occup Ther* 70 (2): 88-96.

Dagfinrud, H., and K. Hagen. 2001. Physiotherapy interventions for ankylosing spondylitis. *Cochrane Database of Systematic Reviews* (4): CD002822.

Daltroy, L.H., C. Robb-Nicholson, M.D. Iversen, E.A. Wright, and M.H. Liang. 1995. Effectiveness of minimally supervised home aerobic training in patients with systemic rheumatic disease. *Br J Rheumatol* 34 (11): 1064-1069.

Decker, J.L. 1983. American Rheumatism Association nomenclature and classification of arthritis and rheumatism (1983). *Arthritis Rheum* 26 (8): 1029-1032.

de Jong, Z., M. Munneke, A.H. Zwinderman, H.M. Kroon, A. Jansen, K.H. Ronday, D. van Schaardenburg, B.A. Dijkmans, C.H. Van den Ende, F.C. Breedveld, T.P. Vliet Vlieland, and J.M. Hazes. 2003. Is a long-term high-intensity exercise program effective and safe in patients with rheumatoid arthritis? Results of a randomized controlled trial. *Arthritis Rheum* 48 (9): 2415-2424.

Dexter, P.A. 1992. Joint exercises in elderly persons with symptomatic osteoarthritis of the hip or knee. Performance patterns, medical support patterns, and the relationship between exercising and medical care. *Arthritis Care Res* 5 (1): 36-41.

Deyle, G.D., N.E. Henderson, R.L. Matekel, M.G. Ryder, M.B. Garber, and S.C. Allison. 2000. Effectiveness of manual physical therapy and exercise in osteoarthritis of the knee. A randomized, controlled trial. *Ann Intern Med* 132 (3): 173-181.

Deyo, R.A. 1982. Compliance with therapeutic regimens in arthritis: Issues, current status, and a future agenda. *Semin Arthritis Rheum* 12 (2): 233-244.

Ekblom, B. 1975. Effect of short-term physical training on patients with rheumatoid arthritis. a six-month follow-up study. *Scand J Rheumatol* 4 (2): 87-91.

Ekblom, B., O. Lovgren, M. Alderin, M. Fridstrom, and G. Satterstrom. 1975. Effect of short-term physical training on patients with rheumatoid arthritis I. *Scand J Rheumatol* 4 (2): 80-86.

Ekdahl, C., S.I. Andersson, U. Moritz, and B. Svensson. 1990. Dynamic versus static training in patients with rheumatoid arthritis. *Scand J Rheumatol* 19 (1): 17-26.

Ekdahl, C., R. Ekman, I. Petersson, and B. Svensson. 1994. Dynamic training and circulating neuro*Peptides* in patients with rheumatoid arthritis: A comparative study with healthy subjects. *Int J Clin Pharmacol Res* 14 (2): 65-74.

Escalante, A., L. Miller, and T.D. Beardmore. 1993. Resistive exercise in the rehabilitation of polymyositis/dermatomyositis. *J Rheumatol* 20 (8): 1340-1344.

Ettinger, W.H. Jr., R. Burns, S.P. Messier, W. Applegate, W.J. Rejeski, T. Morgan, S. Shumaker, M.J. Berry, M. O'Toole, J. Monu, and T. Craven. 1997. A randomized trial comparing aerobic exercise and resistance exercise with a health education program in older adults with knee osteoarthritis. The Fitness Arthritis and Seniors Trial (FAST). *JAMA* 277 (1): 25-31.

Fisher, N.M., D.R. Pendergast, G.E. Gresham, and E. Calkins. 1991. Muscle rehabilitation: Its effect on muscular and functional performance of patients with knee osteoarthritis. *Arch Phys Med Rehabil* 72 (6): 367-374.

Fransen, M., J. Crosbie, and J. Edmonds. 2001. Physical therapy is effective for patients with osteoarthritis of the knee: A randomized controlled clinical trial. *J Rheumatol* 28 (1): 156-164.

Garfinkel, M.S., H.R. Schumacher Jr., A. Husain, M. Levy, and R.A. Reshetar. 1994. Evaluation of a yoga based regimen for treatment of osteoarthritis of the hands. *J Rheumatol* 21 (12): 2341-2343.

Gecht, M.R., K.J. Connell, J.M. Sinacore, and T.R. Prohaska. 1996. A survey of exercise beliefs and exercise habits among people with arthritis. *Arthritis Care Res* 9 (2): 82-88.

Gerber, L.H. 1990. Exercise and arthritis. *Bull Rheum Dis* 39 (6): 1-9.

Gerber, L.H., and J.E. Hicks. 1990. Exercise in rheumatic disease. In *Therapeutic exercise*, ed. J.V. Basmajian and S.L. Wolf. Baltimore: Williams & Wilkins.

Godin, G. 1987. Importance of the emotional aspect of attitude to predict intention. *Psychol Rep* 61 (3): 719-723.

Green, J., F. McKenna, E.J. Redfern, and M.A. Chamberlain. 1993. Home exercises are as effective as outpatient hydrotherapy for osteoarthritis of the hip. *Br J Rheumatol* 32 (9): 812-815.

Hakkinen, A., K. Hakkinen, and P. Hannonen. 1994. Effects of strength training on neuromuscular function and disease activity in patients with recent-onset inflammatory arthritis. *Scand J Rheumatol* 23 (5): 237-242.

Hakkinen, A., T. Sokka, A. Kotaniemi, and P. Hannonen. 2001. A randomized two-year study of the effects of dynamic strength training on muscle strength, disease activity, functional capacity, and bone mineral density in early rheumatoid arthritis. *Arthritis Rheum* 44 (3): 515-522.

Hakkinen, A., T. Sokka, A. Kotaniemi, H. Kautiainen, I. Jappinen, L. Laitinen, and P. Hannonen. 1999. Dynamic strength training in patients with early rheumatoid arthritis increases muscle strength but not bone mineral density. *J Rheumatol* 26 (6): 1257-1263.

Hall, J., S.M. Skevington, P.J. Maddison, and K. Chapman. 1996. A randomized and controlled trial of hydrotherapy in rheumatoid arthritis. *Arthritis Care Res* 9 (3): 206-215.

Hansen, T.M., G. Hansen, A.M. Langgaard, and J.O. Rasmussen. 1993. Long-term physical training in rheumatoid arthritis. A randomized trial with different training programs and blinded observers. *Scand J Rheumatol* 22 (3): 107-112.

Harkcom, T.M., R.M. Lampman, B.F. Banwell, and C.W. Castor. 1985. Therapeutic value of graded aerobic exercise training in rheumatoid arthritis. *Arthritis Rheum* 28 (1): 32-39.

Harris, E. D. Jr. 1990. Rheumatoid arthritis. Pathophysiology and implications for therapy. *N Engl J Med* 322 (18): 1277-1289.

Hayes, K.W. 1996. Heat and cold in the management of rheumatoid arthritis. In *Rehabilitation of persons with rheumatoid arthritis*, ed. R.W. Chang. Gaithersburg, Maryland: Aspen.

Hicks, J.E. 1985. Compliance: A major factor in the successful treatment of rheumatic disease. *Compr Ther* 11 (4): 31-37.

Hicks, J.E. 1994. Exercise in rheumatoid arthritis. *Phys Med Rehabil Clin of N Am* 5: 701-727.

Hicks, J.E., F. Miller, P. Plotz, T.H. Chen, and L. Gerber. 1993. Isometric exercise increases strength and does not produce sustained creatinine phosphokinase increases in a patient with polymyositis. *J Rheumatol* 20 (8): 1399-1401.

Hidding, A., S. van der Linden, M. Boers, X. Gielen, L. de Witte, A. Kester, B. Dijkmans, and D. Moolenburgh. 1993. Is group physical therapy superior to individualized therapy in ankylosing spondylitis? A randomized controlled trial. *Arthritis Care Res* 6 (3): 117-125.

Hidding, A., S. van der Linden, X. Gielen, L. de Witte, B. Dijkmans, and D. Moolenburgh. 1994. Continuation of group physical therapy is necessary in ankylosing spondylitis: Results of a randomized controlled trial. *Arthritis Care Res* 7 (2): 90-96.

Hoenig, H., G. Groff, K. Pratt, E. Goldberg, and W. Franck. 1993. A randomized controlled trial of home exercise on the rheumatoid hand. *J Rheumatol* 20 (5): 785-789.

Hopman-Rock, M., and M.H. Westhoff. 2000. The effects of a health educational and exercise program for older adults with osteoarthritis of the hip or knee. *J Rheumatol* 27 (8): 1947-1954.

Hurley, M.V., and D.L. Scott. 1998. Improvements in quadriceps sensorimotor function and disability of patients with knee osteoarthritis following a clinically practicable exercise regime. *Br J Rheumatol* 37 (11): 1181-1187.

Iversen, M.D., A.H. Fossel, and L.H. Daltroy. 1999. Rheumatologist-patient communication about exercise and physical therapy in the management of rheumatoid arthritis. *Arthritis Care Res* 12 (3): 180-192.

Iverson, D.C., J.E. Fielding, R.S. Crow, and G.M. Christenson. 1985. The promotion of physical activity in the United States population: The status of programs in medical, worksite, community, and school settings. *Public Health Rep* 100 (2): 212-224.

Jensen, G.M., and C.D. Lorish. 1994. Promoting patient cooperation with exercise programs: Linking research, theory, and practice. *Arthritis Care Res* 7 (4): 181-189.

Komatireddy, G.R., R.W. Leitch, K. Cella, G. Browning, and M. Minor. 1997. Efficacy of low load resistive muscle training in patients with rheumatoid arthritis functional class II and III. *J Rheumatol* 24 (8): 1531-1539.

Kovar, P.A., J.P. Allegrante, C.R. MacKenzie, M.G. Peterson, B. Gutin, and M.E. Charlson. 1992. Supervised fitness walking in patients with osteoarthritis of the knee. A randomized, controlled trial. *Ann Intern Med* 116 (7): 529-534.

Kraag, G., B. Stokes, J. Groh, A. Helewa, and C. Goldsmith. 1990. The effects of comprehensive home physiotherapy and supervision on patients with ankylosing spondylitis: A randomized controlled trial. *J Rheumatol* 17 (2): 228-233.

Kraag, G., B. Stokes, J. Groh, A. Helewa, and C.H. Goldsmith. 1994. The effects of comprehensive home physiotherapy and supervision on patients with ankylosing spondylitis: An 8-month follow-up. *J Rheumatol* 21 (2): 261-263.

Lawrence, R.C., M.C. Hochberg, J.L. Kelsey, F.C. McDuffie, T.A. Medsger Jr., W.R. Felts, and L.E. Shulman. 1989. Estimates of the prevalence of selected arthritic and musculoskeletal diseases in the United States. *J Rheumatol* 16 (4): 427-44.

Leivseth, G., J. Torstensson, and O. Reikeras. 1989. Effect of passive muscle stretching in osteoarthritis of the hip. *Clin Sci (Lond)* 76 (1): 113-137.

Lyngberg, K., B. Danneskiold-Samsoe, and O. Halskov. 1988. The effect of physical training on patients with rheumatoid arthritis: Changes in disease activity, muscle strength and aerobic capacity. A clinically controlled minimized cross-over study. *Clin Exp Rheumatol* 6 (3): 253-20.

Lyngberg, K.K., B.U. Ramsing, A. Nawrocki, M. Harreby, and B. Danneskiold-Samsoe. 1994. Safe and effective isokinetic knee extension training in rheumatoid arthritis. *Arthritis Rheum* 37 (5): 623-628.

Mangione, K.K., K. McCully, A. Gloviak, I. Lefebvre, M. Hofmann, and R. Craik. 1999. The effects of high-intensity and low-intensity cycle ergometry in older adults with knee osteoarthritis. *J Gerontol A Biol Sci Med Sci* 54 (4): M184-M190.

McMeeken, J., B. Stillman, I. Story, P. Kent, and J. Smith. 1999. The effects of knee extensor and flexor muscle training on the timed-up-and-go test in individuals with rheumatoid arthritis. *Physiother Res Int* 4 (1): 55-67.

Minor, M.A., J.E. Hewett, R.R. Webel, S.K. Anderson, and D.R. Kay. 1989. Efficacy of physical conditioning exercise in patients with rheumatoid arthritis and osteoarthritis. *Arthritis Rheum* 32 (11): 1396-1405.

Nordemar, R., B. Ekblom, L. Zachrisson, and K. Lundqvist. 1981. Physical training in rheumatoid arthritis: A controlled long-term study. I. *Scand J Rheumatol* 10 (1): 17-23.

Nordesjo, L.O., B. Nordgren, A. Wigren, and K. Kolstad. 1983. Isometric strength and endurance in patients with severe rheumatoid arthritis or osteoarthrosis in the knee joints. A comparative study in healthy men and women. *Scand J Rheumatol* 12 (2): 152-156.

O'Reilly, S.C., K.R. Muir, and M. Doherty. 1999. Effectiveness of home exercise on pain and disability from osteoarthritis of the knee: A randomised controlled trial. *Ann Rheum Dis* 58 (1): 15-19.

Penninx, B.W., S.P. Messier, W.J. Rejeski, J.D. Williamson, M. DiBari, C. Cavazzini, W.B. Applegate, and M. Pahor. 2001. Physical exercise and the prevention of disability in activities of daily living in older persons with osteoarthritis. *Arch Intern Med* 161 (19): 2309-2316.

Perlman, S.G., K.J. Connell, A. Clark, M.S. Robinson, P. Conlon, M. Gecht, P. Caldron, and J.M. Sinacore. 1990. Dance-based aerobic exercise for rheumatoid arthritis. *Arthritis Care Res* 3 (1): 29-35.

Petrella, R.J., and C. Bartha. 2000. Home based exercise therapy for older patients with knee osteoarthritis: A randomized clinical trial. *J Rheumatol* 27 (9): 2215-2221.

Philbin, E.F., G.D. Groff, M.D. Ries, and T.E. Miller. 1995. Cardiovascular fitness and health in patients with end-stage osteoarthritis. *Arthritis Rheum* 38 (6): 799-805.

Quilty, B., M. Tucker, R. Campbell, and P. Dieppe. 2003. Physiotherapy, including quadriceps exercises and patellar taping, for knee osteoarthritis with predominant patello-femoral joint involvement: Randomized controlled trial. *J Rheumatol* 30 (6): 1311-1317.

Rall, L.C., S.N. Meydani, J.J. Kehayias, B. Dawson-Hughes, and R. Roubenoff. 1996. The effect of progressive resistance training in rheumatoid arthritis. Increased strength without changes in energy balance or body composition. *Arthritis Rheum* 39 (3): 415-426.

Ramsey-Goldman, R., E.M. Schilling, D. Dunlop, C. Langman, P. Greenland, R.J. Thomas, and R.W. Chang. 2000. A pilot study on the effects of exercise in patients with systemic lupus erythematosus. *Arthritis Care Res* 13 (5): 262-269.

Rejeski, W.J., L. R. Brawley, W. Ettinger, T. Morgan, and C. Thompson. 1997. Compliance to exercise therapy in older participants with knee osteoarthritis: Implications for treating disability. *Med Sci Sports Exerc* 29 (8): 977-985.

Robb-Nicholson, L.C., L. Daltroy, H. Eaton, V. Gall, E. Wright, L.H. Hartley, P.H. Schur, and M.H. Liang. 1989. Effects of aerobic conditioning in lupus fatigue: A pilot study. *Br J Rheumatol* 28 (6): 500-505.

Rogind, H., B. Bibow-Nielsen, B. Jensen, H.C. Moller, H. Frimodt-Moller, and H. Bliddal. 1998. The effects of a physical training program on patients with osteoarthritis of the knees. *Arch Phys Med Rehabil* 79 (11): 1421-1427.

Schilke, J.M., G.O. Johnson, T.J. Housh, and J.R. O'Dell. 1996. Effects of muscle-strength training on the functional status of patients with osteoarthritis of the knee joint. *Nurs Res* 45 (2): 68-72.

Sell, S., J. Zacher, and S. Lack. 1993. [Disorders of proprioception of the arthrotic knee joint]. *Z Rheumatol* 52 (3): 150-155.

Semble, E.L. 1995. Rheumatoid arthritis: New approaches for its evaluation and management. *Arch Phys Med Rehabil* 76 (2): 190-201.

Semble, E.L., R.F. Loeser, and C.M. Wise. 1990. Therapeutic exercise for rheumatoid arthritis and osteoarthritis. *Semin Arthritis Rheum* 20 (1): 32-40.

Sharma, L. 2001. Local factors in osteoarthritis. *Curr Opin Rheumatol* 13 (5): 441-446.

Sharma, L., D.D. Dunlop, S. Cahue, J. Song, and K.W. Hayes. 2003. Quadriceps strength and osteoarthritis progression in malaligned and lax knees. *Ann Intern Med* 138 (8): 613-619.

Sharma, L., Y.C. Pai, K. Holtkamp, and W.Z. Rymer. 1997. Is knee joint proprioception worse in the arthritic knee versus the unaffected knee in unilateral knee osteoarthritis? *Arthritis Rheum* 40 (8): 1518-1525.

Slemenda, C., K.D. Brandt, D.K. Heilman, S. Mazzuca, E.M. Braunstein, B.P. Katz, and F. D. Wolinsky. 1997. Quadriceps weakness and osteoarthritis of the knee. *Ann Intern Med* 127 (2): 97-104.

Smedstad, L.V., and M.H. Liang. 1997. Psychosocial management of rheumatic diseases. In *Textbook of rheumatology*, ed. W.N. Kelley, T. Harris, S. Ruddy and C.B. Sledge. Philadelphia: W.B. Saunders.

Stamm, T.A., K.P. Machold, J.S. Smolen, S. Fischer, K. Redlich, W. Graninger, W. Ebner, and L. Erlacher. 2002. Joint protection and home hand exercises improve hand function in patients with hand osteoarthritis: A randomized controlled trial. [comment]. *Arthritis Rheum* 47 (1): 44-49.

Stenstrom, C.H. 1994. Therapeutic exercise in rheumatoid arthritis. *Arthritis Care Res* 7 (4): 190-197.

Stenstrom, C.H. 1997. Home exercise and compliance in inflammatory rheumatic diseases--a prospective clinical trial. *J Rheumatol* 24 (3): 470-476.

Stenstrom, C.H., B. Arge, and A. Sundbom. 1996. Dynamic training versus relaxation training as home exercise for patients with inflammatory rheumatic diseases. A randomized controlled study. *Scand J Rheumatol* 25 (1): 28-33.

Stenstrom, C.H., B. Lindell, E. Swanberg, P. Swanberg, K. Harms-Ringdahl, and R. Nordemar. 1991. Intensive dynamic training in water for rheumatoid arthritis functional class II: A long-term study of effects. *Scand J Rheumatol* 20 (5): 358-365.

Steultjens, M.P., J. Dekker, and J.W. Bijlsma. 2002. Avoidance of activity and disability in patients with osteoarthritis of the knee: The mediating role of muscle strength. *Arthritis Rheum* 46 (7): 1784-1788.

Sweeney, S., G. Taylor, and A. Calin. 2002. The effect of a home based exercise intervention package on outcome in ankylosing spondylitis: A randomized controlled trial. *J Rheumatol* 29 (4): 763-766.

Tench, C.M., J. McCarthy, I. McCurdie, P.D. White, and D.P. D'Cruz. 2003. Fatigue in systemic lupus erythematosus: A randomized controlled trial of exercise. *Rheumatology* 42 (9): 1050-1054.

Uhrin, Z., S. Kuzis, and M.M. Ward. 2000. Exercise and changes in health status in patients with ankylosing spondylitis. *Arch Intern Med* 160: 2969-2975.

van Baar, M.E., W.J. Assendelft, J. Dekker, R.A. Oostendorp, and J.W. Bijlsma. 1999. Effectiveness of exercise therapy in patients with osteoarthritis of the hip or knee: A systematic review of randomized clinical trials. *Arthritis Rheum* 42 (7): 1361-1369.

van Baar, M.E., J. Dekker, R.A. Oostendorp, D. Bijl, T.B. Voorn, J.A. Lemmens, and J.W. Bijlsma. 1998. The effectiveness of exercise therapy in patients with osteoarthritis of the hip or knee: A randomized clinical trial. *J Rheumatol* 25 (12): 2432-2439.

van den Ende, C.H., F.C. Breedveld, S. le Cessie, B.A. Dijkmans, A.W. de Mug, and J.M. Hazes. 2000. Effect of intensive exercise on patients with active rheumatoid arthritis: A randomised clinical trial. *Ann Rheum Dis* 59 (8): 615-621.

van den Ende, C.H., J.M. Hazes, S. le Cessie, W.J. Mulder, D.G. Belfor, F.C. Breedveld, and B.A. Dijkmans. 1996. Comparison of high and low intensity training in well controlled rheumatoid arthritis. Results of a randomised clinical trial. *Ann Rheum Dis* 55 (11): 798-805.

van Tubergen, A., R. Landewe, D. van der Heijde, A. Hidding, N. Wolter, M. Asscher, A. Falkenbach, E. Genth, H.G. The, and S. van der Linden. 2001. Combined spa-exercise therapy is effective in patients with ankylosing spondylitis: A randomized controlled trial. *Arthritis Rheum* 45 (5): 430-438.

Wegener, L., C. Kisner, and D. Nichols. 1997. Static and dynamic balance responses in persons with bilateral knee osteoarthritis. *J Orthop Sports Phys Ther* 25 (1): 1318.

Westby, M.D., J.P. Wade, K.K. Rangno, and J. Berkowitz. 2000. A randomized controlled trial to evaluate the effectiveness of an exercise program in women with rheumatoid arthritis taking low dose prednisone. *J Rheumatol* 27 (7): 1674-1680.

Wiesinger, G.F., M. Quittan, M. Graninger, A. Seeber, G. Ebenbichler, B. Sturm, K. Kerschan, J. Smolen, and W. Graninger. 1998. Benefit of 6 months long-term physical training in polymyositis/dermatomyositis patients. *Br J Rheumatol* 37 (12): 1338-1342.

CHAPTER 12

Agre, J.C., and A.A. Rodriquez. 1991. Intermittent isometric activity: Its effect on muscle fatigue in postpolio subjects. *Arch Phys Med Rehabil* 72: 971-975.

Aitkens, S.G., M.A. McCrory, D.D. Kilmer, and E.M. Bernauer. 1993. Moderate resistance exercise program: Its effect in slowly progressive neuromuscular disease. *Arch Phys Med Rehabil* 74: 711-715.

Appell, H.J. 1990. Muscular atrophy following immobilisation. *Sports Med* 10: 42-58.

Armstrong, R.B., G.L. Warren, and J.A. Warren. 1991. Mechanisms of exercise-induced muscle fibre injury. *Sports Med* 12: 184-207.

Bar-Or, O. 1996. Role of exercise in the assessment and management of neuromuscular disease in children. *Med Sci Sports Exerc* 28: 421-427.

Bennett, R.L., and G.C. Knowlton. 1958. Overwork weakness in partially denervated skeletal muscle. *Clin Orthop* 12: 22-29.

Bonilla, E., C.E. Samitt, A.F. Miranda, A.P. Hays, G. Salviati, S. DiMauro, L.M. Kunkel, E.P. Hoffman, and L.P. Rowland. 1988. Duchenne muscular dystrophy: Deficiency of dystrophin at the muscle cell surface. *Cell* 54: 447-452.

Bonsett, C.A. 1963. Pseudohypertrophic muscular dystrophy: Distribution of degenerative features as revealed by anatomic study. *Neurology* 13: 728-738.

Borg, K., J. Borg, L. Edstrom, and L. Grimby. 1988. Effects of excessive use of remaining muscle fibers in prior polio and LV lesion. *Muscle Nerve* 11: 1219-1230.

Brouwer, O.F., G.W. Padberg, R.J. van der Ploeg, C.J. Ruys, and R. Brand. 1992. The influence of handedness on the distribution of muscular weakness of the arm in facioscapulohumeral muscular dystrophy. *Brain* 115: 1587-1598.

Brown, R.H. 1997. Dystrophin-associated proteins and the muscular dystrophies. *Ann Rev Med* 48: 457-466.

Carroll, J.E., J.M. Hagberg, M.H. Brooke, and J.B. Shumate. 1979. Bicycle ergometry and gas exchange measurements in neuromuscular diseases. *Arch Neurol* 36: 457-461.

Carter, G.T., R.T. Abresch, W.M. Fowler Jr., E.R. Johnson, D.D. Kilmer, and C.M. McDonald. 1995a. Profiles of neuromuscular diseases: Spinal muscular atrophy. *Am J Phys Med Rehabil* 74: S150-S159.

Carter, G.T., R.T. Abresch, W.M. Fowler Jr., E.R. Johnson, D.D. Kilmer, and C.M. McDonald. 1995b. Profiles of neuromuscular diseases: Hereditary motor and sensory neuropathy, types I and II. *Am J Phys Med Rehabil* 74: S140-S149.

Casperson, C.J. 1989. Physical activity epidemiology: Concepts, methods, and applications to exercise science. In *Exercise and sport sciences reviews*. Vol. 17, ed. K. Pandolf, 423-473. Baltimore: Williams & Wilkins.

Clarkson, P.M., and M.J. Hubal. 2002. Exercise-induced muscle damage in humans. *Am J Phys Med Rehabil* 81: S52-S69.

Clarkson, P.M., K. Nosaka, and B. Braun. 1992. Muscle function after exercise-induced muscle damage and rapid adaptation. *Med Sci Sports Exerc* 24: 512-520.

Cooper, B.J. 1989. Animal models of Duchenne and Becker muscular dystrophy. *Br Med Bull* 45: 703-718.

Dolmage, T., and E. Cafarelli. 1991. Rate of fatigue during repeated submaximal contractions of human quadriceps muscle. *Can J Physiol Pharmacol* 69: 1410-1415.

Edwards, R.H.T., D.A. Jones, D.J. Newham, and S.J. Chapman. 1984. Role of mechanical damage in pathogenesis of proximal myopathy in man. *Lancet* 8376: 548-551.

Ervasti, J.M., and K.P. Campbell. 1993. A role for the dystrophin-glycoprotein complex as a transmembrane linker between laminin and actin. *J Cell Biol* 122: 809-823.

Fenichel, G.M., J.M. Florence, A. Pestronk, J.R. Mendell, R.T. Moxley III, R.C. Griggs, M.H. Brooke, J.P. Miller, J. Robison, W. King, L. Signore, S. Pandya, J. Schierbecker, and B. Wilson. 1991. Long-term benefit from prednisone therapy in Duchenne muscular dystrophy. *Neurology* 41: 1874-1877.

Florence, J.M., M.H. Brooke, J.M. Hagberg, and J.E. Carroll. 1984. Endurance exercise in neuromuscular disease. In *Neuromuscular diseases,* ed. G. Serratrice, 577-581. New York: Raven Press.

Fowler, W.M. Jr., R.T. Abresch, T.R. Koch, M.L. Brewer, R.K. Bowden, and R.L. Wanlass. 1997. Employment profiles in neuromuscular diseases. *Am J Phys Med Rehabil* 76: 26-37.

Franco, A. Jr., and J.B. Lansman. 1990. Calcium entry through stretch-inactivated ion channels in mdx myotubes. *Nature* 344: 670-673.

Friden, J., and R.L. Lieber. 1992. Structural and mechanical basis of exercise-induced muscle injury. *Med Sci Sports Exerc* 24: 521-530.

Haller, R.G., and S.F. Lewis. 1984. Pathophysiology of exercise performance in muscle disease. *Med Sci Sports Exerc* 16: 456-459.

Haller, R.G., S.F. Lewis, J.D. Cook, and C.G. Blomqvist. 1983. Hyperkinetic circulation during exercise in neuromuscular disease. *Neurology* 33: 1283-1287.

Hoffman, E.P., R.H. Brown Jr., and L.M. Kunkel. 1987. Dystrophin: The protein product of the Duchenne muscular dystrophy locus. *Cell* 51: 919-928.

Jacobs, S.C., A.L. Bootsma, P.W. Willems, P.R. Bar, and J.H. Wokke. 1996. Prednisone can protect against exercise-induced muscle damage. *J Neurol* 243: 410-416.

Jejurikar, S.S., and W.M. Kuzon Jr. 2003. Satellite cell depletion in degenerative skeletal muscle. *Apoptosis* 8: 573-578.

Johnson, E.R., R.T. Abresch, G.T. Carter, D.D. Kilmer, W.M. Fowler Jr., B.J. Sigford, and R.L. Wanlass. 1995. Profiles of neuromuscular diseases: Myotonic dystrophy. *Am J Phys Med Rehabil* 74: S104-S116.

Johnson, E.W., and R. Braddom. 1971. Over-work weakness in facioscapulohumeral dystrophy. *Arch Phys Med Rehabil* 52: 333-336.

Kilmer, D.D. 1996. Functional anatomy of skeletal muscle. In *Physical Medicine Rehabilitation State of the Art Reviews* 10: 3, ed. K. Shankar, 413-426. Philadelphia: Hanley & Belfus.

Kilmer, D.D., R.T. Abresch, M.A. McCrory, G.T. Carter, W.M. Fowler Jr., E.R. Johnson, and C.M. McDonald. 1995. Profiles of neuromuscular diseases: Facioscapulohumeral muscular dystrophy. *Am J Phys Med Rehabil* 74: S131-S139.

Kilmer, D.D., M.A. McCrory, N.C. Wright, S.A. Aitkens, and E.M. Bernauer. 1994. The effect of a high resistance exercise program in slowly progressive neuromuscular disease. *Arch Phys Med Rehabil* 75: 560-563.

Kilmer, D.D., M.A. McCrory, N.C. Wright, R.A. Rosko, H.R. Kim, and S.A. Aitkens. 1997. Reliability of hand-held dynamometry in persons with neuropathic weakness. *Arch Phys Med Rehabil* 78: 1364-1368.

Kilmer, D.D., and C.M. McDonald. 1995. Childhood progressive neuromuscular disease. In *Sports and exercise for children with chronic health conditions,* ed. B. Goldberg, 109-121. Champaign, IL: Human Kinetics.

Leon, A.S., and J. Connett. 1991. Physical activity and 10.5 year mortality in the Multiple Risk Factor Intervention Trial (MRFIT). *Int J Epidemiology* 20: 690-697.

Lieber, R.L., and J. Friden. 1993. Muscle damage is not a function of muscle force but active muscle strain. *J Appl Physiol* 74: 520-526.

Lieber, R.L., L.E. Thornell, and J. Friden. 1996. Muscle cytoskeletal disruption occurs within the first 15 min of cyclic eccentric contraction. *J Appl Physiol* 80: 278-284.

Lindeman, E., P. Leffers, J. Reulen, F. Spaans, and J. Drukker. 1994. Reduction of knee torques and leg-related functional abilities in hereditary motor and sensory neuropathy. *Arch Phys Med Rehabil* 75: 1201-1205.

Lindeman, E., P. Leffers, F. Spaans, J. Drukker, J. Reulen, M. Kerckhoffs, and A. Koke. 1995. Strength training in patients with myotonic dystrophy and hereditary motor and sensory neuropathy: A randomized clinical trial. *Arch Phys Med Rehabil* 76: 612-20.

Mankodi, A., and C.A. Thornton. 2002. Myotonic syndromes. *Curr Opin Neurol* 15: 545-552.

McCartney, N., D. Moroz, S.H. Garner, and A.J. McComas. 1988. The effects of strength training in patients with selected neuromuscular disorders. *Med Sci Sports Exerc* 20: 362-368.

McCrory, M.A., H.R. Kim, N.C. Wright, C.A. Lovelady, S. Aitkens, and D.D. Kilmer. 1998. Energy expenditure, physical activity and body composition of ambulatory adults with hereditary neuromuscular disease. *Am J Clin Nutr* 67: 1162-1169.

McDonald, C.M., R.T. Abresch, G.T. Carter, W.M. Fowler Jr., E.R. Johnson, and D.D. Kilmer. 1995a. Profiles of neuromuscular diseases: Becker's muscular dystrophy. *Am J Phys Med Rehabil* 74: S93-S103.

McDonald, C.M., R.T. Abresch, G. T. Carter, W.M. Fowler Jr., E.R. Johnson, D.D. Kilmer, and B.J. Sigford. 1995b. Profiles of neuromuscular diseases: Duchenne muscular dystrophy. *Am J Phys Med Rehabil* 74: S70-S92.

McHugh, M.P. 2003. Recent advances in the understanding of the repeated bout effect: The protective effect against muscle damage from a single bout of eccentric exercise. *Scand J Med Sci Sports* 13: 88-97.

Milner-Brown, H.S., and R.G. Miller. 1988. Muscle strengthening through high-resistance weight training in patients with neuromuscular disorders. *Arch Phys Med Rehabil* 69: 14-19.

Moens, P., P.H. Baatsen, and G. Marechal. 1993. Increased susceptibility of EDL muscles from mdx mice to damage induced by contractions with stretch. *J Muscle Res Cell Motil* 14: 446-451.

Mujika, I., and S. Padilla. 2000. Muscular characteristics of detraining in humans. *Med Sci Sports Exerc* 33: 1297-1303.

Murakami, T., C.A. Garcia, L.T. Reiter, and J.R. Lupski. 1996. Charcot-Marie-Tooth disease and related inherited neuropathies. *Medicine* 75: 233-250.

Perry, J., G. Barnes, and J.K. Gronley. 1988. The postpolio syndrome: An overuse phenomenon. *Clin Orthop* 233: 145-162.

Petrof, B.J. 1998. The molecular basis of activity-induced muscle injury in Duchenne muscular dystrophy. *Mol Cell Biochem* 179: 111-123.

Petrof, B.J. 2002. Molecular pathophysiology of myofiber injury in deficiencies of the dystrophin-glycoprotein complex. *Am J Phys Med Rehabil* 81: S162-S174.

Petrof, B., J.B. Shrager, H.H. Stedman, A.M. Kelly, and H.L. Sweeney. 1993. Dystrophin protects the sarcolemma from stresses developed during muscle contraction. *Proc Natl Acad Sci* 90: 3710-3714.

Sanjak, M., D. Paulson, R. Sufit, W. Reddan, D. Beaulieu, L. Erickson, A. Shug, and B.R. Brooks. 1987. Physiologic and metabolic response to progressive and prolonged exercise in amyotrophic lateral sclerosis. *Neurology* 37: 1217-1220.

Sharma, K.R., J.A. Kent-Braun, S. Majumdar, Y. Huang, M. Mynhier, M.W. Weiner, and R.G. Miller. 1995. Physiology of fatigue in amyotrophic lateral sclerosis. *Neurology* 45: 733-740.

Sharma, K.R., and R.G. Miller. 1996. Electrical and mechanical properties of skeletal muscle underlying increased fatigue in patients with amyotrophic lateral sclerosis. *Muscle Nerve* 19: 1391-1400.

Sockolov, R., B. Irwin, R.H. Dressendorfer, and E.M. Bernauer. 1977. Exercise performance in 6-to-11-year-old boys with Duchenne muscular dystrophy. *Arch Phys Med Rehabil* 58: 195-201.

Spector, S.A., P.L. Gordon, I.M. Feuerstein, K. Sivakumar, B.F. Hurley, and M.C. Dalakas. 1996. Strength gains without muscle injury after strength training in patients with postpolio muscular atrophy. *Muscle Nerve* 19: 1282-1290.

Stedman, H.H., H.L. Sweeney, J.B. Shrager, H.C. Maguire, R.A. Panettieri, B. Petrof, M. Narusawa, J.M. Leferovich, J.T. Sladky, and A.M. Kelly. 1991. The mdx mouse diaphragm reproduces the degenerative changes of Duchenne muscular dystrophy. *Nature* 352: 536-539.

Taivassalo, T., N. DeStefano, J. Chen, G. Karpati, D.L. Arnold, and Z. Argov. 1999. Short-term aerobic training response in chronic myopathies. *Muscle Nerve* 22: 1239-1243.

Tollback, A., S. Eriksson, A. Wredenberg, G. Jenner, R.Vargas, K. Borg, and T. Ansved. 1999. Effects of high resistance training in patients with myotonic dystrophy. *Scand J Rehabil Med* 31: 9-16.

Turner, P.R., P.Y. Fong, W.F. Denetclaw, and R.A. Steinhardt. 1991. Increased calcium influx in dystrophic muscle. *J Cell Biol* 115: 1701-1712.

Vignos, P.J. Jr. 1983. Physical models of rehabilitation in neuromuscular disease. *Muscle Nerve* 6: 323-338.

Vignos, P.J. Jr., and M.P. Watkins. 1966. Effect of exercise in muscular dystrophy. *JAMA* 197: 843-848.

Weller, B., G. Karpati, and S. Carpenter. 1990. Dystrophin-deficient mdx muscle fibers are preferentially vulnerable to necrosis induced by experimental lengthening contractions. *J Neurol Sci* 100: 9-13.

Wright, N.C., D.D. Kilmer, M.A. McCrory, S.A. Aitkens, B.J. Holcomb, and E.M. Bernauer. 1996. Aerobic walking in slowly progressive neuromuscular disease: Effect of a 12-week program. *Arch Phys Med Rehabil* 77: 64-69.

CHAPTER 13

Ahn, S.H., H.W. Park, B.S. Lee, H.W. Moon, S.H. Jang, J. Sakong, and J.H. Bae. 2003. Gabapentin effect on neuropathic pain compared among patients with spinal cord injury and different durations of symptoms. *Spine* 28: 341-346.

Aksnes, A.K., N. Hjeltnes, E.W. Wahlstrom, A. Katz, J.R. Zierath, and H. Wallberg-Henriksson. 1996. Intact glucose transport in morphologically altered denervated skeletal muscle from quadriplegic patients. *Am J Physiol* 271: E593-E600.

Andersen, J.L., T. Mohr, F. Biering-Sorensen, H. Galbo, and M. Kjaer. 1996. Myosin heavy chain isoform transformation in single fibres from m. vastus lateralis in spinal cord injured individuals: Effects of long-term functional electrical stimulation (FES). *Pflugers Arch* 431: 513-518.

Ballinger, D.A., D.H. Rintala, and K.A. Hart. 2000. The relation of shoulder pain and range-of-motion problems to functional limitations, disability, and perceived health of men with spinal cord injury: a multifaceted longitudinal study. *Arch Phys Med Rehabil* 81: 1575-1581.

Barbeau, H., K. Norman, J. Fung, M. Visintin, and M. Ladouceur. 1998. Does neurorehabilitation play a role in the recovery of walking in neurological populations? *Ann N Y Acad Sci* 860: 377-392.

Barber, D.B., and N.G. Gall. 1991. Osteonecrosis: An overuse injury of the shoulder in paraplegia: case report. *Paraplegia* 29: 423-426.

Barstow, T.J., A.M. Scremin, D.L. Mutton, C.F. Kunkel, T.G. Cagle, and B.J. Whipp. 1995. Gas exchange kinetics during functional electrical stimulation in subjects with spinal cord injury. *Med Sci Sports Exerc* 27: 1284-1291.

Barstow, T.J., A.M. Scremin, D.L. Mutton, C.F. Kunkel, T.G. Cagle, and B.J. Whipp. 1996. Changes in gas exchange kinetics with training in patients with spinal cord injury. *Med Sci Sports Exerc* 28: 1221-1228.

Basso, D.M. 2000. Neuroanatomical substrates of functional recovery after experimental spinal cord injury: implications of basic science research for human spinal cord injury. *Phys Ther* 80: 808-817.

Bauman, W.A., R.H. Adkins, A.M. Spungen, R. Herbert, C. Schechter, D. Smith, B.J. Kemp, R. Gambino, P., Maloney, and R.L. Waters. 1999a. Is immobilization associated with an abnormal lipoprotein profile? Observations from a diverse cohort. *Spinal Cord* 37: 485-493.

Bauman, W.A., R.H. Adkins, A.M. Spungen, and R.L. Waters. 1999b. The effect of residual neurological deficit on oral glucose tolerance in persons with chronic spinal cord injury. *Spinal Cord* 37: 765-771.

Bauman, W.A., N.N. Kahn, D.R. Grimm, and A.M. Spungen. 1999c. Risk factors for atherogenesis and cardiovascular autonomic function in persons with spinal cord injury. *Spinal Cord* 37: 601-616.

Bauman, W.A., M. Raza, A.M. Spungen, and J. Machac. 1994. Cardiac stress testing with thallium-201 imaging reveals silent ischemia in individuals with paraplegia. *Arch Phys Med Rehabil* 75: 946-950.

Bauman, W.A., and A.M. Spungen. 1994. Disorders of carbohydrate and lipid metabolism in veterans with paraplegia or quadriplegia: a model of premature aging. *Metabolism* 43: 749-756.

Bauman, W.A., and A.M. Spungen. 2000. Metabolic changes in persons after spinal cord injury. *Phys Med Rehabil Clin N Am* 11: 109-140.

Bauman, W.A., A.M. Spungen, R.H. Adkins, and B.J. Kemp. 1999d. Metabolic and endocrine changes in persons aging with spinal cord injury. *Assist Technol* 11: 88-96.

Bauman, W.A., A.M. Spungen, M. Raza, J. Rothstein, R.L. Zhang, Y.G. Zhong, M. Tsuruta, R. Shahidi, R.N. Pierson Jr., J. Wang, et al. 1992. Coronary artery disease: Metabolic risk factors and latent disease in individuals with paraplegia. *Mt Sinai J Med* 59(2): 163-168.

Bayley, J.C., T.P. Cochran, and C.B. Sledge. 1987. The weight-bearing shoulder. The impingement syndrome in paraplegics. *J Bone Joint Surg (Am)* 69: 676-678.

BeDell, K.K., A.M. Scremin, K.L. Perell, and C.F. Kunkel. 1996. Effects of functional electrical stimulation-induced lower extremity cycling on bone density of spinal cord-injured patients. *Am J Phys Med Rehabil* 75: 29-34.

Bloomfield, S.A., R.D. Jackson, and W.J. Mysiw. 1994. Catecholamine response to exercise and training in individuals with spinal cord injury. *Med Sci Sports Exerc* 26: 1213-1219.

Bloomfield, S.A., W.J. Mysiw, and R.D. Jackson. 1996. Bone mass and endocrine adaptations to training in spinal cord injured individuals. *Bone* 19: 61-68.

Bostom, A.G., M.M. Toner, W.D. McArdle, T. Montelione, C.D. Brown, and R.A. Stein. 1991. Lipid and lipoprotein profiles relate to peak aerobic power in spinal cord injured men. *Med Sci Sports Exerc* 23: 409-414.

Boudaoud, L., J. Roussi, S. Lortat-Jacob, B. Bussel, O. Dizien, and L. Drouet. 1997. Endothelial fibrinolytic reactivity and the risk of deep venous thrombosis after spinal cord injury. *Spinal Cord* 35: 151-157.

Brackett, N.L., M.S. Nash, and C.M. Lynne. 1996. Male fertility following spinal cord injury: facts and fiction. *Phys Ther* 76: 1221-1231.

Bregman, B.S., P.S. Diener, M. McAtee, H.N. Dai, and C. James. 1997. Intervention strategies to enhance anatomical plasticity and recovery of function after spinal cord injury. *Adv Neurol* 72: 257-275.

Brissot, R., P. Gallien, M.P. Le Bot, A. Beaubras, D. Laisne, J. Beillot, and J. Dassonville. 2000. Clinical experience with functional electrical stimulation-assisted gait with Parastep in spinal cord-injured patients. *Spine* 25: 501-508.

Bryden, A.M., W.D. Memberg, and P.E. Crago. 2000. Electrically stimulated elbow extension in persons with C5/C6 tetraplegia: A functional and physiological evaluation. *Arch Phys Med Rehabil* 81: 80-88.

Burnham, R., T. Martin, R. Stein, G. Bell, L. MacLean, and R. Steadward. 1997. Skeletal muscle fibre type transformation following spinal cord injury. *Spinal Cord* 35: 86-91.

Burnham, R.S., L. May, E. Nelson, R. Steadward, and D.C. Reid. 1993. Shoulder pain in wheelchair athletes. The role of muscle imbalance. *Am J Sports Med* 21: 238-242.

Burstein, R., G. Zeilig, M. Royburt, Y. Epstein, and A. Ohry. 1996. Insulin resistance in paraplegics—effect of one bout of acute exercise. *Int J Sports Med* 17: 272-276.

Calancie, B., B. Needham-Shropshire, P. Jacobs, K. Willer, G. Zych, and B.A. Green. 1994. Involuntary stepping after chronic spinal cord injury. Evidence for a central rhythm generator for locomotion in man. *Brain* 117 (Pt 5): 1143-1159.

Cameron, T., J.G. Broton, B. Needham-Shropshire, and K.J. Klose. 1998. An upper body exercise system incorporating resistive exercise and neuromuscular electrical stimulation (NMS). *J Spinal Cord Med* 21: 1-6.

Campagnolo, D.I., J.A. Bartlett, and S.E. Keller. 2000. Influence of neurological level on immune function following spinal cord injury: a review. *J Spinal Cord Med* 23: 121-128.

Cardenas, D.D., C.A. Warms, J.A. Turner, H. Marshall, M.M. Brooke, and J.D. Loeser. 2002. Efficacy of amitriptyline for relief of pain in spinal cord injury: Results of a randomized controlled trial. *Pain* 96: 365-373.

Castro, M.J., D.F. Apple Jr., E.A. Hillegass, and G.A. Dudley. 1999a. Influence of complete spinal cord injury on skeletal muscle cross-sectional area within the first 6 months of injury. *Eur J Appl Physiol Occup Physiol* 80: 373-378.

Castro, M.J., D.F. Apple Jr., S. Rogers, and G.A. Dudley. 2000. Influence of complete spinal cord injury on skeletal muscle mechanics within the first 6 months of injury. *Eur J Appl Physiol Occup Physiol* 81: 128-131.

Castro, M.J., D.F. Apple Jr., R.S. Staron, G.E. Campos, and G.A. Dudley. 1999b. Influence of complete spinal cord injury on skeletal muscle within 6 mo of injury. *J Appl Physiol* 86: 350-8.

Chancellor, M.B., M.J. Erhard, I.H. Hirsch, and W.E. Stass Jr. 1994. Prospective evaluation of terazosin for the treatment of autonomic dysreflexia. *J Urol* 151: 111-113.

Chantraine, A., B. Nusgens, and C.M. Lapiere. 1986. Bone remodeling during the development of osteoporosis in paraplegia. *Calcif Tissue Int* 38: 323-327.

Colombo, G., M. Wirz, and V. Dietz. 2001. Driven gait orthosis for improvement of locomotor training in paraplegic patients. *Spinal Cord* 39: 252-255.

Comarr, A.E., and I. Eltorai. 1997. Autonomic dysreflexia/hyperreflexia. *J Spinal Cord Med* 20: 345-354.

Cooney, M.M., and J.B. Walker. 1986. Hydraulic resistance exercise benefits cardiovascular fitness of spinal cord injured. *Med Sci Sports Exerc* 18: 522-525.

Cooper, G. IV, and R.J. Tomanek. 1982. Load regulation of the structure, composition, and function of mammalian myocardium. *Circ Res* 50: 788-798.

Cowell, L.L., W.G. Squires, and P.B. Raven. 1986. Benefits of aerobic exercise for the paraplegic: A brief review. *Med Sci Sports Exerc* 18: 501-508.

Cruse, J.M., R.E. Lewis, S. Dilioglou, D.L. Roe, W.F. Wallace, and R.S. Chen. 2000. Review of immune function, healing of pressure ulcers, and nutritional status in patients with spinal cord injury. *J Spinal Cord Med* 23: 129-135.

Curtis, K.A., G.A. Drysdale, R.D. Lanza, M. Kolber, R.S. Vitolo, and R. West. 1999a. Shoulder pain in wheelchair users with tetraplegia and paraplegia. *Arch Phys Med Rehabil* 80: 453-457.

Curtis, K.A., S. McClanahan, K.M. Hall, D. Dillon, and K.F. Brown. 1986. Health, vocational, and functional status in spinal cord injured athletes and nonathletes. *Arch Phys Med Rehabil* 67: 862-865.

Curtis, K.A., T.M. Tyner, L. Zachary, G. Lentell, D. Brink, T. Didyk, K. Gean, J. Hall, M. Hooper, J. Klos, S. Lesina, and B. Pacillas. 1999b. Effect of a standard exercise protocol on shoulder pain in long-term wheelchair users. *Spinal Cord* 37: 421-429.

Dallmeijer, A.J. 1998. Spinal cord injury and physical activity: Wheelchair performance in rehabilitation and sports. Doctoral dissertation. Faculty of Human Movement Sciences. Amsterdam, The Netherlands, Vrijr Universiteit (Free University).

Davis, G.M. 1993. Exercise capacity of individuals with paraplegia. *Med Sci Sports Exerc* 25: 423-432.

Davis, G.M., and R.J. Shephard. 1988. Cardiorespiratory fitness in highly active versus inactive paraplegics. *Med Sci Sports Exerc* 20: 463-468.

Davis, G.M., and R.J. Shephard. 1990. Strength training for wheelchair users. *Br J Sports Med*. 24(1): 25-30.

Dearwater, S.R., R.E. LaPorte, R.J. Robertson, G. Brenes, L.L. Adams, and D. Becker. 1986. Activity in the spinal cord-injured patient: an epidemiologic analysis of metabolic parameters. *Med Sci Sports Exerc* 18: 541-544.

Demirel, G., H. Yilmaz, N. Paker, and S. Onel. 1998. Osteoporosis after spinal cord injury. *Spinal Cord* 36: 822-825.

DeVivo, M.J., K.J. Black, and S.L. Stover. 1993. Causes of death during the first 12 years after spinal cord injury. *Arch Phys Med Rehabil* 74: 248-254.

DeVivo, M.J., B.K. Go, and A.B. Jackson. 2002. Overview of the national spinal cord injury statistical center database. *J Spinal Cord Med* 25: 335-358.

DeVivo, M.J., R.M. Shewchuk, S.L. Stover, K.J. Black, and B.K. Go. 1992. A cross-sectional study of the relationship between age and current health status for persons with spinal cord injuries. *Paraplegia* 30: 820-827.

DiCarlo, S.E. 1988. Effect of arm ergometry training on wheelchair propulsion endurance of individuals with quadriplegia. *Phys Ther* 68: 40-44.

Dietz, V., G. Colombo, L. Jensen, and L. Baumgartner. 1995. Locomotor capacity of spinal cord in paraplegic patients. *Ann Neurol* 37: 574-582.

Dietz, V., R. Muller., and G. Colombo. 2002. Locomotor activity in spinal man: significance of afferent input from joint and load receptors. *Brain* 125: 2626-2634.

Dietz, V., M. Wirz, G. Colombo, and A. Curt. 1998. Locomotor capacity and recovery of spinal cord function in paraplegic patients: a clinical and electrophysiological evaluation. *Electroencephalogr Clin Neurophysiol* 109: 140-153.

Dietz, V., M. Wirz, and Jensen, L. 1997. Locomotion in patients with spinal cord injuries. *Phys Ther* 77: 508-516.

Ditunno, J.F., J.W. Little, A. Tessler, and A.S. Burns. 2004. Spinal shock revisited: a four-phase model. *Spinal Cord* 42: 383-395.

Ditunno, J.F. Jr., S.L. Stover, M.M. Freed, and J.H. Ahn. 1992. Motor recovery of the upper extremities in traumatic quadriplegia: a multicenter study. *Arch Phys Med Rehabil* 73: 431-436.

Dobkin, B.H., S. Harkema, P. Requejo, and V.R. Edgerton. 1995. Modulation of locomotor-like EMG activity in subjects with complete and incomplete spinal cord injury. *J Neurol Rehabil* 9: 183-190.

Drory, Y., A. Ohry, M.E. Brooks, D. Dolphin, and J.J. Kellermann. 1990. Arm crank ergometry in chronic spinal cord injured patients. *Arch Phys Med Rehabil* 71: 389-92.

Duckworth, W.C., Solomon, S.S., Jallepalli, P., C. Heckemeyer, J. Finnern, and A. Powers. 1980. Glucose intolerance due to insulin resistance in patients with spinal cord injuries. *Diabetes* 29: 906-910.

Dudley, G.A., M.J. Castro, S. Rogers, and D.R. Apple Jr. 1999. A simple means of increasing muscle size after spinal cord injury: a pilot study. *Eur J Appl Physiol Occup Physiol* 80: 394-396.

Erickson, R.P. 1980. Autonomic hyperreflexia: pathophysiology and medical management. *Arch Phys Med Rehabil* 61: 431-440.

Escobedo, E.M., J.C. Hunter, M.C. Hollister, R.M. Patten, and B. Goldstein. 1997. MR imaging of rotator cuff tears in individuals with paraplegia. *AJR Am J Roentgenol* 168: 919-923.

Field-Fote, E.C. 2001. Combined use of body weight support, functional electric stimulation, and treadmill training to improve walking ability in individuals with chronic incomplete spinal cord injury. *Arch Phys Med Rehabil* 82: 818-824.

Field-Fote, E.C. 2004. Electrical stimulation modifies spinal and cortical neural circuitry. *Exerc Sc Sports Rev* 32(4): 155-160.

Field-Fote, E.C., and D. Tepavac. 2002. Improved intralimb coordination in people with incomplete spinal cord injury following training with body weight support and electrical stimulation. *Phys Ther* 82: 707-715.

Figoni, S.F. 1984. Cardiovascular and haemodynamic responses to tilting and to standing in tetraplegic patients: a review. *Paraplegia* 22: 99-109.

Figoni, S.F. 1997. Spinal cord injury. In *Exercise management for persons with chronic diseases and disabilities,* ed. J.L. Durstine. Champaign, IL: Human Kinetics.

Franklin, B.A. 1985. Exercise testing, training and arm ergometry. *Sports Med* 2: 100-119.

Gardner, M.B., M.K. Holden, J.M. Leikauskas, and R.L. Richard. 1998. Partial body weight support with treadmill locomotion to improve gait after incomplete spinal cord injury: a single-subject experimental design. *Phys Ther* 78: 361-374.

Garland, D.E., R.H. Adkins, N.N. Matsuno, and C.A. Stewart. 1999. The effect of pulsed electromagnetic fields on osteoporosis at the knee in individuals with spinal cord injury. *J Spinal Cord Med* 22: 239-245.

Gass, G.C., and E.M. Camp. 1984. The maximum physiological responses during incremental wheelchair and arm cranking exercise in male paraplegics. *Med Sci Sports Exerc* 16: 355-359.

Gass, G.C., E.M. Camp, E.R. Nadel, T.H. Gwinn, and P. Engel. 1988. Rectal and rectal vs. esophageal temperatures in paraplegic men during prolonged exercise. *J Appl Physiol* 64: 2265-2271.

Gass, G.C., J. Watson, E.M. Camp, H.J. Court, L.M. McPherson, and P. Redhead. 1980. The effects of physical training on high level spinal lesion patients. *Scand J Rehabil Med* 12: 61-65.

Gellman, H., I. Sie, and R.L. Waters. 1988. Late complications of the weight-bearing upper extremity in the paraplegic patient. *Clin Orthop Relat Res* 233: 132-135.

Gerhart, K.A., E. Bergstrom, S.W. Charlifue, R.R. Menter, and G.G. Whiteneck. 1993. Long-term spinal cord injury: functional changes over time. *Arch Phys Med Rehabil* 74: 1030-1034.

Gerrits, H.L., A. de Haan, A.J. Sargeant, H. van Langen, and M.T. Hopman. 2001. Peripheral vascular changes after electrically stimulated cycle training in people with spinal cord injury. *Arch Phys Med Rehabil* 82: 832-839.

Gettman, L.R., J.J. Ayres, M.L. Pollock, and A. Jackson. 1978. The effect of circuit weight training on strength, cardiorespiratory function, and body composition of adult men. *Med Sci Sports* 10: 171-176.

Glaser, R.M. 1994. Functional neuromuscular stimulation. Exercise conditioning of spinal cord injured patients. *Int J Sports Med* 15: 142-258.

Goldstein, B., J. Young, and E.M. Escobedo. 1997. Rotator cuff repairs in individuals with paraplegia. *Am J Phys Med Rehabil* 76: 316-322.

Graupe, D. 2002. An overview of the state of the art of noninvasive FES for independent ambulation by thoracic level paraplegics. *Neurol Res* 24: 431-442.

Graupe, D., and K.H. Kohn. 1997. Transcutaneous functional neuromuscular stimulation of certain traumatic complete thoracic paraplegics for independent short-distance ambulation. *Neurol Res* 19: 323-333.

Graupe, D., and K.H. Kohn. 1998. Functional neuromuscular stimulator for short-distance ambulation by certain thoracic-level spinal-cord-injured paraplegics. *Surg Neurol* 50: 202-207.

Green, D., R.D. Hull, E.F Mammen, G.J. Merli, S.I. Weingarden, and J.S. Yao. 1992. Deep vein thrombosis in spinal cord injury. Summary and recommendations. *Chest* 102: 633S-635S.

Greve, J.M., R. Muszkat, B. Schmidt, J. Chiovatto, T.E. Barros Filho, and L.R. Batisttella. 1993. Functional electrical stimulation (FES): muscle histochemical analysis. *Paraplegia* 31: 764-770.

Grundy, S.M. 1995. Atherogenic dyslipidemia: lipoprotein abnormalities and implications for therapy. *Am J Cardiol* 75: 45B-52B.

Hart, D.M., E. Farish, C.D. Fletcher, J.F. Barnes, H. Hart, D. Nolan, and K. Spowak. 1999. Long-term effects of continuous combined HRT on bone turnover and lipid metabolism in postmenopausal women. *Osteoporos Int* 8: 326-332.

Hartkopp, A., R.J. Murphy, T. Mohr, M. Kjaer, and F. Biering-Sorensen. 1998. Bone fracture during electrical stimulation of the quadriceps in a spinal cord injured subject. *Arch Phys Med Rehabil* 79: 1133-1136.

Hashimoto, R., H. Adachi, M. Tsuruta, H. Tashiro, and H. Toshima. 1995. Association of hyperinsulinemia and serum free fatty acids with serum high density lipoprotein-cholesterol. *J Atheroscler Thromb* 2: 53-59.

Hjeltnes, N. 1977. Oxygen uptake and cardiac output in graded arm exercise in paraplegics with low level spinal lesions. *Scand J Rehabil Med* 9: 107-113.

Hjeltnes, N. 1986. Cardiorespiratory capacity in tetra- and paraplegia shortly after injury. *Scand J Rehabil Med* 18: 65-70.

Hjeltnes, N., A.K. Aksnes, K.I. Birkeland, J. Johansen, A. Lannem, and Wallberg-Henriksson. 1997. Improved body composition after 8 wk of electrically stimulated leg cycling in tetraplegic patients. *Am J Physiol* 273: R1072-R1079.

Hjeltnes, N., D. Galuska, M. Bjornholm, A.K. Aksnes, A. Lannem, J.R. Zierath, and H. Wallberg-Henriksson. 1998. Exercise-induced overexpression of key regulatory proteins involved in glucose uptake and metabolism in tetraplegic persons: molecular mechanism for improved glucose homeostasis. *FASEB J* 12: 1701-1712.

Hoffman, M.D. 1986. Cardiorespiratory fitness and training in quadriplegics and paraplegics. *Sports Med* 3: 312-330.

Hooker, S.P., S.F. Figoni, R.M. Glaser, M.M Rodgers, B.N. Ezenwa, and P.D. Faghri. 1990. Physiologic responses to prolonged electrically stimulated leg-cycle exercise in the spinal cord injured. *Arch Phys Med Rehabil* 71: 863-869.

Hooker, S.P., A.M. Scremin, D.L. Mutton, C.F. Kunkel, and G. Cagle. 1995. Peak and submaximal physiologic responses following electrical stimulation leg cycle ergometer training. *J Rehabil Res Dev* 32: 361-366.

Hooker, S.P., and C.L. Wells. 1989. Effects of low- and moderate-intensity training in spinal cord-injured persons. *Med Sci Sports Exerc* 21: 18-22.

Hopman, M.T., M. Monroe, C. Dueck, W.T. Phillips, and J.S. Skinner. 1998. Blood redistribution and circulatory responses to submaximal arm exercise in persons with spinal cord injury. *Scand J Rehabil Med* 30: 167-174.

Hopman, M.T., B. Oeseburg, and R.A. Binkhorst. 1992a. Cardiovascular responses in paraplegic subjects during arm exercise. *Eur J Appl Physiol* 65: 73-78.

Hopman, M.T., B. Oeseburg, and R.A. Binkhorst. 1992b. The effect of an anti-G suit on cardiovascular responses to exercise in persons with paraplegia. *Med Sci Sports Exerc* 24: 984-990.

Hopman, M.T., B. Oeseburg, and R.A. Binkhorst. 1993a. Cardiovascular responses in persons with paraplegia to prolonged arm exercise and thermal stress. *Med Sci Sports Exerc* 25: 577-583.

Hopman, M.T., M. Pistorius, I.C. Kamerbeek, and R.A. Binkhorst. 1993b. Cardiac output in paraplegic subjects at high exercise intensities. *Eur J Appl Physiol* 66: 531-535.

Hopman, M.T., W.N. van Asten, and B. Oeseburg. 1996. Changes in blood flow in the common femoral artery related to inactivity and muscle atrophy in individuals with long-standing paraplegia. *Adv Exp Med Biol* 388: 379-383.

Houtman, S., J.J. Thielen, R.A. Binkhorst, and M.T. Hopman. 1999. Effect of a pulsating anti-gravity suit on peak exercise performance in individuals with spinal cord injuries. *Eur J Appl Physiol* 79: 202-204.

Hughes, J.T. 1988. The Edwin Smith Surgical Papyrus: an analysis of the first case reports of spinal cord injuries. *Paraplegia* 26: 71-82.

Ishii, K., M. Yamasaki, S. Muraki, T. Komura, K. Kikuchi, T. Satake, T. Miyagawa, S. Fujimoto, and K. Maeda. 1995. Effects of upper limb exercise on thermoregulatory responses in patients with spinal cord injury. *Appl Human Sci* 14: 149-154.

Jacobs, P.L., E.T. Mahoney, M.S. Nash, and B.A. Green. 2002a. Circuit resistance training in persons with complete paraplegia. *J Rehabil Res Dev* 39: 21-28.

Jacobs, P.L., E.T. Mahoney, A. Robbins, and M. Nash. 2002b. Hypokinetic circulation in persons with paraplegia. *Med Sci Sports Exerc* 34: 1401-1407.

Jacobs, P.L., M.S. Nash, K.J. Klose, R.S. Guest, B.M. Needham-Shropshire, and B.A. Green. 1997. Evaluation of a training program for persons with SCI paraplegia using the Parastep 1 ambulation system: part 2. Effects on physiological responses to peak arm ergometry. *Arch Phys Med Rehabil* 78: 794-798.

Jacobs, P.L., M.S. Nash, and J.W. Rusinowski. 2001. Circuit training provides cardiorespiratory and strength benefits in persons with paraplegia. *Med Sci Sports Exerc* 33: 711-717.

Jaeger, R.J. 1992. Lower extremity applications of functional neuromuscular stimulation. *Assist Technol* 4: 19-30.

Janssen, T.W., C.A. van Oers, H.E. Veeger, A.P. Hollander, L.H. van der Woude, and R.H. Rozendal. 1994. Relationship between physical strain during standardised ADL tasks and physical capacity in men with spinal cord injuries. *Paraplegia* 32: 844-859.

Jeppesen, J., F.S. Facchini, and G.M. Reaven. 1998. Individuals with high total cholesterol/HDL cholesterol ratios are insulin resistant. *J Intern Med* 243: 293-298.

Kantrowitz, A. 1960. *Electronic physiologic aids: A report of the Maimonides Hospital,* pp. 4-5. Brooklyn, NY: Maimonides Hospital).

Karlsson, A.K. 1999. Insulin resistance and sympathetic function in high spinal cord injury. *Spinal Cord* 37: 494-500.

Karlsson, A.K., S. Attvall, P.A. Jansson, L. Sullivan, and P. Lonnroth. 1995. Influence of the sympathetic nervous system on insulin sensitivity and adipose tissue metabolism: a study in spinal cord-injured subjects. *Metabolism* 44: 52-58.

Kessler, K.M., I. Pina, B. Green, B. Burnett, M. Laighold, M. Bilsker, A.R. Palomo, and R.J. Myerburg. 1986. Cardiovascular findings in quadriplegic and paraplegic patients and in normal subjects. *Am J Cardiol* 58: 525-530.

King, M.L., D.M. Freeman, J.T. Pellicone, E.R. Wanstall, and L.D. Bhansali. 1992. Exertional hypotension in thoracic spinal cord injury: case report. *Paraplegia* 30: 261-266.

King, M.L., S.W. Lichtman, J.T. Pellicone, R.J. Close, and P. Lisanti. 1994. Exertional hypotension in spinal cord injury. *Chest* 106: 1166-1171.

Kirshblum, S. 1999. Treatment alternatives for spinal cord injury related spasticity. *J Spinal Cord Med* 22: 199-217.

Klefbeck, B., E. Mattsson, and J. Weinberg. 1996. The effect of trunk support on performance during arm ergometry in patients with cervical cord injuries. *Paraplegia* 34: 167-172.

Klose, K.J., P.L. Jacobs, J.G. Broton, R.S. Guest, B.M. Needham-Shropshire, N. Lebwohl, M.S. Nash, and B.A. Green. 1997. Evaluation of a training program for persons with SCI paraplegia using the Parastep 1 ambulation system: part 1. Ambulation performance and anthropometric measures. *Arch Phys Med Rehabil* 78: 789-793.

Kocina, P. 1997. Body composition of spinal cord injured adults. *Sports Med* 23: 48-60.

Krause, J.S., B. Kemp, and J. Coker. 2000. Depression after spinal cord injury: relation to gender, ethnicity, aging, and socioeconomic indicators. *Arch Phys Med Rehabil* 81: 1099-1109.

Kuhne, S., H.M. Hammon, R.M. Bruckmaier, C. Morel, Y. Zbinden, and J.W. Blum. 2000. Growth performance, metabolic and endocrine traits, and absorptive capacity in neonatal calves fed either colostrum or milk replacer at two levels. *J Anim Sci* 78: 609-620.

Ladouceur, M., and H. Barbeau. 2000. Functional electrical stimulation-assisted walking for persons with incomplete spinal injuries: longitudinal changes in maximal overground walking speed. *Scand J Rehabil Med* 32: 28-36.

Lal, S. 1998. Premature degenerative shoulder changes in spinal cord injury patients. *Spinal Cord* 36: 186-189.

Laskin, J.J., E.A. Ashley, L.M. Olenik, R. Burnham, D.C. Cumming, R.D. Steadward, and G.D. Wheeler. 1993. Electrical stimulation-assisted rowing exercise in spinal cord injured people. A pilot study. *Paraplegia* 31: 534-541.

Lazo, M.G., P. Shirazi, M. Sam, A. Giobbie-Hurder, M.J. Blacconiere, and M. Muppidi. 2001. Osteoporosis and risk of fracture in men with spinal cord injury. *Spinal Cord* 39: 208-214.

Leeds, E.M., K.J. Klose, W. Ganz, A. Serafini, and B.A. Green. 1990. Bone mineral density after bicycle ergometry training. *Arch Phys Med Rehabil* 71: 207-209.

Levi, R., C. Hultling, M.S. Nash, and A. Seiger. 1995. The Stockholm spinal cord injury study: 1. Medical problems in a regional SCI population. *Paraplegia* 33: 308-315.

Levy, M., J. Mizrahi, and Z. Susak. 1990. Recruitment, force and fatigue characteristics of quadriceps muscles of paraplegics isometrically activated by surface functional electrical stimulation. *J Biomed Eng* 12: 150-156.

Lockette, K.F., and A.M. Keyes. 1994. *Conditioning with physical disabilities.* Champaign, IL: Human Kinetics.

Lopes, P., S.F. Figoni, and I. Perkash. 1984. Upper limb exercise effect on tilt tolerance during orthostatic training of patients with spinal cord injury. *Arch Phys Med Rehabil* 65: 251-253.

Lundqvist, C., A. Siosteen, L. Sullivan, C. Blomstrand, B. Lind, and M. Sullivan. 1997. Spinal cord injuries: a shortened measure of function and mood. *Spinal Cord* 35: 17-21.

Maki, K.C., E.R. Briones, W.E. Langbein, A. Inman-Felton, B. Nemchausky, M. Welch, and J. Burton. 1995. Associations between serum lipids and indicators of adiposity in men with spinal cord injury. *Paraplegia* 33: 102-109.

Marino, R.J., J.F. Ditunno Jr., W.H. Donovan, and F. Maynard Jr. 1999. Neurologic recovery after traumatic spinal cord injury: data from the Model Spinal Cord Injury Systems. *Arch Phys Med Rehabil* 80: 1391-1396.

McKinley, W.O., A.B. Jackson, D.D. Cardenas, and M.J. DeVivo. 1999. Long-term medical complications after traumatic spinal cord injury: a regional model systems analysis. *Arch Phys Med Rehabil* 80: 1402-1410.

Minaire, P. 1989. Immobilization osteoporosis: a review. *Clin Rheumatol* 8 Suppl 2: 95-103.

Mohr, T., F. Dela, A. Handberg, F. Biering-Sorensen, H. Galbo, and M. Kjaer. 2001. Insulin action and long-term electrically induced training in individuals with spinal cord injuries. *Med Sci Sports Exerc* 33: 1247-1252.

Mohr, T., J. Podenphant, F. Biering-Sorensen, H. Galbo, G. Thamsborg, and M. Kjaer. 1997. Increased bone mineral density after prolonged electrically induced cycle training of paralyzed limbs in spinal cord injured man. *Calcif Tissue Int* 61: 22-25.

Mukand, J., L. Karlin, K. Barrs, and P. Lublin. 2001. Midodrine for the management of orthostatic hypotension in patients with spinal cord injury: A case report. *Arch Phys Med Rehabil* 82: 694-696.

Mulcahey, M.J., R.R. Betz, B.T. Smith, A.A. Weiss, and S.E. Davis. 1997. Implanted functional electrical stimulation hand system in adolescents with spinal injuries: an evaluation. *Arch Phys Med Rehabil* 78: 597-607.

Muraki, S., M. Yamasaki, K. Ishii, K. Kikuchi, and K. Seki. 1995. Effect of arm cranking exercise on skin blood flow of lower limb in people with injuries to the spinal cord. *Eur J Appl Physiol Occup Physiol* 71: 28-32.

Muraki, S., M. Yamasaki, K. Ishii, K. Kikuchi, and K. Seki. 1996. Relationship between core temperature and skin blood flux in lower limbs during prolonged arm exercise in persons with spinal cord injury. *Eur J Appl Physiol* 72: 330-334.

Murphy, R.J., A. Hartkopp, P.F. Gardiner, M. Kjaer, and L. Beliveau. 1999. Salbutamol effect in spinal cord injured individuals undergoing functional electrical stimulation training. *Arch Phys Med Rehabil* 80: 1264-1267.

Mutton, D.L., A.M. Scremin, T.J. Barstow, M.D. Scott, C.F. Kunkel, and T.G. Cagle. 1997. Physiologic responses during functional electrical stimulation leg cycling and hybrid exercise in spinal cord injured subjects. *Arch Phys Med Rehabil* 78: 712-718.

Nash, M.S. 1997. Exercise reconditioning of the heart and peripheral circulation after spinal cord injury. *Top Spinal Cord Inj Rehabil* 3: 1-15.

Nash, M.S. 2000. Known and plausible modulators of depressed immune functions following spinal cord injuries. *J Spinal Cord Med* 23: 111-120.

Nash, M.S. 2002. Cardiovascular fitness after spinal cord injuries. In *Spinal cord medicine,* ed. V. Lin. New York: Demos Medical.

Nash, M.S., M.S. Bilsker, H.M. Kearney, J.N. Ramirez, B. Applegate, and B.A. Green. 1995. Effects of electrically-stimulated exercise and passive motion on echocardiographically-derived wall motion and cardiodynamic function in tetraplegic persons. *Paraplegia* 33: 80-89.

Nash, M.S., S. Bilsker, A.E. Marcillo, S.M. Isaac, L.A. Botelho, K.J. Klose, B.A. Green, M.T. Rountree, and J.D. Shea. 1991. Reversal of adaptive left ventricular atrophy following electrically-stimulated exercise training in human tetraplegics. *Paraplegia* 29: 590-599.

Nash, M.S., and J.A. Horton. 2002. Recreational and therapeutic exercise after SCI. In *Spinal cord injury medicine,* eds. S. Kirshbaum, D.I. Campagnolo, and J.S. DeLisa. Philadelphia: Lippincott Williams & Wilkins.

Nash, M.S., P.L. Jacobs, A.J. Mendez, and R.B. Goldberg. 2001. Circuit resistance training improves the atherogenic lipid profiles of persons with chronic paraplegia. *J Spinal Cord Med* 24: 2-9.

Nash, M.S., P.L. Jacobs, B.M. Montalvo, K.J. Klose, R.S. Guest, and B.M. Needham-Shropshire. 1997. Evaluation of a training program for persons with SCI paraplegia using the Parastep 1 ambulation system: part 5. Lower extremity blood flow and hyperemic responses to occlusion are augmented by ambulation training. *Arch Phys Med Rehabil* 78: 808-814.

Nash, M.S., P.L. Jacobs, J.M. Woods, J.E. Clark, T.A. Pray, and A.E. Pumarejo. 2002. A comparison of 2 circuit exercise training techniques for eliciting matched metabolic responses in persons with paraplegia. *Arch Phys Med Rehabil* 83: 201-209.

Nash, M.S., B.M. Montalvo, and B. Applegate. 1996. Lower extremity blood flow and responses to occlusion ischemia differ in exercise-trained and sedentary tetraplegic persons. *Arch Phys Med Rehabil* 77: 1260-1265.

Nash, M.S., J. Tehranzadeh, B.A. Green, M.T. Rountree, and J.D. Shea. 1994. Magnetic resonance imaging of osteonecrosis and osteoarthrosis in exercising quadriplegics and paraplegics. *Am J Phys Med Rehabil* 73: 184-192.

Needham-Shropshire, B.M., J.G. Broton, K.J. Klose, N. Lebwohl, R.S. Guest, and P.L. Jacobs. 1997. Evaluation of a training program for persons with SCI paraplegia using the Parastep 1 ambulation system: part 3. Lack of effect on bone mineral density. *Arch Phys Med Rehabil* 78: 799-803.

Nichols, P.J., P.A. Norman, and J.R. Ennis. 1979. Wheelchair user's shoulder? Shoulder pain in patients with spinal cord lesions. *Scand J Rehabil Med* 11: 29-32.

Nilsson, S., P.H. Staff, and E.D. Pruett. 1975. Physical work capacity and the effect of training on subjects with long-standing paraplegia. *Scand J Rehabil Med* 7: 51-56.

Noreau, L., R.J. Shephard, C. Simard, G. Pare, and P. Pomerleau. 1993. Relationship of impairment and functional ability to habitual activity and fitness following spinal cord injury. *Int J Rehabil Res* 16: 265-275.

Olenik, L.M., J.J. Laskin, R. Burnham, G.D. Wheeler, and R.D. Steadward. 1995. Efficacy of rowing, backward wheeling and isolated scapular retractor exercise as remedial strength activities for wheelchair users: application of electromyography. *Paraplegia* 33: 148-152.

Peckham, P.H., and G.H. Creasey. 1992. Neural prosthesis: Clinical applications of functional electrical stimulation in spinal cord injury. *Paraplegia* 30: 96-101.

Pentland, W.E., and L.T. Twomey. 1991. The weight-bearing upper extremity in women with long term paraplegia. *Paraplegia* 29: 521-530.

Pentland, W.E., and L.T. Twomey. 1994. Upper limb function in persons with long term paraplegia and implications for independence: Part I. *Paraplegia* 32: 211-218.

Petrofsky, J.S., and C.A. Phillips. 1984. The use of functional electrical stimulation for rehabilitation of spinal cord injured patients. *Cent Nerv Syst Trauma* 1: 57-74.

Phillips, C.A. 1987. Medical criteria for active physical therapy. Physician guidelines for patient participation in a program of functional electrical rehabilitation. *Am J Phys Med* 66: 269-286.

Phillips, C.A., J.J. Gallimore, and D.M. Hendershot. 1995. Walking when utilizing a sensory feedback system and an electrical muscle stimulation gait orthosis. *Med Eng Phys* 17: 507-513.

Phillips, W.T., B.J. Kiratli, M. Sarkarati, G. Weraarchakul, J. Myers, B.A. Franklin, I. Parkash, and V. Froelicher. 1998. Effect of spinal cord injury on the heart and cardiovascular fitness. *Curr Probl Cardiol* 23: 641-716.

Pinter, M.M., and M.R. Dimitrijevic. 1999. Gait after spinal cord injury and the central pattern generator for locomotion. *Spinal Cord* 37: 531-537.

Powers, C.M., C.J. Newsam, J.K. Gronley, C.A. Fontaine, and J. Perry. 1994. Isometric shoulder torque in subjects with spinal cord injury. *Arch Phys Med Rehabil* 75: 761-765.

Price, M.J., and I.G. Campbell. 1999. Thermoregulatory responses of spinal cord injured and able-bodied athletes to prolonged upper body exercise and recovery. *Spinal Cord* 37: 772-779.

Priebe, M.M., A.M. Sherwood, J.I. Thornby, N.F. Kharas, and J. Markowski. 1996. Clinical assessment of spasticity in spinal cord injury: a multidimensional problem. *Arch Phys Med Rehabil* 77: 713-716.

Protas, E.J., S.A. Holmes, H. Qureshy, A. Johnson, D. Lee, and Sherwood, A.M. 2001. Supported treadmill ambulation training after spinal cord injury: a pilot study. *Arch Phys Med Rehabil* 82: 825-831.

Ragnarsson, K.T. 1993. The cardiovascular system. In *Aging with spinal cord injury.* New York: Demos.

Ragnarsson, K.T., S. Pollack, W. O'Daniel Jr., R. Edgar, J. Petrofsky, and M.S. Nash. 1988. Clinical evaluation of computerized functional electrical stimulation after spinal cord injury: a multicenter pilot study. *Arch Phys Med Rehabil* 69: 672-677.

Ragnarsson, K.T., and G.H. Sell. 1981. Lower extremity fractures after spinal cord injury: a retrospective study. *Arch Phys Med Rehabil* 62: 418-423.

Raymond, J., G.M. Davis, M. Climstein, and J.R. Sutton. 1999. Cardiorespiratory responses to arm cranking and electrical stimulation leg cycling in people with paraplegia. *Med Sci Sports Exerc* 31: 822-828.

Robinson, M.D., R.W. Hussey, and C.Y. Ha. 1993. Surgical decompression of impingement in the weightbearing shoulder. *Arch Phys Med Rehabil* 74: 324-327.

Rochester, L., M.J. Barron, C.S. Chandler, R.A. Sutton, S. Miller, and M.A. Johnson. 1995a. Influence of electrical stimulation of the tibialis anterior muscle in paraplegic subjects. 2. Morphological and histochemical properties. *Paraplegia* 33: 514-522.

Rochester, L., C.S. Chandler, M.A. Johnson, R.A. Sutton, and S. Miller. 1995b. Influence of electrical stimulation of the tibialis anterior muscle in paraplegic subjects. 1. Contractile properties. *Paraplegia* 33: 437-449.

Rodgers, M.M., R.M. Glaser, S.F. Figoni, S.P. Hooker, B.N. Ezenwa, S.R. Collins, T. Mathews, A.G. Suryaprasad, and S.C. Gupta. 1991. Musculoskeletal responses of spinal cord injured individuals to functional neuromuscular stimulation-induced knee extension exercise training. *J Rehabil Res Dev* 28: 19-26.

Sawka, M.N., W.A. Latzka, and K.B. Pandolf. 1989. Temperature regulation during upper body exercise: able-bodied and spinal cord injured. *Med Sci Sports Exerc* 21: S132-S140.

Schmid, A., M. Huonker, J.M. Barturen, F. Stahl, A. Schmidt-Trucksass, D. Konig, D. Grathwohl, M. Lehmann, and J. Keul. 1998a. Catecholamines, heart rate, and oxygen uptake during exercise in persons with spinal cord injury. *J Appl Physiol* 85: 635-641.

Schmid, A., M. Huonker, F. Stahl, J.M. Barturen, D. Konig, M. Heim, M. Lehmann, and J. Keul. 1998b. Free plasma catecholamines in spinal cord injured persons with different injury levels at rest and during exercise. *J Auton Nerv Syst* 68: 96-100.

Schmidt-Trucksass, A., A. Schmid, C. Brunner, N. Scherer, G. Zach, J. Keul, and M. Huonker. 2000. Arterial properties of the carotid and femoral artery in endurance-trained and paraplegic subjects. *J Appl Physiol* 89: 1956-1963.

Schneider, D.A., D.A. Sedlock, E. Gass, and G. Gass. 1999. VO_2peak and the gas-exchange anaerobic threshold during incremental arm cranking in able-bodied and paraplegic men. *Eur J Appl Physiol* 80: 292-297.

Scremin, A.M., L. Kurta, A. Gentili, B. Wiseman, K. Perell, C. Kunkel, and O.U. Scremin. 1999. Increasing muscle mass in spinal cord injured persons with a functional electrical stimulation exercise program. *Arch Phys Med Rehabil* 80: 1531-1536.

Segatore, M. 1995a. The skeleton after spinal cord injury. Part 1. Theoretical aspects. *SCI Nurs* 12: 82-86.

Segatore, M. 1995b. The skeleton after spinal cord injury. Part 2: management of sublesional osteoporosis. *SCI Nurs* 12: 115-120.

Shields, R.K. 2002. Muscular, skeletal, and neural adaptations following spinal cord injury. *J Orthop Sports Phys Ther* 32: 65-74.

Shields, R.K., L.F. Law, B. Reiling, K. Sass, and J. Wilwert. 1997. Effects of electrically induced fatigue on the twitch and tetanus of paralyzed soleus muscle in humans. *J Appl Physiol* 82: 1499-1507.

Sie, I.H., R.L. Waters, R.H. Adkins, and H. Gellman. 1992. Upper extremity pain in the postrehabilitation spinal cord injured patient. *Arch Phys Med Rehabil* 73: 44-48.

Signorile, J.F., K. Banovac, M. Gomez, D. Flipse, J.F. Caruso, and I. Lowensteyn. 1995. Increased muscle strength in paralyzed patients after spinal cord injury: effect of beta-2 adrenergic agonist. *Arch Phys Med Rehabil* 76: 55-58.

Silfverskiold, J., and R.L. Waters. 1991. Shoulder pain and functional disability in spinal cord injury patients. *Clin Orthop Relat Res* 272: 141-145.

Solomonow, M., E. Reisin, E. Aguilar, R.V. Baratta, R. Best, and R. D'Ambrosia. 1997. Reciprocating gait orthosis powered with electrical muscle stimulation (RGO II). Part II: Medical evaluation of 70 paraplegic patients. *Orthopedics* 20: 411-418.

Spungen, A.M., W.A. Bauman, J. Wang, and R.N. Pierson Jr. 1995. Measurement of body fat in individuals with tetraplegia: a comparison of eight clinical methods. *Paraplegia* 33: 402-408.

Stein, R.B., M. Belanger, G. Wheeler, M. Wieler, D.B. Popovic, A. Prochazka, and L.A. Davis. 1993. Electrical systems for improving locomotion after incomplete spinal cord injury: an assessment. *Arch Phys Med Rehabil* 74: 954-959.

Subbarao, J.V., J. Klopfstein, and R. Turpin. 1995. Prevalence and impact of wrist and shoulder pain in patients with spinal cord injury. *J Spinal Cord Med* 18: 9-13.

Talmadge, R.J., M.J. Castro, D.F. Apple Jr., and G.A. Dudley. 2002. Phenotypic adaptations in human muscle fibers 6 and 24 wk after spinal cord injury. *J Appl Physiol* 92: 147-154.

Talmadge, R.J., R.R. Roy, and V.R. Edgerton. 1995. Prominence of myosin heavy chain hybrid fibers in soleus muscle of spinal cord-transected rats. *J Appl Physiol* 78: 1256-1265.

Taricco, M., R. Adone, C. Pagliacci, and E. Telaro. 2000. Pharmacological interventions for spasticity following spinal cord injury. *Cochrane Database Syst Rev* CD001131.

Taylor, A.W., E. McDonell, and L. Brassard. 1986. The effects of an arm ergometer training programme on wheelchair subjects. *Paraplegia* 24: 105-114.

Taylor, P.N., D.J. Ewins, B. Fox, D. Grundy, and I.D. Swain. 1993. Limb blood flow, cardiac output and quadriceps muscle bulk following spinal cord injury and the effect of training for the Odstock functional electrical stimulation standing system. *Paraplegia* 31: 303-310.

Trimble, M.H., C.G. Kukulka, and A.L. Behrman. 1998. The effect of treadmill gait training on low-frequency depression of the soleus H-reflex: comparison of a spinal cord injured man to normal subjects. *Neurosci Lett* 246: 186-188.

Triolo, R.J., C. Bieri, J. Uhlir, R. Kobetic, A. Scheiner, and E.G. Marsolais. 1996. Implanted functional neuromuscular stimulation systems for individuals with cervical spinal cord injuries: clinical case reports. *Arch Phys Med Rehabil* 77: 1119-1128.

Uebelhart, D., B. Demiaux-Domenech, M. Roth, and A. Chantraine. 1995. Bone metabolism in spinal cord injured individuals and in others who have prolonged immobilisation. A review. *Paraplegia* 33: 669-673.

Vaidyanathan, S., B.M. Soni, P. Sett, J.W. Watt, T. Oo, and J. Bingley. 1998. Pathophysiology of autonomic dysreflexia: long-term treatment with terazosin in adult and paediatric spinal cord injury patients manifesting recurrent dysreflexic episodes. *Spinal Cord* 36: 761-770.

van Baak, M.A., L.H. Mayer, R.E. Kempinski, and F. Hartgens. 2000. Effect of salbutamol on muscle strength and endurance performance in nonasthmatic men. *Med Sci Sports Exerc* 32: 1300-1306.

Van Loan, M.D., S. McCluer, J.M. Loftin, and R.A. Boileau. 1987. Comparison of physiological responses to maximal arm exercise among able-bodied, paraplegics and quadriplegics. *Paraplegia* 25: 397-405.

Vestergaard, P., K. Krogh, L. Rejnmark, and L. Mosekilde. 1998. Fracture rates and risk factors for fractures in patients with spinal cord injury. *Spinal Cord* 36: 790-6.

Washburn, R.A., and S.F. Figoni. 1998. Physical activity and chronic cardiovascular disease prevention in spinal cord injury: a comprehensive literature review. *Top Spinal Cord Inj Rehabil* 3: 16-32.

Washburn, R.A., and S.F. Figoni. 1999. High density lipoprotein cholesterol in individuals with spinal cord injury: the potential role of physical activity. *Spinal Cord* 37: 685-695.

Webborn, A.D. 1999. "Boosting" performance in disability sport. *Br J Sports Med* 33: 74-75.

Wernig, A., A. Nanassy, and S. Muller. 1999. Laufband (treadmill) therapy in incomplete paraplegia and tetraplegia. *J Neurotrauma* 16: 719-726.

Whiteneck, G. 1992. Learning from empirical investigations. In *Perspectives on aging with spinal cord injury,* R. Menter and G. Whiteneck. New York: Demos.

Widerstrom-Noga, E.G., and D.C. Turk. 2003. Types and effectiveness of treatments used by people with chronic pain associated with spinal cord injuries: influence of pain and psychosocial characteristics. *Spinal Cord* 41: 600-609.

Winther, K., G. Gleerup, K. Snorrason, and F. Biering-Sorensen. 1992. Platelet function and fibrinolytic activity in cervical spinal cord injured patients. *Thromb Res* 65: 469-474.

Wirz, M., G. Colombo, and V. Dietz. 2001. Long term effects of locomotor training in spinal humans. *J Neurol Neurosurg Psychiatry* 71: 93-96.

Yim, S.Y., K.J. Cho, C.I. Park, T.S. Yoon, D.Y. Han, S.K. Kim, and H.L. Lee. 1993. Effect of wheelchair ergometer training on spinal cord-injured paraplegics. *Yonsei Med J* 34: 278-286.

Zlotolow, S.P., E. Levy, and W.A. Bauman. 1992. The serum lipoprotein profile in veterans with paraplegia: the relationship to nutritional factors and body mass index. *J Am Paraplegia Soc* 15: 158-162.

CHAPTER 14

Aisen, F.L., H.I. Krebs, N. Hogan, F. McDowell, and B.T. Volpe. 1997. The effect of robot-assisted therapy and rehabilitative training on motor recovery following stroke. *Arch Neurol* 54: 443-e46.

American Heart Association. 2003. *Heart disease and stroke statistics 2003 update*. Dallas: American Heart Association.

Asanuma, C. 1991. Mapping movements within a moving motor map. *Trends Neurosci* 14: 217-218.

Badics, E., A. Wittman, M. Rupp, B. Stabauer, and U.A. Zifko. 2002. Systematic muscle building exercises in the rehabilitation of stroke patients. *Neurorehabilitation* 17: 211-214.

Balliet, R., K.B. Harbst, D. Kim, and R.V. Stewart. 1987. Retraining of functional gait through the reduction of upper extremity weightbearing in chronic cerebellar ataxia. *Int Rehabil Med* 8: 149-153.

Barbeau, H., and M. Visintin. 2003. Optimal outcomes obtained with body-weight support combined with treadmill training in stroke subjects. *Arch Phys Med Rehabil* 84(10): 1458-1465.

Basmajian, J.V., C. Gowland, M.E. Brandstater, L. Swanson, and J. Trotter. 1982. EMG feedback treatment of upper limb in hemiplegic stroke patients: A pilot study. *Arch Phys Med Rehabil* 63: 613-616.

Basmajian, J.V., C.A. Gowland, M.A. Finlayson, A.L. Hall, L.R. Swanson, P.W. Stratford, J.E. Trotter, and M.E. Brandstater. 1987. Stroke treatment: Comparison of integrated behavioral-physical therapy vs traditional physical therapy programs. *Arch Phys Med Rehabil* 68: 267-272.

Basmajian, J.V., C.G. Kukulka, M.G. Narayan, and K. Takebe. 1975. Biofeedback treatment of foot-drop after stroke compared with standard rehabilitation technique: Effects on voluntary control and strength. *Arch Phys Med Rehabil* 56: 231-236.

Bethel, A., J.R. Kirsch, R.C. Koehler, S.P. Finklestein, and R.J. Traystman. 1997. Intravenous basic fibroblast growth factor decreased brain injury resulting from focal ischemia in cats. *Stroke* 28: 609-615.

Bobath, B. 1990. *Adult hemiplegia: Evaluation and treatment.* 3rd ed., 60-61. Oxford, England: Butterworth Heinemann.

Bogataj, U., N. Gros, M. Kljajic, R. Acimovic, and M. Malezic. 1995. The rehabilitation of gait in patients with hemiplegia: A comparison between conventional therapy and multichannel functional electrical stimulation therapy. *Phys Ther* 75: 490-502.

Bohannon, R.W. 1995. Standing balance, lower extremity muscle strength, and walking performance of patients referred for physical therapy. *Percept Mot Skills* 80: 379-385.

Bohannon, R.W., and A.W. Andrews. 1990. Correlation of knee extensor muscle torque and spasticity with gait speed in patients with stroke. *Arch Phys Med Rehabil* 71: 330-333.

Bohannon, R.W., P.A. Larkin, M.B. Smith, and M.G. Horton. 1987. Relationship between static muscle strength deficits and spasticity in stroke patients with hemiparesis. *Phys Ther* 67: 1068-1071.

Bohannon, R.W., and M.B. Smith. 1987. Upper extremity strength deficits in hemiplegic stroke patients: Relationship between admission and discharge assessment and time since onset. *Arch Phys Med Rehabil* 68: 155-157.

Bourbonnais, D., S. Bilodeau, Y. Lepage, N. Beaudoin, D. Gravel, and R. Forget. 2002. Effect of force-feedback treatments in patients with chronic motor deficits after a stroke. *Am J Phys Med Rehabil* 18: 890-897.

Bowman, B.R., L.L. Baker, and R.L. Waters. 1979. Positional feedback and electrical stimulation: An automated treatment for the hemiplegic wrist. *Arch Phys Med Rehabil* 60: 492-502.

Bradley, L., B.B. Hart, S. Mandan, K. Flowers, M. Riches, and P. Sanderson. 1998. Electromyographic biofeedback for gait training after stroke. *Clin Rehabil* 12: 11-22.

Bronner, L.L., D.S. Kanter, and J.E. Manson. 1995. Primary prevention of stroke. *N Engl J Med* 333: 1392-1400.

Brooke, M.H., and W.K. Engel. 1969. The histographic analysis of human muscle biopsies with regard to fiber types. Part 2. Diseases of the upper and lower motor neuron. *Neurology* 19: 378-393.

Brown, D.A., and S.A. Kautz. 1998. Increased workload enhances force output during pedaling exercise in persons with post-stroke hemiplegia. *Stroke* 29: 598-606.

Browne, T.R. III, and D.C. Poskanzer. 1969. Treatment of strokes. *N Engl J Med* 281: 594-602.

Burnside, I.G., S. Tobias, and D. Bursill. 1982. Electromyographic feedback in the remobilization of stroke patients: A controlled trial. *Arch Phys Med Rehabil* 63: 217-222.

Butefisch, C., H. Hummelsheim, P. Densler, and K. Mauritz. 1995. Repetitive training of isolated movements improves the outcome of motor rehabilitation of the centrally paretic hand. *J Neurol Sci* 130: 59-68.

Chae, J. 2003. Neuromuscular electrical stimulation for motor relearning in hemiparesis. *Phys Med Rehabil Clin N Am* 14(1 Suppl.): S93-S109.

Chae, J., F. Bethoux, T. Bohine, L. Dobos, T. Davis, and A. Friedl. 1998. Neuromuscular stimulation for upper extremity motor and functional recovery in acute hemiplegia. *Stroke* 29: 975-979.

Cheng, P.T., S.H. Wu, M.Y. Liaw, A.M. Wong, and F.T. Tang. 2001. Symmetrical body-weight distribution training in stroke patients and its effect on fall prevention. *Arch Phys Med Rehabil* 82: 1650-1654.

Clark, W.M., S.J. Warach, and L.C. Pettigrew, R.E. Gammans, and L.A. Sabounjian. 1997. A randomized dose-response trial of citicoline in acute ischemic stroke patients. *Neurology* 49: 671-678.

Colborne, G.R., S.J. Olney, and M.P. Griffin. 1993. Feedback of ankle joint angle and soleus electromyography in the rehabilitation of hemiplegic gait. *Arch Phys Med Rehabil* 74: 1100-1106.

Colebatch, J.G., and S.C. Gandevia.1989. The distribution of muscular weakness in upper motor neuron lesions affecting the arm. *Brain* 112: 749-763.

Cotman, C.W., and N.C. Berchtold. 2002. Exercise: A behavioral intervention to enhance brain health and plasticity. *Trends Neurosci* 25(6): 295-301.

Cozean, C.D., W.S. Pease, and S.I. Hubbell. 1988. Biofeedback and functional electric stimulation in stroke rehabilitation. *Arch Phys Med Rehabil* 69: 401-05.

Cramer, S.C., G. Nelles, R.R. Benson, J.D. Kaplan, R.A. Parker, K.K. Kwong, D.N. Kennedy, S.P. Finklestein, and B.R. Rosen. 1997. A functional MRI study of subjects recovered from hemiparetic stroke. *Stroke* 28: 2518-27.

Crisostomo, E.A., P.W. Duncan, M. Propst, D.V. Dawson, and J.N. Davis. 1988. Evidence that amphetamine with physical therapy promotes recovery of motor function in stroke patients. *Ann Neurol* 23: 94-97.

Crow, J.L., N.B. Lincoln, F.M. Nouri, and W. DeWeerdt. 1989. The effectiveness of EMG biofeedback in the treatment of arm function after stroke. *Int Disabil Studies* 11: 155-160.

Dattola, R., P. Girlanda, G. Vita, M. Santoro, M.L. Roberto, A. Toscano, C. Venuto, A. Baradello, and C. Messina. 1993. Muscle rearrangement in patients with hemiparesis after stroke: An electrophysiological and morphological study. *Eur Neurol* 33: 109-114.

Davis, A.E., and R.G. Lee. 1980. EMG biofeedback in patients with motor disorders: An aid for coordinating activity in antagonistic muscle groups. *Can J Neurol Sci* 7: 199-206.

Dean, C.M., and R.B. Shepherd. 1997. Task-related training improves performance of seated reaching tasks after stroke. A randomized controlled trial. *Stroke* 28: 722-728.

DeBow, S.B., M.L. Davies, H.L. Clarke, and F. Coulborne. 2003. Constraint-induced movement therapy and rehabilitation exercises lessen motor deficits and volume of brain injury after striatal hemorrhagic stroke in rats. *Stroke* 34: 1021-1026.

de Kroon, J.R., J.H. van der Lee, M.J. Ijzerman, and G.J. Lankhorst. 2002. Therapeutic electrical stimulation to improve motor control and functional abilities of the upper extremity after stroke: A systematic review. *Clin Rehabil* 16: 350-360.

Dickstein, R., S. Hocherman, T. Pillar, and R. Shaham. 1986. Stroke rehabilitation. Three exercise therapy approaches. *Phys Ther* 66: 1233-1238.

Dietz, V., U. Ketelsen, W. Berger, and J. Quintern. 1986. Motor unit involvement in spastic paresis. *J Neurol Sci* 75: 89-103.

Disler, P.B., and D.T. Wade. 2003. Should all stroke rehabilitation be home based? *Am J Phys Med Rehabil* 82: 733-735.

Dobkin, B., E. Fowler, and R. Gregor. 1991. A strategy to train locomotion in patients with chronic hemiplegic stroke. *Ann Neurol* 30: 278.

Dobrovolny, C.L., F.M. Ivey, M.A. Rogers, J.D. Sorkin, and R.F. Macko. 2003. Reliability of treadmill exercise testing in older patients with chronic hemiparetic stroke. *Arch Phys Med Rehabil* 84: 1308-1312.

Dromerick, A.W., D.F. Edwards, and M. Hahn. 2000. Does the application of constraint-induced movement therapy during acute rehabilitation reduce arm impairment after stroke? *Stroke* 31: 2984-2988.

Duncan, P., L. Richards, D. Wallace, J. Stoker-Yates, P. Pohl, C. Luchies, A. Ogle, and S. Studenski. 1998. A randomized, controlled pilot study of a home-based exercise program for individuals with mild and moderate stroke. *Stroke* 29: 2055-2060.

Duncan, P., S. Studenski, L. Richards, S. Gollub, S.M. Lai, D. Reker, S. Perera, J. Yates, V. Koch, S. Rigler, and D. Johnson. 2003. Randomized clinical trial of therapeutic exercise in subacute stroke. *Stroke* 34: 2173-2180.

Dursun, E., N. Hamamci, S. Donmez, O. Tuzunalp, and A. Cakci. 1996. Angular biofeedback device for sitting balance of stroke patients. *Stroke* 27: 1354-57.

Eng, J.J., K.S. Chu, C.M. Kim, A.S. Dawson, A. Carswell, and K.E. Hepburn. 2003. A community-based group exercise program for persons with chronic stroke. *Med Sci Sports Exerc* 35: 1271-1278.

Engardt, M. 1994. Rising and sitting down in stroke patients. Auditory feedback and dynamic strength training to enhance symmetrical body weight distribution. *Scand J Rehabil Med* (Suppl.) 31: 1-57.

Engardt, M., E. Knutsson, M. Jonsson, and M. Sternhag. 1995. Dynamic muscle strength training in stroke patients: Effects on knee extension torque, electromyographic activity, and motor function. *Arch Phys Med Rehabil* 76: 419-425.

Engardt, M., T. Ribbe, and E. Olsson. 1993. Vertical ground reaction force feedback to enhance stroke patients' symmetrical bodyweight distribution while rising/sitting down. *Scand J Rehabil Med* 25: 41-48.

Evans, R.L., R.T. Connis, R.D. Hendricks, and J.K. Haselkorn. 1995. Multidisciplinary rehabilitation versus medical care: A metaanalysis. *Soc Sci Med* 40: 1699-1706.

Faghri, P.D., M.M. Rodgers, R.M. Glaser, J.G. Bors, C. Ho, and P. Akuthota. 1994. The effects of functional electrical stimulation on shoulder subluxation, arm function recovery, and shoulder pain in hemiplegic stroke patients. *Arch Phys Med Rehabil* 75: 73-79.

Fasoli, S.E., H.I. Krebs, J. Stein, W.R. Frontera, and N. Hogan. 2003. Effects of robotic therapy on motor impairment and recovery in chronic stroke. *Arch Phys Med Rehabil* 84: 477-482.

Fasoli, S.E., H.I. Krebs, J. Stein, W.R. Frontera, R. Hughes, and N. Hogan. 2004. Robotic therapy for chronic motor impairments after stroke: Follow-up results. *Arch Phys Med Rehabil* 85(7): 1106-1111.

Feeney, D.M., A. Gonzales, and W. Law. 1982. Amphetamine, haloperidol and experience interact to affect rate of recovery after motor cortex injury. *Science* 217: 855-857.

Feigin, L., B. Sharon, B. Czaczkes, and A.J. Rosin. 1996. Sitting equilibrium 2 weeks after a stroke can predict the walking ability after 6 months. *Gerontology* 42: 348-353.

Ferguson, J.M., and C.A. Trombly. 1997. The effect of added-purpose and meaningful occupation on motor learning. *Am J Occup Ther* 51(7): 508-515.

Ferraro, M., J.J. Palazzolo, J. Krol, H.I. Krebs, N. Hogan, and B.T. Volpe. 2003. Robot-aided sensorimotor arm training improves outcome in patients with chronic stroke. *Neurology* 61: 1604-1607.

Fields, R.W. 1987. Electromyographically triggered electrical muscle stimulation for chronic hemiplegia. *Arch Phys Med Rehabil* 68: 407-414.

Fisher, C.M. 1992. Concerning the mechanism of recovery in stroke hemiplegia. *Can J Neurol Sci* 19: 57-63.

Fisher, M., and W. Schaebitz. 2000. An overview of acute stroke therapy: Past, present, and future. *Arch Intern Med* 160: 3196-3206.

Francisco, G., J. Chae, H. Chawla, S. Kirshblum, R. Zorowitz, G. Lewis, and S. Pang. 1998. Electromyogram-triggered neuromuscular stimulation for improving the arm function of acute stroke survivors: A randomized pilot study. *Arch Phys Med Rehabil* 79: 570-575.

Frontera, W.R., L. Grimby, and L. Larsson. 1997. Firing rate of the lower motoneuron and contractile properties of its muscle fibers after upper motoneuron lesion in man. *Muscle Nerve* 20: 938-947.

Geiger, R.A., J.B. Allen, J. O'Keefe, and R.R. Hicks. 2001. Balance and mobility following stroke: Effects of physical therapy interventions with and without biofeedback/forceplate training. *Phys Therapy* 81: 995-1005.

Gemperline, J.J., S. Allen, D. Walk, and W.Z. Rymer. 1995. Characteristics of motor unit discharge in subjects with hemiparesis. *Muscle Nerve* 18: 1101-1114.

Gill-Body, K.M., R.A. Popat, S.W. Parker, and D.E. Krebs. 1997. Rehabilitation of balance in two patients with cerebellar dysfunction. *Phys Ther* 77: 534-552.

Gillum, R.F., M.E. Mussolino, and D.D. Ingram. 1996. Physical activity and stroke incidence in women and men: The NHANES I epidemiologic follow-up study. *Am J Epidemiol* 143: 860-869.

Glanz, M., S. Klawansky, W. Stason, C. Berkey, and T.C. Chalmers. 1996. Functional electrostimulation in poststroke rehabilitation: A meta-analysis of the randomized controlled trials. *Arch Phys Med Rehabil* 77: 549-553.

Glanz, M., S. Klawansky, W. Stason, C. Berkey, H. Phan, and N. Shah. 1995. Biofeedback therapy in poststroke rehabilitation: A meta-analysis of the randomized controlled trials. *Arch Phys Med Rehabil* 76: 508-515.

Glasser, L. 1986. Effects of isokinetic training on the rate of movement during ambulation in hemiparetic patients. *Phys Ther* 66: 673-676.

Glees, P. 1980. Functional reorganization following hemispherectomy in man and after small experimental lesions in primates. In *Recovery of function: Theoretical considerations for brain injury rehabilitation,* ed. P. Bach-y-Rita. Baltimore: University Park Press.

Goldstein, L.B., and the Sygen in Acute Stroke Study Investigators. 1995. Common drugs may influence motor recovery after stroke. *Neurology* 45: 865-871.

Gowland, C. 1982. Recovery of motor function following stroke: Profile and predictors. *Physiotherapy* 34: 77-84.

Grade, C., B. Redford, J. Chrostowski, L. Toussaint, and B. Blackwell. 1998. Methylphenidate in early poststroke recovery: A double-blind, placebo-controlled study. *Arch Phys Med Rehabil* 79: 1047-1050.

Greenberg, S., and R.S. Fowler Jr. 1980. Kinesthetic biofeedback: A treatment modality for elbow range of motion in hemiplegia. *Am J Occup Ther* 34: 738-743.

Guercio, J., R. Chittum, and M. McMorrow. 1997. Self-management in the treatment of ataxia: A case study in reducing ataxic tremor through relaxation and biofeedback. *Brain Injury* 11: 353-362.

Hamdy, R.C., G. Krishnaswamy, V. Cancellaro, K. Whalen, and L. Harvill. 1993. Changes in bone mineral content and density after stroke. *Am J Phys Med Rehabil* 72: 188-191.

Hamdy, R.C., S.W. Moore, V.A. Cancellaro, and L.M. Harvill. 1995. Long-term effects of strokes on bone mass. *Am J Phys Med Rehabil* 74: 351-356.

Hamrin, E., G. Eklund, A.K. Hillgren, O. Borges, J. Hall, and O. Hellstrom. 1982. Muscle strength and balance in poststroke patients. *Upsala J Med Sci* 87: 11-26.

Hertzer, N.R., J.R. Young, E.G. Beven, R.A. Graor, P.J. O'Hara, W.F. Ruschhaupt, V.G. de Wolfe, and L.C. Maljovec. 1985. Coronary angiography in 506 patients with extracranial cerebrovascular disease. *Arch Intern Med* 145: 849-852.

Hesse, S., C. Bertelt, M.T. Jahnke, A. Schaffrin, P. Baake, M. Malezic, and K.H. Maurtitz. 1995. Treadmill training with partial body weight support compared with physiotherapy in nonambulatory hemiparetic patients. *Stroke* 26: 976-981.

Hesse, S., C. Bertelt, A. Schaffrin, M. Malezic, and K.H. Mauritz. 1994. Restoration of gait in nonambulatory hemiparetic patients by treadmill training with partial bodyweight support. *Arch Phys Med Rehabil* 75: 1087-1093.

Hesse, S.A., M.T. Jahnke, C.M. Bertelt, C. Schreiner, D. Lucke, and K.H. Mauritz. 1994. Gait outcome in ambulatory hemiparetic patients after a 4-week comprehensive rehabilitation program and prognostic factors. *Stroke* 25: 1999-2004.

Hesse, S., D. Uhlenbrock, and T. Sarkodie-Gyan. 1999. Gait pattern of several disabled hemiparetic subjects on a new controlled gait trainer as compared to assisted treadmill walking with partial body weight support. *Clin Rehabil* 12: 401-410.

Hesse, S., C. Werner, D. Uhlenbrock, S. von Frankenberg, A. Bardeleben, and B. Brandl-Hesse. 2001. An electromechanical gait trainer for restoration of gait in hemiparetic stroke patients: Preliminary results. *Neurorehabil Neural Repair* 15: 39-50.

Hocherman, S., R. Dickstein, and T. Pillar. 1984. Platform training and postural stability in hemiplegia. *Arch Phys Med Rehabil* 65: 588-592.

Holden, M.K., A. Dettwiler, T. Dyar, G. Niemann, and E. Bizzi. 2001. Retraining movement in patients with acquired brain injury using a virtual environment. *Stud Health Technol Inform* 81: 192-198.

Hovda, D.A., and D.M. Feeney. 1984. Amphetamine and experience promote recovery of locomotor function after unilateral frontal cortex injury in the cat. *Brain Res* 298: 358-361.

Hsieh, C.L., D.L. Nelson, D.A. Smith, and C.Q. Peterson. 1996. A comparison of performance in added-purpose occupations and rote exercise for dynamic standing balance in persons with hemiplegia. *Am J Occup Ther* 50(1): 10-6.

Hummelsheim, H., M.L. Maier-Loth, and C. Eickhof. 1997. The functional value of electrical muscle stimulation for the rehabilitation of the hand in stroke patients. *Scand J Rehabil Med* 29: 3-10.

Hurd, W.W., V. Pegram, and C. Nepomuceno. 1980. Comparison of actual and simulated EMG biofeedback in the treatment of hemiplegic patients. *Am J Phys Med* 59: 73-82.

Inaba, M., E. Edberg, J. Montgomery, and M.K. Gillis. 1973. Effectiveness of functional training, active exercise, and resistive exercise for patients with hemiplegia. *Phys Ther* 53: 28-35.

Indredavik, B., S.A. Slordahl, F. Bakke, R. Rokseth, and L.L. Haheim. 1997. Stroke unit treatment: Longterm effects. *Stroke* 28: 1861-1866.

Inglis, J., M.W. Donald, T.N. Monga, M. Sproule, and M.J. Young. 1984. Electromyographic biofeedback and physical therapy of the hemiplegic upper limb. *Arch Phys Med Rehabil* 65: 755-759.

Intiso, D., V. Santilli, M.G. Grasso, R. Rossi, and I. Caruso. 1994. Rehabilitation of walking with electromyographic biofeedback in footdrop after stroke. *Stroke* 25: 1189-1192.

Jack, D., R. Boian, A.S. Merians, M. Tremaine, G.C. Burdea, S.V. Adamovich, M. Recce, and H. Poizner. 2001. Virtual reality enhanced stroke rehabilitation. *IEEE Trans Neural Systems Rehabil Eng* 9: 308-318.

Jacobs, K.M., and J.P. Donoghue. 1991. Reshaping the cortical motor map by unmasking latent intracortical connections. *Science* 251: 944-947.

Jakobsson, F., L. Edstrom, L. Grimby, and L.E. Thornell. 1991. Disuse of anterior tibial muscle during locomotion and increased proportion of type II fibers in hemiplegia. *J Neurol Sci* 105: 49-56.

Johansson, B.B. 1996. Functional outcome in rats transferred to an enriched environment 15 days after focal brain ischemia. *Stroke* 27: 324-326.

Johansson, K., I. Lindgren, H. Widner, I. Wiklund, and B.B. Johansson. 1993. Can sensory stimulation improve the functional outcome in stroke patients? *Neurology* 43: 2189-2192.

John, J. 1986. Failure of electrical myofeedback to augment the effects of physiotherapy in stroke. *Int J Rehabil Res* 9: 35-45.

Jones, T.A., and T. Schallert. 1994. Use-dependent growth of pyramidal neurons after neocortical damage. *J Neurosci* 14: 2140-2152.

Jongbloed, L., S. Stacey, and C. Brighton. 1989. Stroke rehabilitation: Sensorimotor integrative treatment versus functional treatment. *Am J Occup Ther* 43: 391-397.

Jorgensen, L., and B.K. Jacobsen. 2001. Changes in muscle mass, fat mass, and bone mineral content in the legs after stroke: A 1 year prospective study. *Bone* 28: 655-659.

Kaas, J.H., L.A. Krubitzer, Y.M. Chino, A.L. Langston, E.H. Polley, and N. Blair. 1990. Reorganization of retinotopic cortical maps in adult mammals after lesions of the retina. *Science* 248: 229-231.

Kalra, L., P. Dale, and P. Crome. 1993. Improving stroke rehabilitation: A controlled study. *Stroke* 24: 1462-1467.

Kalra, L., and J. Eade. 1995. Role of stroke rehabilitation units in managing severe disability after stroke. *Stroke* 26: 2031-2034.

Kaste, M., H. Palomaki, and S. Sarna. 1995. Where and how should elderly stroke patients be treated? A randomized trial. *Stroke* 26: 249-253.

Katz-Leurer, M., M. Shochina, E. Carmeli, and Y. Friedlander. 2003. The influence of early aerobic training on the functional capacity in patients with cerebrovascular accident at the subacute stage. *Arch Phys Med Rehabil* 84: 1609-1614.

Kawamata, T., E.K. Speliotes, and S.P. Finklestein. 1997. The role of polypeptide growth factors in recovery from stroke. *Adv Neurol* 73: 377-382.

Keith, R.A., D.B. Wilson, and P. Gutierrez. 1995. Acute and subacute rehabilitation for stroke: A comparison. *Arch Phys Med Rehabil* 76: 495-500.

Kiely, D.K., P.A. Wolf, L.A. Cupples, A.S. Beiser, and W.B. Kannel. 1994. Physical activity and stroke risk: The Framingham Study. *Am J Epidemiol* 140: 608-620.

King, A.J., and D.R. Moore. 1991. Plasticity of auditory maps in the brain. *Trends Neurosci* 14: 21-27.

Kosak, M.C., and M.J. Reding. 2000. Comparison of partial body weight-supported treadmill gait training versus aggressive bracing assisted walking post stroke. *Neurorehabil Neural Repair* 14: 13-19.

Kozak, J.J., P.A. Hancock, E.J. Arthur, and S.T. Chrysler. 1993. Transfer of training from virtual reality. *Ergonomics* 36: 777-784.

Kozlowski, D.A., C.D. James, and T. Schallert. 1996. Use-dependent exaggeration of neuronal injury after unilateral sensorimotor cortex lesions. *J Neurosci* 16: 4776-4786.

Kraft, G.H., S.S. Fitts, and M.C. Hammond. 1992. Techniques to improve function of the arm and hand in chronic hemiplegia. *Arch Phys Med Rehabil* 73: 220-227.

Kramer, A.M., J.F. Steiner, R.E. Schlenker, T.B. Eilertsen, C.A. Hrincevich, D.A. Tropea, L.A. Ahmad, and E.G. Eckhoff. 1997. Outcomes and costs after hip fracture and stroke: A comparison of rehabilitation settings. *JAMA* 277: 396-404.

Kunkel, A., B. Kopp, G. Muller, K. Villringer, A. Villringer, E. Taub, and H. Flor. 1999. Constraint-induced movement therapy for motor recovery in chronic stroke patients. *Arch Phys Med Rehabil* 80: 624-628.

Kwakkel, G., B.J. Kollen, and R.C. Wagenaar. 2002. Long term effects of intensity of upper and lower limb training after stroke: A randomised trial. *J Neurol Neurosurg Psych* 72: 473-479.

Kwakkel, G., R.C. Wagenaar, T.W. Koelman, G.J. Lankhorst, and J.C. Koetsier. 1997. Effects of intensity of rehabilitation after stroke. A research synthesis. *Stroke* 28: 1550-1556.

Kwakkel, G., R.C. Wagenaar, J.W. Twisk, G.J. Lankhorst, and J.C. Koetsier. 1999. Intensity of leg and arm training after primary middle-cerebral-artery stroke: A randomised trial. *Lancet* 354(9174): 191-196.

Landin, S., L. Hagenfeldt, B. Saltin, and J. Wahren. 1977. Muscle metabolism during exercise in hemiparetic patients. *Clin Sci Mol Med* 53: 257-269.

Langhorne, P., R. Wagenaar, and C. Partridge. 1996. Physiotherapy after stroke: More is better? *Physiother Res Int* 1: 75-88.

Lee, C.D., A.R. Folsom, and S.N. Blair. 2003. Physical activity and stroke risk: A meta-analysis. *Stroke* 34: 2475-2482.

Lehmann, J.F., B.J. Delatuer, and R.S. Fowler Jr., C.G. Warren, R. Arnhold, G. Schertzer, R. Hurka, J.J. Whitmore, A.J. Masock, and K.H. Chambers. 1975. Stroke: Does rehabilitation affect outcome? *Arch Phys Med Rehabil* 56: 375-382.

LeLorier, J., G. Gregoire, A. Benhaddad, J. Lapierre, and F. Derderian. 1997. Discrepancies between meta-analyses and subsequent large randomized controlled trials. *N Engl J Med* 337: 536-542.

Levin, M.F., and C.W.Y. Hui-Chan. 1992. Relief of hemiparetic spasticity by TENS is associated with improvement in reflex and voluntary motor functions. *Electroencephelogr Clin Neurophysiol* 85: 131-142.

Levy, C.E., D.S. Nichols, P.M. Schmalbrock, P. Keller, and D.W. Chakeres. 2001. Functional MRI evidence of cortical reorganization in upper-limb stroke hemiplegia treated with constraint-induced movement therapy. *Am J Phys Med Rehabil* 80: 4-12.

Liepert, J., H. Bauder, H.R. Wolfgang, W.H. Miltner, E. Taub, and C. Weiller. 2000. Treatment-induced cortical reorganization after stroke in humans. *Stroke* 31: 1210-1216.

Logigian, M.K., M.A. Samuels, and J.F. Falconer. 1983. Clinical exercise trial for stroke patients. *Arch Phys Med Rehabil* 64: 364-367.

Lomo, T. 1989. Long term effects of altered activity on skeletal muscle. *Biomed Biochim Acta* 48: S432-S444.

Lord, J.P., and K. Hall. 1986. Neuromuscular reeducation versus traditional programs for stroke rehabilitation. *Arch Phys Med Rehabil* 67: 88-91.

Luft, A.R., S. McCombe-Waller, J. Whitall, L.W. Forrester, R. Macko, J.D. Sorkin, J.B. Shulz, A.P. Goldberg, and D.F. Hanley. 2004. Repetition bilateral arm training and motor cortex activation in chronic stroke: A randomized controlled trial. *JAMA* 292: 1853-1861.

Lum, P.S., C.G. Burgar, P.C. Shor, M. Majmundar, and M. Van der Loos. 2002. Robot-assisted movement training compared with conventional therapy techniques for the rehabilitation of upper-limb motor function after stroke. *Arch Phys Med Rehabil* 83: 952-959.

Ma, H.I., and C.A. Trombly. 2001. The comparison of motor performance between part and whole tasks in elderly persons. *Am J Occup Ther* 55(1): 62-67.

Ma, H.I., and C.A. Trombly. 2002. A synthesis of the effects of occupational therapy for persons with stroke, part II: Remediation of impairments. *Am J Occup Ther* 56: 260-274.

MacKay-Lyons, M.J., and L. Makrides. 2002a. Cardiovascular stress during a contemporary stroke rehabilitation program: Is the intensity adequate to induce a training effect? *Arch Phys Med Rehabil* 83: 1378-1383.

MacKay-Lyons, M.J., and L. Makrides. 2002b. Exercise capacity early after stroke. *Arch Phys Med Rehabil* 83: 1697-1702.

Macko, R.F., L.I. Katzel, A. Yataco, L.D. Tretter, C.A. DeSouza, D.R. Dengel, G.V. Smith, and K.H. Silver. 1997. Low velocity graded treadmill stress testing in hemiparetic stroke patients. *Stroke* 28: 988-992.

Macko, R.F., G.V. Smith, C.L. Dobrovolny, J.D. Sorkin, A.P. Goldberg, and K.H. Silver. 2001. Treadmill training improves fitness reserve in chronic stroke patients. *Arch Phys Med Rehabil* 82(7): 879-884.

Magnusson, M., K. Johansson, and B.B. Johansson. 1994. Sensory stimulation promotes normalization of postural control after stroke. *Stroke* 25: 1176-1180.

Mandel, A.R., N.J. Nymark, S.J. Balmer, D.M. Grinnell, and M.D. O'Riain. 1990. Electromyographic versus rhythmic positional biofeedback in computerized gait retraining with stroke patients. *Arch Phys Med Rehabil* 71: 649-654.

Martinsson, L., and N.G. Wahlgren. 2003. Safety of dexamphetamine in acute ischemic stroke: A randomized, double-blind, controlled dose-escalation study. *Stroke* 34: 475-481.

Matsumoto, N., J.P. Whisnant, L.T. Kurland, and H. Okazaki. 1973. Natural history of stroke in Rochester, Minnesota, 1955 through 1969: An extension of a previous study, 1945 through 1954. *Stroke* 4: 20-29.

Maulucci, R.A., and R.H. Eckhouse. 2001. Retraining reaching in chronic stroke with real-time auditory feedback. *NeuroRehabilitation* 16: 171-182.

McCrea, P.H., J.J. Eng, and A.J. Hodgson. 2003. Time and magnitude of torque generation is impaired in both arms following stroke. *Muscle Nerve* 28(1): 46-53.

Merians, A.S., D. Jack, R. Boian, M. Tremaine, G.C. Burdea, S.V. Adamovich, M. Recce, and H. Poizner. 2002. Virtual reality-augmented rehabilitation for patients following stroke. *Phys Ther* 82: 898-915.

Merletti, R., F. Zelaschi, D. Latella, M. Galli, S. Angeli, and M.B. Sessa. 1978. A control study of muscle force recovery in hemiparetic patients during treatment with functional electrical stimulation. *Scand J Rehabil Med* 10: 147-154.

Miller, G.J., and K.E. Light. 1997. Strength training in spastic hemiparesis: Should it be avoided? *NeuroRehabilitation* 9: 17-28.

Miltner, W.H., H. Bauder, M. Sommer, C. Dettmers, and E. Taub. 1999. Effects of constraint-induced movement therapy on patients with chronic motor deficits after stroke: A replication. *Stroke* 30: 586-592.

Moldover, J.R., M.C. Daum, and J.A. Downey. 1984. Cardiac stress testing of hemiparetic patients with a supine bicycle ergometer: Preliminary study. *Arch Phys Med Rehabil* 65: 470-476.

Monga, T.N., D.A. Deforge, J. Williams, and L.A. Wolfe. 1988. Cardiovascular responses to acute exercise in patients with cerebrovascular accidents. *Arch Phys Med Rehabil* 69: 937-940.

Monger, C., J.H. Carr, and V. Fowler. 2002. Evaluation of a home-based exercise and training programme to improve sit-to-stand in patients with chronic stroke. *Clin Rehabil* 16: 361-367.

Moreland, J., and M.A. Thomson. 1994. Efficacy of electromyographic biofeedback compared with conventional physical therapy for upper extremity function in patients following stroke: A research overview and metaanalysis. *Phys Ther* 74: 534-543.

Morgan, M.H. 1975. Ataxia and weights. *Physiotherapy* 61: 332-334.

Morris, M.E., T.A. Matyas, T.M. Bach, and P.A. Goldie. 1992. Electrogoniometric feedback: Its effect on genu recurvatum in stroke. *Arch Phys Med Rehabil* 73: 1147-1154.

Moseley, A.M., A. Stark, I.D. Cameron, and A. Pollock. 2003. Treadmill training and body weight support for walking after stroke. *Cochrane Database of Systematic Reviews* (3): CD002840.

Mroczek, N., D. Halpern, and R. McHugh. 1978. Electromyographic feedback and physical therapy for neuromuscular retraining in hemiplegia. *Arch Phys Med Rehabil* 59: 258-267.

Mulder, T., W. Hulstijn, and J. Van der Meer. 1986. EMG feedback and the restoration of motor control. A controlled group study of 12 hemiparetic patients. *Am J Phys Med* 65: 173-188.

Naeser, M.A., M.P. Alexander, D. Stiassny-Eder, V. Galler, J. Hobbs, and D. Bachman. 1992. Real versus sham acupuncture in the treatment of paralysis in acute stroke patients: A CT scan lesion site study. *J Neuro Rehabil* 6: 163-173.

Nakamura, R., T. Hosokawa, and I. Tsuji. 1985. Relationship of muscle strength for knee extension to walking capacity in patients with spastic hemiparesis. *Tohoku J Experimental Med* 145: 335-340.

National Institute for Neurological Disorders and Stroke rt-PA Stroke Study Group. 1995. Tissue plasminogen activator for acute ischemic stroke. *N Engl J Med* 333: 1581-1587.

Nelson, D.L., K. Konosky, K. Fleharty, R. Webb, K. Newer, V.P. Hazboun, C. Fontane, and B.C. Licht. 1996. The effects of an occupationally embedded exercise on bilaterally assisted supination in persons with hemiplegia. *Am J Occup Ther* 50: 639-646.

Nilsson, L., J. Carlsso, A. Danielsson, A. Fugl-Meyer, K. Hellstron, L. Kristensen, B. Sjolund, K.S. Sunnerhagen, and G. Grimby. 2001. Walking training of patients with hemiparesis at an early stage after stroke: A comparison of walking training on a treadmill with body weight support and walking training on the ground. *Clin Rehabil* 15: 515-527.

Nudo, R.J., and G.W. Milliken. 1996. Reorganization of movement representations in primary motor cortex following focal ischemic infarcts in adult squirrel monkeys. *J Neurophysiol* 75: 2144-2149.

Nudo, R.J., G.W. Milliken, W.M. Jenkins, and M.M. Merzenich. 1996. Use-dependent alterations of movement representations in primary motor cortex of adult squirrel monkeys. *J Neurosci* 16: 785-807.

Nudo, R.J., B.M. Wise, F. SiFuentes, and G.W. Milliken. 1996. Neural substrates for the effects of rehabilitative training on motor recovery after ischemic infarct. *Science* 272: 1791-1794.

Nugent, J.A., K.A. Schurr, and R.D. Adams. 1994. A dose-response relationship between amount of weightbearing exercise and walking outcome following cerebrovascular accident. *Arch Phys Med Rehabil* 75: 399-402.

Nyberg-Hansen, R., and E. Rinvik. 1963. Some comments on the pyramidal tract, with special reference to its individual variations in man. *Acta Neurol Scand* 39: 1-30.

Ohlsson, AL., and B.B. Johansson. 1995. The environment influences functional outcome of cerebral infarction in rats. *Stroke* 26: 644-649.

Ouellette, M.M., N.K. LeBrasseur, J. Bean, E. Phillips, J. Stein, W.R. Frontera, and R.A. Fielding. 2004. High-intensity resistance training improves muscle strength, self-reported function and disability in long-term stroke survivors. *Stroke* 35: 1404-1409.

Outcome Service Trialists. 2003. Therapy-based rehabilitation services for stroke patients at home. *Cochrane Database of Systematic Reviews* CD002925.

Page, S.J., S. Sisto, M.V. Johnston, P. Levine, and M. Hughes. 2002a. Modified constraint-induced therapy in subacute stroke: A case report. *Arch Phys Med Rehabil* 83: 286-290.

Page, S.J., S.A. Sisto, and P. Levine. 2002b. Modified constraint-induced therapy in chronic stroke. *Am J Phys Med Rehabil* 81: 870-875.

Pascual-Leone, A., J. Grafman, and M. Hallett. 1994. Modulation of cortical motor output maps during development of implicit and explicit knowledge. *Science* 263: 1287-1289.

Pette, D., and G. Vrbova. 1992. Adaptation of mammalian skeletal muscle fibers to chronic electrical stimulation. *Rev Physiol Biochem Pharmacol* 120: 115-202.

Pohl, M., J. Mehrholz, C. Ritschel, and S. Ruckriem. 2002. Speed-dependent treadmill training in ambulatory hemiparetic stroke patients: A randomized controlled trial. *Stroke* 33: 553-558.

Pons, T.P., P.E. Garraghty, and M. Mishkin. 1988. Lesion-induced plasticity in the second somatosensory cortex of adult macaques. *Proc Natl Acad Sci* 85: 5279-5281.

Potempa, K., L.T. Braun, T. Tinknell, and J. Popovich. 1996. Benefits of aerobic exercise after stroke. *Sports Med* 21: 337-346.

Potempa, K., M. Lopez, L.T. Braun, J.P. Szidon, L. Fogg, and T. Tincknell. 1995. Physiological outcomes of aerobic exercise training in hemiparetic stroke patients. *Stroke* 26: 101-105.

Prevo, A.J., S.L. Visser, and T.W. Vogelaar. 1982. Effect of EMG feedback on paretic muscles and abnormal cocontraction in the hemiplegic arm, compared with conventional physical therapy. *Scand J Rehabil Med* 14: 121-131.

Retchin, S.M., R.S. Brown, S-C.J. Yeh, D. Chu, and L. Moreno. 1997. Outcomes for stroke patients in Medicare fee for service and managed care. *JAMA* 278: 119-124.

Richards, C.L., F. Malouin, S. Wood-Dauphinee, J.I. Williams, J.P. Bouchard, and D. Brunet. 1993. Task-specific physical therapy for optimization of gait recovery in acute stroke patients. *Arch Phys Med Rehabil* 74: 612-620.

Rimmer, J.H., B. Riley, T. Creviston, and T. Nicola. 2000. Exercise training in a predominantly African-American group of stroke survivors. *Med Sci Sports Exerc* 32(12): 1990-1996.

Rodriquez, A.A., P.O. Black, K.A. Kile, J. Sherman, B. Stellberg, J. McCormick, J. Roszkowski, and E. Swiggum. 1996. Gait training efficacy using a home-based practice model in chronic hemiplegia. *Arch Phys Med Rehabil* 77: 801-805.

Rohrer, B., S. Fasoli, H.I. Krebs, R. Hughes, B. Volpe, W.R. Frontera, J. Stein, and N. Hogan. 2002. Movement smoothness changes during stroke recovery. *J Neurosci* 22(18): 8297-8304.

Roth, E.J. 1993. Heart disease in patients with stroke: Incidence, impact, and implications for rehabilitation. Part 1: Classification and prevalence. *Arch Phys Med Rehabil* 74: 752-760.

Sabatini, U., D. Toni, P. Pantano, G. Brughitta, A. Padovani, L. Bozzao, and G.L. Lenzi. 1994. Motor recovery after early brain damage. *Stroke* 25: 514-517.

Salmons, S., and F.A. Sreter. 1976. Significance of impulse activity in the transformation of skeletal muscle type. *Nature* 263: 30-34.

Scelsi, R., S. Lotta, G. Lommi, P. Poggi, and C. Marchetti. 1984. Hemiplegic atrophy. *Acta Neuropathol* 62: 324-331.

Schaechter, J.D. 2004. Motor rehabilitation and brain plasticity after hemiparetic stroke. *Progress in Neurobiology* 73(1): 61-72.

Schallert, T., D.A. Kozlowski, J.S. Humm, and R.R. Cocke. 1997. Use-dependent structural events in recovery of function. *Adv Neurol* 73: 229-238.

Scheidtmann, K., W. Fries, F. Muller, and E. Koenig. 2001. Effect of levodopa in combination with physiotherapy on functional motor recovery after stroke: A prospective, randomised, double-blind study. *Lancet* 358(9284): 787-790.

Schleenbaker, R.E., and A.G. Mainous. 1993. Electromyographic biofeedback for neuromuscular reeducation in the hemiplegic stroke patient: A meta-analysis. *Arch Phys Med Rehabil* 74: 1301-1304.

Seitz, R.H., K.E. Allred, M.E. Backus, and J.A. Hoffman. 1987. Functional changes during acute rehabilitation in patients with stroke. *Phys Ther* 67: 1685-1690.

Sharp, S.A., and B.J. Brouwer. 1997. Isokinetic strength training of the hemiparetic knee: Effects on function and spasticity. *Arch Phys Med Rehabil* 78: 1231-1236.

Shiavi, R.G., S.A. Champion, F.R. Freeman, and H.J. Bugel. 1979. Efficacy of myofeedback therapy in regaining control of lower extremity musculature following stroke. *Am J Phys Med* 58: 185-194.

Shinton, R. 1997. Lifelong exposures and the potential for stroke prevention: The contribution of cigarette smoking, exercise, and body fat. *J Epidemiol Community Health* 51: 138-143.

Shumway-Cook, A., D. Anson, and S. Haller. 1988. Postural sway biofeedback: Its effect on reestablishing stance stability in hemiplegic patients. *Arch Phys Med Rehabil* 69: 395-400.

Sivenius, J., K. Pyorala, O.P. Heinonen, J.T. Salonen, and P. Riekkinen. 1985. The significance of intensity of rehabilitation of stroke: A controlled trial. *Stroke* 16: 928-931.

Slager, U.T., J.D. Hsu, and C. Jordan. 1985. Histochemical and morphometric changes in muscles of stroke patients. *Clin Orthop* 199: 159-168.

Sliwa, J.A., S. Thatcher, and J. Jet. 1994. Paraneoplastic subacute cerebellar degeneration: Functional improvement and the role of rehabilitation. *Arch Phys Med Rehabil* 75: 355-357.

Smith, D.S., E. Goldenberg, A. Ashburn, G. Kinsella, K. Sheikh, P.J. Brennan, T.W. Meade, D.W. Zutshi, J.D. Perry, and J.S. Reebacket. 1981. Remedial therapy after stroke: A randomized controlled trial. *BMJ* 282: 517-520.

Sonde, L., M. Nordstrom, C.G. Nilsson, J. Lokk, and M. Viitanen. 2001. A double-blind placebo-controlled study of the effects of amphetamine and physiotherapy after stroke. *Cerebrovasc Dis* 12: 253-257.

Stein, J., H.I. Krebs, W.R. Frontera, S.E. Fasoli, R. Hughes, and N. Hogan. 2004. Comparison of the techniques of robot-aided upper limb exercise training after stroke. *Am J Phys Med Rehabil* 83: 720-728.

Stern, P.H., F. McDowell, J.M. Miller, and M. Robinson. 1970. Effects of facilitation exercise techniques in stroke rehabilitation. *Arch Phys Med Rehabil* 51: 526-531.

Sterr, A., and S. Freivogel. 2003. Motor-improvement following intensive training in low-functioning chronic hemiparesis. *Neurology* 61: 842-844.

Stevens, R.S., N.R. Ambler, and M.D. Warren. 1984. A randomised controlled trial of a stroke rehabilitation ward. *Age Ageing* 13: 65-75.

Strand, T., K. Asplund, S. Eriksson, E. Hagg, F. Lithner, and P.O. Wester. 1985. A non-intensive stroke unit reduced functional disability and the need for long-term hospitalisation. *Stroke* 16: 29-34.

Stroke Unit Trialists' Collaboration. 1997. Collaborative systematic review of the randomized trials of organized inpatient (stroke unit) care after stroke. *BMJ* 314: 1151-1159.

Sullivan, K.J., B.J. Knowlton, and B.H. Dobkin. 2002. Step training with body weight support: Effect of treadmill speed and practice paradigms on poststroke locomotor recovery. *Arch Phys Med Rehabil* 83: 683-691.

Sunderland, A., D. Fletcher, L. Bradley, D. Tinson, R.L. Hewer, and T.D. Wade. 1994. Enhanced physical therapy for arm function after stroke: A one year follow up study. *J Neurol Neurosurg Psych* 57: 856-858.

Sunderland, A., D. Tinson, L. Bradley, and R.L. Hewer. 1989. Arm function after stroke. An evaluation of grip strength as a measure of recovery and a prognostic indicator. *J Neurolog Neurosurg Psych* 52: 1267-1272.

Sunnerhagen, K.S., U. Svantesson, L. Lonn, M. Krotkiewski, and G. Grimby. 1999. Upper motor neuron lesions: Their effect on muscle performance and appearance in stroke patients with minor motor impairment. *Arch Phys Med Rehabil* 80: 155-161.

Sze, F.K., E. Wong, K.K. Or, J. Lau, and J. Woo. 2002a. Does acupuncture improve motor recovery after stroke? A meta-analysis of randomized controlled trials. *Stroke* 33: 2604-2619.

Sze, F.K., E. Wong, X. Yi, and J. Woo. 2002b. Does acupuncture have additional value to standard poststroke motor rehabilitation? *Stroke*: 33: 186-194.

Tangeman, P.T., D.A. Banaitis, and A.K. Williams. 1990. Rehabilitation of chronic stroke patients: Changes in functional performance. *Arch Phys Med Rehabil* 71: 876-880.

Taub, E., N.E. Miller, T.A. Novack, E.W. Cook, W.C. Fleming, C.S. Nepomuceno, J.S. Connell, and J.E. Crago. 1993. Technique to improve chronic motor deficit after stroke. *Arch Phys Med Rehabil* 74: 347-354.

Taub, E., and S.L. Wolf. 1997. Constraint induced movement techniques to facilitate upper extremity use in stroke patients. *Top Stroke Rehabil* 3: 38-61.

Teixeira-Salmela, L.F., S. Nadeau, I. Mcbride, and S.J. Olney. 2001. Effects of muscle strengthening and physical conditioning training on temporal, kinematic and kinetic variables during gait in chronic stroke survivors. *J Rehabil Med* 33: 53-60.

Teixeira-Salmela, L.F., S.J. Olney, S. Nadeau, and B. Brouwer. 1999. Muscle strengthening and physical conditioning to reduce impairment and disability in chronic stroke survivors. *Arch Phys Med Rehabil* 80: 1211-1218.

Trombly, C.A., and L.A. Quintana. 1983. The effects of exercise on finger extension of CVA patients. *Am J Occup Ther* 37: 195-202.

Trombly, C.A., L. Thayer-Nason, G. Bliss, C.A. Girard, L.A. Lyrist, and A. Brexa-Hooson. 1986. The effectiveness of therapy in improving finger extension in stroke patients. *Am J Occup Ther* 40: 612-617.

Trombly, C.A., and C.Y. Wu. 1999. Effect of rehabilitation tasks on organization of movement after stroke. *Am J Occup Ther* 53(4): 333-344.

Urbsheit, N.L., and B.S. Oremland. 1990. Cerebellar dysfunction. In *Neurological rehabilitation*, 2nd ed., ed. D.A. Umphred, 597-618. St. Louis: Mosby.

van der Lee, J.H. 2001. Constraint-induced therapy for stroke: More of the same or something completely different? *Curr Opin Neurol* 14: 741-744.

van der Lee, J.H., I.A. Snels, H. Beckerman, G.J. Lankhorst, R.C. Wagenaar, and L.M. Bouter. 2001. Exercise therapy for arm function in stroke patients: A systematic review of randomized controlled trials. *Clin Rehabil* 15: 20-31.

van der Lee, J.H., R.C. Wagenaar, G.J. Lankhorst, T.W. Vogelaar, W.L. Deville, and L.M. Bouter. 1999. Forced use of the upper extremity in chronic stroke patients: Results from a single-blind randomized clinical trial. *Stroke* 30: 2369-2375.

Veizovic, T., J.S. Beech, R.P. Stroemer, W.P. Watson, and H. Hodges. 2001. Resolution of stroke deficits following contralateral grafts of conditionally immortal neuroepithelial stem cells. *Stroke* 32: 1012-1019.

Visintin, M., H. Barbeau, N. Korner-Bitensky, and N.E. Mayo. 1998. A new approach to retrain gait in stroke patients through body weight support and treadmill stimulation. *Stroke* 29: 1122-1128.

Volpe, B.T., H.I. Krebs, N. Hogan, L. Edelstein, C.M. Diels, and M.L. Aisen. 1999. Robot training enhanced motor outcome in patients with stroke maintained over 3 years. *Neurology* 53(8): 1874-1876.

Volpe, B.T., H.I Krebs, N. Hogan, L. Edelstein, C. Diels, and M. Aisen. 2000. A novel approach to stroke rehabilitation: Robot-aided sensorimotor stimulation. *Neurology* 54(10): 1938-1944.

Wade, D.T., F.M. Collen, G.F. Robb, and C.P. Warlow. 1992. Physiotherapy intervention late after stroke and mobility. *BMJ* 304: 609-13.

Wagenaar, R.C., O.G. Meijer, P.C. van Wieringen, D.J. Kuik, G.J. Hazenberg, J. Lindeboom, F. Wichers, and H. Rijswijk. 1990. The functional recovery of stroke: A comparison between neurodevelopmental treatment and the Brunnstrom method. *Scand J Rehabil Med* 22: 1-8.

Walker-Batson, D., P. Smith, S. Curtis, H. Unwin, and R. Greenlee. 1995. Amphetamine paired with physical therapy accelerates motor recovery after stroke. Further evidence. *Stroke* 26: 2254-9.

Weiss, A., T. Suzuki, J. Bean, and R.A. Fielding. 2000. High intensity strength training improves strength and functional performance after stroke. *Am J Phys Med Rehabil* 79: 369-376.

Werner, C., S. Von Frankenberg, T. Treig, M. Konrad, and S. Hesse. 2002. Treadmill training with partial body weight support and an electromechanical gait trainer for restoration of gait in subacute stroke patients: A randomized crossover trial. *Stroke* 33: 2895-2901.

Werner, R.A., and S. Kessler. 1996. Effectiveness of an intensive outpatient rehabilitation program for postacute stroke patients. *Am J Phys Med Rehabil* 75: 114-20.

Winchester, P., J. Montgomery, B. Bowman, and H. Hislop. 1983. Effects of feedback stimulation training and cyclical electrical stimulation on knee extension in hemiparetic patients. *Phys Ther* 63: 1096-1103.

Winstein, C.J., E.R. Gardner, D.R. McNeal, P.S. Barto, and D.E. Nicholson. 1989. Standing balance training: Effect on balance and locomotion in hemiparetic adults. *Arch Phys Med Rehabil* 70: 755-62.

Winstein, C.J., J.P. Miller, S. Blanton, E. Taub, G. Uswatte, D. Morris, D. Nichols, and S. Wolf. 2003. Methods for a multisite randomized trial to investigate the effect of constraint-induced movement therapy in improving upper extremity function among adults recovering from a cerebrovascular stroke. *Neurorehabil Neural Repair* 17: 137-152.

Wolf, S.L., and S.A. Binder-Macleod. 1983a. Electromyographic biofeedback applications to the hemiplegic patient: Changes in upper extremity neuromuscular and functional status. *Phys Ther* 63: 1393-1403.

Wolf, S.L., and S.A. Binder-Macleod. 1983b. Electromyographic biofeedback applications to the hemiplegic patient: Changes in lower extremity neuromuscular and functional status. *Phys Ther* 63: 1404-13.

Wolf, S.L., D.E. LeCraw, L.A. Barton, and B.B. Jann. 1989. Forced use of hemiplegic upper extremities to reverse the effect of learned nonuse among chronic stroke and head-injured patients. *Exp Neurol* 104: 125-32.

Wu, C., C.A. Trombly, K. Lin, and L. Tickle-Degnen. 2000. A kinematic study of contextual effects on reaching performance in persons with and without stroke: Influences of object availability. *Arch Phys Med Rehabil* 81(1): 95-101.

CHAPTER 15

Aloia, J.F., S.H. Cohn, T. Babu, C. Abesamis, N. Kalici, and K. Ellis. 1978. Skeletal mass and body composition in marathon runners. *Metabolism* 27: 1793-1796.

Aloia, J.F., S.H. Cohn, J.A. Ostuni, R. Cane, and K. Ellis. 1978. Prevention of involutional bone loss by exercise. *Ann Intern Med* 89: 356-358.

Aloia, J.F., A. Vaswani, J. Yeh, and S. Cohn. 1988. Premenopausal bone mass is related to physical activity. *Arch Intern Med* 148: 121-123.

American College of Sports Medicine. 1995. Position stand on osteoporosis and exercise. *Med Sci Sports Exerc* 27: 1-7.

American College of Sports Medicine. 1998. Position stand on exercise and physical activity for older adults. *Med Sci Sports Exerc* 30: 992-1008.

Ayalon, J., A. Simkin, I. Leichter, and S. Raifmann. 1987. Dynamic bone loading exercises for postmenopausal women: Effect on the density of the distal radius. *Arch Phys Med Rehabil* 68: 280-283.

Baecker, N., A. Tomic, C. Mika, A. Gotzmann, P. Platen, R. Gerzer, and M. Heer. 2003. Bone resorption is induced on the second day of bed rest: Results of a controlled crossover trial. *J Appl Physiol* 95: 977-982.

Bakker, I., J.W.R. Twisk, W. VanMechelen, J.C. Roos, and H.C.G. Kemper. 2003. Ten-year longitudinal relationship between physical activity and lumbar bone mass in (young) adults. *J Bone Miner Res* 18: 325-332.

Ballard, J.E., B.C. McKeown, H.M. Graham, and S.A. Zinkgraf. 1990. The effect of high level physical activity (8.5 METs or greater) and estrogen replacement therapy upon bone mass in postmenopausal females, aged 50-68 years. *Int J Sports Med* 11: 208-214.

Bass, S., G. Pearce, M. Bradney, E. Hendrich, P.D. Delmas, A. Harding, and E. Seeman. 1998. Exercise before puberty may confer residual benefits in bone density in adulthood: Studies in active prepubertal and retired female gymnasts. *J Bone Miner Res* 13: 500-507.

Bass, S.L., L. Saxon, R.M. Daly, C.H. Turner, A.G. Robling, E. Seeman, and S. Stuckey. 2002. The effect of mechanical loading on the size and shape of bone in pre-, peri-, and post-pubertal girls: A study in tennis players. *J Bone Miner Res* 17: 2274-2280.

Bassey, E.J., and S.J. Ramsdale. 1994. Increase in femoral bone density in young women following high-impact exercise. *Osteoporos Int* 4: 72-75.

Bassey, E.J., and S.J. Ramsdale. 1995. Weight-bearing exercise and ground reaction forces: A 12-month randomized controlled trial of effects on bone mineral density in healthy postmenopausal women. *Bone* 16: 469-476.

Bassey, E.J., M.C. Rothwell, J.J. Littlewood, and D.W. Pye. 1998. Pre- and postmenopausal women have different bone mineral density responses to the same high-impact exercise. *J Bone Miner Res* 13: 1805-1813.

Bevier, W.C., R.A. Wiswell, G. Pyka, K.C. Kozak, K.M. Newhall, and R. Marcus. 1989. Relationship of body composition, muscle strength, and aerobic capacity to bone mineral density in older men and women. *J Bone Miner Res* 4: 421-432.

Bilanin, J.E., M.S. Blanchard, and E. Russek-Cohen. 1989. Lower vertebral bone density in male long distance runners. *Med Sci Sports Exerc* 21: 66-70.

Blimkie, C.J.R., S. Rice, C.E. Webber, J. Martin, D. Levy, and C.L. Gordon. 1996. Effects of resistance training on bone mineral content and density in adolescent females. *Can J Physiol Pharmacol* 74: 1025-1033.

Bonjour, J.P., G. Theintz, B. Buchs, D. Slosman, and R. Rizzoli. 1991. Critical years and stages of puberty for spinal and femoral bone mass accumulation during adolescence. *J Clin Endocrinol Metab* 73: 555-563.

Bouxsein, M.L., and R. Marcus. 1994. Overview of exercise and bone mass. *Rheum Dis Clin North Am* 20: 787-802.

Bravo, G., P. Gauthier, R.-M. Roy, H. Payette, P. Gaulin, M. Harvey, L. Peloquin, and M.-F. Dubois. 1996. Impact of a 12-month exercise program on the physical and psychological health of osteopenic women. *J Am Geriatr Soc* 44: 756-762.

Cavanaugh, D.J., and C.E. Cann. 1988. Brisk walking does not stop bone loss in postmenopausal women. *Bone* 9: 201-204.

Chandler, J.M., S.I. Zimmerman, C.J. Girman, A.R. Martin, W. Hawkes, J.R. Hebel, P.D. Sloane, L. Holder, and J. Magaziner. 2000. Low bone mineral density and risk of fracture in white female nursing home residents. *JAMA* 284: 972-977.

Chow, R., J.E. Harrison, C.F. Brown, and V. Hajek. 1986. Physical fitness effect on bone mass in postmenopausal women. *Arch Phys Med Rehabil* 67: 231-234.

Chow, R., J.E. Harrison, and C. Notarius. 1987. Effect of two randomized exercise programmes on bone mass of healthy postmenopausal women. *Br Med J* 295: 1441-1444.

Conroy, B.P., W.J. Kraemer, C.M. Maresh, S. Fleck, M.H. Stone, A.C. Fry, P.D. Miller, and G.P. Dalsky. 1993. Bone mineral density in elite junior Olympic weightlifters. *Med Sci Sports Exerc* 25: 1103-1109.

Consensus Development Conference. 1993. Diagnosis, prophylaxis, and treatment of osteoporosis. *Am J Med* 94: 646-650.

Cooper, C., M. Cawley, A. Bhalla, P. Egger, F. Ring, L. Morton, and D. Barker. 1995. Childhood growth, physical activity, and peak bone mass in women. *J Bone Miner Res* 10: 940-947.

Cummings, S.R., D.M. Black, and S.M. Rubin. 1989. Lifetime risks of hip, Colles' or vertebral fracture and coronary heart disease among white postmenopausal women. *Arch Intern Med* 149: 2445-2448.

Cummings, S.R., M.C. Nevitt, W.S. Browner, K. Stone, K.M. Fox, K.E. Engrud, J. Cauley, D. Black, and T.M. Vogt for the Study of Osteoporotic Fractures Research Group. 1995. Risk factors for hip fracture in white women. *N Engl J Med* 332: 767-773.

Dalsky, G.P., K.S. Stocke, A.A. Ehsani, E. Slatopolsky, W.C. Lee, and S.J. Birge Jr. 1988. Weight-bearing exercise training and lumbar bone mineral content in postmenopausal women. *Ann Intern Med* 108: 824-828.

Davee, A.M., C.J. Rosen, and R.A. Adler. 1990. Exercise patterns and trabecular bone density in college women. *J Bone Miner Res* 5: 245-250.

del Puente, A., N. Pappone, M.G. Mandes, D. Mantova, R. Scarpa, and P. Oriente. 1996. Determinants of bone mineral density in immobilization: A study on hemiplegic patients. *Osteoporos Int* 6: 50-54.

Dhesi, J.K., L.M. Bearne, C. Moniz, M.V. Hurley, S.H.D. Jackson, C.G. Swift, and T.J. Allain. 2002. Neuromuscular and psychomotor function in elderly subjects who fall and the relationship with vitamin D status. *J Bone Miner Res* 17: 891-897.

DiPietro, L. 2001. Physical activity in aging: Changes in patterns and their relationship to health and function. *J Gerontol* Series A 56A: 13-22.

Drinkwater, B.L., K. Nilson, C.H. Chesnut III, W. Bremner, S. Shainholtz, and M.B. Southworth. 1984. Bone mineral content of amenorrheic and eumenorrheic athletes. *N Engl J Med* 311: 277-281.

Drinkwater, B.L., K. Nilson, S. Ott, and C.H. Chesnut III. 1986. Bone mineral density after resumption of menses in amenorrheic athletes. *JAMA* 256: 380-282.

Ernst, E. 1998. Exercise for female osteoporosis: A systematic review of controlled clinical trials. *Sports Med* 25(6): 359-368.

Fehling, P.C., L. Alekel, J. Clasey, A. Rector, and R.J. Stillman. 1995. A comparison of bone mineral densities among female athletes in impact loading and active loading sports. *Bone* 17: 205-210.

Fiatarone, M.A., E.F. O'Neill, N.D. Ryan, K. Clements, G.R. Solares, M.E. Nelson, S.B. Roberts, J.J. Kehayias, L.A. Lipsitz, and W.J. Evans. 1994. Exercise training and nutritional supplementation for physical frailty in very elderly people. *N Engl J Med* 330: 1769-1775.

Fisher, E.C., M.E. Nelson, W.R. Frontera, R.N. Turksoy, and W.J. Evans. 1986. Bone mineral content and levels of gonadotropins and estrogens in amenorrheic running women. *J Clin Endocrinol Metab* 62: 1232-1236.

Flodgren, G., H. Hedelin, and K. Henriksson-Larsen. 1999. BMD in flatwater sprint kayakers. *Calcif Tissue Int* 64: 374-379.

Friedlander, A.L., H.K. Genant, S. Sadowsky, N.N. Byl, and C.C. Gluer. 1995. A two-year program of aerobics and weight training enhances bone mineral density of young women. *J Bone Miner Res* 10: 574-585.

Fuchs, R.K., J.J. Bauer, and C.M. Snow. 2001. Jumping improves hip and lumbar spine bone mass in prepubescent children: A randomized controlled trial. *J Bone Miner Res* 16: 148-156.

Gardner, M.M., M.C. Robertson, and A.J. Campbell. 2000. Exercise in preventing falls and fall-related injuries in older people: A review of randomized controlled trials. *Br J Sports Med* 34: 7-17.

Gerdham, P., K.A.M. Ringsberg, K. Akesson, and K.J. Obrant. 2003. Influence of muscle strength, physical activity and weight on bone mass in a population-based sample of 1004 elderly women. *Osteoporos Int* 14: 768-772.

Giangregorio, L., and C.J.R Blimkie. 2002. Skeletal adaptations to alterations in weight-bearing activity: A comparison of models of disuse osteoporosis. *Sports Med* 32: 459-476.

Gleeson, P.B., E.J. Protas, A.D. LeBlanc, V.S. Schneider, and H.J. Evans. 1990. Effects of weight lifting on bone mineral density in premenopausal women. *J Bone Miner Res* 5: 153-158.

Goemaere, S., M. Van Laere, P. DeNeve, and J.M. Kaufman. 1994. Bone mineral status in paraplegic patients who do or do not perform standing. *Osteoporos Int* 4: 138-143.

Greendale, G.A., E. Barrett-Connor, S. Edelstein, S. Ingles, and R. Haile. 1995. Lifetime leisure exercise and osteoporosis. The Rancho Bernardo study. *Am J Epidemiol* 141: 951-959.

Greenspan, S.L., E.R. Myers, D.P. Kiel, R.A. Parker, W.C. Hayes, and N.M. Resnick. 1998. Fall direction, bone mineral density, and function: Risk factors for hip fracture in frail nursing home elderly. *Am J Med* 104: 539-545.

Greenspan, S.L., E.R. Myers, L.A. Maitland, N.M. Resnick, and W.C. Hayes. 1994. Fall severity and bone mineral density as risk factors for hip fracture in ambulatory elderly. *JAMA* 271: 128-133.

Gregg, E.W., M.A. Pereira, and C.J. Casperen. 2000. Physical activity, falls and fractures among older adults: A review of the epidemiologic evidence. *J Am Geriatr Soc* 48: 883-893.

Grisso, J.A., J.L. Kelsey, B.L. Strom, G.Y. Chiu, G. Maislin, L.A. O'Brien, S. Hoffman, F. Kaplan, and the Northeast Hip Fracture Study Group. 1991. Risk factors for falls as a cause of hip fracture in women. *N. Engl J Med* 324: 1326-1331.

Grove, K.A., and B.R. Londeree. 1992. Bone density in postmenopausal women: High impact vs. low impact exercise. *Med Sci Sports Exerc* 24: 1190-1194.

Gutin, B., and M.J. Kasper. 1992. Can vigorous exercise play a role in osteoporosis prevention? A review. *Osteoporos Int* 2: 55-69.

Haapasalo, H., P. Kannus, H. Sievanen, M. Pasanen, K. Uusi-Rasi, A. Heinonen, P. Oja, and I. Vuori. 1998. Effect of long-term unilateral activity on bone mineral density of female junior tennis players. *J Bone Miner Res* 13: 310-319.

Haapasalo, H., H. Sievanen, P. Kannus, A. Heinonen, P. Oja, and I. Vuori. 1996. Dimensions and estimated mechanical characteristics of the humerus after long-term tennis loading. *J Bone Miner Res* 11: 864-872.

Halioua, L., and J.J.B. Anderson. 1989. Lifetime calcium intake and physical activity habits: Independent and combined effects on the radial bone of healthy premenopausal women. *Am J Clin Nutr* 49: 534-41.

Hamdy, R.C., J.S. Anderson, K.E. Whalen, and L.M. Harvill. 1994. Regional differences in bone density in young men involved in different exercises. *Med Sci Sports Exerc* 26: 884-888.

Hatori, M., A. Hasegawa, H. Adachi, A. Shinozaki, R. Hayashi, H. Okamo, H. Mizunuma, and K. Murata. 1993. The effects of walking at the anaerobic threshold level on vertebral bone loss in postmenopausal women. *Calcif Tissue Int* 52: 411-414.

Heinonen, A., P. Kannus, H. Sievanen, P. Oja, M. Pasanen, M. Rinne, K. Uusi-Rasi, and I. Vuori. 1996. Randomized controlled trial of effect of high-impact exercise on selected risk factors for osteoporotic fractures. *Lancet* 348: 1343-1347.

Heinonen, A., P. Oja, P. Kannus, H. Sievanen, H. Haapasalo, A. Manttari, and I. Vuori. 1995. Bone mineral density in female athletes representing sports with different loading characteristics of the skeleton. *Bone* 17: 197-203.

Heinonen, A., P. Oja, P. Kannus, H. Sievanen, A. Manttari, and I. Vuori. 1993. Bone mineral density of female athletes in different sports. *Bone Miner* 23: 1-14.

Heinonen, A., P. Oja, H. Sievanen, M. Pasanen, and I. Vuori. 1998. Effect of two training regimens on bone mineral density in healthy perimenopausal women: A randomized controlled trial. *J Bone Miner Res* 13: 483-490.

Heinonen, A., H. Sievanen, P. Kannus, P. Oja, M. Pasanen, and I. Vuori. 2000. High-impact exercise and bones of growing girls: A 9-month controlled trial. *Osteoporos Int* 11: 1010-1017.

Heinrich, C.H., S.B. Going, R.W. Pamenter, C.D. Perry, T.W. Boynden, and T.G. Lohman. 1990. Bone mineral content of cyclically menstruating female resistance and endurance trained athletes. *Med Sci Sports Exerc* 22: 558-563.

Hetland, M.L., J. Haarbo, and C. Christiansen. 1993. Low bone mass and high bone turnover in male long distance runners. *J Clin Endocrinol Metab* 77: 770-775.

Hirota, T., M. Nara, M. Ohguri, E. Manago, and K. Hirota. 1992. Effect of diet and lifestyle on bone mass in Asian young women. *Am J Clin Nutr* 55: 1168-1173.

Huddleston, A.L., D. Rockwell, D. Kulund, and R.B. Harrison. 1980. Bone mass in lifetime tennis athletes. *JAMA* 244: 1107-1109.

Hughes, V.A., W.R. Frontera, G.E. Dallal, K.J. Lutz, E.C. Fisher, and W.J. Evans. 1995. Muscle strength and body composition: Associations with bone density in older subjects. *Med Sci Sports Exer* 27: 967-974.

Humphries, B., R.U. Newton, R. Bronks, S. Marshall, J. McBride, T. Triplett-McBride, K. Hakkinen, W.J. Kraemer, and N. Humphries. 2000. Effect of exercise intensity on bone density, strength, and calcium turnover in older women. *Med Sci Sports Exerc* 32: 1043-1050.

Iuliano-Burns, S., L. Saxon, G. Naughton, K. Gibbons, and S.L. Bass. 2003. Regional specificity of exercise and calcium during skeletal growth in girls: A randomized controlled trial. *J Bone Miner Res* 18: 156-162.

Iwamoto, J., T. Takeda, T. Otani, and Y. Yabe. 1998. Effect of increased physical activity on bone mineral density in postmenopausal osteoporotic women. *Keio J Med* 47: 157-161.

Jacobson, P.C., W. Beaver, S.A. Grubb, T.N. Taft, and R.V. Talmage. 1984. Bone density in women: College athletes and older athletic women. *J Orthop Res* 2: 328-332.

Johnell, O., B. Gullberg, J.A. Kanis, E. Allander, L. Elffors, J. Dequcker, G. Dilsen, C. Gennari, A.L. Vaz, G. Lyritis, G. Mazzuoli, L. Miravet, M. Passeri, R.P. Cano, A. Rapado, and C. Ribot. 1995. Risk factors for hip fracture in European women: The MEDOS study. *J Bone Miner Res* 10: 1802-1815.

Jones, H.H., J.D. Priest, W.C. Hayes, C.C. Tichenor, and D.A. Nagel. 1977. Humeral hypertrophy in response to exercise. *J Bone Joint Surg* 59A: 204-208.

Kanis, J.A., L.J. Melton III, C. Christiansen, C.C. Johnston, and N. Khaltaev. 1994. The diagnosis of osteoporosis. *J Bone Miner Res* 9: 1137-1141.

Kannus, P., H. Haapasalo, M. Sankelo, H. Sievanen, M. Paganen, A. Heinonen, P. Oja, and I. Vuori. 1995. Effect of starting age of physical activity on bone mass in the dominant arm of tennis and squash players. *Ann Intern Med* 123: 27-31.

Karlsson, M. 2002. Does exercise reduce the burden of fractures: A review. *Acta Orthop Scand* 73: 691-705.

Karlsson, M.K., O. Johnell, and K.J. Obrant. 1993a. Bone mineral density in professional ballet dancers. *Bone Miner* 21: 163-169.

Karlsson, M.K., O. Johnell, and K.J. Obrant. 1993b. Bone mineral density in weight lifters. *Calcif Tissue Int* 52: 212-215.

Kelley, G.A. 1998. Exercise and regional bone mineral density in postmenopausal women: A meta-analytic review of randomized trials. *Am J Phys Med Rehabil* 77: 76-87.

Kelly, G.A., K.S. Kelly, and Z.V. Tran. 2001. Resistance training and bone mineral density in women: A meta-analysis of controlled trials. *Am J Phys Med Rehabil* 80: 65-77.

Kerr, D., T. Ackland, B. Maslen, A. Morton, and R. Prince. 2001. Resistance training over 2 years increases bone mass in calcium-replete postmenopausal women. *J Bone Miner Res* 16: 175-181.

Khan, K.M., R.M. Green, A. Saul, K.L. Bennell, K.J. Crichton, J.L. Hopper, and J.D. Wark. 1996. Retired elite female ballet dancers and nonathletic controls have similar bone mineral density at weight-bearing sites. *J Bone Miner Res* 11: 1566-1574.

Kirk, S., C.F. Sharp, N. Elbaum, D.B. Enders, S.M. Simons, J.G. Mohler, and R.K. Rude. 1989. Effect of long distance running on bone mass in women. *J Bone Miner Res* 4: 515-522.

Klesges, R.C., K.D. Ward, M.L. Shelton, W.B. Applegate, E.D. Cantler, G.M.A. Palmieri, K. Harmon, and J. Davis. 1996. Changes in bone mineral content in male athletes: Mechanism of action and intervention effects. *JAMA* 276: 226-230.

Kohrt, W.M., A.A. Ehsani, and S.J. Birge Jr. 1997. Effects of exercise involving predominantly either joint-reaction or ground-reaction forces on bone mineral density in older women. *J Bone Miner Res* 12: 1253-1261.

Kontulainen, S., H. Sievanen, P. Kannus, M. Pasanen, and I. Vuori. 2003. Effect of long-term impact loading on mass, size, and estimated strength of humerus and radius of female racquet-sports players: A peripheral quantitative computed tomography study between young and old starters and controls. *J Bone Miner Res* 18: 352-359.

Kroger, H., A. Kotaniemi, L. Kroger, and E. Alhava. 1993. Development of bone mass and bone density of the spine and femoral neck: A prospective study of 65 children and adolescents. *Bone Miner* 23: 171-182.

Krolner, B., and B. Toft. 1983. Vertebral bone loss: An unheeded side effect of therapeutic bedrest. *Clin Sci* 64: 537-540.

Krolner, B., B. Toft, S.P. Nielsen, and T. Tondevold. 1983. Physical activity as prophylaxis against involutional vertebral bone loss: A controlled trial. *Clin Sci* 64: 541-546.

Lane, N.E., D.A. Bloch, H.H. Jones, W.H. Marshall Jr., P.D. Wood, and J.F. Fries. 1986. Long distance running, bone density and osteoarthritis. *JAMA* 255: 1147-1151.

Lanyon, L.E. 1996. Using functional loading to influence bone mass and architecture: Objectives, mechanisms, and relationship with estrogen of the mechanically adaptive process in bone. *Bone* 18(Suppl.): 37-43.

Lau, E.M.C., J. Woo, P.C. Leung, R. Swaminathan, and D. Leung. 1992. The effects of calcium supplementation and exercise on bone density in elderly Chinese women. *Osteoporos Int* 2: 168-173.

Lohman, T., S. Going, R. Pamenter, M. Hall, T. Boyden, L. Houtkooper, C. Ritenbaugh, L. Bare, A. Hill, and M. Aickin. 1995. Effects of resistance training on regional and total bone mineral density in premenopausal women: A randomized prospective study. *J Bone Miner Res* 10: 1015-1024.

Lord, S.R., J.A. Ward, and P. Williams. 1996. Exercise effect on dynamics stability in older women: A randomized controlled trial. *Arch Phys Med Rehabil* 77: 232-236.

MacDougall, J.D., C.E. Webber, J. Martin, S. Ormerod, A. Chesley, E.V. Younglai, C.L. Gordon, and C.J.R. Blimkie. 1992. Relationship among running mileage, bone density, and serum testosterone in male runners. *J Appl Physiol* 73: 1165-1170.

MacKelvie, K.J., H.A. McKay, K. Khan, and P.R.E. Crocker. 2001. A school-based exercise intervention augments bone mineral accrual in early pubertal girls. *J Pediatr* 139: 501-507.

MacKelvie, K.J., H.A. McKay, M.A. Petit, O. Moran, and K.M. Khan. 2002. Bone mineral response to a 7-month randomized controlled, school-based jumping intervention in 121 prepubertal boys: Associations with ethnicity and body mass index. *J Bone Miner Res* 17: 834-844.

Maddalozzo, G.F., and C.M. Snow. 2000. High intensity resistance training: Effects on bone in older men and women. *Calcif Tissue Int* 66: 399-404.

Madsen, O.R., O. Schaadt, H. Bliddal, C. Egsmose, and J. Sylvest. 1993. Relationship between quadriceps strength and bone mineral density of the proximal tibia and distal forearm in women. *J Bone Miner Res* 12: 1439-1444.

Marcus, R., C. Cann, P. Madvig, J. Minkoff, M. Goddard, M. Bayer, M. Martin, L. Gaudiani, W. Haskel, and H. Genant. 1985. Menstrual function and bone mass in elite women distance runners: Endocrine and metabolic features. *Ann Intern Med* 102: 158-163.

Marcus, R., B. Drinkwater, G. Dalsky, J. Dufek, D. Rabb, C. Slemenda, and C. Snow-Harter. 1992. Osteoporosis and exercise in women. *Med Sci Sports Exerc* 24(Suppl.): 301-307.

Martin, D., and M. Notelovitz. 1993. Effect of aerobic training on bone mineral density of postmenopausal women. *J Bone Miner Res* 8: 931-936.

Matkovic, V., T. Jelic, G.M. Wardlaw, J.Z. Ilich, P.K. Goel, J.K. Wright, M.B. Andon, K.T. Smith, and R.P. Heaney. 1994. Timing of peak bone mass in Caucasian females and its implication for the prevention of osteoporosis. Inference from a cross-sectional model. *J Clin Invest* 93: 799-808.

Mazess, R.B., and H.S. Barden. 1991. Bone density in premenopausal women: Effects of age, dietary intake, physical activity, smoking, and birth-control pills. *Am J Clin Nutr* 53: 132-142.

McCulloch, R.G., D.A. Bailey, C.S. Houston, and B.L. Dodd. 1990. Effects of physical activity, dietary calcium intake and selected lifestyle factors on bone density in young women. *Can Med Assoc J* 142: 221-227.

McKay, H., M. Petit, R.W. Schultz, J.C. Prior, S. Barr, and K. Khan. 2000. Augmented trochanteric bone mineral density after modified physical education classes: A randomized school-based exercise intervention study in prepubescent and early pubescent children. *J Pediatr* 136: 156-162.

Melton, L.J. III. 1993. Hip fractures. A worldwide problem today and tomorrow. *Bone* 14(Suppl.): 1-8.

Melton, L.J. III, E.A. Chrischilles, C. Cooper, A.W. Lane, and B.L. Riggs. 1992. How many women have osteoporosis? *J Bone Miner Res* 9: 1005-1010.

Melton, L.J. III, M. Thamer, N.F. Ray, J.K. Chan, C.H. Chestnut III, T.A. Einhorn, C.C. Johnston, L.G. Raise, S.L. Silverman, and E.S. Siris. 1997. Factors attributable to osteoporosis: Report from the National Osteoporosis Foundation. *J Bone Miner Res* 12: 16-23.

Metz, J.A., J.J.B. Anderson, and P.N. Gallagher Jr. 1993. Intakes of calcium, phosphorus, and protein, and physical-activity level are related to radial bone mass in young adult women. *Am J Clin Nutr* 58: 537-542.

Michel, B.A., D.A. Bloch, and J.F. Fries. 1989. Weight-bearing exercise, overexercise, and lumbar bone density over age 50 years. *Arch Intern Med* 149: 2325-2329.

Michel, B.A., N.E. Lane, D.A. Bloch, H.H. Jones, and J.F. Fries. 1991. Effect of changes in weight-bearing exercise on lumbar bone mass after age fifty. *Ann Med* 23: 397-401.

Myburgh, K.H., L.K. Bachrach, B. Lewis, K. Kent, and R. Marcus. 1993. Low bone mineral density at axial and appendicular sites in amenorrheic athletes. *Med Sci Sports Exerc* 25: 1197-1202.

Myburgh, K.H., J. Hutchins, A.B. Fataar, S.F. Hough, and T.D. Noakes. 1990. Low bone density is an etiologic factor for stress fractures in athletes. *Ann Intern Med* 113: 754-759.

Nelson, M.E., M.A. Fiatarone, C.M. Morganti, I. Trice, R.A. Greenberg, and W.J. Evans. 1994. Effects of high-intensity strength training on multiple risk factors for osteoporotic fractures: A randomized controlled trial. *JAMA* 272: 1909-1914.

Nelson, M.E., E.C. Fisher, F.A. Dilmanian, G.E. Dallal, and W.J. Evans. 1991. A 1-year walking program and increased dietary calcium in postmenopausal women: Effects on bone. *Am J Clin Nutr* 53: 1304-1311.

Nelson, M.E., C.N. Meredith, B. Dawson-Hughes, and W.J. Evans. 1988. Hormone and bone mineral status in endurance-trained and sedentary postmenopausal women. *J Clin Endocrinol Metab* 66: 927-933.

NIH Consensus Development Panel on Osteoporosis Prevention, Diagnosis and Therapy. 2001. Osteoporosis prevention, diagnosis, and therapy. *JAMA* 285: 785-795.

Nilsson, B.E., and N.E. Westlin. 1971. Bone density in athletes. *Clin Orthop* 77: 179-182.

Notelovitz, M., D. Martin, R. Tesar, F.Y. Khan, C. Probart, C. Fields, and L. McKenzie. 1991. Estrogen therapy and variable-resistance weight training increase bone mineral in surgically menopausal women. *J Bone Miner Res* 6: 583-590.

Nurmi-Lawton, J.A., A.D. Baxter-Jones, R.L. Mirwald, J.A. Bishop, P. Taylor, C. Cooper, and S.A. New. 2004. Evidence of sustained skeletal benefits from impact-loading exercise in young females: A 3-year longitudinal study. *J Bone Miner Res* 19: 314-322.

O'Connor, J.A., L.E. Lanyon, and H. MacFie. 1982. The influence of strain rate on adaptive bone remodeling. *J Biomech* 15: 767-781.

Peterson, S.E., M.D. Peterson, G. Raymond, C. Gilligan, M.M. Checovich, and E.L. Smith. 1991. Muscular strength and bone density with weight training in middle-aged women. *Med Sci Sports Exerc* 23: 499-504.

Petit, M.A., H.A. McKay, K.J. MacKelvie, A. Heinonen, K.M. Khan, and T.J. Beck. 2002. A randomized school-based jumping intervention confers site and maturity-specific benefits on bone structural properties in girls: A hip structural analysis study. *J Bone Miner Res* 17: 363-372.

Pettersson, U., H. Alfredson, P. Nordstrom, K. Henriksson-Larsen, and R. Lorentzon. 2000a. Bone mass in female cross-country skiers: Relationship between muscle strength and different BMD sites. *Calcif Tissue Int* 67: 199-206.

Pettersson, U., H. Alfredson, P. Nordstrom, K. Henriksson-Larsen, and R. Lorentzon. 2000b. Effect of high impact activity in bone mass and size in adolescent females: A comparative study between two different types of sports. *Calcif Tissue Int* 67: 207-214.

Picard, D., L.G. Ste-Marie, D. Coutu, L. Carrieri, R. Chartrand, R. Lepage, P. Fugere, and P.D. Armour. 1988. Premenopausal bone mineral content relates to height, weight and calcium intake during early adulthood. *Bone Miner* 4: 299-309.

Pocock, N.A., J.A. Eisman, M.G. Yeates, P.N. Sambrook, and S. Eberl. 1986. Physical fitness is a major determinant of femoral neck and lumbar spine bone mineral density. *J Clin Invest* 78: 618-621.

Prince, R., A. Devine, I. Dick, A. Criddle, D. Kerr, N. Kent, R. Price, and A. Randell. 1995. The effects of calcium supplementation (milk powder or tablets) and exercise on bone density in postmenopausal women. *J Bone Miner Res* 10: 1068-1075.

Prince, R.L., M. Smith, I. Dick, R.I. Price, P.G. Webb, N.K. Henderson, and M.M. Harris. 1991. Prevention of postmenopausal osteoporosis: A comparative study of exercise, calcium supplementation, and hormone replacement therapy. *N Engl J Med* 325: 1189-1195.

Province, M.A., E.C. Hadley, M.C. Hornbrook, L.A. Lipsitz, J.P. Miller, C.D. Mulrow, M.G. Ory, R.W. Sattin, M.E. Tinetti, and S.L. Wolf for the FICSIT Group. 1995. The effects of exercise on falls in elderly patients: A preplanned meta-analysis of the FICSIT trials. *JAMA* 273: 1341-1347.

Pruitt, L.A., R.D. Jackson, R.L. Bartels, and H.J. Lehnhard. 1992. Weight-training effects on bone mineral density in early postmenopausal women. *J Bone Miner Res* 7: 179-185.

Pruitt, L.A., D.R. Taaffe, and R. Marcus. 1995. Effects of a one-year high-intensity versus low-intensity resistance training program on bone mineral density in older women. *J Bone Miner Res* 10: 1788-1795.

Rambaut, P.C., and A.W. Goode. 1985. Skeletal changes during space flight. *Lancet* 2: 1050-1052.

Ramnemark, A., L. Nyberg, R. Lorentzon, U. Englund, and Y. Gustafson. 1999. Progressive hemiosteoporosis on the paretic side and increased bone mineral density in the non-paretic arm in the first year after stroke. *Osteoporos Int* 9: 269-275.

Ray, N.F., J.K. Chan, M. Thaemer, and L.J. Melton III. 1997. Medical expenditures for the treatment of osteoporotic fractures in the United States in 1995: Report from the National Osteoporosis Foundation. *J Bone Miner Res* 12: 24-35.

Recker, R.R., K.M. Davies, S.M. Hinders, R.P. Heaney, M.R. Stegman, and D.B. Kimmel. 1992. Bone gain in young adult women. *JAMA* 268: 2403-2408.

Reid, I.R., R. Ames, M.C. Evans, S. Sharpe, G. Gamble, J.T. France, T.M.T. Lim, and T.F. Cundy. 1992. Determinants of total body and regional bone mineral density in normal postmenopausal women: A key role for fat mass. *J Clin Endocrinol Metab* 75: 45-51.

Reid, I.R., L.D. Plank, and M.C. Evans. 1992. Fat mass is an important determinant of whole body bone density in premenopausal women but not in men. *J Clin Endocrinol Metab* 75: 779-782.

Rencken, M.L., C.H. Chestnut III, and B.L. Drinkwater. 1996. Bone density at multiple skeletal sites in amenorrheic athletes. *JAMA* 276: 238-240.

Revel, M., M.A. Mayoux-Benhamou, J.P. Rabourdin, F. Bagheri, and C. Roux. 1993. One-year psoas training can prevent lumbar bone loss in postmenopausal women: A randomized controlled trial. *Calcif Tissue Int* 53: 307-311.

Riggs, B.L., and L.J. Melton III. 1986. Involutional osteoporosis. *N Engl J Med* 314: 1676-1686.

Robinson, T.L., C. Snow-Harter, D.R. Taaffe, D. Gillis, J. Shaw, and R. Marcus. 1995. Gymnasts exhibit higher bone mass than runners despite similar prevalence of amenorrhea and oligomenorrhea. *J Bone Miner Res* 10: 26-35.

Rockwell, J.C., A.M. Sorensen, S. Baker, D. Leahey, J.L. Stock, J. Michaels, and D.T. Baran. 1990. Weight training decreases vertebral bone density in premenopausal women: A prospective study. *J Clin Endocrinol Metab* 71: 988-993.

Rodin, A., B. Murby, M.A. Smith, M. Caleffi, I. Fentiman, M.G. Chapman, and I. Fogelman. 1990. Premenopausal bone loss in the lumbar spine and neck of femur: A study of 225 Caucasian women. *Bone* 11: 1-5.

Rubenstein, L.Z., K.R. Josephson, and A.S. Robbins. 1994. Falls in the nursing home. *Ann Intern Med* 121: 442-451.

Rubin, C.T., and L.E. Lanyon. 1985. Regulation of bone mass by mechanical strain magnitude. *Calcif Tissue Int* 37: 411-417.

Rundgren, A., A. Aniansson, P. Ljungberg, and H. Wetterqvist. 1984. Effects of a training programme for elderly people on mineral content of the heel bone. *Arch Gerontol Geriatr* 3: 243-248.

Sandler, R.B., J.A. Cauley, D.L. Hom, D. Sashin, and A.M. Kriska. 1987. The effects of walking on the cross-sectional dimensions of the radius in postmenopausal women. *Calcif Tissue Int* 41: 65-69.

Sandstrom, P., P. Jonsson, R. Lorentzon, and K. Thorsen. 2000. Bone mineral density and muscle strength in female ice hockey players. *Int J Sports Med* 21: 524-528.

Sattin, R.W. 1992. Falls among older persons: A public health perspective. *Annu Rev Public Health* 13: 489-508.

Schwarz, A.J., J.A. Brasel, R.L. Hintz, S. Mohan, and D.M. Cooper. 1996. Acute effect of brief low- and high-intensity exercise on circulating insulin-like growth factor (IGF) I, II and IGF-binding protein-3 and its proteolysis in young healthy men. *J Clin Endocrinol Metab* 81: 3492-3497.

Sinaki, M. 2003. Nonpharmacologic interventions: Exercise, fall prevention, and role of physical medicine. *Clin Geriatr Med* 19: 337-359.

Sinaki, M., M.C. McPhee, S.F. Hodgson, J.M. Merritt, and K.P. Offord. 1986. Relationship between bone mineral density of spine and strength of back extensors in healthy postmenopausal women. *Mayo Clin Proc* 61: 116-122.

Sinaki, M., and K.P. Offord. 1988. Physical activity in postmenopausal women. Effect on back muscle strength and bone mineral density of the spine. *Arch Phys Med Rehabil* 69: 277-280.

Sinaki, M., J.L. Opitz, and H.W. Wahner. 1974. Bone mineral content: Relationship to muscle strength in normal subjects. *Arch Phys Med Rehabil* 55: 508-512.

Sinaki, M., H.W. Wahner, E.J. Bergstrall, S.F. Hodgson, K.P. Offord, R.W. Squires, R.G. Swee, and P.C. Kao. 1996. Three-year controlled randomized trial of the effect of dose-specified loading and strengthening exercises on bone mineral density of spine and femur in nonathletic, physically active women. *Bone* 19: 233-244.

Sinaki, M., H.W. Wahner, K.P. Offord, and S.F. Hodgson. 1989. Efficiency of non-loading exercises in prevention of vertebral bone loss in postmenopausal women: A controlled trial. *Mayo Clin Proc* 64: 762-769.

Slemenda, C.W., and C.C. Johnston. 1993. High intensity activities in young women: Site specific bone mass effects among female figure skaters. *Bone Miner* 20: 125-132.

Slemenda, C.W., J.Z. Miller, S.L. Hui, T.K. Reister, and C.C. Johnston Jr. 1991. Role of physical activity in the development of skeletal mass in children. *J Bone Miner Res* 6: 1227-1233.

Slemenda, C.W., T.K. Reister, S.L. Hui, J.Z. Miller, J.C. Christian, and C.C. Johnston Jr. 1994. Influences on skeletal mineralization in children and adolescents: Evidence for varying effects of sexual maturation and physical activity. *J Pediatr* 125: 201-207.

Smidt, G.L., S-Y. Lin, K.D. O'Dwyer, and P.R. Blanpied. 1992. The effect of high-intensity trunk exercise on bone mineral density of postmenopausal women. *Spine* 17: 280-285.

Smith, E.L., C. Gilligan, M. McAdam, C. Ensign, and P. Smith. 1989. Deterring bone loss by exercise intervention in premenopausal and postmenopausal women. *Calcif Tissue Int* 44: 312-321.

Smith, R., and O.M. Rutherford. 1993. Spine and total body bone mineral density and serum testosterone levels in male athletes. *Eur J Appl Physiol* 67: 330-334.

Snow, C.M., J.M. Shaw, and C.C. Matkin. 1996. Physical activity and risk for osteoporosis. In *Osteoporosis,* ed. R. Marcus, D. Feldman, and J. Kelsey. San Diego: Academic Press.

Snow-Harter, C., M.L. Bouxsein, B.T. Lewis, D.R. Carter, and R. Marcus. 1992. Effects of resistance and endurance exercise on bone mineral status of young women: A randomized exercise intervention trial. *J Bone Miner Res* 7: 761-769.

Snow-Harter, C., M.L. Bouxsein, B.T. Lewis, S. Charette, P. Weinstein, and R. Marcus. 1990. Muscle strength as a predictor of bone mineral density in young women. *J Bone Miner Res* 5: 589-595.

Soderman, K., E. Bergstrom, R. Lorentzon, and H. Alfredson. 2000. Bone mass and muscle strength in young female soccer players. *Calcif Tissue Int* 67: 297-303.

Sudarsky, L. 1990. Gait disturbances in the elderly. *N Engl J Med* 322: 1441-1446.

Taaffe, D.R., T.L. Robinson, C.M. Snow, and R. Marcus. 1997. High-impact exercise promotes bone gain in well-trained female athletes. *J Bone Miner Res* 12: 255-260.

Taaffe, D.R., C. Snow-Harter, D.A. Connolly, T.L. Robinson, M.D. Brown, and R. Marcus. 1995. Differential effects of swimming versus weight-bearing activity on bone mineral status of eumenorrheic athletes. *J Bone Miner Res* 10: 586-593.

Tinetti, M.E. 2003. Preventing falls in elderly persons. *N Engl J Med* 348: 42-49.

Tinetti, M.E., D.I. Baker, G. McAvay, E.B. Claus, P. Garrett, M. Gottschalk, M.L. Koch, K. Trainor, and R.I. Horwitz. 1994. A multifactorial intervention to reduce the risk of falling among elderly people living in the community. *N Engl J Med* 331: 821-827.

Tinetti, M.E., M. Speechley, and S.F. Ginter. 1988. Risk factors for falls among elderly persons living in the community. *N Engl J Med* 319: 1701-1707.

Torgerson, D.J., M.K. Campbell, and D.M. Reid. 1995. Life-style, environmental and medical factors influencing peak bone mass in women. *Br J Rheumatol* 34: 620-624.

Uusi-Rasi, K., H. Sievanen, M. Pasanen, P. Oja, and I. Vuori. 2002. Associations of calcium intake and physical activity with bone density and size in premenopausal and postmenopausal women: A peripheral quantitative computed tomography study. *J Bone Miner Res* 17: 544-552.

Uusi-Rasi, K., H. Sievanen, I. Vuori, M. Pasanen, A. Heinonen, and P. Oja. 1998. Associations of physical activity and calcium intake with bone mass and size in healthy women at different ages. *J Bone Miner Res* 13: 133-142.

Vico, L., P. Collet, A. Guignandon, M.-H. Lafage-Proust, T. Thomas, M. Rehailia, and C. Alexandre. 2000. Effects of long-term microgravity exposure on cancellous and cortical weight-bearing bones of cosmonauts. *Lancet* 355: 1607-1611.

Vico, L., J.F. Pouget, P. Calmels, J.C. Chatard, M. Rehailia, P. Minaire, A. Geyssant, and C. Alexandre. 1995. The relations between physical ability and bone mass in women aged over 65 years. *J Bone Miner Res* 10: 374-383.

Virvidakis, K., E. Georgiou, A. Korkotsidis, K.N. Talles, and C. Provkakis. 1990. Bone mineral content of junior competitive weightlifters. *Int J Sports Med* 11: 244-246.

Vuori, I.M. 2001. Dose-response of physical activity and low back pain, osteoarthritis, and osteoporosis. *Med Sci Sports Exer* 33(6 Suppl.): 551-586.

Wallace, B.A., and R.G. Cumming. 2000. Systematic review of randomized trials of the effect of exercise on bone mass in pre- and postmenopausal women. *Calcif Tissue Int* 67: 10-18.

Welten, D.C., H.C.G. Kemper, G.B. Post, W. Van Mechelen, J. Twisk, P. Lips, and G.J. Teule. 1994. Weight-bearing activity during youth is a more important factor for peak bone mass than calcium intake. *J Bone Miner Res* 9: 1089-1096.

West, R.V. 1998. The female athlete: The triad of disordered eating, amenorrhoea and osteoporosis. *Sports Med* 26: 63-71.

Williams, J.A., J. Wagner, R. Wasnick, and L. Heilbrun. 1984. The effect of long-distance running upon appendicular bone mineral content. *Med Sci Sports Exerc* 16: 223-227.

Winters, K.M., and C.M. Snow. 2000. Detraining reverses positive effects of exercise on the musculoskeletal system in premenopausal women. *J Bone Miner Res* 15: 2495-2503.

Witzke, K.A., and C.M. Snow. 2000. Effects of plyometric jump training on bone mass in adolescent girls. *Med Sci Sports Exerc* 32: 1051-1057.

Wolff, I., J.J. van Croonenborg, H.C.G. Kemper, P.J. Kostense, and J.W.R. Twisk. 1999. The effect of exercise training programs on bone mass: A meta-analysis of published controlled trials in pre- and postmenopausal women. *Osteoporos Int* 9: 1-12.

Young, N., C. Formica, G. Szmukler, and E. Seeman. 1994. Bone density at weightbearing and nonweightbearing sites in ballet dancers: The effects of exercise, hypogonadism, and body weight. *J Clin Endocrinol Metab* 78: 449-454.

Zanker, C.L., L. Gannon, C.B. Cooke, K.L. Gee, B. Oldroyd, and J.G. Truscott. 2003. Difference in bone density, body composition, physical activity and diet between child gymnasts and untrained children 7-8 years of age. *J Bone Miner Res* 18: 1043-1050.

CHAPTER 16

Agin, D., D. Gallagher, J. Wang, S.B. Heymsfield, R.N. Pierson Jr., and D.P. Kotler. 2001. Effects of whey protein and resistance exercise on body cell mass, muscle strength, and quality of life in women with HIV. *AIDS* 15(18): 2431-2440.

Angel, J.B., B.M. Saget, S.P. Walsh, T.F. Greten, C.A. Dinarello, P.R. Skolnik, and S. Endres. 1995. Rolipram, a specific type IV phosphodiesterase inhibitor, is a potent inhibitor of HIV-1 replication. *AIDS* 9(10): 1137-1144.

Behrens, G., A. Dejam, H. Schmidt, H.J. Balks, G. Braband, T. Korner, M. Stoll, and R.E. Schmidt. 1999. Impaired glucose tolerance, beta cell function and lipid metabolism in HIV patients under treatment with protease inhibitors. *AIDS* 13(10): F63-70.

Bhasin, S., T.W. Storer, M. Javanbakht, N. Berman, K.E. Yareshseski, J. Philips, M. Dike, I. Sinha-Hikim, R. Shen, R.D. Haya, and G. Beall. 2000. Testosterone replacement and resistance exercise in HIV-infected men with weight loss and low testosterone levels. *JAMA* 283: 763-670.

Bjorntorp, P. 1988. The associations between obesity, adipose tissue distribution and disease. *Acta Med Scand* (Suppl 723) 8: 121-134.

Cade, W.T., L. Peralta, and R.E. Keyser. 2002. Aerobic capacity in late adolescents infected with HIV and controls. *Pediatr Rehabil* 5(3): 161-169.

Cannon, J.G. 1993. Exercise and resistance to infection. *J Appl Physiol* 74(3): 973-981.

Cannon, J.G., and M.J. Kluger. 1983. Endogenous pyrogen activity in human plasma after exercise. *Science* 220(4597): 617-619.

Carr, A., K. Samara, A. Thorisdottir, G.R. Kaufmann, D.J. Chisholm, and D.A. Cooper. 1999. Diagnosis, prediction, and natural course of HIV-1 protease-inhibitor associated lipodystrophy, hyperlipidaemia, and diabetes mellitus: A cohort study. *Lancet* 353(9170): 2093-2099.

Centers for Disease Control. 1987. Revision of the CDC surveillance definition for acquired immunodeficiency syndrome. *MMWR* 36(Suppl 1S): 3S-15S.

Centers for Disease Control. 2002. *HIV/AIDS Surveillance Report. Volume* 14. Available online at www.cdc.gov/hiv/STATS/hasr1402/technotes.htm. Accessed April 27, 2005.

Cohen, S., D.A. Tyrrell, and A.P. Smith. 1991. Psychological stress and susceptibility to the common cold. *N Engl J Med* 325(9): 606-612.

Corless, I., E. Bunch, J.K. Kemppainen, W.L. Holzemer, K.M. Nokes, L. Sanzero Eller, C.J. Portillo, E. Butensky, P.K. Nicholas, C.A. Bain, S. Davis, K.M. Kirksey, and F. Chou. 2002. Self-care for fatigue in patients with HIV. *Oncol Nurs Forum* 29(5): E60-E69. Available online at www.ons.org/publications/journals/ONF/Volume29/Issue5/290560.asp. Accessed April 27, 2005.

Driscoll, S.D., G.E. Meininger, M.T. Lareau, S.E. Dolan, K.M. Killilea, C. Hadigan, D.M. Lloyd-Jones, A. Klibanski, W.R. Frontera, and S. Grinspoon. 2004a. Effects of exercise training and metformin on body composition and cardiovascular indices in HIV infected patients. *AIDS* 18(3): 465-473.

Driscoll, S.D., G.E. Meininger, K. Ljungquist, C. Hadigan, M. Torriani, A. Klibanski, W.R. Frontera, and S. Grinspoon. 2004b. Differential effects of metformin and exercise on muscle adiposity and metabolic indices in HIV infected patients. *J Clin Endocrinol Metab* 89(5): 2171-2178.

Fielding, R.A., T.J. Manfredi, W. Ding, M.A. Fiatarone, W.J. Evand, and J.G. Cannon. 1993. Acute phase response in exercise. III. Neutrophil and IL-1 beta accumulation in skeletal muscle. *Am J Physiol* 265(1 Pt 2): R166-172.

Franz, M.J., E.S. Horton Sr., J.P. Bantle, C.A. Beebe, J.D. Brunzell, A.M. Coulston, R.R. Henry, B.J. Hoogwerf, and P.W. Stacpoole. 1994. Nutrition principles for the management of diabetes and related complications. *Diabetes Care* 17(5): 490-518.

Friedl, A.C., B. Ledergerber, M. Flepp, B. Hirschel, A. Telenti, H. Furrer, H.C. Bucher, E. Bernasconi, and R. Weber. 2001. Response to first protease inhibitor and efavirenz containing antiretroviral combination therapy. The Swiss HIV Cohort Study. *AIDS* 15(14): 1793-1800.

Fujioka, S., Y. Matsuzawa, K. Tokunaga, and S. Tarui. 1987. Contribution of intra-abdominal fat accumulation to the impairment of glucose and lipid metabolism in human obesity. *Metabolism* 36: 54-59.

Gavrila, A., Tsiodras, S., Doweiko, J., G.S. Nagy, Brodovicz, K., W. Hsu, Karchmer, A.W., Mantzoros, C.S. 2003. Exercise and vitamin E intake are independently associated with metabolic abnormalities in human immunodeficiency virus-positive subjects: A cross-sectional study. *Clin Infect Dis* 36(12): 1593-1601.

Granowitz, E.V., B.M. Saget, Angel, J.B., M.Z. Wang, A. Wang, C.A. Dinarello, and P.R. Skolnik. 1996. Soluble tumor necrosis factor receptors inhibit phorbol myristate acetate and cytokine-induced HIV-1 expression in chronically infected U1 cells. *J Acq Imm Def Syndr Hum Retrovirol* 11(5): 430-437.

Granowitz, E.V., B.M. Saget, M.Z. Wang, C.A. Dinarello, and P.R. Skolnik. 1995. Interleukin 1 induces HIV-1 expression in chronically infected U1 cells: Blockade by interleukin 1 receptor antagonist and tumor necrosis factor binding protein type 1. *Mol Med* 1(6): 667-677.

Grinspoon, S., C. Corcoran, K. Parlman, M. Costello, D. Rosenthal, E. Anderson, T. Stanley, Schoenfeld, D., B. Burrows, D. Hayden, N. Basgoz, and A. Klibanski. 2000. Effects of testosterone and progressive resistance training in eugonadal men with AIDS wasting. *Ann Int Med* 133: 348-355.

Grinspoon, S., C. Corcoran, D. Rosenthal, T. Stanley, K. Parlman, M. Costello, M. Treat, S. Davis, B. Burrows, N. Basgoz, and A. Klibanski. 1999. Quantitative assessment of cross-sectional muscle area, functional status and muscle strength in men with the AIDS wasting syndrome. *J Clin Endocrinol Metab* 84: 201-206.

Guenter, P., N. Muurahainen, G. Simons, A. Kosok, G.R. Cohan, R. Rudenstein, and J.L. Turner. 1993. Relationships among nutritional status, disease progression, and survival in HIV infection. *J Acq Imm Def Syndr* 6(10): 1130-1138.

Jones, S.P., D.A. Doran, P.B. Leatt, B. Maher, and M. Pirmohamed. 2001. Short-term exercise training improves body composition and hyperlipidaemia in HIV-positive individuals with lipodystrophy. *AIDS* 15(15): 2049-2051.

Lichtenstein, K.A., D.J. Ward, A.C. Moorman, K.M. Delaney, B. Young, F.J. Pallela Jr., P.H. Rhodes, K.C. Wood, S.D. Holmberg, and HIV Outpatient Study Investigators. 2001. Clinical assessment of HIV-associated lipodystrophy in an ambulatory population. *AIDS* 15(11): 1389-1398.

Lo, J.C., K. Mulligan, V.W. Tai, H. Algren, and M. Schambelan. 1998. "Buffalo hump" in men with HIV-infection. *Lancet* 351: 871-875.

MacArthur, R.D., S.D. Levine, and T.J. Birk. 1993. Supervised exercise training improves cardiopulmonary fitness in HIV infected persons. *Med Sci Sports Med* 25: 684-688.

Matsuzawa, Y., T. Nakamura, I. Shimomura, and K. Kotani. 1995. Visceral fat accumulation and cardiovascular disease. *Obes Res* 3(Suppl 5): 645S-647S.

Moore, R.D., and R.E. Chaisson. 1999. Natural history of HIV infection in the era of combination antiretroviral therapy. *AIDS* 13(14): 1933-1942.

Mustafa, T., F.S. Sy, C.A. Macera, S.J. Thompson, K.L. Jackson, A. Selassie, and L.L. Dean. 1999. Association between exercise and HIV disease progression in a cohort of homosexual men. *Ann Epidemiol* 9(2): 127-131.

National Cholesterol Education Program. 2001. Executive summary of the third report of the National Cholesterol Education Program (NCEP) Expert Panel on Detection, Evaluation, and Treatment of High Blood Cholesterol in Adults (Adult Treatment Panel III). 2001. *JAMA* 285(19): 2486-2497.

Neidig, J.L., B.A. Smith, D.E. Brashers. 2003. Aerobic exercise training for depressive symptom management in adults living with HIV infection. *J Assoc Nurses AIDS Care* 14(2): 30-40.

Nieman, D.C. 1997. Immune response to heavy exertion. *J Appl Physiol* 82(5): 1385-1394.

Nieman, D.C., L.M. Johanssen, J.W. Lee, and K. Arabatzis. 1990. Infectious episodes in runners before and after the Los Angeles Marathon. *J Sports Med Phys Fitness* 30(3): 316-328.

Orlando, G., G. Guaraldi, R. Murri, A. Wu, G. Nardini, B. Beghetto, G.K. Sterrantino, S. Sbaragli, M. Borderi, S. Talo, C. Grosso, C. Erba, A.M. Cattelan, A. Aninori, and R. Esposito. 2002. Does lipodystrophy affect quality of life? XIV International AIDS Conference, Barcelona, Spain.

Palenicek, J.P., N.M.H. Graham, Y.D. He, D.A. Hoover, J.S. Oishi, L. Kingsley, and A.J. Saah. 1995. Weight loss prior to clinical AIDS as a predictor of survival. *J Acq Imm Def Syndr* 10: 366-373.

Perna, F.M., A. LaPerriere, N. Klimas, G. Ironson, A. Perry, J. Pavone, A. Goldstein, P. Majors, D. Makemson, C. Talutto, N. Schneiderman, M.A. Fletcher, O.G. Meijer, and L. Koppes. 1999. Cardiopulmonary and CD4 cell changes in response to exercise training in early symptomatic HIV infection. *Med Sci Sports Exerc* 31(7): 973-979.

Power, R., H.L. Tate, S.M. McGill, and C. Taylor. 2003. A qualitative study of the psychosocial implications of lipodystrophy syndrome on HIV positive individuals. *Sexually Trans Inf* 79(2): 137-141.

Rigsby, L.W., R.K. Dishman, A.W. Jackson, G.S. Maclean, and P.B. Raven. 1992. Effects of exercise training on men seropositive for human immunodeficiency virus-1. *Med Sci Sports Exerc* 24(1): 6-12.

Roge, B.T., J.A. Calbet, K. Moller, H. Ullum, H.W. Hendel, J. Gerstoft, and B.K. Pedersen. 2002. Skeletal muscle mitochondrial function and exercise capacity in HIV-infected patients with lipodystrophy and elevated p-lactate levels. *AIDS* 16(7): 973-982.

Rohde, T., H. Ullum, J.P. Rasmussen, J.H. Kristensen, E. Newsholme, and B.K. Pedersen. 1995. Effects of glutamine on the immune system: Influence of muscular exercise and HIV infection. *J Appl Physiol* 79: 146-150.

Roubenoff, R., L.W. Abad, and N. Lundgren. 2001. Effect of acquired immune deficiency syndrome wasting on the protein metabolic response to acute exercise. *Metabolism* 50(3): 288-292.

Roubenoff, R., A. McDermott, L. Weiss, J. Suri, M. Wood, R. Bloch, and S. Gorbach. 1999a. Short-term progressive resistance training increases strength and lean body mass in adults infected with human immunodeficiency virus. *AIDS* 13: 231-239.

Roubenoff, R., H. Schmitz, L. Bairos, J. Layne, E. Potts, G.J. Cloutier, and F. Denry. 2002. Reduction of abdominal obesity in lipodystrophy associated with human immunodeficiency virus infection by means of diet and exercise: Case report and proof of principle. *Clin Infect Dis* 34(3): 390-393.

Roubenoff, R., P.R. Skolnik, A. Shevitz, L. Snydman, A. Wang, S. Melanson, and S. Gorbach. 1999b. Effect of a single bout of acute exercise on plasma human immunodeficiency virus RNA levels. *J Appl Physiol* 86(4): 1197-1201.

Roubenoff, R., Weiss, L., A. McDermott, T. Heflin, G.J. Cloutier, M. Wood, and S. Gorbach. 1999c. A pilot study of exercise training to reduce trunk fat in adults with HIV-associated fat redistribution. *AIDS* 13(11): 1373-1375.

Sattler, F.R., S.V. Jaque, E.T. Schroeder, C. Olson, M.P. Dube, C. Martinez, W. Briggs, R. Horton, and S. Azen. 1999. Effects of pharmacological doses of nandrolone decanoate and progressive resistance training in immunodeficiency patients infected with human immunodeficiency virus. *J Clin Endocrinol Metab* 84: 1268-1276.

Sattler, F.R., E.T. Schroeder, M.P. Dube, S.V. Jaque, C. Martinez, P.J. Blanche, S. Azen, and R.M. Krauss. 2002. Metabolic effects of nandrolone decanoate and resistance training in men with HIV. *Am J Physiol Endocrinol Metab* 283(6): E1214-1222.

Schwenk, A., A. Beisenherz, K. Romer, G. Kremer, B. Salzberger, and M. Elia. 2000. Phase angle from bioelectrical impedance analysis remains an independent predictive marker in HIV-infected patients in the era of highly active antiretroviral treatment. *Am J Clin Nutr* 72(2): 496-501.

Smith, B.A., J.L. Neidig, J.T. Nickel, G.L. Mitchell, M.F. Para, and R.J. Fass. 2001. Aerobic exercise: Effects on parameters related to fatigue, dyspnea, weight and body composition in HIV-infected adults. *AIDS* 15(6): 693-701.

Spence, D.W., M.L. Galantino, K.A. Mossberg, and S.O. Zimmerman. 1990. Progressive resistance exercise: Effect on muscle function and anthropometry of a select AIDS population. *Arch Phys Med Rehabil* 71: 644-648.

Strawford, A., T. Barbieri, M. Van Loan, E. Parks, D. Catlin, N. Barton, R. Neese, M. Christiansen, J. King, and M.K. Hellerstein. 1999. Resistance exercise and supraphysiologic androgen therapy in eugonadal men with HIV-related weight loss. *JAMA* 281: 1282-1290.

Stringer, W.W., M. Berezovska, W.A. O'Brien, C.K. Beck, and R. Casaburi. 1998. The effect of exercise training on aerobic fitness, immune indices and quality of life in HIV+ patients. *Med Sci Sports Exerc* 30: 11-16.

Suttmann, U., J. Ockenga, O. Selberg, L. Hoogestraat, H. Deicher, and M.J. Muller. 1995. Incidence and prognostic value of malnutrition and wasting in human immunodeficiency virus-infected outpatients. *J Acq Imm Def Syndr* 8: 239-246.

Terry, L., E. Sprinz, and J.P. Ribeiro. 1999. Moderate and high intensity exercise training in HIV-1 seropositive individuals: A randomized trial. *Int J Sports Med* 20(2): 142-146.

Thiebaut, R., D. Malvy, C. Marimoutou, and F. Davis. 2000. Anthropometric indices as predictors of survival in AIDS adults. Aquitaine Cohort, France, 1985-1997. Groupe d'Epidemiologie Clinique du Sida en Aquitaine (GECSA). *Eur J Epidemiol* 16(7): 633-639.

Thoni, G.J., C. Fedou, J.F. Brun, J. Fabre, E. Renard, J. Reynes, A. Varray, and J. Mercier. 2002. Reduction of fat accumulation and lipid disorders by individualized light aerobic training in human immunodeficiency virus infected patients with lipodystrophy and/or dyslipidemia. *Diabetes Metab* 28(5): 397-404.

Ullum, H., J. Palmo, J. Halkjaer-Kristensen, M. Diamant, M. Klokker, A. Kruuse, A. LaPerriere, and B.K. Pedersen. 1994. The effect of acute exercise on lymphocyte subsets, natural killer cells, proliferative responses, and cytokines in HIV-seropositive persons. *J Acq Imm Def Syndr* 7(11): 1122-1133.

Wagner, G., J. Rabkin, and R. Rabkin. 1998. Exercise as a mediator of psychological and nutritional effects of testosterone therapy in HIV+ men. *Med Sci Sports Exerc* 30(6): 811-817.

Wanke, C., M. Silva, T. Knox, J. Forrester, D. Speigelman, and S. Gorbach. 2000. Weight loss and wasting remain common complications in individuals infected with HIV in the era of highly active antiretroviral therapy. *Clin Inf Dis* 31: 803-805.

Wheeler, D.A., C.L. Gibert, C.A. Launer, N. Muurahainen, R.A. Elion, D.I. Abrams, and G.E. Bartsch. 1998. Weight loss as a predictor of survival and disease progression in HIV infection. Terry Beirn Community Programs for Clinical Research on AIDS. *J Acq Imm Def Syndr Hum Retrovirol* 18(1): 80-85.

Yarasheski, K.E., P. Tebas, B. Stanerson, S. Claxton, D. Marin, K. Bae, M. Kennedy, W. Tantisiriwat, and W.G. Powderly. 2001. Resistance exercise training reduces hypertriglyceridemia in HIV-infected men treated with antiviral therapy. *J Appl Physiol* 90(1): 133-138.

CHAPTER 17

Astrup, A., L. Breum, and S. Toubro. 1995. Pharmacological and clinical studies of ephedrine and other thermogenic agents. *Obes Res* 3: 537-540S.

Ballor, D., J. Harvey-Berion, P. Ades, J. Cryan, and J. Callews-Escandon. 1996. Contrasting effects of resistance and aerobic training on body composition and metabolism after diet-induced weight loss. *Metabolism* 45: 179-183.

Ballor, D.L., and E.T. Poehlman. 1994. Exercise-training enhances fat-free mass preservation during diet-induced weight loss: A meta-analytical finding. *Int J Obes* 18: 35-40.

Broader, C., K. Burrhus, L. Svanevik, and J. Wilmore. 1992. The effects of either high-intensity resistance or endurance training on resting metabolic rate. *Am J Clin Nutr* 55: 801-810.

Campbell, W., M. Crim, V. Young, and W. Evans. 1994. Increased energy requirements and changes in body composition with resistance training in older adults. *Am J Clin Nutr* 60: 167-175.

Coakley, E.H., E.B. Rimm, G. Colditz, I. Kawachi, and W. Willett. 1998. Predictors of weight change in men: Results from the Health Professionals Follow-Up Study. *Int J Obes* 22: 89-96.

Cohn, S.H., D. Vartsky, and S. Yasumura. 1980. Compartmental body composition based on the body nitrogen, potassium and calcium. *Am J Physiol* 239: E192-200.

Colditz, G.A., W.C. Willett, A. Rotnizky, and J.E. Manson. 1995. Weight gain as a risk factor for clinical diabetes mellitus in women. *Ann Intern Med* 122: 481-486.

Dash, A., A. Agrawal, N. Venkat, J. Moxham, and J. Ponte. 1994. Effect of oral theophylline on resting energy expenditure in normal volunteers. *Thorax* 49: 1116-1120.

Davies, P.S.W., J.M. Day, and A. Lucas. 1991. Energy expenditure in early infancy and later fatness. *Int J Obesity* 15: 727-731.

Forbes, G. 1987. *Human body composition: Growth, aging, nutrition, and activity.* New York: Springer-Verlag.

Fox, A., J. Thompson, G. Butterfield, U. Gylfadottir, S. Moynihan, and G. Spiller. 1996. Effects of diet and exercise on common cardiovascular disease risk factors in moderately obese older women. *Am J Clin Nutr* 63: 225-233.

Gardner, A.W., and E.T. Poehlman. 1993. Physical activity is a significant predictor of body density in women. *Am J Clin Nutr* 57: 8-14.

Gardner, A.W., and E.T. Poehlman. 1994. Leisure time physical activity is a significant predictor of body density in men. *J Clin Epidemiol* 47: 283-291.

Griffiths, M., and P.R. Payne. 1976. Energy expenditure in small children of obese and non-obese parents. *Nature* 260: 698-700.

Griffiths, M., P.R. Payne, A.J. Stunkard, J.P.W. Rivers, and M. Cox. 1990. Metabolic rate and physical development in children at risk of obesity. *Lancet* 336: 76-78.

Hubert, H.B., M. Feinleib, P.M. McNamara, and W.P. Castelli. 1983. Obesity an independent risk factor for cardiovascular disease: A 26-year follow-up of participants in the Framingham Heart Study. *Circulation* 67: 968-977.

Jakicic, J., and K. Gallagher. 2003. Exercise considerations for the sedentary, overweight adult. *Exerc Sport Sci Rev* 31: 91-95.

Jakicic, J.M., C. Winters, W. Lang, and R.R. Wing. 1999. Effect of intermittent exercise and use of home exercise equipment on adherence, weight loss, and fitness in overweight women: A randomized trial. *JAMA* 286: 1554-1560.

Jeffery, R.W., and S.A. French. 1997. Preventing weight gain in adults: Design, methods and one year results from the Pound of Prevention study. *Int J Obes Rel Metab Disord* 21: 457-464.

Jeffery, R.W., R.R. Wing, N.E. Sherwood, and D.F. Tate. 2003. Physical activity and weight loss: Does prescribing higher physical activity improve outcomes? *Am J Clin Nutr* 78: 684-689.

Katzel, L.I., E.R. Bleecker, E.G. Colman, E.M. Rogus, J.D. Sorkin, and A.P. Goldberg. 1995. Effects of weight loss vs. aerobic exercise training on risk factors for coronary disease in healthy, obese, middle-aged and older men. *JAMA* 274: 1915-1921.

King, N.A., A. Tremblay, and J.E. Blundell. 1997. Effects of exercise on appetite control: Implications for energy balance. *Med Sci Sports Exerc* 29: 1076-1089.

Klem, M.L., R.R. Wing, M.T. McGuire, H.M. Seagle, and J.O. Hill. 1997. A descriptive study of individuals successful at long-term maintenance of substantial weight loss. *Am J Clin Nutr* 66: 239-246.

Korner, J., and L.J. Aronne. 2003. The emerging science of body weight regulation and its impact on obesity treatment. *J Clin Invest* 111: 565-570.

Leibel, R.L., M. Rosenbaum, and J. Hirsch. 1995. Changes in energy expenditure resulting from altered body weight. *N Engl J Med* 332: 621-628.

Leon, A.S., J. Conrad, D.B. Hunninghake, and R. Serfass. 1979. Effects of a vigorous walking program on body composition, and carbohydrate and lipid metabolism of obese young men. *Am J Clin Nutr* 32(9): 1776-1783.

Meredith, C.N., W.R. Frontera, E.C. Fisher, V.A. Hughes, J.C. Herland, and W.J. Evans. 1989. Peripheral effects of endurance training in young and old subjects. *J Appl Physiol* 66: 2844-2849.

Metropolitan Life Insurance Company. 1980. *The 1979 Build Study.* Chicago: Society of Actuaries and Association of Life Insurance Medical Directors of America.

Micossi, M.S., and T.M. Harris. 1990. Age variations in the relation of body mass index to estimates of body fat and muscle mass. *Am J Phys Anthrop* 81: 375-379.

Miller, W.C., D.M. Koceja, and E.J. Hamilton. 1997. A meta-analysis of the past 25 years of weight loss research using diet, exercise, or diet plus exercise intervention. *Int J Obes Rel Metab Disord* 21: 941-947.

Nelson, M.E. 1998. *Strong women stay slim.* New York: Bantam Books.

NHLBI Obesity Education Initiative Expert Panel on the Identification, Evaluation, and Treatment of Overweight and Obesity in Adults. 1998. *Clinical guidelines on the identification, evaluation, and treatment of overweight and obesity in adults. The evidence report.* Bethesda, MD: National Institutes of Health.

Nieman, D.C., and L.M. Onasch. 1990. The effect of moderate exercise training on nutrient intake in mildly obese women. *J Am Diet Assoc* 90: 1557-1562.

Owens, J.F., K.A. Matthews, and R.R. Wing. 1992. Can physical activity mitigate the effects of aging in middle-aged women? *Circulation* 85: 1265-1270.

Pace, N., and E.N. Rathburn. 1945. Studies of body composition. III. The body water and chemically combined nitrogen content in relation to fat content. *J Biol Chem* 158: 685-691.

Pavlou, K.N., S. Krey, and W.P. Steffee. 1989. Exercise as an adjunct to weight loss and maintenance in moderately obese subjects. *Am J Clin Nutr* 49: 1115-1123.

Pi-Sunyer, F.X., and R. Wood. 1985. Effect of exercise on food intake in human subjects. *Am J Clin Nutr* 42: 983-990.

Pritchard, J.E., C.A. Nowson, and J.D. Wark. 1997. A worksite program for overweight middle-aged men achieves lesser weight loss with exercise than with dietary change. *J Am Diet Assoc* 97: 37-42.

Racette, S.B., D.A. Schoeller, R.F. Kushner, and K.M. Neil. 1995. Exercise enhances dietary compliance during moderate energy restriction in obese women. *Am J Clin Nutr* 62: 345-349.

Rall, L., S. Meydani, J. Kehayias, B. Dawson-Hughes, and R. Roubenoff. 1996. The effect of progressive resistance training in rheumatoid arthritis: Increased strength without changes in energy balance or body composition. *Arthr Rheum* 39: 415-426.

Ravussin, E., S. Lillioja, and W.C. Knowler. 1988. Reduced rate of energy expenditure as a risk factor for body-weight gain. *New Engl J Med* 318: 467-472.

Rising, L.R., I.T. Harper, A.M. Fontvielle, R.T. Ferraro, M. Spraul, and E. Ravussin. 1994. Determinants of total daily energy expenditure: Variability in physical activity. *Am J Clin Nutr* 59: 800-804.

Roberts, S.B. 1989. Use of the doubly labeled water method for measurement of energy expenditure, total body water, water intake, and metabolizable energy intake in humans and small animals. *Can J Physiol Pharmacol* 67: 1190-1198.

Roberts, S.B., W. Dietz, T. Sharp, G.E. Dallal, and J.O. Hall. 1995. Multiple laboratory comparison of the doubly labeled water technique. *Obes Res* 3(Suppl. 2): 155S-163S.

Roberts, S.B., P. Fuss, M.B. Heyman, G.E. Dallal, and V.R. Young. 1996. Effects of age on energy expenditure and substrate oxidation during experimental underfeeding in healthy men. *J Gerontol* 51A: B158-B166.

Roberts, S.B., J. Savage, W.A. Coward, B. Chew, and A. Lucas. 1988. Energy expenditure and energy intake in infants born to lean and overweight mothers. *N Engl J Med* 318: 461-466.

Roubenoff, R., G.E. Dallal, and P.W.F. Wilson. 1995. Predicting body fatness: The body mass index vs. estimation by bioelectrical impedance. *Am J Pub Health* 85: 726-728.

Roubenoff, R., and J.J. Kehayias. 1991. The meaning and measurement of lean body mass. *Nutr Rev* 46: 163-175.

Sahakian, B.J., P. Trayhurm, M. Wallace, R. Deeley, P. Winn, T.W. Robbins, and B.J. Everitt. 1983. Increased weight gain and reduced activity in brown adipose tissue produced by depletion of hypothalamic noradrenaline. *Neurosci Lett* 39: 321-326.

Saltzman, E., and S.B. Roberts. 1995. The role of energy expenditure in energy regulation: Findings from a decade of research. *Nutr Rev* 53: 209-220.

Saltzman, E., and S.B. Roberts. 1996. Effects of energy imbalance on energy expenditure and respiratory quotient in young and older men: A summary of data from two metabolic studies. *Aging Clin Exp Res* 8: 370-378.

Saris, W.H.M., M.C. Koenders, D.L.E. Pannemans, and M.A. van Baak. 1992. Outcome of a multicenter outpatient weight-management program including very-low calorie diet and exercise. *Am J Clin Nutr* 56: 294-296S.

Schoeller, D. 1998. Balancing energy expenditure and body weight. *Am J Clin Nutr* 68: 956S-961S.

Schoeller, D.A., K. Shay, and R.F. Kushner. 1997. How much physical activity is needed to minimize weight gain in previously obese women? *Am J Clin Nutr* 66: 551-556.

Schulz, L.O., and D.A. Schoeller. 1994. A compilation of total daily energy expenditures and body weights in healthy adults. *Am J Clin Nutr* 60: 676-681.

Schwartz, M.W., S.C. Woods, R.J. Seeley, G.S. Barsh, D.G. Baskin, and R.L. Leibel. 2003. Is the energy homeostasis system inherently biased toward weight gain? *Diabetes* 52: 232-238.

Schwartz, R. 1987. The independent effects of dietary weight loss and aerobic training on high density lipoproteins and apolipoprotein A-1 concentrations in obese men. *Metabolism* 36: 165-171.

Sweeney, M.E., J.O. Hill, P.A. Heller, R. Baney, and M. DiGirolamo. 1993. Severe vs. moderate energy restriction with and without exercise in the treatment of obesity: Efficiency of weight loss. *Am J Clin Nutr* 57: 127-134.

Vallejo, E.A. 1957. La dieta de hambre a disas alternos in la almentacion de los viejos. *Rev Clin Exp* 63: 25.

Van Etten, L., K. Westerterp, F. Verstappen, B. Boon, and W. Saris. 1997. Effect of an 18-wk weight-training program on energy expenditure and physical activity. *J Appl Physiol* 82: 298-304.

Van Pelt, R., K. Davy, E. Stevenson, T. Wilson, P. Jones, and D. Seals. 1998. Smaller differences in total and regional adiposity with age in women who regularly perform endurance exercise. *Am J Clin Nutr* 42: 983-990.

Weigle, D.S., K.J. Sande, P.-H. Iverisu, E.R. Monsen, and J.D. Brunzell. 1988. Weight loss leads to a marked decrease in non-resting energy expenditure in ambulatory human subjects. *Metabolism* 37: 930-936.

Welle, S., R.G. Schwartz, and M. Statt. 1991. Reduced metabolic rate during beta-adrenergic blockade in humans. *Metabolism* 40: 619-622.

Williamson, D.F. 1993. Descriptive epidemiology of body weight and weight change in U.S. adults. *Ann Intern Med* 119: 646-649.

Williamson, D.F. 1996. Dietary intake and physical activity as "predictors" of weight gain in observational, prospective studies of adults. *Nutr Rev* 54: S101-S109.

Williamson, D.F., J. Madans, R.F. Anda, J.C. Kleinman, H.S. Kahn, and T. Byers. 1993. Recreational physical activity and ten-year weight change in a U.S. national cohort. *Int J Obes* 17: 279-286.

Wilmore, J., P. Stanforth, L. Hudspeth, J. Gagnon, E. Daw, A. Leon, D. Rao, J. Skinner, and C. Bouchard. 1998. Alterations in resting metabolic rate as a consequence of 20 wk of endurance training: The HERITAGE Family Study. *Am J Clin Nutr* 68: 66-71.

Wood, P.D., M.L. Stefanick, D.M. Dreon, B. Frey-Hewitt, S.C. Garay, P.T. Williams, H.R. Superko, S.P. Fortmann, J.J. Albers, K.M. Vranizan, N.M. Ellsworth, R.M. Terry, and W.L. Haskell. 1988. Changes in plasma lipids and lipoproteins in overweight men during weight loss through dieting as compared with exercise. *N Engl J Med* 319: 1173-1179.

Wood, P.D., M.L. Stefanick, P.T. Williams, and W.L. Haskell. 1991. The effects on plasma lipoproteins of a prudent weight-reducing diet, with or without exercise, in overweight men and women. *N Engl J Med* 325: 461-466.

Yale, J.-F., L.A. Leiter, and E.B. Marliss. 1989. Metabolic responses to intense exercise in lean and obese subjects. *J Clin Endocrinol Metab* 68: 438.

CHAPTER 18

American Cancer Society. 2004. *Cancer facts & figures 2004.* Atlanta: American Cancer Society.

American College of Sports Medicine. 1998. Position stand. The recommended quantity and quality of exercise for developing and maintaining cardiorespiratory and muscular fitness, and flexibility in healthy adults. *Med Sci Sports Exerc* 30(6): 975-991.

Battiato, L.A., and V.S. Wheeler. 2000. Biotherapy. In *Cancer nursing: Principles and practice,* 5th ed., pp. 543-579, eds. C.H. Yarbro, M. Goodman, M.H. Frogge, and S.L. Groenwald. Sudbury, MA: Jones & Bartlett.

Brown, J.K., T. Byers, C. Doyle, K.S. Courneya, W. Demark-Wahnefried, L.H. Kushi, A. McTieman, C.L. Rock, N. Aziz, A.S. Bloch, B. Eldridge, K. Hamilton, C. Katzin, A. Koonce, J. Main, C. Mobley, M.E. Morra, M.S. Pierce, K.A. Sawyer, and American Cancer Society. 2003. Nutrition and physical activity during and after cancer treatment: An American Cancer Society guide for informed choices. *CA Cancer J Clin* 53(5): 268-291.

Burnham, T.R., and A. Wilcox. 2002. Effects of exercise on physiological and psychological variables in cancer survivors. *Med Sci Sports Exerc* 34(12): 1863-1867.

Camp-Sorrell, D. 2000. Chemotherapy: Toxicity management. In *Cancer nursing: Principles and practice,* 5th ed., pp. 444-486, eds. C.H. Yarbro, M. Goodman, M.H. Frogge, and S.L. Groenwald. Sudbury, MA: Jones & Bartlett.

Coleman, E.A., S. Coon, J. Hall-Barrow, K. Richards, D. Gaylor, and B. Stewart. 2003. Feasibility of exercise during treatment for multiple myeloma. *Cancer Nurs* 26(5): 410-419.

Courneya, K.S. 2003. Exercise in cancer survivors: An overview of research. *Med Sci Sports Exerc* 35(11): 1846-1852.

Courneya, K.S., and C.M. Friedenreich. 1997a. Relationship between exercise during cancer treatment and current quality of life in survivors of breast cancer. *J Psychosoc Oncol* 5: 120-127.

Courneya, K.S., and C.M. Friedenreich. 1997b. Relationship between exercise pattern across the cancer experience and current quality of life in colorectal cancer survivors. *J Alternative Complementary Med* 3: 215-226.

Courneya, K.S., and C.M. Friedenreich. 1997c. Determinants of exercise during colorectal cancer treatment: An application of the theory of planned behavior. *Oncol Nurs Forum* 24(10): 1715-1723.

Courneya, K.S., and C.M. Friedenreich. 1999. Utility of the theory of planned behavior for understanding exercise during breast cancer treatment. *Psychooncology* 8(2): 112-122.

Courneya, K.S., and C.M. Friedenreich. 2001. Framework PEACE: An organizational model for examining physical exercise across the cancer experience. *Ann Behav Med* 23(4): 263-272.

Courneya, K.S., C.M. Friedenreich, H.A. Quinney, A.L. Fields, L.W. Jones, and A.S. Fairey. 2003a. A randomized trial of exercise and quality of life in colorectal cancer survivors. *Eur J Cancer Care* 12: 347-357.

Courneya, K.S., C.M. Friedenreich, R.A. Sela, H.A. Quinney, R.E. Rhodes, and M. Handman. 2003b. The group psychotherapy and home-based physical exercise (group-hope) trial in cancer survivors: Physical fitness and quality of life outcomes. *Psychooncology* 12(4): 357-374.

Courneya, K.S., J.R. Mackey, G.J. Bell, L.W. Jones, C.J. Field, and A.S. Fairey. 2003c. Randomized controlled trial of exercise training in postmenopausal breast cancer survivors: Cardiopulmonary and quality of life outcomes. *J Clin Oncol* 21(9): 1660-1668.

Courneya, K.S., J.R. Mackey, and L.W. Jones. 2000. Coping with cancer: Can exercise help? *Phys Sportsmed* 28: 49-73.

Courneya, K.S., J.R. Mackey, and D.C. McKenzie. 2002a. Exercise for breast cancer survivors: Research evidence and clinical guidelines. *Phys Sportsmed* 30: 33-42.

Courneya, K.S., J.R. Mackey, and H.A. Quinney. 2002b. Neoplasms. In *American College of Sports Medicine's resources for clinical exercise physiology: Musculoskeletal, neuromuscular, neoplastic, immunologic, and hematologic conditions,* pp. 179-191, eds. J.N. Myers, W.G. Herbert, and R. Humphrey. Baltimore: Lippincott Williams & Wilkins.

Dimeo, F., S. Fetscher, W. Lange, R. Mertelsmann, and J. Keul. 1997. Effects of aerobic exercise on the physical performance and incidence of treatment-related complications after high-dose chemotherapy. *Blood* 90(9): 3390-3394.

Dimeo, F., S. Schwartz, T. Fietz, T. Wanjura, D. Boning, and E. Thiel. 2003. Effects of endurance training on the physical performance of patients with hematological malignancies during chemotherapy. *Support Care Cancer* 11(10): 623-628.

Fairey, A.S., K.S. Courneya, C.J. Field, G.J. Bell, L.W. Jones, and J.R. Mackey. 2003. Effects of exercise training on fasting insulin, insulin resistance, insulin-like growth factors, and insulin-like growth factor binding proteins in postmenopausal breast cancer survivors: A randomized controlled trial. *Cancer Epidemiol Biomarkers Prev* 12(8): 721-727.

Ferlay, J. F. Bray, P. Pisani, and D.M. Parkin. 2004. *Globocan 2002: Cancer incidence, mortality and prevalence worldwide.* IARC CancerBase No. 5. Version 2.0. Lyon, France: IARC-*Press.* Available online at http: //www-dep.iarc.fr. Accessed May 12, 2005.

Frogge, M.H., and S.M. Cunning. 2000. Surgical therapy. In *Cancer nursing: Principles and practice,* 5th ed., pp. 272-285, eds. C.H. Yarbro, M. Goodman, M.H. Frogge, and S.L. Groenwald. Sudbury, MA: Jones & Bartlett.

Gribbon, J., and L.J. Loescher. 2000. Biology of cancer. In *Cancer nursing: Principles and practice,* 5th ed., pp. 17-34, eds. C.H. Yarbro, M. Goodman, M.H. Frogge, and S.L. Groenwald. Sudbury, MA: Jones & Bartlett.

Hayes, S., P.S. Davies, T. Parker, and J. Bashford. 2003a. Total energy expenditure and body composition changes following peripheral blood stem cell transplantation and participation in an exercise programme. *Bone Marrow Trans* 31(5): 331-338.

Hayes, S.C., D. Rowbottom, P.S. Davies, T.W. Parker, and J. Bashford. 2003b. Immunological changes after cancer treatment and participation in an exercise program. *Med Sci Sports Exerc* 35(1): 2-9.

Hilderley, L.J. 2000. Principles of radiation therapy. In *Cancer nursing: Principles and practice,* 5th ed., pp. 286-299, eds. C.H. Yarbro, M. Goodman, M.H. Frogge, and S.L. Groenwald. Sudbury, MA: Jones & Bartlett.

Jones, L.W., and K.S. Courneya. 2002. Exercise counseling and programming preferences of cancer survivors. *Cancer Pract* 10(4): 208-215.

Kolden, G.G., T.J. Strauman, A. Ward, J. Kuta, T.E. Woods, K.L. Schneider, E. Heerey, L. Sanborn, C. Burt, L. Millbrandt, N.H. Kalin, J.A. Stewart, and B. Mullen. 2002. A pilot study of group exercise training (GET) for women with primary breast cancer: Feasibility and health benefits. *Psychooncology* 11(5): 447-456.

Maher, K.E. 2000. Radiation therapy: Toxicities and management. In *Cancer nursing: Principles and practice,* 5th ed., pp. 323-351, eds. C.H. Yarbro, M. Goodman, M.H. Frogge, and S.L. Groenwald. Sudbury, MA: Jones & Bartlett.

McKenzie, D.C., and A.L. Kalda. 2003. Effect of upper extremity exercise on secondary lymphedema in breast cancer patients: A pilot study. *J Clin Oncol* 21(3): 463-466.

Nelson, J.P. 1991. Perceived health, self-esteem, health habits, and perceived benefits and barriers to exercise in women who have and who have not experienced stage I breast cancer. *Oncol Nurs Forum* 18(7): 1191-1197.

Oldervoll, L.M., S. Kaasa, H. Knobel, and J.H. Loge. 2003. Exercise reduces fatigue in chronic fatigued Hodgkins disease survivors—results from a pilot study. *Eur J Cancer* 39(1): 57-63.

Parkin, D.M., F. Bray, J. Ferlay, and P. Pisani. 2001. Estimating the world cancer burden: Globocan 2000. *Int J Cancer* 94(2): 153-156.

Pinto, B.M., M.M. Clark, N.C. Maruyama, and S.I. Feder. 2003. Psychological and fitness changes associated with exercise participation among women with breast cancer. *Psychooncology* 12(2): 118-126.

Pinto, B.M., J.J. Trunzo, P. Reiss, and S.Y. Shiu. 2002. Exercise participation after diagnosis of breast cancer: Trends and effects on mood and quality of life. *Psychooncology* 11(5): 389-400.

Segal, R., W. Evans, D. Johnson, J. Smith, S. Colletta, J. Gayton, S. Woodard, G. Wells, and R. Reid. 2001. Structured exercise improves physical functioning in women with stages I and II breast cancer: Results of a randomized controlled trial. *J Clin Oncol* 19(3): 657-665.

Segal, R., R.D. Reid, K.S. Courneya, S.C. Malone, M.B. Parliament, C.G. Scott, P.M. Venner, H.A. Quinney, L.W. Jones, M.E. D'Angelo, and G.A. Wells. 2003. Resistance exercise in men receiving androgen deprivation therapy for prostate cancer. *J Clin Oncol* 21(9): 1653-1659.

Winningham, M.L., M.G. MacVicar, M. Bondoc, J.I. Andrerson, and J.P. Minton. 1989. Effect of aerobic exercise on body weight and composition in patients with breast cancer on adjuvant chemotherapy. *Oncol Nurs Forum* 16: 683-689.

Young-McCaughan, S., M.Z. Mays, S.M. Arzola, L.H. Yoder, S.A. Dramiga, K.M. Leclerc, J.R. Caton, R.L. Sheffler, and M.U. Nowlin. 2003. Research and commentary: Change in exercise tolerance, activity and sleep patterns, and quality of life in patients with cancer participating in a structured exercise program. *Oncol Nurs Forum* 30(3): 441-454; discussion 441-454.

Young-McCaughan, S., and D.L. Sexton. 1991. A retrospective investigation of the relationship between aerobic exercise and quality of life in women with breast cancer. *Oncol Nurs Forum* 18(4): 751-757.

CHAPTER 19

AHA Science Advisory. 2000. Assessment of functional capacity in clinical and research applications. An advisory from the committee on Exercise, Rehabilitation and Prevention, Council on Clinical Cardiology, American Heart Association. *Circulation* 102: 1591-1597.

Akiba, T., N. Matsui, S. Shinohar, H. Fujiwara, T. Nomura, and F. Marumo. 1995. Effects of recombinant erythropoeitin and exercise training on exercise capacity in hemodialysis patients. *Artif Organs* 19(12): 1262-1268.

Basset, D.R., and E.T. Howley. 2000. Limiting factors for maximum oxygen uptake and determinants of endurance performance. *Med Sci Sports Exerc* 32(1): 70-84.

Beddhu, S., L.M. Pappas, N. Ramkumar, and M. Samore. 2003. Effects of body size and body composition on survival in hemodialysis patients. *J Am Soc Nephrol* 14(9): 2366-2372.

Bevan, M. 2000. The older person with renal failure. *Nursing Standard* 14: 48-52.

Bhatnagar, V. 1998. Ethical issues involved in dialysis for the elderly. *Ger Nephrol Urol* 8(2): 111-114.

Blake, K., M.B. Codd, A. Cassidy, and Y.M. O'Meara. 2000. Physical function, employment and quality of life in end stage renal disease. *J Nephrol* 13: 15-22.

Bommer, J. 1992. Medical complications of the long term dialysis patient. In *Oxford textbook of clinical nephrology,* eds. S. Cameron, A. Davidson, J.P. Grufeld, D. Kerr, and E. Ritz. New York: Oxford University Press.

Bradley, R.J., J.R. Anderson, D.B. Evans, and A.J. Cowley. 1990. Impaired nutritive skeletal muscle blood flow in patients with chronic renal failure. *Clin Sci* 79: 239-245.

Brautbar, N. 1983. Skeletal myopathy in uremia: Abnormal energy metabolism. *Kidney Int* 16: S81-S86.

Cappy, S.C., J. Jablonka, and E.T. Schroeder. 1999. The effects of exercise during hemodialysis on physical performance and nutrition assessment. *J Ren Nutr* 9(2): 63-70.

Carnney, R.M., B. Templeton, B.A. Hong, H.R. Harter, J.M. Hagberg, K.B. Schechtman, and A.P. Goldberg. 1987. Exercise training reduces depression and increases the performance of pleasant activities in hemodialysis patients. *Nephron* 47: 194-198.

Castaneda, C., P.L. Gordon, K.L. Uhlin, A.S. Levey, J.J. Kehayias, J.T. Dwyer, R.A. Fielding, R. Roubenoff, and M.F. Singh. 2001. Resistance training to counteract the catabolism of a low-protein diet in patients with chronic renal insufficiency: A randomized, controlled trial. *Ann Intern Med* 135(11): 965-976.

Chester, A.C., T.A. Rakowski, and W.P. Argy. 1979. Haemodialysis in the eighth and ninth decades of life. *Arch Intern Med* 139: 1001-1005.

Deligiannis, A., E. Kouidi, and A. Tourkantonis. 1999a. Effects of physical training on heart rate variability in patients on hemodialysis. *Am J Cardiol* 84(15): 197-202.

Deligiannis, A., E. Kouidi, E. Tassoulas, P. Gigis, A. Tourkantonis, and A. Coats. 1999b. Cardiac effects of exercise rehabilitation in hemodialysis patients. *Int J Cardiol* 70: 253-266.

Department of Health Renal Team. 2004. *National service framework for renal services part one: Dialysis and transplantation.* London: Department of Health.

DePaul, V., J. Moreland, T. Eager, and C.M. Clase. 2002. The effectiveness of aerobic and muscle strength training in patients receiving hemodialysis and EPO: A randomised controlled trial. *Am J Kidney Dis* 40(6): 1229-1229.

Diaz-Buxo, J., E.G. Lowrie, N.L. Lew, H. Zhang, and J.M. Lazarus. 2000. Quality of life evaluation using short form 36: Comparison in hemodialysis and peritoneal dialysis patients. *Am J Kidney Dis* 35(2): 293-300.

Diesel, W., M. Emms, B.K. Knight, T.D. Noakes, C. Swanepoel, R. van Zyl Smit, R.O.C. Kascula, and C.C. Sinclair-Smith. 1993. Morphologic features of the myopathy associated with chronic renal failure. *Am J Kidney Dis* 22(5): 677-684.

Diesel, W., T. Noakes, C. Swanepoel, and M. Lambert. 1990. Isokinetic muscle strength predicts maximum exercise tolerance in renal patients on chronic haemodialysis. *Am J Kidney Dis* 16: 109-114.

Evans, R.W., D.L. Manninen, L.P. Garrison, L.G. Hart, C.R. Blagg, R.A. Gutman, A.R. Hull, and E.G. Lowrie. 1985. The quality of life of patients with end stage renal disease. *N Engl J Med* 312: 553-559.

Gleeson, N.P., P.F. Naish, J.E. Wilcock, and T.H. Mercer. 2002. Reliability of indices of neuromuscular leg performance in end-stage renal disease. *J Rehab Med* 34(6): 273-277.

Goldberg, P.A., E.M. Geltman, J.M. Hagberg, J.R. Gavin, J.A. Delmez, R.M. Carney, A. Naumowicz, M.H. Oldfield, and H.R. Harter. 1983. Therapeutic benefits of exercise training for haemodialysis patients. *Kidney Int* 16: S303-S309.

Greene, M.C., P.M. Zabetakis, G.W. Gleim, F.L. Pasternak, A.J. Saratini, M.F. Michelis, and J.A. Nicholas. 1979. Effect of exercise on lipid metabolism and dietary intake in hemodialysis patients. *Proc Dial Transplant Forum* 9: 80-85.

Hagberg, J.M., A.P. Goldberg, A.A. Ehsani, G.W. Heath, J.A. Delmez, and H.R. Harter. 1983. Exercise training improves hypertension in hemodialysis patients. *Am J Nephrol* 3: 209-212.

Headley, A., M. Germain, P. Mailloux, J. Mulhern, B. Ashworth, J. Burris, B. Brewer, B. Nindl, M. Coughlin, R. Welles, and M. Jones. 2002. Resistance training improves strength and functional measures in patients with end stage renal disease. *Am J Kidney Dis* 40(2): 355-364.

Heiwe, S., A. Tollback, and N. Clyne. 2001. Twelve weeks of exercise training increases muscle function and walking capacity in elderly predialysis patients and healthy subjects. *Nephron* 88: 48-56.

Horber, F.F., H. Hoppeler, D. Herren, H. Claassen, H. Howald, C. Gerber, and F.J. Frey. 1986. Altered skeletal muscle ultrastructure in renal transplant patients on prednisone. *Kidney Int* 30(3): 411-416.

Johansen, K.L., G.M. Chertow, A.V. Ng, K. Mulligan, S. Carey, P.Y. Schoenfeld, and J.A. Kent-Braun. 2000. Physical activity levels in patients on hemodialysis and healthy sedentary controls. *Kidney Int* 57(6): 2564-2570.

Johansen, K.L., G.M. Chertow, M. DaSilva, S. Carey, and P. Painter. 2001. Determinants of physical performance in ambulatory patients on hemodialysis. *Kidney Int* 60: 1586-1591.

Johansen, K.L., T. Schubert, J. Doyle, B. Soher, G.K. Sakkas, and J.A. Kent-Braun. 2003. Muscle atrophy in patients receiving haemodialysis: Effects on muscle strength, muscle quality and physical function. *Kidney Int* 63: 291-297.

Kemp, G.J., A.V. Crowe, H.K.I. Anijeet, Q.Y. Gong, W.E. Bimson, S.P. Frostick, J.M. Bone, G.M. Bell, and J.N. Roberts. 2004. Abnormal mitochondrial function and muscle wasting but normal contractile efficiency in haemodialysed patients studied non-invasively in-vivo. *Nephrol Dial Transplant* 19(6): 1520-1527.

Konstantinidou, E., G. Koukouvou, E. Kouidi, A. Deligiannis, and A. Tourkantonis. 2002. Exercise training in patients with end stage renal disease on hemodialysis: Comparison of three rehabilitation programs. *J Rehab Med* 34: 40-45.

Kopple, J.D. 1999. Pathophysiology of protein-energy wasting in chronic renal failure. *J Nutr* 129: 247S-251S

Koufaki, P. 2001. *The effect of erythropoietin therapy and exercise rehabilitation on the cardiorespiratory performance of patients with end stage renal disease*. PhD thesis. The Manchester Metropolitan University.

Koufaki, P., T.H. Mercer, and P.F. Naish. 2001. Dialysis mode does not affect exercise intolerance of patients with end stage renal disease. *Clin Exerc Physiol* 3: 154-160.

Koufaki, P., T.H. Mercer, and P.F. Naish. 2002a. Effects of exercise training on aerobic and functional capacity of end stage renal disease patients. *Clin Physiol Funct Im* 22: 115-124.

Koufaki, P., T.H. Mercer, and P.F. Naish. 2002b. Evaluation of efficacy of exercise training in patients with chronic disease. *Med Sci Sports Exerc* 34(8): 1234-1241.

Kouidi, E., M. Albanis, K. Natsis, A. Megalopoulos, P. Gigis, O. Tziampiri, A. Tourkantonis, and A. Deligiannis. 1998. The effects of exercise training on muscle atrophy in haemodialysis patients. *Nephrol Dial Transplant* 13: 685-699.

Kouidi, E., D. Grekas, A. Deligiannis, and A. Tourkantonis. 2004. Outcomes of long term exercise training in dialysis patients: Comparison of two training programs. *Clin Nephrol* 61: S31-S38.

Kouidi, E., A. Iacovides, P. Iordanidis, S. Vassiliou, A. Deligiannis, C. Ierodiakonou, and A. Tourkantonis. 1997. Exercise renal rehabilitation program: Psychosocial effects. *Nephron* 77: 152-158.

Kutner, N., D., Brogan, and B. Fielding. 1997. Physical and psychosocial resource variables related to long-term survival in older dialysis patients. *Ger Nephrol Urol* 6: 81-88.

Lo, C., L. Li, W.K. Lo, M.L. Chan, E. So, S. Tang, M.C. Yuen, I.K. Cheng, and T.M. Chan. 1998. Benefits of exercise training in patients on continuous ambulatory peritoneal dialysis. *Am J Kidney Dis* 32(6): 1011-1018.

Mercer, T.H. 2001. Reproducibility of blood lactate-anchored ratings of perceived exertion. *Eur J Appl Physiol* 85(5): 496-499.

Mercer, T.H., P. Koufaki, and P.F. Naish. 2004. Nutritional status, functional capacity and exercise rehabilitation in end stage renal disease. *Clin Nephrol S1* 61(1): S54-S59.

Mercer, T.H., P.F. Naish, N.P. Gleeson, and C. Crawford. 2002. Low volume exercise rehabilitation improves functional capacity and self reported functional status of dialysis patients. *Am J Phys Med Rehab* 81: 162-167.

Mercer, T.H., P.F. Naish, N.P. Gleeson, J.E. Wilcock, and C. Crawford. 1998. Development of a walking test for the assessment of functional capacity in non-anaemic maintenance dialysis patients. *Nephrol Dial Transplant* 13: 2023-2026.

Meyer, K. 2001. Exercise training in heart failure: Recommendations based on current research. *Med Sci Sports Exerc* 33(4): 525-531.

Miller, B.W., C.L. Cress, M.E. Johnson, D.H. Nichols, and M.A. Schnitzler. 2002. Exercise during hemodialysis decreases the use of antihypertensive medications. *Am J Kidney Dis* 39(4): 828-833.

Moore, G.E. 2000. Integrated gas exchange response: Chronic renal failure. In *Pulmonary and peripheral gas exchange in health and disease,* pp. 649-684, eds. J. Roca, R. Rodriguez-Roisin, and P.D. Wagner. Lung Biology in Health and Disease, C. Lenfant (series ed.), vol. 148. New York: Marcel Dekker.

Moore, G.E., L.A. Bertocci, and P.L. Painter. 1993a. ^{31}P-Magnetic resonance spectroscopy assessment of subnormal oxidative metabolism in skeletal muscle of renal failure patients. *J Clin Inves* 91: 420-424.

Moore, G.E., K.R. Brinker, J. Stray-Gundersen, and J.H. Mitchell. 1993b. Determinants of VO_2peak in patients with end stage renal disease: On and off dialysis. *Med Sci Sports Exerc* 25(1): 18-23.

Moore, G.E., D.B. Parsons, J.S. Gundersen, P.L. Painter, K.R. Brinker, and J.H. Mitchell. 1993c. Uraemic myopathy limits aerobic capacity in haemodialysis patients. *Am J Kidney Dis* 22(2): 277-287.

Myers, J., M. Prakash, V. Froelicher, D. Dot, S. Partington, and J.E. Atwood. 2002. Exercise capacity and mortality among men referred for exercise testing. *N Engl J Med* 346(11): 793-801.

Naish, P.F., T.H. Mercer, P. Koufaki, and J.E. Wilcock. 2000. VO_2peak underestimates physical dysfunction in elderly dialysis patients. *Med Sci Sports Exerc* 32(5): S160.

National Kidney Foundation. 2002. KDOQI clinical practice guidelines for chronic kidney disease: Evaluation, classification, and stratification. Kidney Disease Outcome Quality Initiative. *Am J Kidney Dis* 39(2 Suppl. 2): S1-S246.

Ota, S., K. Takashashi, H. Suzuki, S. Nishimura, H. Makino, Z. Ota, K. Taniai, and T. Kaneshige. 1996. Exercise rehabilitation for elderly patients on chronic hemodialysis. *Ger Nephrol Urol* 5: 157-165.

Painter, P. 1993. End-stage renal disease. In *Exercise testing and prescription for special cases,* 2nd ed., pp. 352-362, ed. J.S. Skinner. Baltimore: Williams & Wilkins.

Painter, P. 1999. Exercise after renal transplantation. *Adv Ren Replace Ther* 6(2): 159-164.

Painter, P., L. Carlson, S. Carey, S.P. Paul, and J. Myll. 2000. Physical functioning and health related quality of life changes with exercise training in haemodialysis patients. *Am J Kidney Dis* 35(3): 482-492.

Painter, P., D. Messer-Rehak, P. Hanson, S.W. Zimmerman, and N.R. Glass. 1986a. Exercise capacity in hemodialysis, CAPD, and renal transplant patients. *Nephron* 42: 47-51.

Painter, P., J.N. Nelson-Worel, M.M. Hill, D.R. Thornbery, R. Shelp, A.R. Harrington, and A.B. Weinstein. 1986b. Effects of exercise training during haemodialysis. *Nephron* 43: 87-92.

Porter, M.M., A.A. Vandervoort, and J. Lexell. 1995. Aging of human muscle: Structure, function and adaptability. *Scand J Med Sci Sports* 5: 129-142.

Rayner, H.C., R.L. Pisoni, J. Bommer, B. Canaud, E. Hecking, F. Locatelli, L. Piera, J.L. Bragg-Gresham, H.I. Feldman, D.A. Goodkin, B. Gillespie, R.A. Wolfe, P.J. Held, and F.K. Port. 2004. Mortality and hospitalization in haemodialysis patients in five European countries: Results from the Dialysis Outcomes and Practice Patterns Study (DOPPS). *Nephrol Dial Transplant* 19(1): 108-112.

Sakkas, G.K., D. Ball, T.H. Mercer, A.J. Sargeant, K. Tolfrey, and P.F. Naish. 2003a. Atrophy of non-locomotor muscle in patients with end-stage renal failure. *Nephrol Dial Transplant* 18(10): 2074-2078.

Sakkas, G.K., A.J. Sargeant, T.H. Mercer, D. Ball, P. Koufaki, C. Karatzaferi, and P.F. Naish. 2003b. Changes in muscle morphology in dialysis patients after 6 months of aerobic exercise training. *Nephrol Dial Transplant* 18(9): 1854-1861.

Sietsema, K.E., E.R. Hiatt, A. Esler, S.G. Adler, A. Amato, and E.P. Brass. 2002. Clinical and demographic predictors of exercise capacity in end stage renal disease. *Am J Kidney Dis* 39(1): 76-85.

Sietsema, K.E., A. Amato, S.G. Adler, and E.P. Brass. 2004. Exercise capacity as a predictor of survival among ambulatory patients with end stage renal disease. *Kidney Int* 65: 719-724.

Sims, R.J.A., M.J.D. Cassid, and T. Masud. 2003. The increasing numbers of older patients with renal disease. *Brit Med J* 327: 463-464.

Stack, A.G., and J.M. Messana. 2000. Renal replacement therapy in the elderly: Medical, ethical and psychosocial considerations. *Adv Ren Replace Ther* 7(1): 52-62.

Stephens, R., A. Williams, T. McKnight, and S. Dodd. 1991. Effects of self-monitored exercise on selected blood chemistry parameters of end stage renal disease patients. *Am J Phys Med Rehabil* 70(3): 149-153.

Sugawara, J., M. Myachi, K.L. Moreau, F.A. Dinenno, C.A. DeSouza, and H. Tanaka. 2002. Age-related reduction in appendicular skeletal muscle mass: Association with habitual physical activity. *Clin Physiol Funct Im* 22: 169-172.

Tawney, K.W., P.J.W. Tawney, G. Hladik, S.L. Hogan, R.J. Falk, C. Weaver, D.T. Moore, and M.Y. Lee. 2000. The life readiness program: A physical rehabilitation program for patients on haemodialysis. *Am J Kidney Dis* 36(3): 581-591.

Tawney, K.W., P.J.W. Tawney, and J. Kovach. 2003. Disablement and rehabilitation in end-stage renal disease. *Sem Dial* 16(6): 447-452.

U.K. Renal Registry. 2002. *UK Renal Registry, fourth annual report,* eds. D. Ansell, T. Feest, and C. Byrne. Bristol, UK: U.K. Renal Registry.

U.S. Renal Data System. 2001. USRDS 2001 annual data report: Atlas of end-stage renal disease in the United States. Bethesda, MD: National Institutes of Health, National Institute of Diabetes and Digestive and Kidney Diseases.

U.S. Renal Data System. 2002. United States Renal Data System Web site. Point prevalence rates of reported end-stage renal disease, adjusted. Available online at www.usrds.org/2002/pdf/a.pdf. Accessed March 12, 2005.

Winearls, C. 1999. Crisis in renal replacement service provision. *Brit J Ren Med* 4(1): 1-6.

Zabetakis, P.M., G.W. Gleim, F.L. Pasternack, A. Saraniti, J.A. Nicholas, and M.F. Michelis. 1982. Long duration submaximal exercise conditioning in hemodialysis patients. *Clin Nephrol* 18(1): 17-22.

CHAPTER 20

Ades, P.A., D.L. Ballor, T. Ashikaga, J.L. Utton, and K. Sreekumaran. 1996. Weight training improves walking endurance in healthy elderly persons. *Ann Int Med* 124: 568-572.

Alexander, N., A.B. Schultz, and D.N. Warwick. 1991. Rising from a chair: Effects of age and functional ability on performance biomechanics. *J Gerontol* 46: M91-M98.

American College of Sports Medicine. 1998. Position Stand: Exercise and physical activity for older adults. *Med Sci Sports Exerc* 30(6): 992-1008.

Anderson, K., and L. Hermansen. 1965. Aerobic work capacity in middle-aged Norwegian men. *J Appl Physiol* 20: 432-436.

Aniansson, A., G. Grimby, and A. Rundgren. 1980. Isometric and isokinetic quadriceps muscle strength in 70-year old men and women. *Scand J Rehab Med* 12: 161-168.

Bassey, E.J., M.A. Fiatarone, E.F. O'Neil, M. Kelly, W.J. Evans, and L.A. Lipsitz. 1992. Leg extensor power and functional erformance in very old men and women. *Clin Sci* 82: 321-327.

Bean, J.F., S. Herman, D.K. Kiely, D. Callahan, K. Mizer, W.R. Frontera, and R.A. Fielding. 2002a. Weighted stair climbing in mobility limited elders: A pilot study. *J Am Geriatr Soc* 50: 663-670.

Bean, J.F., S. Herman, D.K. Kiely, I.C. Frey, S.G. Leveille, R.A. Fielding, and W.R. Frontera. 2003a. Increased velocity exercise specific to task (InVEST) training: A pilot study exploring effects on leg power, balance and mobility in community-dwelling older women. *J Am Geriatr Soc* 52(5): 799-804.

Bean, J.F., D.K. Kiely, S. Herman, S.G. Leveille, K. Mizer, W.R. Frontera, and R.A. Fielding. 2002b. The relationship between leg power and physical performance in mobility limited elders. *J Am Geriatr Soc* 50: 461-467.

Bean, J.F., S.G. Leveille, D.K. Kiely, S. Bandinelli, J.M. Guralnik, and L. Ferrucci. 2003b. A comparison of leg power and leg strength within the InCHIANTI study: Which influences mobility more? *J Gerontol Med Sci* 58A(8): 728-733.

Bean, J.F., A. Vora, and W.R. Frontera. 2004. The benefits of exercise for community-dwelling older adults. *Arch Phys Med Rehabil* 85(7 Suppl 3): S31-S42.

Beniamini, Y., J.J. Rubenstein, A.D. Faigenbaum, A.H. Lichtenstein, and M.C. Crim. 1999. High-intensity strength training of patients enrolled in an outpatient cardiac rehabilitation program. *J Cardiopulm Rehabil* 19(1): 8-17.

Beniamini, Y., J.J. Rubenstein, and L.D. Zaichowsky. 1997. Effects of high-intensity strength training on quality-of-life parameters in cardiac rehabilitation patients. *Am J Cardiol* 80: 841-846.

Bevier, W., R. Wiswell, G. Pyka, K. Kozak, K. Newhall, and R. Marcus. 1989. Relationship of body composition, muscle strength, and aerobic capacity to bone mineral density in older men and women. *J Bone Miner Res* 4: 421-432.

Borg, G. 1998. *Borg's perceived exertion and pain scales*. Champaign, IL: Human Kinetics.

Borkan, G., and A. Norris. 1977. Fat redistribution and the changing body dimensions of the adult male. *Human Biol* 49: 495-514.

Bortz, W.M. 1989. Redefining human aging. *J Am Geriatr Soc* 37: 1092-1096.

Brown, A.B., N. McCartney, and D.G. Sale. 1990. Positive adaptations to weight-lifting training in the elderly. *J Appl Physiol* 69: 1725-1733.

Brown, M., D.R. Sinacore, and H. Host. 1995. The relationship of strength to function in the older adult. *J Gerontol* 50A: 55-59.

Buchner, D.M. 1993. Understanding variability in studies of strength training in older adults: A meta-analytic perspective. *Top Geriatr Rehabil* 8: 1.

Buchner, D.M., S.A. Beresford, E.B. Larson, A.Z. LaCroix, and E.H. Wagner. 1992. Effects of physical activity on health status in older adults II: Intervention studies. *Annu Rev Publ Health* 13: 469-488.

Buchner, D.M., M.E. Cress, B.J. de Lateur, P.C. Esselman, A.J. Margherita, R. Price, and E.H. Wagner. 1997. The effect of strength and endurance training on gait, balance, fall risk, and health services use in community-living older adults. *J Gerontol A Biol Soc Med Sci* 52(4): M218-M224.

Buchner, D.M., and B.J. de Lateur. 1991. The importance of skeletal muscle strength to physical function in older adults. *Ann Behav Med* 13: 91-98.

Buchner, D.M., E.B. Larson, E.H. Wagner, T.D. Koepsell, and B.J. de Lateur. 1996. Evidence for a non-linear relationship between leg strength and gait speed. *Age Ageing* 25: 386-391.

Campion, E.W. 1994. The oldest old. *N Engl J Med* 330: 1819-1820.

Cartee, G.D. 1994. Aging skeletal muscle: Response to exercise. In *Exercise and sports sciences review,* ed. T.H. Grayson. Baltimore: Williams & Wilkins.

Castaneda, C., P.L. Gordon, K.L. Uhlin, A.S. Levey, J.J. Kehayias, J.T. Dwyer, R.A. Fielding, R. Roubenoff, and M.F. Singh. 2001. Resistance training to counteract the catabolism of a °low-protein diet in patients with chronic renal insufficiency: A randomized, controlled trial. *Ann Intern Med* 135(11): 965-976.

Centers for Disease Control and Prevention. 2003. Trends in aging—United States and worldwide. *MMWR* 52(6): 101-106.

Chandler, J.M., P.W. Duncan, G. Kochersberger, and S. Studenski. 1998. Is lower extremity strength gain associated with improvement in physical performance and disability in frail, community-dwelling elders? *Arch Phys Med Rehabil* 79(1): 24-30.

Cohn, S.H., D. Vartsky, S. Yasumura, A. Sawitsky, I. Zanzi, A. Vaswani, and K.J. Ellis. 1980. Compartmental body composition based on total-body, potassium, and calcium. *Am J Physiol* 239(6): E524-E530.

Commonwealth Fund Commission. 1988. Aging alone: Profiles and projections. In *The Commonwealth Fund Commission on Elderly People Living Alone*. New York: Commonwealth Fund Commission.

Cress, M.E., D.M. Buchner, K.A. Questad, P.C. Esselman, B.J. de Lateur, and R.S. Schwartz. 1999. Exercise: Effects on physical functional performance in independent older adults. *J Gerontol A Biol Sci Med Sci* 54(5): M242-M248.

Crippen, D.L. 2001. "Prescription drugs and Medicare financing." Statement before the Committee on Finance, U.S. Senate, 107th Congress, 1st Session, March 22, 2001. Available online www.cbo.gov/showdoc.cfm?index=2760&sequence=0. Accessed June 13, 2005.

Cunningham, D., P. Rechnitzer, M.E. Pearce, and A.P. Donner. 1982. Determinants of self-selected walking pace across ages 19-66. *J Gerontol* 37: 560-564.

Dalsky, G.P., K.S. Stocke, A.A. Ehsani, E. Slatopolsky, W.C. Lee, and S.J. Birge Jr. 1988. Weight-bearing exercise training and lumbar bone mineral content in postmenopausal women. *Ann Intern Med* 108(6): 824-828.

Damush, T.M., and J.G. Damush Jr. 1999. The effects of strength training on strength and health-related quality of life in older adult women. *Gerontologist* 39: 705-710.

Dean, C.M., C.L. Richards, and F. Malouin. 2000. Task-related circuit training improves performance of locomotor tasks in chronic stroke: A randomized, controlled pilot trial. *Arch Phys Med Rehabil* 81(4): 409-417.

Dean, C.M., and R.B. Shepherd 1997. Task-related training improves performance of seated reaching tasks after stroke. A randomized controlled trial. *Stroke* 28(4): 722-728.

Dishman, R. 1989. Determinants of physical activity and exercise for persons 65 years of age and older. In *Physical activity and aging,* ed. W. Spirduso and H. Eckert. Champaign, IL: Human Kinetics.

Dishman, R.K. 1994. Motivating older adults to exercise. *S Med J* 87: S79-S82.

Dorup, I., K. Skajaa, T. Clausen, and K. Kjeldsen. 1988. Reduced concentrations of potassium, magnesium, and sodium-potassium pumps in human skeletal muscle during treatment with diuretics. *Br Med J* 296: 455-458.

Earles, D.R., J.O. Judge, and O.T. Gunnarsson. 2001. Velocity training induces power-specific adaptations in highly functioning older adults. *Arch Phys Med Rehabil* 82(7): 872-878.

Ettinger, W.H. Jr., R. Burns, S.P. Messier, W. Applegate, W.J. Rejeski, T. Morgan, S. Shumaker, M.J. Berry, M. O'Toole, J.

Monu, and T. Craven. 1997. A randomized trial comparing aerobic exercise and resistance exercise with a health education program in older adults with knee osteoarthritis. The Fitness Arthritis and Seniors Trial (FAST). *JAMA* 277(1): 25-31.

Evans, W.J. 1995. Effects of exercise on body composition and functional capacity of the elderly. *J Gerontol* 50A(Special Issue): 147-150.

Evans, W.J. 2000. Exercise strategies should be designed to increase muscle power. *J Gerontol Med Sci* 55A(6): M309-M310.

Evans, W.J., and W.W. Campbell. 1993. Sarcopenia and age-related changes in body composition and functional capacity. *J Nutr* 123: 465-468.

Fiatarone, M.A., E.C. Marks, N.D. Ryan, C.N. Meredith, L.A. Lipsitz, and W.J. Evans. 1990. High-intensity strength training in nonagenarians. *JAMA* 263: 3029-3034.

Fiatarone, M.A., E.F. O'Neill, N.D. Ryan, K.M. Clements, G.R. Solares, M.E. Nelson, S.B. Roberts, J.J. Kehayias, L.A. Lipsitz, and W.J. Evans. 1994. Exercise training and nutritional supplementation for physical frailty in very elderly people. *N Engl J Med* 330: 1769-1775.

Fiatarone-Singh, M.A. 2002. Exercise comes of age: Rationale and recommendations for a geriatric exercise prescription. *J Gerontol Med Sci* 57A: M262-M282.

Fielding, R.A., N.K. LeBrasseur, A. Cuoco, J. Bean, K. Mizer, M.A. Fiatarone-Singh. 2002. High-velocity power training increases skeletal muscle strength and power in community-dwelling older women. *J Am Geriatr Soc* 50(4): 655-662.

Fisher, N.M., D.R. Pendergast, and E. Calkins. 1991. Muscle rehabilitation in impaired elderly nursing home residents. *Arch Phys Med Rehabil* 72: 181-185.

Foldvari, M., M. Clark, L.C. Laviolette, M.A. Bernstein, D. Kaliton, C. Castaneda, C.T. Pu, J.M. Hausdorff, R.A. Fielding, and M.A. Singh. 2000. Association of muscle power with functional status in community-dwelling elderly women. *J Gerontol A Biol Sci Med Sci* 55(4): M192-M199.

Forbes, G.B. 1999. Longitudinal changes in adult fat-free mass: Influence of body weight. *Am J Clin Nutr* 70(6): 1025-1031.

Frontera, W.R., and J.F. Bean. 2004. *Strength and power training: A guide for adults of all ages*. Stamford, CT: Harvard Medical School.

Frontera, W.R., V.A. Hughes, K.J. Lutz, and W.J. Evans. 1991. A cross-sectional study of muscle strength and mass in 45- to 78-yr-old men and women. *J Appl Physiol* 71: 644-650.

Frontera, W.R., C.N. Meredith, K.P. O'Reilly, H.G. Knuttgen, and W.J. Evans. 1988. Strength conditioning in older men: Skeletal muscle hypertrophy and improved function. *J Appl Physiol* 64(3): 1038-1044.

Frontera, W.R., D. Suh, L.S. Krivickas, V.A. Hughes, R. Goldstein, and R. Roubenoff. 2000. Skeletal muscle fiber quality in older men and women. *Am J Physiol Cell Physiol* 279(3): C611-C618.

Galbo, H. 1983. *Hormonal and metabolic adaptations to exercise*. New York: Thieme Verlag.

Gallagher, D., E. Ruts, M. Visser, S. Heshka, R.N. Baumgartner, J. Wang, R.N. Pierson, F.X. Pi-Sunyer, and S.B. Heymsfield. 2000. Weight stability masks sarcopenia in elderly men and women. *Am J Physiol Endocrinol Metab* 279(2): E366-E375.

Ghilarducci, L., R. Holly, and E.A. Amsterdam. 1989. Effects of high resistance training in coronary artery disease. *Am J Cardiol* 64: 866-870.

Gill, T.M., D.I. Baker, M. Gottschalk, E.A. Gahbauer, P.A. Charpentier, P.T. de Regt, and S.J. Wallace. 2003. A prehabilitation program for physically frail community-living older persons. *Arch Phys Med Rehabil* 84(3): 394-404.

Gill, T.M., D.I. Baker, M. Gottschalk, P.N. Peduzzi, H. Allore, and A. Byers. 2002. A program to prevent functional decline in physically frail, elderly persons who live at home. *N Engl J Med* 347(14): 1068-1074.

Gill, T.M., C.S. Williams, and M.E. Tinetti. 1995. Assessing risk for the onset of functional dependence among older adults: The role of physical performance. *J Am Geriatr Soc* 43: 603-609.

Green, J.S., and S.F. Crouse. 1995. The effects of endurance training on functional capacity in the elderly: A meta-analysis. *Med Sci Sports Exerc* 27: 920-926.

Grembowski, D., D. Patrick, P. Diehr, M. Durham, S. Beresford, E. Kay, and J. Hecht. 1993. Self-efficacy and health behavior among older adults. *J Health Soc Behav* 34: 89-104.

Grimby, G., and B. Saltin. 1966. Physiological analysis of physically well trained middle-aged and old athletes. *J Appl Physiol* 179: 513-526.

Guralnik, J.M., L. Ferrucci, C.F. Pieper, S.G. Leveille, K.S. Markides, G.V. Ostir, S. Studenski, L.F. Berkman, and R.B. Wallace. 2000. Lower extremity function and subsequent disability: Consistency across studies, predictive models, and value of gait speed alone compared with the short physical performance battery. *J Gerontol Med Sci* 55A(4): M221-M231.

Guralnik, J.M., L. Ferrucci, E.M. Simonsick, M.E. Salive, and R.B. Wallace. 1995. Lower-extremity function in persons over the age of 70 years as a predictor of subsequent disability. *N Engl J Med* 332: 556-561.

Guralnik, J.M., A. LaCroix, L.G. Branch, S.V. Kasl, and R.B. Wallace. 1991. Morbidity and disability in older persons in the years prior to death. *Am J Publ Health* 81: 443-447.

Guralnik, J.M., E.M. Simonsick, L. Ferrucci, R.J. Glynn, L.F. Berkman, D.G. Blazer, P.A. Scherr, and R.B. Wallace. 1994. A short physical performance battery assessing lower extremity function: Association with self-reported disability and prediction of mortality and nursing home admission. *J Gerontol* 29: M85-M94.

Hagberg, J. 1987. Effect of training on the decline of VO_2max with aging. *Fed Proc* 46: 1830.

Hakkinen, K., W.J. Kraemer, R.U. Newton, and M. Alen. 2001. Changes in electromyographic activity, muscle fibre and force production characteristics during heavy resistance/power strength training in middle-aged and older men and women. *Acta Physiol Scand* 171(1): 51-62.

Haley, S.M., A.M. Jette, W.J. Coster, J.T. Kooyoomjian, S. Levenson, T. Heeren, and J. Ashba. 2002. Late life function and disability instrument: II. Development and evaluation of the function component. *J Gerontol A Biol Sci Med Sci* 57(4): M217-M222.

Harman, D. 2001. Aging: Overview. *Ann NY Acad Sci* 928: 1-21.

Harper, C.M., and Y.M. Lyles. 1988. Physiology and complications of bed rest. *J Am Geriatr Soc* 36: 1047-1054.

Harridge, S., G. Magnussen, and B. Saltin. 1997. Life-long endurance-trained elderly men have high aerobic power but have similar muscle strength to non-active elderly men. *Aging Clin Exp Res* 9: 80-87.

Heath, G.W., J.M. Hagberg, A.A. Ehsani, and J.O. Holloszy. 1981. A physiological comparison of young and older endurance athletes. *J Appl Physiol* 51: 634-640.

Hopp, J.F. 1993. Effects of age and resistance training on skeletal muscle: A review. *Phys Ther* 73: 361-373.

Hubert, H., D. Bloch, and J.A. Fries. 1993. Risk factors for physical disability in an aging cohort: The NHANES I epidemiologic follow-up study. *J Rheumatol* 20: 480-488.

Hughes, V.A., W.R. Frontera, R. Roubenoff, W.J. Evans, and M.A. Singh. 2002. Longitudinal changes in body composition in older men and women: Role of body weight change and physical activity. *Am J Clin Nutr* 76(2): 473-81.

Jette, A.M. 1997. Disablement outcomes in geriatric rehabilitation. *Med Care* 35(6): JS28-JS37.

Jette, A.M., and L.G. Branch. 1981. The Framingham disability study: II physical disability among the aging. *Am J Publ Health* 71: 1211-1216.

Jette, A.M., S.M. Haley, W.J. Coster, J.T. Kooyoomjian, S. Levenson, T. Heeren, and J. Ashba. 2002. Late life function and disability instrument: I. Development and evaluation of the disability component. *J Gerontol A Biol Sci Med Sci* 57(4): M209-M216.

Jette, A.M., B.A. Harris, L. Sleeper, M.E. Lachman, D. Heislan, M. Giorgetti, and C. Levenson. 1996. A home-based exercise program for nondisabled older adults. *J Am Geriatr Soc* 44: 644-649.

Jette, A.M., M. Lachman, M.M. Giorgetti, S.F. Assmann, B.A. Harris, C. Levenson, M. Wernick, and D. Krebs. 1999. Exercise—it's never too late: The strong-for-life program. *Am J Public Health* 89(1): 66-72.

Jozsi, A.C., W.W. Campbell, L. Joseph, S.L. Davey, and W.J. Evans. 1999. Changes in power with resistance training in older and younger men and women. *J Gerontol A Biol Sci Med Sci* 54(11): M591-M596.

Judge, J.O., C. Lindsey, M. Underwood, and D. Winsemius. 1993. Balance improvements in older women: Effects of exercise training. *Phys Ther* 73: 254-264.

Judge, J.O., M. Underwood, and T. Gennosa. 1992. Exercise to improve gait velocity in older persons. *Arch Phys Med Rehabil* 74(4): 400-406.

Judge, J.O., R.H. Whipple, and L.I. Wolfson. 1994. Effects of resistive and balance exercises on isokinetic strength in older persons. *J Am Geriatr Soc* 42(9): 937-946.

Kehayias, J.J., M.A. Fiatarone, H. Zhuang, and R. Roubenoff. 1997. Total body potassium and body fat: Relevance to aging. *Am J Clin Nutr* 66(4): 904-910.

Kemper, P., and C. Murtaugh. 1991. Lifetime use of nursing home care. *N Engl J Med* 324: 595-600.

Keysor, J.J., and A.M. Jette. 2001. Have we oversold the benefit of late-life exercise? *J Gerontol A Biol Sci Med Sci* 56(7): M412-M423.

King, A.C., L.A. Pruitt, W. Phillips, R. Oka, A. Rodenburg, and W.L. Haskell. 2000. Comparative effects of two physical activity programs on measured and perceived physical functioning and other health-related quality of life outcomes in older adults. *J Gerontol A Biol Sci Med Sci* 55(2): M74-M83.

Klitgaard, H., M. Mantoni, S. Schiaffino, S. Ausoni, L. Gorza, C. Laurent-Winter, and P. Schnohr. 1990. Function, morphology and protein expression of ageing, skeletal muscle: A cross sectional study of elderly men with different training backgrounds. *Acta Physiol Scand* 140: 41-54.

Kohrt, W., M. Malley, A.R. Coggan, R.J. Spina, T. Ogawa, A.A. Ehsani, R.E. Bourney, W.H. Martin, and J.O. Holloszy. 1991. Effects of gender, age, and fitness level on response of VO_2max to training in 60 to 71-yr-olds. *J Appl Physiol* 71: 2004-2011.

Kovar, P.A., J.P. Allegrante, C.R. MacKenzie, M.G. Peterson, B. Gutin, and M.E. Charlson. 1992. Supervised fitness walking in patients with osteoarthritis of the knee: A randomized, controlled trial. *Ann Intern Med* 116(7): 529-534.

Lakatta, E. 1990. Changes in cardiovascular function with aging. *Eur Heart J* 11(Suppl C): 22.

Larsson, L. 1982. Physical training effects on muscle morphology in sedentary males at different ages. *Med Sci Sports Exerc* 14: 203-206.

Larsson, L., G. Grimby, and J. Karlsson. 1979. Muscle strength and speed of movement in relation to age and muscle morphology. *J Appl Physiol* 46: 451-456.

Latham, N.K., D.A. Bennett, C.M. Stretton, and C.S. Anderson. 2004. Systematic review of progressive resistance strength training in older adults. *J Gerontol A Biol Sci Med Sci* 59(1): 48-61.

Layne, J.E., and M.E. Nelson. 1999. The effects of progressive resistance training on bone density: A review. *Med Sci Sports Exerc* 31(1): 25-30.

Lazowski, D.A., N.A. Ecclestone, A.M. Myers, D.H. Paterson, C. Tudor-Locke, C. Fitzgerald, G. Jones, N. Shima, and D.A. Cunningham. 1999. A randomized outcome evaluation of group exercise programs in long-term care institutions. *J Gerontol A Biol Sci Med Sci* 54(12): M621-M628.

Levy, W.C., M.D. Cerqueira, I.B. Abrass, R.S. Schwartz, and J.R. Stratton. 1993. Endurance exercise training augments diastolic filling at rest and during exercise in healthy young and older men. *Circulation* 88: 116-126.

Lexell, J., K. Henriksson-Larsen, and M. Sjostrom. 1983a. Distribution of different fibre types in human skeletal muscles. 2. A study of cross sections of whole m. vastus lateralis. *Acta Physiol Scand* 117: 115-122.

Liao, Y., D.L. McGee, G. Cao, and R.S. Cooper. 2001. Recent changes in the health status of the older U.S. population: findings from the 1984 and 1994 supplement on aging. *J Am Geriatr Soc* 49(4): 443-449.

Limacher, M.C. 1994. Aging and cardiac function: Influence of exercise. *S Med J* 87: S13-S16.

Lord, S.R., D.G. Lloyd, M. Nirui, J. Raymond, P. Williams, and R.A. Stewart. 1996a. The effect of exercise on gait patterns in older women: A randomized controlled trial. *J Gerontol* 51A: M64-M70.

Lord, S.R., J.A. Ward, and P. Williams. 1996b. Exercise effect on dynamic stability in older women: A randomized controlled trial. *Arch Phys Med Rehabil* 77: 232-236.

Lord, S.R., J. Ward, P. Williams, and M. Strudwick. 1995. The effect of a 12-month exercise trial on balance, strength, and falls in older women: A randomized controlled trial. *J Am Geriatr Soc* 43: 1198-1206.

MacDougall, J. 1986. Adaptability of muscle to strength training: A cellular approach. In *Biochemistry of exercise VI,* ed. B. Saltin. Champaign, IL: Human Kinetics.

Marcell, T.J. 2003. Sarcopenia: Causes, consequences, and preventions. *J Gerontol A Biol Sci Med Sci* 58(10): M911-M916.

McMurdo, M.E., and R. Johnstone. 1995. A randomized controlled trial of a home exercise programme for elderly people with poor mobility. *Age Ageing* 24(5): 425-428.

Meredith, C., W. Frontera, E.C. Fisher, V.A. Hughes, J.C. Herland, J. Edwards, and W.J. Evans. 1989. Peripheral effects of endurance training in young and old subjects. *J Appl Physiol* 66: 2844-2849.

Metter, E.J., R. Conwit, J. Tobin, and J.L. Fozard. 1997. Age associated loss of power and strength in the upper extremities in women and men. *J Gerontol A Bio Sci Med Sci* 52(5): B267-B276.

Miller, R.A. 1994. The biology of aging and longevity. In *Principles of geriatric medicine and gerontology,* eds. W.R. Hazzard J.P. Glass, J.B. Halter, J.G. Ouslander, and M. Tinetti. New York: McGraw-Hill.

Minor, M.A., J.E. Hewett, R.R. Webel, S.K. Anderson, and D.R. Kay. 1989. Efficacy of physical conditioning exercise in patients with rheumatoid arthritis and osteoarthritis. *Arthritis Rheum* 32(11): 1396-1405.

Miszko, T.A., M.E. Cress, J.M. Slade, C.J. Covey, S.K. Agrawal, and C.E. Doerr. 2003. Effect of strength and power training on physical function in community-dwelling older adults. *J Gerontol A Biol Sci Med Sci* 58(2): 171-175.

Monger, C., J.H. Carr, and V. Fowler. 2002. Evaluation of a home-based exercise and training programme to improve sit-to-stand in patients with chronic stroke. *Clin Rehabil* 16(4): 361-367.

Morley, J.E. 2003. Mobility performance: A high-tech test for geriatricians. *J Gerontol A Biol Sci Med Sci* 58(8): 712-714.

Morris, J.N., M. Fiatarone, D.K. Kiely, P. Belleville-Taylor, K. Murphy, S. Littlehale, W.L. Ooi, E. O'Neill, and N. Doyle. 1999. Nursing rehabilitation and exercise strategies in the nursing home. *J Gerontol A Biol Sci Med Sci* 54(10): M494-M500.

Muller, E.A. 1970. Influence of training and of inactivity on muscle strength. *Arch Phys Med Rehabil* 51: 449-461.

Nagi, S.Z. 1965. Some conceptual issues in disability and rehabilitation. In *Sociology and rehabilitation,* ed. M.B. Sussman. Washington, DC: American Sociological Society.

National Institute on Aging. 1999. *Exercise: A guide from the National Institute on Aging.* Bethesda, MD: National Institute on Aging, National Institute of Health.

Nelson, M.E., M.A. Fiatarone, C.M. Morganti, I. Trice, R.A. Greenberg, and W.J. Evans. 1994. Effects of high-intensity strength training on multiple risk factors for osteoporotic fractures. *JAMA* 272: 1909-1914.

Ogawa, T., R.J. Spina, W.H. Martin III, W.M. Kohrt, K.B. Schectman, J.O. Holloszy, and A.A. Ehsani. 1992. Effects of aging, sex, and physical training on cardiovascular responses to exercise. *Circulation* 86: 494-503.

Orlander, J., and A. Aniansson. 1980. Effects of physical training on skeletal muscle metabolism and ultrastructure in 70 to 75 year old men. *Acta Physiol Scand* 109: 149-154.

Ory, M.G., K.B. Schechtman, P. Miller, E. Hadley, M.A. Fiatarone, M.A. Province, C.L. Arfken, D. Morgan, S. Weiss, and M. Kaplan, for the FICSIT Group. 1993. Frailty and injuries in later life: The FICSIT trials. *J Am Geriatr Soc* 41: 283-296.

Parizkova, J. 1974. Body composition and exercise during growth and development. In *Physical activity: Human growth and development,* ed. G. Rarick. New York: Academic Press.

Penninx, B.W., S.P. Messier, W.J. Rejeski, J.D. Williamson, M. DiBari, C. Cavazzini, W.B. Applegate, and M. Pahor. 2001. Physical exercise and the prevention of disability in activities of daily living in older persons with osteoarthritis. *Arch Intern Med* 161(19): 2309-2316.

Pimentel, A.E., C.L. Gentile, H. Tanaka, D.R. Seals, and P.E. Gates. 2003. Greater rate of decline in maximal aerobic capacity with age in endurance-trained than in sedentary men. *J Appl Physiol* 94(6): 2406-2413.

Pocock, N., J. Eisman, T. Gwinn, P. Sambrook, P. Kelley, J. Friend, and M. Yeates. 1989. Muscle strength, physical fitness and weight but not age predict femoral neck bone mass. *J Bone Miner Res* 4: 441-448.

Pollock, M.L., J.F. Carroll, J.E. Graves, S.H. Leggett, R.W. Braith, M. Limacher, and J.M. Hagberg. 1991. Injuries and adherence to walk/jog and resistance training programs in the elderly. *Med Sci Sports Exerc* 23: 1194-1200.

Pollock, M.L., C. Foster, D. Knapp, J.L. Rod, and D.H. Schmidt. 1987. Effect of age, training, competition on aerobic capacity and body composition of masters athletes. *J Appl Physiol* 62: 725.

Pollock, M.L., J.E. Graves, D.L. Stewart, and D.T. Lowenthal. 1994. Exercise training and prescription for the elderly. *S Med J* 87: S88-S95.

Posner, J.D., K.K. McCully, L.A. Landsberg, L.P. Sands, P. Tycenski, M.T. Hofmann, K.L. Wetterholt, and C.E. Shaw. 1995. Physical determinants of independence in mature women. *Arch Phys Med Rehabil* 76: 373-380.

Province, M.A., E.C. Hadley, M.C. Hornbrook, L.A. Lipsitz, P. Miller, C.D. Mulrow, M.G. Ory, R.W. Sattin, M.E. Tinetti, and S.L. Wolf. 1995. The effects of exercise on falls in elderly patients: A preplanned meta-analysis of the FICSIT Trials. *JAMA* 273: 1341-1347.

Pu, C.T., M.T. Johnson, D.E. Forman, J.M. Hausdorff, R. Roubenoff, M. Foldvari, R.A. Fielding, and M.A. Singh. 2001. Randomized trial of progressive resistance training to counteract the myopathy of chronic heart failure. *J Appl Physiol* 90(6): 2341-2350.

Rantanen, T., J.M. Guralnik, L. Ferrucci, S. Leveille, and L.P. Fried. 1999. Coimpairments: Strength and balance as predictors of severe walking disability. *J Gerontol A Biol Sci Med Sci* 54(4): M172-M176.

Rantanen, T., R. Sakari-Rantala, and E. Heikkinen. 2002. Muscle strength before and mortality after a bone fracture in older people. *Scand J Med Sci Sports* 12(5): 296-300.

Rejeski, W.J., L.R. Brawley, E. McAuley, and S. Rapp. 2000. An examination of theory and behavior change in randomized clinical trials. *Control Clin Trials* 21(5 Suppl): 164S-170S.

Rejeski, W.J., and B.C. Focht. 2002. Aging and physical disability: On integrating group and individual counseling with the promotion of physical activity. *Exerc Sport Sci Rev* 30(4): 166-170.

Rejeski, W.J., M.E. Miller, C. Foy, S. Messier, and S. Rapp. 2001. Self-efficacy and the progression of functional limitations and self-reported disability in older adults with knee pain. *J Gerontol B Psychol Sci Soc Sci* 56(5): S261-S265.

Rodeheffer, R., G. Gerstenblith, L.C. Becker, J.L. Fleg, M.L. Weisfeldt, and E.G. Lakatta. 1984. Exercise cardiac output is maintained with advancing age in healthy human subjects: Cardiac dilation and increased stroke volume compensate for a diminished heart rate. *Circulation* 69(2): 203-213.

Rogers, M.A., J.M. Hagberg, W.H. Martin III, A.A. Ehsani, and J.O. Holloszy. 1990. Decline in VO_2max with aging master athletes and sedentary men. *J Appl Physiol* 68: 2195-2199.

Rooks, D.S., D.P. Kiel, C. Parsons, and W.C. Hayes. 1997. Self-paced resistance training and walking exercise in community-dwelling older adults: Effects on neuromotor performance. *J Gerontol* 52A(3): M161-M168.

Rubenstein, L.Z., K.R. Josephson, P.R. Trueblood, S. Loy, J.O. Harker, F.M. Pietruszka, and A.S. Robbins. 2000. Effects of a group exercise program on strength, mobility, and falls among fall-prone elderly men. *J Gerontol A Biol Sci Med Sci* 55(6): M317-M321.

Sayers, S.P., J.F. Bean, A. Cuoco, N.K. Lebrasseur, A.M. Jette, and R.A. Fielding. 2003. Changes in function and disability after resistance training: Does velocity matter? A pilot study. *Am J Phys Med Rehabil* 82: 605-613.

Schnelle, J.F., C.A. Alessi, S.F. Simmons, N.R. Al-Samarrai, J.C. Beck, and J.G. Ouslander. 2002. Translating clinical research into practice: A randomized controlled trial of exercise and incontinence care with nursing home residents. *J Am Geriatr Soc* 50(9): 1476-1483.

Schnelle, J.F., P.G. MacRae, J.G. Ouslander, S.F. Simmons, and M. Nitta. 1995. Functional Incidental Training, mobility performance, and incontinence care with nursing home residents. *J Am Geriatr Soc* 43(12): 1356-1362.

Schocken, D.D., J.A. Blumenthal, S. Port, P. Hindle, and R.E. Coleman. 1983. Physical conditioning and left ventricular performance in the elderly: Assessment by radionuclide angiocardiography. *Am J Cardiol* 52: 359-364.

Seals, D.R., J.M. Hagberg, B.F. Hurley, A.A. Ehsani, and J.O. Holloszy. 1984. Endurance training in older men and women I: Cardiovascular responses to exercise. *J Appl Physiol* 7: 1024-1029.

Shaw, J.M., and C.M. Snow. 1998. Weighted vest exercise improves indices of fall risk in older women. *J Gerontol Med Sci* 53(1): M53-M58.

Shephard, R.J. 1990. The scientific basis of exercise prescribing for the very old. *J Am Geriat Soc* 38: 62-70.

Sherrington, C., and S.R. Lord. 1997. Home exercise to improve strength and walking velocity after hip fracture: A randomized controlled trial. *Arch Phys Med Rehabil* 78: 208-212.

Skelton, D.A., C.A. Greig, J.M. Davies, and A. Young. 1994. Strength, power and related functional ability of health people aged 65-89 years. *Age and Ageing* 23(5): 371-377.

Skelton, D.A., A. Young, C.A. Greig, and K.E. Malbut. 1995. Effects of resistance training on strength, power, and selected functional abilities of women aged 75 and older. *J Am Geriatr Soc* 43: 1081-1087.

Souminen, H., E. Heikkinen, H. Liesen, D. Michel, and W. Hollman. 1977. Effects of 8 weeks endurance training on skeletal muscle metabolism in 56-70 year old sedentary men. *Eur J Appl Physiol* 37: 173-180.

South-Paul, J.E. 2001. Osteoporosis: Part I. Evaluation and assessment. *Am Fam Physician* 63(5): 897-904, 908.

Spina, R.J. 1999. Cardiovascular adaptations to endurance exercise training in older men and women. *Exerc Sports Sci Rev* 27: 317-332.

Stratton, J.R., M.D. Cerqueira, R.S. Schwartz, W.C. Levy, R.C. Veith, S.E. Kahn, and I. Abrass. 1992. Differences in cardiovascular responses to isopreterenol in relation to age and exercise training in healthy men. *Circulation* 86: 504-512.

Stratton, J.R., W.C. Levy, M.D. Cerqueira, R.S. Schwartz, and I. Abrass. 1994. Cardiovascular responses to exercise: Effects of aging and exercise training in healthy men. *Circulation* 89: 1648-1655.

Studenski, S., S. Perera, D. Wallace, J.M. Chandler, P.W. Duncan, E. Rooney, M. Fox, and J.M. Guralnik. 2003. Physical performance measures in the clinical setting. *J Am Geriatr Soc* 51(3): 314-322.

Suzman, R., D. Willis, and K. Manton. 1992. *The oldest old*. New York: Oxford University Press.

Suzuki, T., J. Bean, and R. Fielding. 2001. Muscle strength and power of the ankle plantar and dorsi flexors predict functional performance in community dwelling older women. *J Am Geriatr Soc* 49: 1161-1167.

Taaffe, D.R., C. Duret, S. Wheeler, and R. Marcus. 1999. Once-weekly resistance exercise improves muscle strength and neuromuscular performance in older adults. *J Am Geriatr Soc* 47(10): 1208-1214.

Tarpenning, K.M., M. Hamilton-Wessler, R.A. Wiswell, and S.A. Hawkins. 2004. Endurance training delays age of decline in leg strength and muscle morphology. *Med Sci Sports Exerc* 36(1): 74-78.

Tinetti, M.E., D. Richman, and L. Powell. 1990. Falls efficacy as a measure of fear of falling. *J Gerontol* 45(6): 239-243.

Tinetti, M.E., and M. Speechley. 1989. Prevention of falls among the elderly. *N Engl J Med* 320: 1055-1059.

United Nations. 2002. Report of the Second World Assembly on Ageing. Madrid, Spain. New York: United Nations. April 8-12, 2002. A/Conf.197/9. Available online at http: /daccessdds.un.org/doc/UNDOC/GEN/N02/397/51/PDF/N02 39751.pdf?OpenElement. Accessed June 13, 2005.

U.S. Department of Health and Human Services. 1996. *Physical activity and health: A report of the Surgeon General*. Atlanta: Centers for Disease Control and Prevention, National Center for Chronic Disease Prevention and Health Promotion.

Welle, S., S. Totterman, and C. Thornton. 1996. Effect of age on muscle hypertrophy induced by resistance training. *J Gerontol* 51A: M270-M275.

Whipple, R.H., L.I. Wolfson, and P.M. Amerman. 1987. The relationship of knee and ankle weakness to falls in nursing home residents: An isokinetic study. *J Am Geriatr Soc* 35: 13-20.

Wolf, S.L., H.X. Barnhart, N.G. Kutner, E. McNeely, C. Coogler, and T. Xu. 1996. Reducing frailty and falls in older persons: An investigation of Tai Chi and computerized balance training. Atlanta FICSIT Group. Frailty and Injuries: Cooperative Studies of Intervention Techniques. *J Am Geriatr Soc* 44(5): 489-497.

Wolf, S.L., C. Coogler, and T. Xu. 1997. Exploring the basis for Tai Chi Chuan as a therapeutic exercise approach. *Arch Phys Med Rehabil* 78(8): 886-892.

Wolfson, L., J. Judge, R. Whipple, and M. King. 1995. Strength is a major factor in balance, gait, and the occurrence of falls. *J Gerontol* 50A: 64-67.

Wolfson, L., R. Whipple, C. Derby, J. Judge, M. King, P. Amerman, J. Schmidt, and D. Smyers. 1996. Balance and strength training in older adults: Intervention gains and Tai Chi maintenance. *J Am Geriatr Soc* 44: 498-506.

Yarasheski, K.E. 2003. Exercise, aging, and muscle protein metabolism. *J Gerontol A Biol Sci Med Sci* 58(10): M918-M922.

Yarasheski, K.E., J.J. Zachweija, and D. Bier. 1993. Acute effects of resistance exercise on muscle protein synthesis rate in young and elderly men and women. *Am J Physiol* 265: E210-E214.

CHAPTER 21

Alexander, M.J.L. 1989. Aspects of performance in wheelchair marathon racing. *Journal de l'ACSEPL* 55: 26-32.

Asato, K.T., R.A. Cooper, F.D. Baldini, and R.N. Robertson. 1992. Training practices of athletes who participated in the National Wheelchair Athletic Association Training Camps. *Adap Phys Act Q* 9: 249-260.

Beck, K. 1992. Evergreen folding camper. *Paraplegia News* 46: 31-32.

Bloomquist, L.E. 1986. Injuries to athletes with physical disabilities: Prevention implications. *Phys Sportsmed* 14: 97-105.

Boninger, M.L., M. Baldwin, R.A. Cooper, A.M. Koontz, and L. Chan. 2000. Manual wheelchair pushrim biomechanics and axle position. *Arch Phys Med Rehabil* 81(5): 608-613.

Boninger, M.L., R.A. Cooper, M.A. Baldwin, S.D. Shimada, and A. Koontz. 1999. Wheelchair pushrim kinetics: Weight and median nerve function. *Arch Phys Med Rehabil* 80(8): 910-915.

Boninger, M.L., B.E. Dicianno, R.A. Cooper, J.D. Towers, A.M. Koontz, and A.L. Souza. 2003. Shoulder injury, wheelchair propulsion, and gender. *Arch Phys Med Rehabil* 84(1): 1615-1620.

Boninger, M.L., R.N. Robertson, M. Wolff, and R.A. Cooper. 1996. Upper limb nerve entrapments in elite wheelchair racers. *Am J Phys Med Rehabil* 75: 170-176.

Boninger, M.L., J.D. Towers, R.A. Cooper, B.E. Dicianno, and M.C. Munin. 2001. Shoulder imaging abnormalities in individuals with paraplegia. *J Rehabil Res Dev* 38(4): 401-408.

Bosscher, R.J. 1993. Running and mixed physical exercises with depressed psychiatric patients. *Int J Sport Psych* 24: 170-184.

Burnham, R.S., and R.D. Steadward. 1994. Upper extremity peripheral nerve entrapments among wheelchair athletes: Prevalence, location, and risk factors. *Arch Phys Med Rehabil* 75: 519-524.

Byrne, A., and D.G. Byrne. 1993. The effect of exercise on depression, anxiety, and other mood states: A review. *J Psychosom Res* 37: 565-574.

Charles, D., K.B. James, and R.B. Stein. 1988. Rehabilitation of musicians with upper limb amputations. *J Rehabil Res Dev* 25: 25-32.

Cook, A.M., and J.G. Webster. 1982. *Therapeutic medical devices: Application and design*. Englewood Cliffs, NJ: Prentice Hall.

Cooper, R.A. 1989a. Racing wheelchair crown compensation. *J Rehabil Res Dev* 26: 25-32.

Cooper, R.A. 1989b. Racing wheelchair rear wheel alignment. *J Rehabil Res Dev* 26: 47-50.

Cooper, R.A. 1989c. An international track wheelchair with a center of gravity directional controller. *J Rehabil Res Dev* 26: 63-70.

Cooper, R.A. 1989d. An arm-powered racing bicycle. *Journal of Assist Technol* 1(3): 71-74.

Cooper, R.A. 1990. Wheelchair racing sports science: A review. *J Rehabil Res Dev* 27: 295-312.

Cooper, R.A. 1992a. Contributions of selected anthropometric and metabolic parameters to 10K performance—a preliminary study. *J Rehabil Res Dev* 29: 29-34.

Cooper, R.A. 1992b. Racing wheelchair roll stability while turning: A simple model. *J Rehabil Res Dev* 29: 23-30.

Cooper R.A., F.D. Baldini, M.L. Boninger, and R. Cooper. 2001. Physiological responses to two wheelchair racing exercise protocols. *Neurorehabil Neural Repair* 15: 191-195.

Cooper, R.A., F.D. Baldini, W.E. Langbein, R.N. Robertson, P. Bennett, and S. Monical. 1993. Prediction of pulmonary function in wheelchair users. *Paraplegia* 31: 560-570.

Cooper, R.A., and J.F. Bedi. 1990. Gross mechanical efficiency of trained wheelchair racers. Paper presented at the 12th Annual International Conference of the IEEE/EMBS. Philadelphia, Pennsylvania.

Cooper, R.A., M.L. Boninger, F.D. Baldini, R.N. Robertson, and R. Cooper. 2003. Wheelchair racing efficiency. *Disabil and Rehabil* 25(4-5): 207-212.

Cooper, R.A., S.M. Horvath, J.F. Bedi, D.M. Drechsler-Parks, and R.E. Williams. 1992. Maximal exercise response of paraplegic wheelchair road racers. *Paraplegia* 30: 573-581.

Cooper, R.A., T.J. O'Connor, R.N. Robertson, W.E. Langbein, and F. Baldini. 1999a. An investigation of the exercise capacity of the Wheelchair Sports USA Team. *Assist Technol* 11: 34-42.

Cooper, R.A., L.A. Quatrano, P.W. Axelson, W. Harlan, M. Stineman, B. Franklin, J.S. Krause, J. Bach, H. Chambers, E.Y.S. Chao, M. Alexander, and P. Painter. 1999b. Research on physical activity and health among people with disabilities: A consensus statement. *J Rehabil Res Dev* 36(2): 142-154.

Coutts, K.D. 1991. Dynamic characteristics of a sport wheelchair. *J Rehabil Res Dev* 28: 45-50.

Curtis, K.A., and D.A. Dillon. 1985. Survey of wheelchair athletic injuries: Common patterns and prevention. *Paraplegia* 23: 170-175.

Curtis, K.A., S. McClanahan, K.M. Hall, D. Dillon, and K.F. Brown. 1986. Health, vocational, and functional status in spinal cord injured athletes and nonathletes. *Arch Phys Med Rehabil* 67: 862-865.

Czerniecki, J.M., A. Gotter, and C. Munro. 1991. Joint moment and muscle power output characteristics of below knee amputees during running: The influence of energy storing prosthetic feet. *J Biomech* 24: 63-75.

Davis, R., and M. Ferrara. 1988. The competitive wheelchair stroke. *J Strength Cond Res* 10: 4-10.

DiGiovine, C.P., R.A. Cooper, M.M. DiGiovine, M.L. Boninger, and R.N. Robertson. 2000. Frequency analysis of kinematics of racing wheelchair propulsion. *IEEE Trans Rehabil Eng* 8(3): 371-384.

Engel, P., and K. Seeliger. 1986. Technological and physiological characteristics of a newly developed hand-lever drive system for wheelchairs. *J Rehabil Res Dev* 23: 37-40.

Ferrara, M.S., W.E. Buckley, B.C. McCann, and T.J. Limbird. 1992. The injury experience of the competitive athlete with a disability: Prevention implications. *Med Sci Sports Exerc* 24: 184-188.

Flowers, W., C. Cullen, and K.P. Tyra. 1990. A preliminary report on the use of a practical biofeedback device for gait training of above-knee amputees. *J Rehabil Res Dev* 23: 7-18.

Gage, J.R., and S. Ounpuu. 1989. Gait analysis in clinical practice. *Semin Orthopedics* 4: 72-87.

Galvin, J.C., and M.J. Scherer. 1996. *Evaluating, selecting, and using appropriate assistive technology*. Gaithersburg, MD: Aspen.

Glaser, R.M. 1989. Arm exercise training for wheelchair users. *Med Sci Sports Exerc* 21: S149-S157.

Glaser, R.M., M.N. Sawka, M.F. Brune, and S.W. Wilde. 1980. Physiological responses to maximal effort wheelchair and arm crank ergometry. *J Appl Physiol* 48: 1060-1064.

Golbranson, F.L., and R.W. Wirta. 1982. *Wheelchair III: Report of a workshop on specially adapted wheelchairs and sports wheelchairs*. Washington, DC: RESNA Press.

Gottschalk, F., B. McClellan, A. Carlton, and V. Mooney. 1985. Early fitting of the amputee with a plastic temporary adjustable below-knee prosthesis. *Proceedings RESNA 8th Annual Conference*. Memphis, TN, 373-375.

Hinkle, J.S. 1992. Aerobic running behavior and psychotherapeutics: Implications for sports counseling and psychology. *J Sport Behav* 15: 263-277.

Horvath, S.M., and E.C. Horvath. 1973. *The Harvard fatigue laboratory: Its history and contributions*. Englewood Cliffs, NJ: Prentice-Hall.

Houtkooper, L. 1986. Nutritional support for muscle weight gain. *J Strength Cond Res* 8: 62-63.

James, W.V. 1991. Principles of limb fitting and prostheses. *Ann R Coll Surg Engl* 73: 158-162.

Janssen, T.W.J., A.J. Dallmeijer, and L.H.V. van der Woude. 2001. Physical capacity and race performance of handcycle users. *J Rehabil Res Dev* 38(1): 33-40.

Janssen, T.W.J., C.A.J.M. van Oers, L.H.V. van der Woude, and P. Hollander. 1994. Physical strain in daily life of wheelchair users with spinal cord injuries. *Med Sci Sports Exerc* 26: 661-670.

King, A.C., C.B. Taylor, and W.L. Haskell. 1993. Effects of differing intensities and formats of 12 months of exercise training on psychological outcomes in older adults. *Health Psychol* 12: 292-300.

Krouskop, T.A., B.L. Goode, D.R. Doughtery, and E.H. Hemmen. 1985. Predicting the loaded shape of an amputee's residual limb. *Proceedings RESNA 8th Annual Conference*. Memphis, TN, 225-227.

Krouskop, T.A., A.L. Muilenberg, D.R. Doughtery, and D.J. Winningham. 1987. Computer-aided design of a prosthetic socket for an above-knee amputee. *J Rehabil Res Dev* 24: 31-38.

Kumar, S., ed. 2003. *Muscle strength*. Philadelphia: Taylor & Francis.

Landsmeer, J.M.F. 1961. Studies in the anatomy of articulation: II. Patterns of movement of bi-muscular, bi-articular systems. *Acta Morphol Neerl Scand* 3: 304-321.

Langbein, W.E., and K.C. Maki. 1995. Predicting oxygen uptake during counterclockwise arm crank ergometry in men with lower limb disabilities. *Arch Phys Med Rehabil* 76: 642-646.

Langbein, W.E., K.C. Maki, L.C. Edwards, M.H. Hwang, P. Sibley, and L. Fehr. 1994. Initial clinical evaluation of a wheelchair ergometer for diagnostic exercise testing: A technical note. *J Rehabil Res Dev* 31: 317-325.

Legro, M.W., G.E. Reiber, J.M. Czerniecki, and B.J. Sangeorzan. 2001. Recreational activities of lower-limb amputees with prostheses. *J Rehabil Res Dev* 38(3): 319-325.

Loverock, P. 1989. The athlete of the future. *Los Angeles Times Magazine,* March 12.

Maarlewski-Probert, B. 1992. The RV industry is meeting the challenge. *Paraplegia News* 46: 21-23.

MacLeish, M.S., R.A. Cooper, J. Harralson, and J.S. Ster. 1993. Design of a composite monocoque frame racing wheelchair. *J Rehabil Res Dev* 30: 233-249.

Malone, L.A., P.L. Gervais, and R.D. Steadward. 2002. Shooting mechanics related to player classification and free throw success in wheelchair basketball. *J Rehabil Res Dev* 39(6): 701-710.

Maresh, C.M., B.G. Sheckley, G.J. Allen, D.N. Camaione, and S.T. Sinatra. 1991. Middle age male distance runners: Physiological and psychological profiles. *J Sports Med Phys Fitness* 31: 461-469.

McArdle, W.D., F.I. Katch, and V.L. Katch. 1991. *Exercise physiology: Energy, nutrition, and human performance*. 3rd ed. Philadelphia/London: Lea & Febiger.

McDonnell, P.M., R.N. Scott, J. Dickison, R.A. Theriault, and B. Wood. 1989. Do artificial limbs become part of the user? New evidence. *J Rehabil Res Dev* 26: 17-24.

Michael, J.W. 1989. Reflections on CAD-CAM in prosthetics and orthotics. *J Prosthet Orthot* 1: 116-121.

National Academy of Sciences. 1989. *Recommended Dietary Allowances*. Washington, DC: National Academy Press.

Nissan, M. 1991. The initiation of gait in lower limb amputees: Some related data. *J Rehabil Res Dev* 28: 1-12.

O'Connor, T.J., R.N. Robertson, and R.A. Cooper. 1998. Three-dimensional kinematic analysis of racing wheelchair propulsion. *Adap Phys Act Q* 15(1): 1-14.

Pappas, G.P., S. Golin, and D.L. Meyer. 1990. Reducing symptoms of depression with exercise. *Psychosomatics* 31: 112-113.

Pelham, T.W., P.D. Campagna, P.G. Ritvo, and W.A. Birnie. 1993. The effects of exercise therapy on clients in a psychiatric rehabilitation program. *Psychosoc Rehabil J* 16: 75-84.

Pinzur, M.S., P. Perona, A. Patwardhan, and R. Havey. 1991. Loading of the contralateral foot in peripheral vascular insufficiency below-knee amputees. *Foot Ankle* 11: 368-371.

Popovic, D., M.N. Oguztoreli, and R.B. Stein. 1991. Optimal control for the active above knee prosthesis. *Ann Biomed Eng* 19: 131-150.

Rick Hansen Centre. 1988. *Proceedings from a national symposium on wheelchair track and road racing department of physical education and sport studies.* Edmonton: University of Alberta Press.

Rodgers, M.M., W. Gayle, S.F. Figoni, M. Kobayashi, J. Lieh, and R.M. Glaser. 1994. Biomechanics of wheelchair propulsion during fatigue. *Arch Phys Med Rehabil* 75: 85-93.

Rozenek, R., and M.H. Stone. 1984. Protein metabolism related to athletes. *J Strength Cond Res* 6: 42-45.

Schneider, K., T. Hart, R.F. Zernicke, Y. Setoguchsi, and W. Oppenheim. 1993. Dynamics of below-knee child amputee gait: SACH foot versus flex foot. *J Biomech* 26: 1191-1204.

Skinner, H.B., and D.J. Effeney. 1985. Gait analysis in amputees. *Am J Phys Med* 64: 82-89.

Snell, F. 1992. Bringing prosthetics into the 21st century. *J Ark Med Soc* 89: 337-338.

Stein, P.N., and R.W. Motta. 1992. Effects of aerobic and nonaerobic exercise on depression and self-concept. *Percept Mot Skills* 74: 79-89.

Steptoe, A., J. Moses, S. Edwards, and A. Mathews. 1993. Exercise and responsivity to mental stress: Discrepancies between the subjective and physiological effects of aerobic training. *Int J Sport Psych* 24: 110-129.

Suzuki, K. 1972. Force plate study on the artificial limb gait. *J Orthop Sci* 46: 503-516.

Topper, A.K., and G.R. Fernie. 1990. An evaluation of computer aided design of below-knee prosthetic sockets. *Prosthet Orthot Int* 14: 136-142.

Torburn, L., J. Perry, E. Ayyappa, and S. Shanfield. 1990. Below-knee amputee gait with dynamic elastic response prosthetic feet: A pilot study. *J Rehabil Res Dev* 27: 369-384.

Torres-Moreno, R., J.B. Morrison, D. Cooper, C.G. Saunders, and J. Foort. 1992. A computer-aided socket design procedure for above-knee prostheses. *J Rehabil Res Dev* 29: 35-44.

University of Illinois at Urbana-Champaign Division of Rehabilitation-Education Services Testing and Training. n.d. Retrieved February 2, 2004, from the Division of Rehabilitation-Education Services, College of Applied Life Studies, the University of Illinois at Urbana-Champaign. www.rehab.uiuc.edu/campuslife/training/techtraining.html.

van der Woude, L.H.V., H.E.J. Veeger, R.H. Rozendal, G.J. van ingen Schenau, E. Rooth, and P. van Nierop. 1988. Wheelchair racing: Effects of rim diameter and speed on physiology and technique. *Med Sci Sports Exerc* 20: 492-500.

Wade, J. 1993. A league of its own. *REHAB Management* 6: 44-51.

Walker, P.S., H. Kurosawa, J.S. Rovick, and R.A. Zimmerman. 1985. External knee joint design based on normal motion. *J Rehabil Res Dev* 22: 9-22.

Wankel, L.M. 1993. The importance of enjoyment to adherent and psychological benefits from physical activity. *Int J Sport Psych* 24: 151-169.

Wirta, R., F. Goldbranson, R. Mason, and K. Calvo. 1990. Analysis of below-knee suspension systems: Effect on gait. *J Rehabil Res Dev* 27: 385-396.

Wirta, R., R. Mason, K. Calvo, and F.L. Goldbranson. 1991. Effect on gait using various prosthetic ankle-foot devices. *J Rehabil Res Dev* 28: 13-24.

SUBJECT INDEX

CITATION INDEX

D

E

I

J

K

L

M

N

T

U

V

ABOUT THE EDITORS

Walter R. Frontera, MD, PhD, is Earle P. and Ida S. Charlton professor and chair of the Department of Physical Medicine and Rehabilitation at Harvard Medical School and Spaulding Rehabilitation Hospital in Boston, Massachusetts. He has a medical specialty of physical medicine and rehabilitation and a PhD in exercise physiology. He has more than 20 years of experience in the practice of physical medicine and rehabilitation and in the use of exercise in various patient populations. He is the secretary general of the International Sports Medicine Federation and the editor in chief of the *American Journal of Physical Medicine and Rehabilitation.*

David M. Slovik, MD, is chief of medicine at Spaulding Rehabilitation Hospital in Boston, Massachusetts, where he has worked for 30 years. He has also served as medical director of the musculoskeletal program at Spaulding. An expert on osteoporosis and related disorders, including the effects of exercise on osteoporosis, he is also an associate professor of medicine at Harvard Medical School, with 30 years of teaching experience. He is a member of the American Society of Bone and Mineral Research.

David M. Dawson, MD, is professor of neurology at Harvard Medical School. He has extensive experience in teaching and in residency supervision and is an expert in clinical neurology with an emphasis on neuromuscular disease and multiple sclerosis. He has served on various boards of the National Multiple Sclerosis Society.

ABOUT THE CONTRIBUTORS

James C. Agre, MD, PhD, is the staff physiatrist with Ministry Medical Group in Rhinelander, Wisconsin. Dr. Agre received his MD from the University of Minnesota and his PhD in physical medicine and rehabilitation, also from the University of Minnesota. He has received numerous professional honors and awards including the Elizabeth and Sidney Licht Award for Excellence in Scientific Writing for 1988. He is a member of the American Academy of Physical Medicine and Rehabilitation and the American College of Sports Medicine. He served on the editorial board of *Archives of Physical Medicine and Rehabilitation.* He has published extensively and authored or coauthored over 40 papers, which have been published in a variety of professional journals.

Susan Aitkens, MS, is a staff research associate in the Department of Physical Medicine and Rehabilitation at the University of California, Davis School of Medicine. She received her master's degree in exercise science from the University of California, Davis. For the past 22 years she has been an active researcher in the areas of physical activity and nutrition related to neuromuscular disease. Her research interests include evaluating the benefits of exercise and nutritional intervention on physical functioning and quality of life, metabolic syndrome in neuromuscular disease, and methods to assess energy intake and expenditure. She is a member of the American College of Sports Medicine and has published in *Medicine and Science in Sports and Exercise, American Journal of Clinical Nutrition, American Journal of Physical Medicine and Rehabilitation, Muscle and Nerve,* and *Pediatric Research.*

Jonathan F. Bean, MD, MS, is an assistant professor in the Department of Physical Medicine and Rehabilitation at Harvard Medical School. He serves as the director of Geriatric Physical Medicine and Rehabilitation at Spaulding Rehabilitation Hospital and medical director of the Spaulding Cambridge Outpatient Center. Dr. Bean directs the Research Center for Lifelong Health and Fitness, which is based at Spaulding Cambridge. He completed a master's degree in exercise physiology from Boston University in 1998 and is currently completing a master's in public health at the Harvard School of Public Health. Dr. Bean has been honored with receipt of the 1998 New Investigator Award from the American Academy of PM&R and the 2002 Dennis W. Jahnigan Career Development Award from the American Geriatrics Society. His work has also been supported by career development awards from the National Institute on Aging. Dr. Bean's research focus is within the areas of geriatric physical medicine and rehabilitation and exercise physiology.

Michael L. Boninger, MD, is a professor and vice chair for research in the Department of Physical Medicine and Rehabilitation and assistant dean for Medical Student Research in the School of Medicine. Dr. Boninger also works as a physician researcher for the Department of Veterans Affairs. Dr. Boninger graduated from Ohio State University with both a medical doctorate and a degree in mechanical engineering. He received his specialty training in physical medicine and rehabilitation at the University of Michigan. Dr. Boninger is the director of the University of Pittsburgh Model Center on Spinal Cord Injury (UPMC-SCI), funded by the National Institutes for Disability and Rehabilitation Research. In addition, Dr. Boninger serves as the medical director of the Human Engineering Research Laboratories, a Department of Veterans Affairs Center of Excellence. He is executive director of the University of Pittsburgh Medical Center's Center for Assistive Technology.

Dr. Boninger has over 100 peer-reviewed journal publications and numerous book chapters and extended abstracts. He has lectured internationally on biomechanics of repetitive strain injury, assistive technology, and wheelchair propulsion. Dr. Boninger also holds two U.S. patents. In 2003 Dr. Boninger won the VA Stars and Stripes Healthcare Network Annual Award for Research Achievement and was elected as a fellow in the American Institute for Medical Biomedical Engineering (AIMBE). In 2002 Dr. Boninger was honored with the Pittsburgh Business Times Health Care Hero Award for Innovation and Research, and in 1998 he won the Young Academician Award of the Association of Academic Physiatrists. Under Dr. Boninger's supervision, medical students, residents, and graduate students have won over 30 national research awards. Dr. Boninger serves on the editorial board of *Archives of Physical Medicine and Rehabilitation* and *Journal of Rehabilitation Research and Development.*

Bartolome R. Celli, MD, graduated from Universidad Central de Venezuela. He completed his training in internal medicine and was chief medical resident at the Boston City Hospital. He was then a clinical and research pulmonary fellow at Boston University where he joined the faculty in 1983. Currently, he is professor of medicine at Tufts University and chief of the Division of Pulmonary and Critical Care at St. Elizabeth's Medical Center in Boston. Author of many publications, his primary research interest is in COPD, pulmonary rehabilitation, exercise, respiratory muscles and control of breathing. He has contributed to many books and is co-editor of *Baum's Textbook of Pulmonary Diseases* and Hodgkin's *Pulmonary Rehabilitation.* He is chairman of the ATS Committee that established the Standards for the Diagnosis and Treatment of Patients with COPD and member of the GOLD executive committee. He is past-chairman of the Clinical Assembly of the ATS and past-president of the Massachusetts Thoracic Society.

Rory A. Cooper, PhD, received his BS and MEng degrees in electrical engineering from California Polytechnic State University, San Luis Obispo in 1985 and 1986, respectively. He received his PhD degree in electrical and computer engineering with a concentration in bioengineering from University of California at Santa Barbara in 1989. He is FISA & Paralyzed Veterans of America (PVA) Chair and distinguished professor of the Department of Rehabilitation Science and Technology, and professor of Bioengineering and Mechanical Engineering at the University of Pittsburgh. He is also a professor in the Departments of Physical Medicine and Rehabilitation and Orthopaedic Surgery at the University of Pittsburgh Medical Center Health System. Dr. Cooper is director and VA Senior Research Career Scientist of the Center for Wheelchairs and Associated Rehabilitation Engineering, a VA Rehabilitation Research and Development Center of Excellence.

Dr. Cooper serves or has served on the editorial board of several prominent peer-reviewed journals in the fields of rehabilitation and bioengineering and has authored or co-authored more than 150 peer-reviewed journal publications. He also has six patents awarded or pending. Dr. Cooper is an elected fellow of the Rehabilitation Engineering and Assistive Technology Society of North America, the Institute of Electrical and Electronics Engineers, and of the American Institute of Medical and Biological Engineering.

Rosemarie Cooper, MPT, received her MPT in physical therapy from University of Pittsburgh in 1998. She is employed as an outpatient physical therapist at the UPMC Rehabilitation Hospital, Pittsburgh, PA. She is currently working as a clinical coordinator at the Human Engineering Research Laboratories and as a wheelchair seating clinician at the UPMC Center for Assistive Technology. She is a RESNA certified Assistive Technology Practitioner (ATP). Preceding her PT studies, she has worked as a research associate for the University of Pittsburgh Medical Center, Division of Physical Medicine & Rehabilitation. Prior to coming to Pittsburgh, she has served as an executive committee member at the National Wheelchair Athletic Association (NWAA) Paralympic Training Camps held in Sacramento, CA, during Spring 1989-1994. Rosemarie Cooper has been an author on several articles on wheelchairs and seating. She is a member of Beta Gamma Sigma, business academic honor society and a member of APTA.

Kerry S. Courneya, PhD, is a professor and Canada Research Chair in physical activity and cancer in the Faculty of Physical Education at the University of Alberta in Edmonton, Canada. He received his BA (1987) and MA (1989) in physical education from the University of Western Ontario (London, Canada) and his PhD (1992) in kinesiology from the University of Illinois (Urbana, IL, USA.). Prof. Courneya's research program focuses on the role of physical activity in cancer control including primary prevention, coping with treatments, rehabilitation after treatments, and secondary prevention and survival. His research interests include both the outcomes and determinants of physical activity for cancer control as well as behavior change interventions. His research program has been funded by the National Cancer Institute of Canada, the Canadian Breast Cancer Research Alliance, the National Institutes of Health (USA), the Alberta Heritage Foundation for Medical Research, and the Alberta Cancer Board.

Carlos J. Crespo, DrPH, MS, is director of the School of Community Health at Portland State University. Previously he was associate professor in the Department of Social and Preventive Medicine of the University at Buffalo and associate research professor at the Roswell Park Cancer Institute. He graduated from the Inter American University of Puerto Rico, and has a master of science in exercise science from Texas Tech University and a Doctor of Public Health from the Loma Linda University School of Public Health. Previous work experience includes working for the Centers for Disease Control and as a public health advisor for the Office of Prevention, Education and Control of the National Heart, Lung, and Blood Institute at NIH. He was an assistant professor in American University in Washington, DC. His main area of research involves the epidemiology of physical activity in the prevention of chronic diseases and research on minority health issues.

He has over 45 peer-review publications in areas of exercise, minority health, obesity, and nutrition. He is also a contributing author to more than 10 government publications, including the Surgeon General's Report on Physical Activity and Health and the Sixth Report on Detection, Evaluation and Treatment of Hypertension. He received the 1997 Secretary of Health Award for Distinguished Service and in 2003 became a Minority Health Scholar from the National Institutes of Health. He was a member of the board of directors of American Council for Exercise and past president of the Mid-Atlantic Chapter of the American College of Sports Medicine.

Susan D. Driscoll, MPH, MSN, is a nurse practitioner who has worked over the last 12 years as an administrator, educator, and health care provider to underserved populations, including men and women living with HIV. She received her MPH at Johns Hopkins University and went on to complete her MSN at the Massachusetts General Hospital, Institute of Health Professions in Boston. Most recently, she worked as a nurse researcher and co-investigator with Steven Grinspoon, MD, director of the Program in Nutritional Metabolism at the Massachusetts General Hospital. Her program of research focused on the use of progressive resistance training as an intervention for those experiencing metabolic complications associated with HIV/AIDS. She has published in *AIDS* and *The Journal of Clinical Endocrinology and Metabolism* and received a Young Academician Scholarship Award to present at the Fifth International Workshop on Adverse Drug Reactions and Lipodystrophy in HIV in July 2003. Currently she lives in Florida and is enjoying her career as a new mother.

Roger A. Fielding, PhD, is currently the director of the Nutrition, Exercise Physiology, and Sarcopenia Laboratory at the Jean Mayer USDA Human Nutrition Research Center on Aging at Tufts University. Dr. Fielding received his BS in applied physiology from Boston University in 1983, his MA in human bioenergetics from Ball State University in 1985, and a PhD in human nutrition from Tufts University in 1993.

From 1993 to 2004, he was a member of the faculty at Boston University, an associate professor in the Department of Health Sciences. He has been the director of the Human Physiology Laboratory since 1999. He is a past recipient of the Brookdale Foundation National Fellowship for potential leadership in aging research and now serves as a member of the Brookdale Institute on Aging. He is a member of the American Physiological Society and the American College of Sports Medicine.

His research interests include the impact of exercise and physical activity on successful human aging, skeletal muscle alterations with advancing age in disabled and non-disabled populations, and age-related alterations in the control of skeletal muscle protein turnover. Dr. Fielding has received support for his research from the National Institute on Aging, the American Federation of Aging Research, private foundations, and industry.

Axel Finckh, MD, MS, is the lead clinical researcher in the Division of Rheumatology at the University of Geneva. He graduated from the University of Geneva, completed training in internal medicine and rheumatology in Paris, Geneva, and Lausanne. He received his MS in epidemiology from Harvard University and completed a postdoctoral fellowship in the Department of Medicine, Brigham and Women's Hospital, Harvard Medical School before joining the faculty at the University of Geneva. Dr. Finckh has received numerous research grants and awards and is the chairman of the Scientific Commission for Rheumatoid Arthritis at the Swiss Society of Rheumatology. His work has appeared in *Arthritis and Rheumatism, Spine, Journal of Rheumatology,* among other publications.

Steven Grinspoon, MD, is an associate professor of medicine at Harvard Medical School and the director of the MGH Program in Nutritional Metabolism. He has published extensively on the endocrine abnormalities in HIV-infected patients and the use of progressive resistance training in this population. He chaired the Health and Human Services Subcommittee on Weight Loss and Wasting.

Bette Ann Harris, DPT, MS, is clinical professor of Graduate Programs in Physical Therapy at MGH Institute of Health Professions in Boston, Massachusetts. She also serves as a clinical consultant for Orthopedics/Outpatient Physical Therapy at the Massachusetts General Hospital. Harris acts as a manuscript reviewer for several professional journals including, *Physiotherapy Research International Journal,* and *Physical Therapy.* She is a lecturer with the Department of Orthopedics at Harvard Medical School. In 1988, she received the Massachusetts Chapter APTA Award in Recognition for outstanding achievement in research and the Nancy T. Watts Award for Teaching Excellence in 2002. She received her BS with certification in physical therapy from Simmons College and her MS and DPT in physical therapy from the MGH Institute of Health Professions in Boston. Her frequent publications have appeared in such magazines as *Journal of Orthopedic and Sports, Physical Therapy,* and *Archives of Physical Medicine and Rehabilitation.*

Gregory W. Heath, DHSc, MPH, is Guerry professor and head of the Department of Health and Human Performance at the University of Tennessee at Chattanooga and director of research at the University of Tennessee College of Medicine, Chattanooga Unit. Dr. Heath was the former lead health scientist in the Physical Activity and Health Branch, Division of Nutrition and Physical Activity with the Centers for Disease Control and Prevention in Atlanta. He received his master's of public health in epidemiology and his doctor of health science in applied physiology from Loma Linda University in California. Among Dr. Heath's numerous awards and honors is the Secretary's Award for Distinguished Service for his 1997 contributions to the Surgeon General's Report on Physical Activity and Health. He is a fellow of the American College of Sports Medicine and a fellow of the Council on Epidemiology and Prevention with the American Heart Association. His work has appeared in *Journal of Applied Physiology, Medicine and Science in Sports and Exercise, American Heart Journal,* and *American Journal of Preventive Medicine.*

Martin D. Hoffman, MD, is a professor of clinical physical medicine and rehabilitation at the University of California, Davis School of Medicine and chief of Physical Medicine and Rehabilitation at the VA Northern California Health Care System. He received his medical degree from St. Louis University School of Medicine and did his residency in physical medicine and rehabilitation with the Medical College of Wisconsin. He served as a team physician with the U.S. Biathlon Team from 1988-1995. He has been a member of the editorial board for *Archives of Physical Medicine and Rehabilitation* since 1996 and a foreign editor for *Science & Sport* since 2000. He is a fellow with both the American College of Sports Medicine and the American Academy of Physical Medicine and Rehabilitation. He has authored or coauthored over 50 articles in professional journals.

Edward S. Horton, MD, is the vice president and director of clinical research at Joslin Diabetes Center in Boston, Massachusetts. He received his medical degree from Harvard Medical School in 1957 where he is now a professor of medicine. His numerous honors and awards include the Robert H. Herman Award from The American Society for Clinical Nutrition in 1990, the Banting Medal for Distinguished Service from the American Diabetes Association in 1991, and the Mizuno Award and Lectureship, which he received in Nara, Japan, in 1994. He has been a member of more than 20 committees, offices, and task forces associated with the American Diabetes Association and served as the Association's vice president from 1988-1989 and president from 1990-1991. He also served as president of The American Society for Clinical Nutrition in 1986. Over the last four decades, he has published over 250 reports and papers in various professional journals.

Maura Daly Iversen, DPT, SD, MPH, is professor and associate director of the Graduate Programs in Physical Therapy at MGH Institute of Health Professions and an instructor in medicine, Department of Medicine, Division of Rheumatology, Immunology and Allergy, Harvard Medical School. She received her BS and Certificate in PT from Simmons College, her MPH from Boston University, and her Doctor of Science from Harvard University and a Doctor of Physical Therapy from MGH Institute. She completed a postdoctoral fellowship in the Department of Medicine, Harvard Medical School. Dr. Iversen has received numerous grants, including a Farnsworth Fellowship, Arthritis Foundation Doctoral Award and New Investigator Award. She is a trustee of the Arthritis Foundation MA chapter, a former member of the Executive Committee of the American College of Rheumatology Executive Committee and past-president of the Association of Rheumatology Health Professions. She received a Clinical Researcher Award in 2004 from the Massachusetts Chapter APTA for outstanding clinical research. She is an associate editor of *Physical Therapy,* special editor for the Current Opinion in Rheumatology edition of *Rehabilitation in Rheumatic Conditions* and is a reviewer for numerous medical journals. She has co-authored over 40 articles. Her articles have appeared in such journals as *New England Journal of Medicine* and *British Journal of Rheumatology.*

Lee W. Jones, PhD, is an assistant professor of medicine in the Division of Medical Oncology at Duke University Medical Center. He received his BS from the University of Brighton in the UK, his MS in kinesiology from Lakehead University in Thunder Bay, Ontario, Canada, and completed his PhD and postdoctoral fellowship in exercise oncology at the University of Alberta, Edmonton, Canada. Dr. Jones's research program focuses on the psychosocial and biological outcomes of exercise as a supportive intervention for cancer patients during and following adjuvant therapy and determining the biological mechanisms underlying these outcomes. Secondary research interests include understanding exercise motivation and designing theoretically-based interventions to promote exercise in cancer patients and survivors. His research program has been supported by the U.S. Department of Defense Breast Cancer Research Program, the Canadian Breast Cancer Research Alliance, the Alberta Cancer Board, and Alberta Heritage Foundation for Medical Research.

David D. Kilmer, MD, is a professor and chair of the Department of Physical Medicine and Rehabilitation at the University of California, Davis School of Medicine. He received his MD from the University of California, Davis, in 1985 and completed residency training at the University's Davis Medical Center in 1989. Dr. Kilmer is a member of the American Academy of Physical Medicine and Rehabilitation and serves as an editor for the organization's journal, *Archives of Physical Medicine and Rehabilitation.* He is also an active member of the American Association of Neuromuscular and Electrodiagnostic Medicine. Dr. Kilmer's research focuses on exercise and functional performance in persons with neuromuscular diseases with funding received through a grant from the National Institute of Disability and Rehabilitation Research. He has published in such professional journals as *Western Journal of Medicine, American Journal of Physical Medicine and Rehabilitation,* and *American Journal of Clinical Nutrition.*

Pelagia Koufaki, PhD, is a research associate at the Division of Metabolic and Cellular Medicine, Faculty of Medicine, University of Liverpool, UK. She received her PhD in clinical exercise physiology from Manchester Metropolitan University, UK. She has extensive experience of the application of exercise physiology and exercise rehabilitation across a wide range of clinical settings and with a number of chronic disease patient sub-populations. She is a member of several professional associations and working groups including the British Association of Sport and Exercise Sciences (Accredited Exercise Physiologist for Research), the American College of Sports Medicine, the European Working Group on Renal Rehabilitation and Exercise Physiology, and the European Working Group on Cardiac Rehabilitation and Exercise Physiology. She has published her research in *Archives of Physical Medicine and Rehabilitation, Clinical Exercise Physiology, Clinical Physiology & Functional Imaging, Clinical Nephrology, Clinical Science, Medicine and Science in Sports and Exercise,* and *Nephrology Dialysis and Transplantation.* Her current research interests include treatment of physical dysfunction in kidney failure and heart failure and factors affecting cardiovascular control during exercise in patients with primary or secondary cardiovascular disease.

Lisa S. Krivickas, MD, is an assistant professor at Harvard Medical School and has clinical appointments in the departments of Physical Medicine and Rehabilitation and Neurology at Spaulding Rehabilitation Hospital, Massachusetts General Hospital, and Brigham and Women's Hospital. She is the director of Electrodiagnostic Services at Spaulding Rehabilitation Hospital and the associate chief of PM&R at Massachusetts General Hospital. Dr. Krivickas received her medical degree from Harvard Medical School in 1991. She is a diplomate of both the American Board of PM&R and the American Board of Electrodiagnostic Medicine. Her current research is in the area of muscle physiology. She has been elected to the Board of Trustees of the American College of Sports Medicine and serves on the Board of Directors for the American Board of Electrodiagnostic Medicine.

Matthew H. Liang, MD, MPH, is professor of medicine at Harvard Medical School and professor of Health Policy and Management at Harvard School of Public Health and is based at the Brigham and Women's Hospital and the Massachusetts Veteran's Epidemiology Research and Information Center (MAVERIC). He is a graduate of Johns Hopkins University in philosophy and chemistry, Harvard Medical School, and the Harvard School of Public Health (HSPH) in tropical public health and epidemiology. He founded and directed the Robert B. Brigham Arthritis and Musculoskeletal Diseases Clinical Research

Center at the Brigham and Women's Hospital between 1977-2002 and is currently its director of Special Projects. He is medical director of Rehabilitation Services at Brigham and Women's Hospital. Dr. Liang is a founding faculty member of the Clinical Effectiveness Program at HSPH and is a member of the BWH Research Institute's Clinical Research Committee.

Dr. Liang also directs the Center for Advanced Methodological Support for Innovative SLE Trials (ASSIST), and is the chief of the Section of Rheumatology at the VA Boston Healthcare System, and a study director in the VA Cooperative Studies Program (CSP). Dr. Liang has served on the Advisory Council of the National Institute of Arthritis, Musculoskeletal and Skin Diseases, and is currently on the Boards of the Alliance for Lupus Research, the Lupus Clinical Trials Consortium, and Rheuminations, Inc. He serves on the editorial boards of *Arthritis and Rheumatism, Lupus, Spine, American Journal of Medicine, Nature Clinical practice Rheumatology, Patient Care,* and *Current Rheumatology Reviews*. He is an active primary care physician and rheumatologist and was named one of the Best Doctors in America.

His current research interests include basic methodologic work in clinimetrics, clinical trials methodology in systemic lupus erythematosus, the epidemiology of rheumatic disease and disability, prevention of Lyme disease, outcomes research, the identification of modifiable risk factors in high risk and disadvantaged populations, clinical decision making, and prevention of osteoarthritis.

John R. Mackey, MD, FRCPC, is a medical oncologist at the Cross Cancer Institute in Edmonton, chair of the Northern Alberta Breast Cancer Program, Canadian Leader of the Breast Cancer International Research Group, medical director of the Translational Cancer Research PolyomX Program, and an associate professor of oncology at the University of Alberta. He was recently appointed as a director of Cancer International Research Group, an academic virtual clinical trials organization with over 7000 patients on randomized intervention studies, with 350 centres located in 54 countries. His clinical trials focus on the systemic and supportive therapy of breast cancer and he chairs or co-chairs four international adjuvant studies. His laboratory researches predictive assays for benefit from systemic therapy of breast cancer, and cellular mechanisms of cytotoxic drug resistance. He has more than 100 scientific publications, including papers in *New England Journal of Medicine, Journal of the National Cancer Institute, Cancer Research, Blood,* and *Journal of Clinical Oncology.*

Tom Mercer, PhD, is the professor of clinical exercise physiology and rehabilitation in the School of Health Sciences at Queen Margaret University College, Edinburgh, UK. He was previously director of research in the School of Sport, Health and Exercise Sciences at the University of Wales, Bangor, UK, and coordinator of the Centre for Health and Exercise at Staffordshire University. He received his BEd (Hons) degree in physical education and biology from Lancaster University, UK, and his MS and PhD degrees in exercise physiology from Lakehead University, Canada, and Staffordshire University, UK, respectively. Dr. Mercer has been a member of both the American College of Sports Medicine and the British Association of Sport and Exercise Sciences (BASES) for over 15 years and has been a BASES research accredited exercise physiologist since 1994. He is an honorary research fellow in the Department of Nephrology at the University Hospital of North Staffordshire, UK, and a charter member of the European Dialysis and Transplantation Association-affiliated European Working Group on Renal Rehabilitation and Exercise Physiology. His peer-reviewed research has appeared in *American Journal of Physical Medicine and Rehabilitation, Archives of Physical Medicine and Rehabilitation, Clinical Nephrology, Clinical Physiology, Clinical Science, European Journal of Applied Physiology, Health Education Research, Journal of Rehabilitation Medicine, Medicine and Science in Sports and Exercise,* and *Sports Medicine*. His current research focuses on limitations to exercise tolerance in, and the trainability of, patients with chronic kidney disease.

Ruy S. Moraes, MD, ScD, is faculty member of the Master and Doctoral Program in Cardiology and Cardiovascular Sciences at the Federal University of Rio Grande do Sul, director of FISICOR Cardiac Rehabilitation Center, and physician at the Cardiovascular Division in the Hospital de Clínicas de Porto Alegre, in Brazil. He received his MD and his ScD from the Federal University of Rio Grande do Sul, and did his cardiology training at the Hospital de Clínicas de Porto Alegre. He has published in a variety of professional journals, with recent publications in the *American Heart Journal, American Journal of Hypertension, Autonomic Neuroscience, Clinical Autonomic Research, Diabetes Care, European Journal of Applied Physiology, Hypertension,* and *Pacing and Clinical Electrophysiology.* His research interest is focused on the study of the autonomic nervous system.

Mark S. Nash, PhD, FACSM, is a tenured associate professor in the Departments of Neurological Surgery, Orthopaedics and Rehabilitaiton, and Physical Therapy at the Miller School of Medicine of the University of Miami. Dr. Nash received his doctoral degree in applied physiology and clinical anatomy from the University of Toledo and the Medical College of Ohio in 1984. Following completion of a fellowship in cardiovascular rehabilitation he was appointed to the Department of Neurological Surgery at the University Of Miami School of Medicine as director of the Functional Electrical Stimulation Laboratory, and project coordinator for the NIDRR-sponsored South Florida Regional Spinal Cord Injury System. When The Miami Project to Cure Paralysis was founded in 1985 Dr. Nash was named a founding principal investigator, a position he holds today. His federally-funded grand awards have focused on pharmacological and exercise strategies to treat cardiovascular disease in persons with SCI. Dr. Nash has published more than 60 juried manuscripts, peer-reviewed monographs, and book chapters on this topic, as well as related themes in rehabilitation of persons with physical disabilities. He is a manuscript reviewer for senior journals in exercise medicine and rehabilitation, and reviews grants for both the federal government and private agencies. Dr. Nash is a fellow of the American College of Sports Medicine, a co-recipient of the 1995 International

Forscheimer Prize in Prosthetics Research, and currently serves as principal investigator and director of Applied Physiology Research for The Miami Project to Cure Paralysis.

Charles T. Pu, MD, CMD, is the associate medical director at Youville Hospital and Rehabilitation Center in Boston. Dr. Pu is the unit chief of the Massachusetts General Hospital's Transitional Care Unit Program in Boston and an instructor in medicine at Harvard Medical School. He received his MD from the Robert Wood Johnson Medical School at the University of Medicine and Dentistry of New Jersey. He completed his clinical and research fellowship in geriatric medicine with the Division on Aging at Harvard Medical School. Dr. Pu is an active member of the American Geriatrics Society, the Gerontologic Society of America, and the American Medical Director's Association where he earned his Certification in Medical Direction (CMD). In 1995, he received the Charles H. Farnsworth Medical Foundation Grant. His research interests include sacopenia, exercise, frailty, heart disease in the elderly and patient safety during transitions in care.

Jorge P. Ribeiro, MD, ScD, is an associate professor at the School of Medicine of the Federal University of Rio Grande do Sul, chief of cardiology at the Hospital Moinhos de Vento, and chief of non-invasive cardiology at the Hospital de Clínicas de Porto Alegre, in Brazil. He received his medical degree from the Federal University of Rio Grande do Sul, did his cardiology training at the Brigham and Women's Hospital, and received his ScD in exercise physiology at Boston University. He has published in a variety of professional journals, with recent publications in the *American Heart Journal, American Journal of Cardiology, Autonomic Neuroscience, Clinical Autonomic Research, Critical Pathways in Cardiology, European Journal of Applied Physiology, Hypertension, International Journal of Cardiology, International Journal of Sports Medicine, Journal of Clinical Epidemiology, Journal of the American College of Cardiology, Obstetrics and Gynecology, Pacing and Clinical Electrophysiology,* and *Platelets*. His research interests include physiology and pathophysiology of exercise.

Ian Rice is currently a doctoral student in The School of Health and Rehabilitation Science at The University of Pittsburgh. He received a BS in psychology from University of Illinois and an MS in occupational therapy from Washington University. Ian has competed professionally in wheelchair racing for seven years. In those seven years he has raced in over 35 marathons, winning the Columbus Marathon, the Chicago Marathon twice, the 10 kilometer road world championships and placing third at the Boston Marathon. In addition, Ian was a member of the 2000 Sydney and 2004 Athens Paralimpic racing team. He has also worked in training wheelchair athletes at various sports camps in Illinois, Michigan, and St. Louis.

Ronenn Roubenoff, MD, MHS, is the senior director of molecular medicine at Millennium Pharmaceuticals; professor of nutrition (adjunct) and associate professor of medicine (adjunct) at Tufts University. Dr. Roubenoff received his MD from Northwestern University, and trained in internal medicine and rheumatology at the Johns Hopkins Hospital, and completed a concurrent fellowship in clinical epidemiology at the Johns Hopkins School of Hygiene and Public Health during his rheumatology fellowship. He then trained in nutrition at Tufts University, and from 1990 to 2002 did pioneering work on the interactions of nutrition, exercise and hormonal and immune regulators of metabolism in aging and chronic disease, including rheumatoid arthritis, osteoarthritis, HIV infection, and aging. He was chief of the Nutrition, Exercise Physiology, and Sarcopenia (NEPS) Laboratory from 1997 to 2002, and director of Human Studies, at the Jean Mayer USDA Human Nutrition Research Center on Aging at Tufts University from 2001 to 2002. He is an adjunct professor of nutrition and associate professor of medicine at Tufts and continues to practice rheumatology and nutrition at Tufts-New England Medical Center. In September 2002, Dr. Roubenoff became senior director of molecular medicine at Millennium Pharmaceuticals, Inc., in Cambridge, MA, where he directs research on biomarkers and personalized medicine. He has co-authored nearly 200 articles and 200 abstracts. He lives in the Boston area with his wife, a physician specializing in HIV medicine, their son, a dog, and two cats.

Sean D. Shimada, PhD, received his BS from the College of Letters & Science at the University of California, Davis in 1992. He continued his education at California State University, Sacramento where he received a MS from the School of Health and Human Services in 1994. He received his PhD from the School of Heath and Rehabilitation Sciences at the University of Pittsburgh in 1998, and a second MS degree in bioengineering from the University in 2000.

Currently, he is the president of Biomechanical Consultants of California, a forensic biomechanics and engineering firm based out of Davis, California. He was formerly an instructor and director of the Biomechanics Laboratory at the California State University, Sacramento in the Department of Kinesiology. His primary area of consulting and research is focused on identifying, determining the likelihood, and prevention of injury.

Dr. Shimada has authored four book chapters, over 15 referred journal publications, over 20 referred conference proceedings, and multiple abstracts in the medical-engineering area. He has presented and conducted a number of research studies at meetings and conferences such as Institute of Electrical and Electronic Engineers-Engineering, Medical, and Biology Society (IEEE-EMBS), Rehabilitation Engineering Society of North America (RESNA), Paralympic Congress (USOC, IOC), Forensic Accident Reconstructionist of Oregon (FARO), and the National Institute of Forensic Studies (NIFS).

Joel Stein, MD, is the medical director of Stroke Rehabilitation and the chief medical officer at Spaulding Rehabilitation Hospital. He also serves as an assistant professor in the Department of Physical Medicine and Rehabilitation at Harvard Medical School and as an associate editor for *The American Journal of Physical Medicine and Rehabilitation*. Dr. Stein is a member of the American College of Physicians, the American Academy of PM&R, and the Association of Academic Physiatrists. He received his BA from Columbia University in 1982 and his MD from the Albert Einstein College of Medicine in

1986. His current research interests include the use of robotic devices in rehabilitation, stroke and exercise, and the use of neuropharmacologic agents to enhance poststroke function.

Mary P. Watkins, DPT, MS, is a clinical associate professor with Graduate Programs in Physical Therapy at MGH Institute of Health Professions in Boston, Massachusetts. She has received the Baethke-Carlin Award for Teaching Excellence from the American Physical Therapy Association and the Achievement Award for Physical Therapy from the Pennsylvania Physical Therapy Association. She serves on the editorial board of the *Journal of Hand Therapy.* She has written numerous articles and several book chapters and coauthored *Foundation of Clinical Research: Application to Practice,* which received an honorable mention for professional and scholarly publishing by the Association of American Book Publishers.

Edith M. Williams, MS, is a doctoral candidate in the Department of Social and Preventive Medicine of the State University of New York at Buffalo, School of Public Health and Health Professions, and postgraduate research associate with the Buffalo Lupus Project. She graduated from the University of North Carolina at Chapel Hill and has an MS in Epidemiology from the State University of New York at Buffalo. Her main area of research involves environmental determinants of health disparities in minority communities, which she has been studying as part of the New York Angler Cohort Study, Eastside Wellness Study, and Buffalo Lupus Project. Currently, she is independently investigating subclinical heart disease in African American women with lupus; her study, the "Breakfast with a Buddy Biomarkers of Lupus Study," includes measures of traditional cardiovascular risk factors, including levels of physical activity, which are postulated to be related to high rates of lupus and other autoimmune diseases in the target population. Ms. Williams has prepared written materials for lay audiences and summarized relevant issues in peer-reviewed journals. Her independent research has included preparation of proposals and summaries for federal agencies and intra-university committees/boards.